PROBLEMS
OF AGEING

This is a volume in the
Arno Press collection

AGING AND OLD AGE

Advisory Editor

Robert Kastenbaum

Editorial Board

Joseph T. Freeman
Gerald J. Gruman
Michel Philibert

See last page of this volume
for a complete list of titles.

PROBLEMS
OF AGEING

Edited by
(Edmund Vincent)
E. V. COWDRY

ARNO PRESS
A New York Times Company
New York • 1979

Editorial Supervision: Joseph Cellini

Reprint Edition 1979 by Arno Press Inc.

Reprinted from a copy in the University of Illinois Library

AGING AND OLD AGE
ISBN for complete set: 0-405-11800-7
See last pages of this volume for titles.

Manufactured in the United States of America

Library of Congress Cataloging in Publication Data

Cowdry, Edmund Vincent, 1888-1975, ed.
    Problems of aging.

    (Aging and old age)
    Reprint of the 1939 ed. published by Williams &
Wilkins, Baltimore.
    Includes index.
    1. Aging. I. Title. II. Series.
QP86.C6 1979   574.3'72   78-22196
ISBN 0-405-11813-9

QP86
.C6
1979

Copy 1

PROBLEMS
OF AGEING

BIOLOGICAL AND MEDICAL ASPECTS

Contributors

Edgar Allen
Lewellys F. Barker
W. B. Cannon
A. J. Carlson
A. E. Cohn
E. V. Cowdry
Macdonald Critchley
William Crocker
John Dewey
Louis I. Dublin
E. T. Engle
Jonas S. Friedenwald
S. R. Guild

G. V. Hamilton
L. O. Howard
A. C. Ivy
H. S. Jennings
E. B. Krumbhaar
Karl Landsteiner
C. M. McCay
Wm. deB. MacNider
Walter R. Miles
Jean Oliver
T. Wingate Todd
Fred D. Weidman
Clark Wissler

A PUBLICATION OF

THE JOSIAH MACY, JR. FOUNDATION

Edited by

E. V. COWDRY

Washington University, St. Louis

BALTIMORE

THE WILLIAMS & WILKINS COMPANY

1939

Composed and Printed at the
WAVERLY PRESS, INC.
for
The Williams & Wilkins Company
Baltimore, Md., U. S. A.

CONTENTS

CHAPTER 1

CHAPTER 2

CHAPTER 3

CHAPTER 4

CHAPTER 5

PREFACE

This volume is a timely and logical development of the survey of the problem of arteriosclerosis[1] which was published by the Josiah Macy, Jr. Foundation in 1933 to summarize existing knowledge on the degenerative changes and ageing of blood vessels. When the present volume was well under way, the Foundation provided for a conference on ageing, jointly sponsored by the Union of American Biological Societies and the National Research Council, at Woods Hole on June 25 and 26, 1937, which was attended by fifteen of the contributors to this volume as well as by other interested persons. The National Research Council also arranged a conference of its Committee on the Biological Processes of Ageing in Washington, D.C. on February 5, 1938 which included in its attendance seven contributors to this volume. Other smaller meetings of contributors, interested in the ageing of the nervous system and of the endocrines, were arranged by the Foundation. Abstracts and complete manuscripts have been circulated widely among the contributors. Consequently, the opportunity to bring to bear on the problem the experience and points of view of many specialists, working together in a constructive way, has been unrivaled. But each contributor is personally responsible for his chapter. There are, as one would expect, some differences of opinion. These foreshadow progress since they will stimulate further investigation. The style is as simple as possible consistent with scientific accuracy. Each chapter concludes with a summary and a bibliography. The editor feels much indebted to Dr. Ludwig Kast, Mr. Lawrence K. Frank and Dr. F. Fremont-Smith of the Josiah Macy, Jr. Foundation for their continued interest and support. To the contributors of this volume he wishes to express his thanks for their coöperation.

E. V. COWDRY.

July 22, 1938.

[1] Arteriosclerosis: A Survey of the Problem. Edited |by Edmund V. Cowdry. The Macmillan Company, 1933, New York.

FOREWORD

This volume on the process of ageing has been sponsored by the Josiah Macy, Jr. Foundation in continuance of its interest in degenerative diseases and in the hope of focusing attention upon a problem which has far-reaching scientific and social implications for a society with a rapidly increasing proportion of older men and women.

In this symposium current knowledge in regard to the ageing process is presented by investigators in different fields who have reviewed the literature and who, in many cases, have reported their own findings. Through such a presentation of interrelated findings and diverse viewpoints, it is hoped to enlist wider interest in a synoptic view of ageing and to further the study of some of the many questions thus revealed. Obviously the whole problem cannot be covered in a single volume; therefore, certain aspects have been selected to indicate the complexity of the problem and to illuminate some of its more significant phases.

Since all living organisms pass through a sequence of changes, characterized by growth, development, maturation and finally senescence, the question of ageing presents a broad biological problem. But both the rate and the expression of ageing vary widely among organisms; some plants, protozoa and insects, for example, do not exhibit the familiar picture of senescence. No general theory of ageing, therefore, is at present available and the question of human or mammalian senescence must for the present be regarded as a distinct problem, within the larger biological question.

Two conflicting views are held today by students of ageing in man. One considers ageing as an involutionary . process which operates cumulatively with the passage of time and which is revealed in different organ systems as inevitable modifications of cells, tissues and fluids; the other view interprets the changes found in aged organs as due to infections, toxins, traumas, and nutritional disturbances or inadequacies which have forced cells, tissues and fluids to respond with degenerative changes and impairments. It appears, however, that at least some of these changes serve to maintain functioning and are therefore protective. The issue becomes sharply focused upon the possibility of distinguishing between the cumulative but physiological involutions that inevitably take place in all individuals as they grow older, and pathological changes that occur in ageing individuals as the result of adverse environmental conditions.

It is evident that ageing cannot be ascribed to any single structural or functional change or failure. Despite the passage of years many organs and tissues retain a capacity for renewal that enables them to function adequately, while others seem to have a potential duration of life greater than that of the organism. Clinical observation shows extraordinary variations in functional activity of organ systems and tissues among individuals of the same chronological age. Common observation alone is sufficient to remind us that ageing, or senescence, occurs frequently in men and women, who, chronologically speaking, are relatively young; likewise delayed ageing is found among men and women of advanced chronological age who exhibit good health and few, if any, signs of impairment or enfeeblement. It is difficult to classify or label this minority of individuals who do not show the changes and impairments that are considered normal for a certain age because found in the majority. Attempts to establish statistically derived norms of ageing are often productive of more confusion than clarity because they may obscure any real insight into the sequence of events which result in "ageing" of different individuals. It may be emphasized here that both the norms of ageing, and the commonly observed, but less carefully defined, variations in ageing of individuals, are derived from random samples of men and women who have experienced deficiencies and insufficiencies of early nurture as well as injuries, stresses, strains and insults in adult life, many of which we now know to be at least partly avoidable.

From study of the earlier stages of the growth process it is being shown that unfavorable conditions and insufficient or deficient nurture may seriously retard the growth and development of the young organism and inflict more or less permanent impairment; but optimum conditions, both in the prenatal and postnatal life, foster better organisms which exceed many of the statistically established norms for "run of the mine," random samples. As knowledge of nurture, especially nutrition, becomes more precise and more widely practiced, some of the better nurtured children may have a senescence that is quite different from the current picture of ageing. Moreover, since the evidence for the selective influence of heredity upon duration of life is also derived from similar random samples of individuals, the heredity factor in ageing may prove to be less controlling than is now believed. Already the growing body of experimental evidence on increased longevity of animals indicates that the length of life, as well as the vitality and functional efficiency, of an organism may be considerably enhanced by more adequate nutrition.

In all studies of growth and of ageing, time is of the greatest significance. It cannot reasonably be expected that a person at 60 should
possess the same functional capacity that he had at 30. It is generally
assumed that members of a species of the same *chronological* age constitute a homogeneous group and may therefore be treated as a uniform
sample; intensive studies, however, of both animals and children
have indicated that individuals grow, develop and mature at different
rates and therefore differ widely even at the same chronological age.
Dr. Alexis Carrel and Dr. Lecomte du Noüy have emphasized this differential time rate within individual organisms in their proposed concepts
of "physiological time" and of "biological time." Prof. H. Dingle
asserts that "time produces no effects—events occur in it but not because of it," with the implications that time is solely a frame of reference for measurement of changes but may be relative to the individual
organism under observation. It seems especially important therefore
to recognize that the same chronological age may have a varying
significance for different individuals; moreover, at different periods in
life of the same individual the passage of time does not influence the
development of senescence at a uniform rate. In the search for a
uniform, general process of ageing there is a risk of neglecting the
various factors, influences or conditions that enter into this differential
rate of ageing in each individual at different periods of his life.

The rapid differentiation and involution of the prenatal period
continues in infancy; as Minot suggested some years ago, ageing is
indeed most rapid in early life. Ordinarily, the decreasing functional
efficiency and the structural alterations associated with ageing occur
only in later life and contrast sharply with this earlier process of involution. Throughout the survey of this problem we are faced repeatedly with the crucial issue of how to distinguish between normal
senescence and the pathology of old age.

Individual differences arise not only from heredity but also from
impact of environmental and cultural influences; the problem of ageing
therefore is not a purely biological question, but has large cultural,
social and psychological implications. When we contrast non-literate
peoples having a maximum birthrate and a relatively small proportion
of their men and women surviving to old age, with other peoples
having a restricted and falling birthrate but a growing proportion of
older men and women and a lengthening expectation of life, the social
aspects and implications of the problem of ageing become more evident.
As the individual passes from infancy through childhood, adolescence,

maturity on to senescence he or she is being acted upon by and is reacting to social life and personal, human relationships with feelings and emotions which, as we are recognizing with increasing clarity, influence bodily functions and may give rise to functional impairment and eventually to structural damage. It is obvious that additional burdens of worry, anxiety, and unhappiness may accelerate functional decline and aggravate the impairments of the later years of life.

These general questions and comments find illustrations in the chapters of this volume which give evidence of progressive alteration frequently involving not the whole organ or tissue, but only a portion thereof and therefore not necessarily interfering seriously with the capacity to maintain life. Such considerations must be viewed in the light of the earlier question of whether these changes represent the process of ageing or rather pathological deviations which conceivably might have been avoided or minimized in earlier years.

In several of the chapters, ageing is presented not only in terms of the changes to be observed in specific organ systems and body fluids, but also in terms of impairments of the total organism, as secondary results of chemical alterations in those organs and fluids. It may be pointed out here that since the bulk of present evidence on ageing is drawn from observations of late or terminal results of age changes in cells, tissues and fluids, very little is known about the early processes that generate those changes. The question insistently arises whether these observed degenerations and atrophies in certain organs are primary senescence or the secondary responses to alterations in body fluids, especially the blood, which may have failed to furnish adequate nutrition for cells or to maintain the chemical equilibrium of the intra-organic environment so necessary for functional efficiency. Simple cause and effect relationships can scarcely be considered in such total organic interactions; they must be supplemented, or perhaps replaced, by a broader conceptual picture of the functioning organism as a "field" (to borrow the term from physics) in which the totality and the parts are dynamically interrelated and therefore are continuously reacting to each other and to the environment. The already demonstrated fruitfulness of the "field" concept in embryology indicates its probable future service in the study of ageing.

Further suggestions arise from some chapters, for experimental approaches to the control of ageing, through deliberate interference with the chemical alterations of the blood and other body fluids in aged; for example, in the control of cholesterol metabolism or of cardiovascular-renal and similar functions. Since the skeleton and the skin have the capacity of reflecting or indicating the organism's progress and are especially sensitive to its ageing, they may be used as indicators in experimental methods for controlling ageing; but it must also be asked whether the disorderly or unregulated growths in skeleton and skin, that occur so frequently in ageing organisms, signify a weakening or breakdown of the "organizer" or controller of organic structure.

A closely related question of large biological import is raised by the discussion of ageing of the nervous system, the eye and the ear, in which the observed alterations and breakdowns appear to be less frequent in the phylogentically older structures. Are the more recently developed tissues and cells more vulnerable and therefore in need of greater protection from strain and injury? Such selective action of ageing is, however, to be contrasted with the interrelated process of ageing exhibited by the interactions of endocrines with environmental factors, such as nutrition and emotional stress, which raises the question of how these reciprocal reactions can be interrupted or modified to prevent the accelerated ageing they so frequently bring to the whole organism.

It is of great importance to know how much the impairments of age arise from or reflect a premature cessation of activity and withdrawal from living that induce a functional atrophy which may then become permanently structured. If just the feeling of being old can lead to a diminution of functional activities, is it possible to delay ageing by continuing life activities and maintaining a feeling of competence for life? Since adequacy depends upon responses to environmental demands appropriate at each period of life, adaptability to the passing years is undoubtedly essential to health and longevity. But little is now known about a way of life for the ageing man and woman that will avoid not only undue demands upon lessening capacity but also premature and unnecessary restrictions upon the full activity appropriate to each individual.

In no other aspect of medicine and health-care is the concept of the psychosomatic unity of the organism more important than in the care of the aged, since the older individual faces life with all the emotional patterns of his past. From present knowledge it seems probable that much of that stubborn resistance to needed changes in the regimen of living, as well as the strong resentments, antagonisms and bitterness so frequently found among the aged, represent a lifelong accumulation of protest against experiences that have warped and twisted the individual personality. It is this very emotional resistance that frequently makes it so difficult, or sometimes impossible, to help older persons.

In the ageing man and woman, therefore, medicine faces a series of perplexing problems, largely because of these extraordinary somatic and psychological differences among individuals and the present inadequacy of scientific knowledge about their relation to the ageing process. Two major questions arise in any consideration of the healthcare of the ageing: how can we prolong human life and how can we lessen, if not eliminate, those malfunctionings and disturbances which *impair* the existing lifetime of so many older individuals? The prolongation of life may appear as a desirable goal regardless of the handicaps and limitations imposed by senescence; but a greater aspiration is the conservation of life and well being, so that the individual may live his full life span without the infirmities and handicaps that so often make his continued existence a prolonged misery.

For those who are seeking definitive answers to the many questions about the ageing process, this volume may be disappointing, since, as previously indicated, few definite and convincing answers are possible in our present state of knowledge. Questions, however, are being asked which open up promising leads for investigation in an area which has much scientific significance as well as human importance. If the present volume serves to summarize some of the existing knowledge and promising leads and to acquaint both the professional and the general reader with the present status of this problem, it will have justified the time and effort that has been expended in its preparation.

To the individual contributors to this volume and to the many other individuals who have helped through advice, counsel and information, the Foundation makes grateful and appreciative acknowledgment. To the editor the Foundation is especially indebted since the plan for the volume was originally conceived by him and has been carried through to completion despite all the delays and difficulties which only editors of similar projects can understand.

For the Foundation, the publication of this volume is an occasion for expressing the hope that these contributions may advance the formulation of that larger conception of health-care to which the Foundation was dedicated from its inception.

LAWRENCE K. FRANK.

Josiah Macy, Jr. Foundation.

INTRODUCTION

It is a common experience that solution of one type of problem brings with it new and unforeseen problems that require for solution a very different approach from that which was earlier employed. This is especially true with problems capable of isolation and dealt with by specialized techniques. The first steps in what is now known as the industrial revolution were, for example, taken simply to produce more cheaply a larger amount of woolen goods. The problem seemed to be a purely technical one and capable of solution by technical improvements in the machinery of spinning and weaving. The final social consequences of the adoption of similar methods in all fields of production were unforeseen and unforeseeable. Yet they were such as to bring about a state of affairs in which more than anything else are rooted all of our present social and political problems, domestic and international.

Upon its face, the problem of saving a greater number of lives was a similar special problem. It was a definitely medical question. It was met by improvements in medical care and by improved dietaries and measures of public sanitation. Just as more efficient methods of manufacturing were the result of new physical scientific knowledge, so the improvements in production of personal and public health were the results of new physiological and chemical knowledge. But it is now becoming evident that the changes which have brought about great reduction of infant mortality and the lengthening of the span of life for those who survive the hazards of infancy have had important social effects so that social conditions have been created which confront civilization with issues of the most serious nature.

For a considerable period, say roughly till the beginning of the present century, the effects of the new methods of industry on one side and of new methods of care of the sick and protection of public health on the other side practically coincided. The result was an immense increase of population in all industrially advanced countries. The birth rate was stimulated by new economic opportunities; more children were kept alive; philanthropic zeal coöperated with new medical knowledge and skill to keep alive the enfeebled who formerly would have perished, and new biological knowledge of the sort represented by Pasteur's epoch-making discoveries checked the ravages of the plagues and infectious diseases that had previously made such inroads upon whole populations. The net effect of all these changes was what the biometricians call the population pyramid: for the distribution of the population by ages could be graphically represented by a pyramid, children forming a broad base gradually tapering off to a narrow apex of a comparatively few aged persons.

Recent years have made a marked change. The present distribution of the population by ages, throughout the western world at least, would be represented by something shaped more like an egg cut off at the base, than by a pyramid. The reduction of infant mortality has proceeded apace. But the birth-rate has steadily declined so that the increased survival of infants and children has not checked the decrease in the ratio borne by the youthful element in the population to the older elements. Concurrently with decrease in the relative number of the young has been a dramatic increase in the span of life. Better medical care and more adequate nutrition have effected the survival of ever larger numbers of older people. As compared with the earlier pyramidic form, we now have a narrowed base, a wider middle aged group and a much enlarged group of the aged at the top.

As the chapters in this volume clearly show, present society in Europe and the United States is now approaching a stabilized, even possibly a declining, total population with a larger older population, both absolutely and relatively, than any country in the world has ever known before. In the United States, with decrease of birth-rate and the limitation of immigration (which had been mainly of the young and vigorous) we now have an unprecedented situation. Over one-third of the total population will soon be over fifty years of age. In 1980 the number of persons over sixty-five will be more than double that today.

The most obvious aspect of the social problem thus created is the economic. It is a matter of common knowledge that persons above fifty are experiencing ever greater difficulty in finding employment and that even those above forty are not immune from the effect of the industrial developments which have put a premium on youthful vigor and a discount upon the experience of those who are older. While the change is a matter of common knowledge rather than of statistics scientifically obtained, yet one record of the latter sort may be noted as typical. Reports of almost half a million of persons who have been subjects of public relief show that individuals between the years of twenty-five and thirty-five have found re-employment and been taken off relief-rolls at the rate of two to one as compared with those of the ages from even as low as thirty-five to forty-five.

That this economic shift has political repercussions is manifest in the general movement for old-age pensions on one side, and on the other side in the efforts, such as legal restrictions on child labor, to hold a larger number of jobs open for persons in the middle years. Even the legal rights and powers of individuals are coming to be defined, both as regards the older and the younger groups of the total population, on an age basis. So far this re-definition is occurring in response to special conditions, but it is not too much to predict that finally it will mean the conscious emergence of new social standards and ideals. Indeed, the recent economic crisis which prevented the normal entrance of the young into industrial and professional employment has already rendered the problem of youth a conscious social problem both economically and educationally. In its political bearings as to the older group, it should be noted that under existing cultural conditions, and probably to some unknown degree biologically, conservatism increases with age, so that in the degree in which the older group expresses itself politically we have the curious and indeed ironic condition that at just the time when measures of social readjustment are most needed, there is an increasing number of those whose habits of mind and action incline them to resist policies of social readjustment.

This latter remark provides a natural transition to consideration of aspects of the new social problem that are less tangible than the economic one; for after all, the population group which is economically handicapped by age is not a statistical affair. It consists of individuals, each one having his or her own individual past career, his or her own temperament, personal needs, and desires, and his or her own special relations to other persons, especially of his or her family group, and, though less directly, to his or her community. The psychological, educational and moral ramifications of this phase of the new social problem are as endless as they are subtle—and as little understood. Many years ago, Mrs. Florence Kelly asked me if I could give any references in literature to the psychology and sociology of growing old. When I was compelled to admit my ignorance, she remarked, "It is strange that the one thing that every person looks forward to is the one thing for which no preparation is made." The situation is not measurably better today save that the importance of the problem is now recognized as it was not a generation ago.

The present volume of studies is itself evidence of the new recognition of the importance of the problem of ageing. No reflective and informed person will question that the foundation of any serious consideration of the problem of ageing and of methods of dealing with the problem is provided by biological and related chemical knowledge. Whatever else human beings are or are not, they are biological creatures whose physiological process, normal and abnormal, can be understood only by means of adequate physical and chemical knowledge. The studies of this nature which are presented in this book are the necessary foundation for attack upon the more intangible psychological and social aspects of the problem. They provide the needed base line, for they disclose basic conditions which in any case must be taken into account. As they continue to develop they will reveal means and methods by which such anomalies and disorders as now exist can be dealt in their causes and not simply as symptoms.

For the purpose of the present discussion, these studies may be interpreted as presenting a problem that forces upon us an investigation of every form of human relation: the problem, namely, of the relation of the biological and the cultural. Take the matter of the increased conservatism that emerges with increased age. While specific studies of a scientific quality are not numerous, this increased conservatism may be taken as a matter of public knowledge. In a general way, it is a reasonable inference that biological factors play some part. For a declining store of physical energy may be expected, on theoretical grounds, to result in lessened initiative and readiness to undertake new lines of activity. But when it is asserted that large past experience and maturity in general tend to render human beings more and more sceptical of the value of innovation and "reforms," we have left the biological ground for the cultural.

For there is no well grounded way of connecting conservatism of this type with any inherent biological processes. We do not know the extent to which growing aversion to the new and to change is a product of the *quality* of past experiences, rather than to the bare fact of experience, nor the exact extent to which that quality is due to conditions provided by the social environment rather than to anything intrinsic, the social conditions being moreover, socially modifiable. There certainly exist exceptions to the rule of fixation of ideas and belief with increased age. Admitting that there are in these cases, special individual genetic conditions favorable to retention of the plasticity and the interest in growth that are characteristic of youth, the important question is what rôle education and other cultural influences play.

I have referred to this matter of increased conservatism simply as an illustration of the general problem. There are aged persons who are repining and querulous and who make life difficult for their families and immediate associates; who live in the past and who get their chief happiness in recalling the good old times that are no more. But there are other aged persons having exactly the opposite traits. Nobody knows how the two groups compare in numbers. But the very existence of these two kinds of old persons is strong reason for believing that the source of the difference may not be wholly biological and fixed, but may be social and cultural and therefore amenable to change, provided changed social and educational conditions are brought to bear.

The preference of employers for the younger group which has been referred to is not wholly a matter of the greater physical vigor, power of endurance and of greater speed on the part of the young. It is also due to conditions of industry which render past experience of little value in machine operations. The latter may be mastered in a short time. In the older hand industry, on the contrary, length of experience was a positive asset, since it meant increase of judgment, skill and taste. Social conditions, in other words, come into play. Now extend the point to include the common belief that individuals tend with age to get into a rut and lose power to adapt themselves to new conditions. If we admit that this tendency is biologically grounded, we reach a highly pessimistic conclusion, for it means that maturing is quite as much a curse as it is a blessing.

The fact that the conclusion is pessimistic is not of itself a sufficient reason for rejecting it. But it is a reason for examining closely into the reasons why increasing age now tends to render individuals less flexible and less adaptable, with all the personal and social loss that is a consequence of this failure. The age-long quest for the fountain of eternal youth, taken merely in its physical form in the past, has failed. Perhaps a happy ending to the search would be better approximated if we turned the quest in another direction. That conditions and methods of education have *something* to do with retention and with loss of power of re-adaptation to changed conditions will not be denied. Just how much it has to do with it we do not now know, and we shall not know until we employ every available experimental resource to find out. And when I say "education" I mean more than schooling, although I think it is demonstrable that much of current schooling tends automatically to artificial production of habits which arrest growth and create inability to readjust and reconstruct.

The emphasis that is placed in contemporary educational schemes upon production of mechanical forms of skill and mechanical reproduction of information is itself a reflex, moreover, of social conditions. In present culture, the dominant interest is upon the whole the economic, and successful pursuit of this interest is conditioned upon the existence of a large body of persons who are operators of machines. In this work, emphasis falls upon accuracy and speed in the performance of repetitious processes. There is not only little call and little chance for personal initiative and judgment, but the mental and physical strains involved are such as to create demand for artificial diversion and "stimulation" in non-working hours: just as children in a mechanically operated school tend to react to the other extreme when they get outside the school walls. For the conditions under which activity is carried on involves strain because it is *contrary* to normal biological demands, so that compensatory activities are evoked.

When this point is applied to the relatively old, it indicates two things. One of them is the failure, which now exists, of the usual conditions of experience to create the interests and the capacities which will occupy later years fruitfully and happily. The other is the positive side of the same problem: the need of study to ascertain and develop the kind of activities in which the older part of the population can engage with satisfaction to themselves and value to the community. I do not think it is too much to say that this whole field is a practical blank at the present time. There are here and there individuals who have managed to work out a solution, but, as far as I can see, such cases are a matter of combination of a fortunate personal temperament and lucky surroundings. They do not exist because of any general social policy which provides conditions for achieving this happy outcome. It may be that when the number of the old was relatively small, the problem was not an urgent one. With the prospect of over a third of the total population above fifty years in age, it is a pressing problem.

To be laid upon the shelf, to find one's self socially useless and hence socially unwanted, even when other members of the family are personally kind and considerate, is a fate which goes contrary to even normal biological conditions. Upon the social side, it means that accumulation of experience is not regarded as a social asset. I take it that the moral of Shaw's Back to Methuselah was that the process of gaining and using experience is now so constantly interrupted by death that human beings do not gain the wisdom which is necessary if human affairs are to be successfully managed. The idea that wisdom would accumulate and would be applied if only the span of life were sufficiently extended stands, however, in ironic contrast with the present situation. For as that is constituted, we have gone far beyond the ancient adage "If youth only knew, and age only could." For there is now no socially organized means by which the aged have (or at least are supposed to have) even the *knowledge* which is relevant to the conditions of social life, much less have the opportunity of applying it.

The underlying problem, both scientifically and philosophically, it seems to me, is that of the relation of ageing and maturing. We are at present more or less in the unpleasant and illogical condition of extolling maturity and deprecating age. It seems obvious without argument that there is some connection between the two; that we cannot separate the processes of maturing from those of ageing even though the two processes are not identical. The split that now exists between the two, in terms of both individual activity and happiness and of social usefulness, would appear to be socially or culturally produced, rather than to be biologically intrinsic. That there should be a gradual wearing down of energies, physical and mental, in the old age period it is reasonable to expect upon biological grounds. That maturing changes, at some particular age, into incapacity for continued growth in every direction is a very different proposition. We may not be able to affirm with the poet

> Grow old with me
> The best is yet to come,

but there is something abnormal in the situation if we are obliged to admit that after a certain period nothing *better* in any direction, individual and social, can occur because of the process of growing old.

In the previous discussion, I have made a certain separation between the problem of the measures that can be socially organized and administered in ameliorating the estate of the aged and the psychological and moral problems presented by the older part of the population. I do not mean, however, that the two things are independent of each other. I think we can safely foresee the extension of old age allowances, together with provision for the young, which will relieve the aged from a burden they now carry. I do not think that it is a sign of undue extension of imagination to anticipate a time when organized administrative care for the aged will extend not only to greater facilities in the way of hospitalization and old-age homes, special nurses and special forms of medical care, including psychiatric; but to special housing, including perhaps provisions for living in especially congenial climates and special recreational facilities.

But such measures, while important and necessary, are mitigative rather than constructive, unless they are accompanied by changes in the cultural social structure which will give the group of older persons a status of moral security and social value as well as material security. The attitude taken toward the aged has at all historic periods been a function of the general social pattern. Today it is largely a function of the economic and educational pattern of present society. External material improvements can be instituted without going far outside the existing social pattern. But I am unable to see how the basic *human* problem can be solved without social changes which ensure first to every individual the continual chance to have intrinsically worthwhile experience, and secondly provide significant socially useful outlets for the maturity and wisdom gained in this experience.

What has been said has probably made it clear to the reader that it is my conviction that the many perplexing problems now attendant upon human old age have a psychological-social origin. Yet the main purpose of these introductory remarks is to call attention to the fact that there is a *problem* and one of a scope having no precedent in human history. Biological processes are at the roots of the problems and of the methods of solving them, but the biological processes take place in economic, political and cultural contexts. They are inextricably interwoven with these contexts so that one reacts upon the other in all sorts of intricate ways. We need to know the ways in which social contexts react back into biological processes as well as to know the ways in which the biological processes condition social life. This is the problem to which attention is invited.

Recognition of the seriousness of the problem as well as application of the knowledge that is already in our possession is impeded by traditional ideas, intellectual habits and institutional customs. There is urgent need for a philosophy of personal and institutional life that is consequent with present knowledge. Biological science has a great contribution to make to formation of the theory and practice of a new pattern of living, aside from what it can do in provision of special techniques. For biology as a science brings to the foreground of attention the significance of Growth in a way which underlying physical sciences do not. The special technical problems of ageing are all connected with processes of growth, but in addition our philosophy of all life and of all social relations demands reconstruction of traditional beliefs upon the basis of Growth as the fundamental category. When we shall envisage social relations and institutions in the light of the contribution they are capable of making to continued growth, when we are capable of criticizing those which exist on the ground of the ways in which they arrest and deflect processes of growth, we shall be on our way to a solution of the moral and psychological problems of human ageing. Science and philosophy meet on common ground in their joint interest in discovering the processes of normal growth and in the institution of conditions which will favor and support ever continued growth.

JOHN DEWEY.

LIST OF CONTRIBUTORS

ALLEN, EDGAR, Ph.D., Sc.D.
Professor of Anatomy, Yale University, New Haven, Connecticut

BARKER, LEWELLYS FRANKLIN, M.D., LL.D.
Emeritus Professor of Medicine, Johns Hopkins University, Baltimore, Maryland

CANNON, WALTER BRADFORD, A.M., M.D., Sc.D., LL.D., Dr.(hon.)
George Higginson Professor of Physiology, Harvard Medical School, Boston, Massachusetts

CARLSON, ANTON JULIUS, LL.D., Ph.D., M.D.
Frank P. Hixon Professor of Physiology and Chairman of the Department, University of Chicago, Chicago, Illinois

COHN, ALFRED EINSTEIN, M.D.
Member of the Rockefeller Institute for Medical Research, New York, New York

COWDRY, EDMUND VINCENT, Ph.D.
Professor of Cytology, Washington University, St. Louis, Missouri

CRITCHLEY, MACDONALD, M.D., F.R.C.P. (London)
Neurologist, King's College Hospital; Physician to Outpatients, National Hospital, Queen Square, London

CROCKER, WILLIAM, Ph.D.
Managing Director Boyce Thompson Institute for Plant Research, Inc., Yonkers, New York

DEWEY, JOHN, LL.D., Ph.D.
Emeritus Professor of Philosophy, Columbia University, New York, New York.

DUBLIN, LOUIS I., Ph.D.
Third Vice President and Statistician, Metropolitan Life Insurance Company, New York, New York

ENGLE, EARL THERON, Ph.D.
Associate Professor of Anatomy, College of Physicians and Surgeons, Columbia University, New York, New York

FRIEDENWALD, JONAS STEIN, M.D.
Associate Professor of Ophthalmology, Johns Hopkins University, Baltimore, Maryland

GUILD, STACY RUFUS, Ph.D.
Associate Professor of Otology and Director of the Otological Research Laboratory, Johns Hopkins University, Baltimore, Maryland

HAMILTON, GILBERT VAN TASSEL, M.D.
    Clinical Psychiatrist, Santa Barbara, California
HOWARD, LELAND OSSIAN, Ph.D., M.D., LL.D., D.Sc.
    Late Chief Entomologist U.S. Department of Agriculture; Honorary Curator U.S. National Museum, Washington, D.C.
IVY, ANDREW CONWAY, M.D., Ph.D.
    Nathan Smith Davis Professor of Physiology and Pharmacology, Northwestern University, Chicago, Illinois
JENNINGS, HERBERT SPENCER, Sc.D., Ph.D., LL.D.
    Henry Walters Professor of Zoology and Director of the Zoological Laboratory, Johns Hopkins University, Baltimore, Maryland
KRUMBHAAR, EDWARD BELL, M.D., Ph.D.
    Professor of Pathology, University of Pennsylvania, Philadelphia, Pennsylvania
McCAY, CLIVE MAINE, Ph.D.
    Professor of Animal Nutrition, Cornell University, Ithaca, New York
MACNIDER, WILLIAM DE BERNIERE, M.D.
    Kenan Research Professor of Pharmacology and Dean of the Medical School, University of North Carolina, Chapel Hill, North Carolina
MILES, WALTER RICHARD, Ph.D.
    Professor of Psychology, Yale University, New Haven, Connecticut
OLIVER, JEAN R., M.D.
    Professor of Pathology, Long Island College of Medicine, Brooklyn, New York
TODD, T. WINGATE, M.B., Ch.B. (Manc.), F.R.C.S. (England)
    Professor of Anatomy, Director of the Hamann Museum of Comparative Anthropology and Anatomy, Chairman Brush Foundation, Director Developmental Health Inquiry Associated Foundations, Western Reserve University, Cleveland, Ohio
WEIDMAN, FRED DEFOREST, M.D.
    Professor of Dermatological Research, University of Pennsylvania, Philadelphia, Pennsylvania
WISSLER, CLARK, Ph.D., LL.D.
    Curator of Anthropology American Museum of Natural History and Professor of Anthropology, Institute of Human Relations, Yale University, New Haven, Connecticut; American Museum of Natural History, New York, New York

CHAPTER 1

AGEING IN PLANTS

WILLIAM CROCKER

New York

It is impossible to discuss ageing in all plants (Benecke-Jost, 1923–1924, v. 2, p. 211–216) under one concept because there is such a range of plants as to life course and life duration. The several groups of plants as to life duration must be discussed separately. The matter of ageing in plants is also rendered complex by the fact that life course and especially life span of a given plant in nature may be modified greatly by growing it under conditions that vary considerably, or in some cases, even slightly, from the conditions it meets in nature.

In the main, plants form an open system (Küster, 1921), that is, they continually develop new growing points whereas animals more often form a closed system. This means that plants in general do not have a definite or even an approximate life span in contrast with animals.

Certain plants are theoretically immortal, that is, they die only because of unfavorable external conditions. This is true of plants in which all the cells remain embryonic instead of differentiating into reproductive and somatic cells. Even some plants that in nature differentiate into somatic and reproductive cells can be grown continuously vegetatively by the proper cultural conditions. Hartmann (1921) grew *Eudorina elegans*, a colonial alga, for 1300 generations, 5 years, without any differentiation of cells. No doubt this could have been continued indefinitely.

The differentiation of cells of seed plants into somatic tissue is marked by great elongation of the cells and the development of a large central vacuole. A marked thickening of the cell wall is another feature of differentiation of plant cells, such as collenchyma, sclerenchyma, sieve tubes, and wood vessels. Under various conditions collenchyma or sclerenchyma cells, as long as they still contain protoplasts, may be induced to become meristematic again.

Wallace (1928) found very low concentrations of ethylene in the air effective in inducing sclerenchyma cells of apple bark to dissolve away the wall thickening followed by cell enlargement and finally cell division.

1

1. GROWTH CONDITIONS MODIFY LIFE CYCLE AND LIFE SPAN

Klebs (1910) pointed out that many potentialities exist in the internal structure of a species of plants and these potentialities can be learned by growing the species under a great variety of conditions. The manner of development of a plant under ordinary conditions is only one of its many possibilities. His work on experimental development extended over various species of fungi, algae, ferns, and flowering plants. Two examples will suffice to illustrate his results, one fungus and one flowering plant.

Saprolegnia mixta (Klebs, 1910) is a branching filamentous fungus commonly found growing on flies in water. When growing on a fly it forms within a few days a halo of branching white filaments about the insect. Zoosporangia then begin forming at the tips of the mycelia. Therefrom asexual spores are soon released in the water to infect other flies. The formation of zoospores takes place again and again on the mycelia for some days. Finally a third stage of development follows, namely the formation of sex organs which result in sexual resting spores. The plant then dies after only a few weeks of development. Klebs asked the question, Is this very regular succession of different stages, each with its special forms and functions, dependent upon internal causes alone or do the external nutrient conditions act with the internal structure to determine the order of development and even the life span? The fungus is easy to grow on culture medium containing albumen, peptone, extract of peas, etc. When the fungus was grown in this condition with care to keep the medium from being exhausted of nutrients and from staling by transferring pieces of the filament repeatedly to fresh medium it continued to grow vegetatively for six years, or the duration of the experiment, without asexual or sexual spore production. Under this condition the fungus is practically immortal. If portions of the mycelium are transferred from the nutrient just mentioned above to distilled water, innumerable zoospores are formed in the course of a few days and the fungus dies. If well-nourished mycelium is transferred to slightly nutrient water, zoospore production will continue as long as the proper but low nutrient level is maintained. Under this condition the organism is apparently immortal but asexual spore production accompanies mycelial growth. If the mycelium is cultivated in a solution of leucin or haemoglobin (haemachrome) mixed with inorganic salts, mycelial growth is rapid at first, followed by sexual reproduction as the nutrients diminish. In this case asexual spore formation does not precede sexual spore reproduction. If mycelia bearing female sex organs are placed in distilled water asexual spore production soon begins following, in this case, sex organ development. It is evident that the life span as well as the course of development of *Saprolegnia mixta* can be adjusted almost at will by the proper modification and regulation of growth conditions.

Starting with rosettes of the house-leek, *Sempervivum funkii*, all derived from one plant, Klebs (1904, 1905) grew them under a great range of conditions and was able to get more than a dozen types of life history with great variation in life span. On one extreme were rosettes that produced a flower stalk with a few flowers at the tip and died the end of the first season after the fruits matured. On the other extreme were rosettes that produced upright stems that grew year after year continuously adding to the size of the stem. He was also able to produce wide variations in the character of the flowers as to color, size, symmetry, and number of flower organs. He could also produce single or double flowers at will, involving the change of sepals to petals, petals to stamens, stamens to petals, stamens to carpels, and carpels to stamens.

In contrast to the plants on which Klebs worked, Hitzer (1935) found *Stellaria media*, our common annual chickweed, varying little in its life course and life span even when grown under a wide range of conditions. He varied the following factors widely, singly and in combination, in his culture of this species: light intensity, daily light duration, moisture supply, temperature, the several inorganic fertilizers, and the pH of the culture medium. He also used Progynon in the culture solution. He could not prevent the plant from flowering under any of these conditions. In soil cultures the plants began to produce flowers after setting 4 to 12 pairs of leaves. In water cultures the flowering was sometimes delayed until after the production of 21 pairs of leaves, but upon the whole, there was little variation in the life cycle of the plant in spite of the wide range in the growth conditions. Hitzer mentions other plants that seem to show internal fixity as to their life duration and course.

While Klebs may have worked on plant forms that are unusually plastic, yet his work illustrates, as do many other researches, some of which are discussed later on in this paper, the great degree to which the life history and life duration of many plants are dependent upon the conditions furnished during growth.

2. PLANTS OF DEFINITE LIFE SPAN

Many plants die after bearing one crop of seeds (Benecke-Jost, 1923–1924). Such plants are known as monocarpic. Of all physiological groups of plants, monocarpic plants come nearest to representing a closed system as regards life span and ageing. The life span may be one season as in the case of many annual plants, summer grains and many weeds, garden plants, etc. Other plants of this type which grow two years are biennial. During the first year of growth storage organs are formed which supply the developing seeds with food for their development during the second year. After the seeds mature the plants die. In this group are burdock, beets, cabbage, celery, and many other wild and cultivated forms. Finally some plants of this group continue their growth over three or more years before producing seeds and finally dying. This is true of some Sempervivums, the century plant, and others. The development of flower stalks in any of these forms may be considered an ageing change which signals the approach of death.

While monocarpic plants as grown in nature seem to have a very definite life course and life span, more recent experimental work shows that the life course can be changed and the life span lengthened indefinitely in many cases or the life span can be shortened in other cases. Both these changes are brought about by the use of proper growth conditions.

Garner and Allard (1920, 1923) have shown that the length of daily illumination determines when many plants develop flower primordia; some plants flower only on short daily illumination and others only on long daily illumination. By using an unfavorable daily period of illumination such monocarpic plants as respond to day length can be prevented from flowering and forced to continue in vegetative growth. In this way their life span may be continued indefinitely and the ageing effects of flower and seed production prevented.

Lyssenko (1932) found that by subjecting various seeds in the partially soaked condition to temperatures just above the freezing point for some months he could shorten the period required for their complete growth. Certain light treatments have similar effects in some cases. He termed this yarovization or vernalization because of its likeness to a spring awakening. He could change winter grains to summer grains by this treatment.

Thompson (1934) finds that biennials (cabbage, beets, celery, etc.)

can be made to set seed the first year and terminate their lives by sub-jecting the seedlings to a considerable period of low temperature, 10°C. or lower. In this way biennials are transformed to annuals resulting in a great shortening of their life span. On the other hand, the same investigator can prevent certain cabbages from flowering the second year by storing the mature heads formed the first year at high rather than low temperatures during the winter. The heads stored at high temperatures form new heads rather than seed stalks as do those stored at low temperatures.

It should be pointed out that many so-called annual plants of the temperate zone are not monocarpic. They grow as annuals here because the freezing of fall and winter kills them. The tomato plant for instance is not killed by the maturing of fruits and seeds but it will continue to set and ripen fruits over a very long period. In the tropics it may grow as a perennial.

In monocarpic plants why does the maturing of fruits and seeds kill the plants? Two different explanations have been offered for this: starvation of the plants due to the heavy draft of food for maturing of fruits and seeds, and poisoning of the plants by compounds formed in the developing and maturing of fruits. Much more detailed study is needed on this point to determine which if either theory is correct. Sperlich (1919) has found that seeds of *Alectorolophus hirsutus* All. plants that mature first have high quality, while those that mature late are of poor quality. If the flowers that mature early are removed at the time of or before fertilization occurs, the late maturing flowers produce good seeds. This may mean that maturing seeds produce toxic materials that injure not only the plant but even later maturing seeds. The other cause, exhaustion of foods, may also be claimed as an explanation.

It must be remembered, however, that many of the monocarpic perennial plants have developed very effective methods of vegetative reproduction. In fact the use of side rosettes, suckers, or cuttings is a common method of reproduction for the agaves, Sempervivums, and Sedums, especially if they are to be kept true to type. This method of reproduction does not involve the so-called rejuvenating effect of the sex act. If figured from the time of reproduction by seeds no doubt many of these plants attain very great age. Later on in this paper the claimed necessity of rejuvenation by the sex act will be discussed in some detail.

From the statements above it is seen that in monocarpic plants which represent the one group of plants having a closed system, the life span can be modified at will by modifying the growth conditions. This lines up with the findings of Klebs and other workers for other groups of plants. On the other hand, regardless of how the life span is modified, the beginning of flowering marks the beginning of ageing and the maturing of the fruits leads to death.

3. PERENNIAL PLANTS THAT SET SEED REPEATEDLY

In all perennial plants except the monocarpic forms the individual lives for years and bears seeds repeatedly without any apparent injury to the plant. In some perennials such as quack grass and iris (Benecke-Jost, 1923-1924) only the underground portion is perennial while the aerial part is annual. The rhizomes of these plants grow at the tip and form branches from time to time and the basal part gradually ages and dies. Of course as soon as the base of the rhizome dies up to a branch two plants result but they both, and perhaps many others, originated from the same seed. Barring disease, insect injury or other detrimental agents, such rhizomes appear to be immortal, though the basal part gradually ages and dies.

In many perennials the parts above the ground also live year after year. Trees are ever-present and very conspicuous examples of such plants. As we know trees in nature, we think of the different ones (Benecke-Jost, 1923-1924) as of rather definite life span. The American hornbeam lives about 150 years, the beech 300 years, Sequoia 3000-4000 years, the baobab of Cape Verde 5000 years, and finally Chamberlain (1932) estimates that the "Big Tree of Tule," a Taxodium mucronatum 250 miles south of the old city of Mexico, is more than 5000 and perhaps 7000 years old.

Dr. Chamberlain has furnished the author the following statement of how he estimated the age of this tree. "I estimated the age at 5000 years. This estimate was made by counting the rings for about one foot on a trunk of the same species about four feet in diameter. You know that the rings get smaller as the plant gets older. Bearing this in mind, and also making some study of the wound tissue around the Humboldt inscription, Doctor Land thought that 7000 years would be nearer the truth. My measurement was fifty feet in diameter, made by measuring the circumference and dividing by 3.1416. Doctor Land and Doctor Barnes made the diameter a little more, and the Mexican government a couple of years ago got a little more than the Land and Barnes measurement. The trunk is not perfectly circular, slightly

elliptical. It would probably be nearer the truth to say that the minimum diameter is fifty feet and the maximum fifty-two or fifty-three."
   Figure 1 shows the picture of the entire tree. This photograph was furnished by Dr. Chamberlain. Figure 2 shows the picture of the trunk of the tree. This photograph was furnished by The American Forestry Association of Washington, D.C.

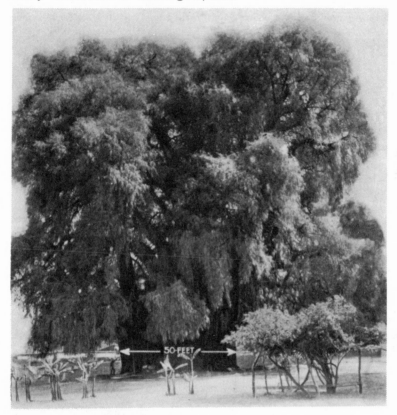

Fig. 1. "Big Tree of Tule," probably about 7000 years old. (Photograph by Dr. C. J. Chamberlain.)

   The annual growth rings of trees are often used to estimate the age of trees. The formation of growth rings depends upon the alternation of a good growing period and a non-growing period during the year. In warm regions this succession is often caused by succession of wet and dry seasons and in the cooler humid temperate zone by succession of summer and winter. The looser structure of the ring is the portion formed in the beginning of the growth season and the more compact portion that formed near the close of the growth season. In the humid temperate zone the loose structure is spring wood and the more compact structure the fall wood. In good growing seasons the rings are of course wide and in poor growing seasons narrow. Poor growth seasons may be due to drought, insect defoliation, fires, or other detrimental factors.

Prof. H. C. Sampson, Botany Department, Ohio State University, has collected many data on the rate of growth of young trees in the deep forest shade in the Adirondack Mountains. He allowed the writer to examine these data and to include a statement concerning them. Such trees show extremely slow growth and very narrow annual wood rings up to the time that the trees reach sufficient

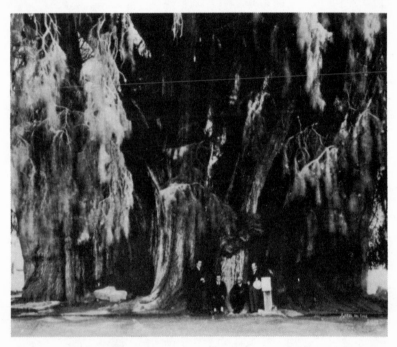

Fig. 2. Trunk of "Big Tree of Tule." (Photograph furnished by The American Forestry Association, Washington, D. C.)

height to lift the crowns into better light. After that the rings increase greatly in diameter. In this case, light intensity is the important factor in determining wood ring width.

Douglas (1919), the foremost student of growth rings and their significance, finds in his studies of trees at Flagstaff and Prescott, Arizona, that rings are not formed some years either in a part or the whole of the circumference of certain trees and that other years two rings may be formed. Methods have been worked out (Glock 1934) for identifying absent and double rings. These two anomalies are caused by drought or peculiar distribution of rainfall. By a method of cross identification of rings of different trees Douglas (1919) worked out the tree ring history at Flagstaff, Arizona, with a high degree of accuracy for the period 1385 to 1906 or for a period of 522 years. He (1934) finds that tree growth gives much information on climatic cycles during past centuries. He says (1919, p. 111): "Certain areas of wet-climate trees in northern Europe give an admirable record of the sunspot numbers and some American wet-climate trees give a similar record, but with their maxima 1 to 3 years in advance of the solar maxima. It is possible to identify living trees giving this remarkable record and to ascertain the exact conditions under which they grow."

Later Douglas (Bryan 1934) turned his attention to the study of growth rings in pieces of timbers found in various Indian pueblo ruins in Arizona and by his cross identification with rings of known date has built up a tree ring calendar from 919 to the present date. By means of this calendar he has approximated the dates on which the various pueblos were built. Douglas' work on tree rings with the tree ring calendar has become a very important tool for both meteorological and archeological sciences. The past and probable future contributions of knowledge of wood rings promise so much in these two sciences that many research institutions in New Mexico and Arizona and some institutions in eastern United States have added tree ring departments to their regular divisions of science.

Figure 3 shows annual wood rings of: (A) small fruited hickory; (B) Burr oak; (C) red oak; and (D) cedar pine. We have no records of when or where these were grown so of course cannot connect them up with known climatic factors, but one can see in them the character and the variations in the wood rings. While in each there is considerable variation in the width of the wood rings, this is most marked in (B) the Burr oak. Near the right of this section there are three series of very narrow rings representing three different periods, each of several years when the growth conditions were very unfavorable.

Does the physiology of the tree determine that it is of limited age or is its age determined by external injurious factors? A tree 150 years old has met many enemies and one 7000 years old has met many more. The roots are subject to the ravages of fungal and bacterial diseases, insects, rodents, and possibly poisonous chemical or other bad soil factors and the tops meet most of these troubles and others such as lightning, cyclones, low temperature, breaking load of ice and snow. We know that the apple trees in many places have a short life span because of root fungi, and black locust in our region falls victim to borers. Barring the continual ravages of these injurious agents and the difficulty of movement of nutrients because of great size, might trees be considered immortal? To this question we would undoubtedly get "No" as the answer of some botanists and "Yes" as the answer of others.

Finally only a very small portion of a big tree is made up of living cells; the cambium layer between the bark and wood, medullary ray cells in the sapwood, certain cells in the bark, and the growing points of the stems and roots. The greater portion of the tree is dead; the pith,

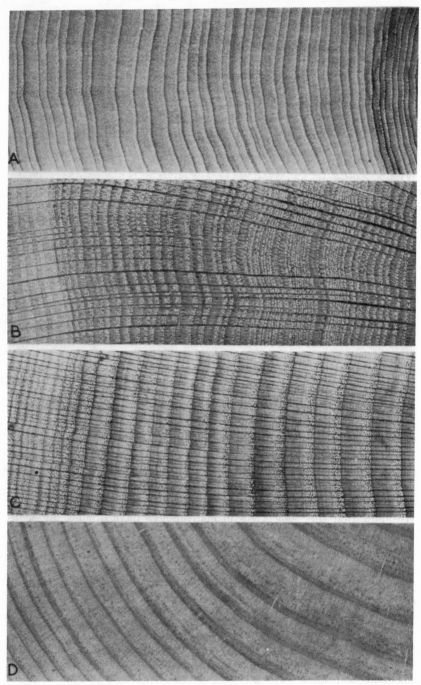

Fig. 3. Wood rings shown in cross sections of (*A*) small fruited hickory; (*B*) Burr oak; (*C*) red oak; (*D*) cedar pine.

10

heartwood, and most cells of the sapwood and bark. Individual cells or tissues are continually differentiating, ageing and dying, but even in death they remain as essential parts of the individual in the way of protective and mechanical tissue. The growing tissues continue to grow on indefinitely.

Many perennials can be propagated from root or stem cuttings. The theory has been offered that the sex act is necessary occasionally for rejuvenation, but the degeneration resulting from continuous vegetative reproduction may be explained by the accumulation of degenerative diseases or by the appearance of bud mutants rather than by innate physiological changes as the next section of this paper shows.

4. DEGENERATION OF PLANTS PROPAGATED VEGETATIVELY

Almost a century and a half ago Knight (1795, 1810), an English horticulturalist, came to the conclusion that any variety of fruit that had to be maintained true to form by vegetative propagation degenerated or became senescent in due time and that in order to keep fruits of high vigor new varieties must be produced from seed. In short, he considered the sex act necessary from time to time to rejuvenate and give vigor to vegetatively propagated varieties. Nearly a century later Zorn, a Hollandish horticulturalist, expressed the same view. Both of these horticulturalists based their conclusions on general observations. They had seen new and often excellent varieties of fruits or vegetables appear, thrive for a while, and later degenerate and become displaced by other new varieties. These views were formerly held rather generally by practical horticulturalists and no doubt they are still held by many.

Senescence due to the lack of the sex act is not the only basis on which degeneration of varieties propagated vegetatively may be explained. Knight stated that new varieties of raspberries from seed degenerate in 20 years. It is now well established that accumulation of virus diseases within the raspberry is a common cause of degeneration of varieties. In regions where the insect vectors are abundant and a source of infection is present, a variety degenerates in a few years. In regions where the vectors are few or absent or a source of infection is not present, the varieties do not degenerate at least within the period studied. It is a common statement that a new variety of potatoes will degenerate in South England after one or two years and in Scotland after 16 to 32 years. This probably corresponds to relative abundance of insect vectors of virus diseases and the nearness and abundance of sources of infection. In various cooler regions of America, certified (virus-free) seed potatoes are produced. Production of virus-free tubers is made possible in such regions by the scarcity of insect vectors and by a system of roguing that removes sources of infection. Potato varieties that are kept free from virus show no degeneration to date. Bushnell (1928) mentions a variety of potato, Long John, that has been grown in Ohio for 90 years with no indication of fall in vigor. Some dahlia varieties (Brierley, 1933) degenerate readily and others persist for years. The first group is greatly injured by virus within the plants and the latter continues to thrive in spite of the presence of the virus in the tissues. The same is true of tulips.

Many plants have been propagated for long periods vegetatively. Stout (1921) states that a thorough search of the literature indicates that no one has ever reported fruit on the single-flowered type of day-lily, *Hemerocallis fulva*. It multiplies exclusively by the formation of new bulbs. He (Stout, 1926) also states that the tiger lily, *Lilium tigrinum*, commonly grown in the United States and Europe, is fruitless and that propagation is entirely by division from the mother bulbs or by bulbils formed in the axils of the leaves. The Lombardy poplar originated as a staminate sport of *Populus nigra* between 1700–1720 (Bailey, 1927, v. 3, p. 2758) and being staminate of course has been propagated vegetatively exclusively since its origin. This tree is relatively short-lived (Reinisch, 1929) as an individual, but it has persisted vegetatively for more than 200 years. The short life of the individual of course may be due to senescence resulting from lack of sex act. On the other hand, this tree is subject to two canker diseases that shorten its life; also there has been no search for other diseases of this tree. It is a well established fact that geographical varieties (Baldwin and Shirley, 1936) of various species of forest trees do poorly if removed to other locations involving only moderate changes in climate. It is an open question whether the short life of the Lombardy poplar is due to senescence, resulting from continuous vegetative reproduction, to diseases accumulated with time, or to poor ecological adaptation.

Many varieties of olives long grown in Italy and Spain are still amongst the better varieties for California. There is no indication that continuous vegetative propagation leads to degeneration in the olive. Eastwood (1930, p. 713) says, "Commercial varieties of bananas do not produce fertile seed, having long since lost the power to reproduce in this way, and consequently the edible banana is now entirely propagated by asexual methods." Viable seeds are so rare in cultivated bananas that perhaps a thousand fruits must be dissected for each viable seed to be used to produce seedlings for breeding.

Geraniums, English ivy, and many other plants are propagated almost exclusively from cuttings.

"Broken tulips," tulips with mottled floral parts, have been known for 350 years and for a considerable time many of them were considered choice varieties. Recently (McKay and Warner, 1933) it has been discovered that the mottling is caused by viruses transmitted by insect vectors. It has also been shown that certain degenerations in foliage and bulbs generally accompany the mottling. Following these discoveries, mottled forms have come to be looked upon with disfavor.

Why does reproduction from seeds reproduce new regenerated varieties from degenerated varieties? Virus diseases with few exceptions are not transmitted through seeds; so rejuvenation may be due to the elimination of virus diseases rather than to overcoming of senescence. The British Isles have been the greatest center for the production of new varieties of potatoes from seeds with the idea at least until lately of overcoming senescence in the Knight sense. It is probable, however, that the vigor of the new varieties is caused by the elimination of virus diseases rather than by overcoming senescence.

Practically all our knowledge of virus diseases in plants has developed during this century and the greater part of it during the last fifteen or twenty years. Because of this the earlier horticulturalists were unable even to recognize virus diseases as a degenerative factor in plants, let alone give a full evaluation of their great destructive effect on plants.

There is a second factor quite aside from physiological ageing that may have led practical horticulturalists of past generations to conclude that plants degenerate under continuous vegetative propagation. The horticulturalists handle many hybrids, and hybrids are likely to produce bud mutants, or sports. The Talisman rose, for example, is a very unstable variety and in its short period of existence has produced dozens of bud sports. If inferior bud sports are used for propagation the variety will of course appear to degenerate but, if buds true to the variety are used, no degeneration will occur except as these may in turn mutate and finally, if superior bud sports are used for propagation, improved varieties are produced.

Shamel and Pomeroy (1937) have shown that various citrus and pomaceous fruits produce occasional bud sports, that some care must be taken in selecting buds or scions for propagation if the variety is to be kept true, and that new desirable varieties can be produced by proper selection of bud sports. They (Shamel and Pomeroy, 1932) record 321 bud variations of apple varieties, many of which surpass the parent in quality and are being grown as distinct strains. By examining 7397 peach trees (Shamel, Pomeroy, and Harmon, 1932) growing in commercial orchards in California, they found 70 distinct limb or entire tree varieties, some of which were improvements over the parent variety. The danger of degenerating rather than improving the variety, if attention is not given to bud selection in propagation, is emphasized by the following quotation from Shamel and Pomeroy (1937, p. 85): "The occurrence of bud mutations is more frequent than has often been realized and undesirable ones are found much oftener than desirable ones." Bregger (1933) gives many examples of the production of improved varieties of fruits, vegetables, and ornamentals through selection of bud mutants.

It is likely that mitotic modifications or mutations accompany or cause bud mutations as we shall find to be the case when seeds produce mutants due to age or heat or X-ray treatment.

Offhand, botanists are likely to assume that hybrids are more profuse producers of bud sports than are species and this may be true. We must remember, however, that plants continuously used in commercial production are much more carefully scrutinized than useless wild species; also it is only recently that horticulturalists have come to realize the frequency of bud sports and the possibilities that they offer for improving varieties. The perverse horticulturalists would also find similar possibility of producing degenerate forms of the variety.

These bud mutant studies show that better as well as poorer varieties of horticultural plants, as measured by the horticulturalist, can be produced by selective vegetative propagation. Knight and other early horticulturalists assume that continual vegetative reproduction in absence of the sex act always leads to degeneration of varieties. Later work shows that selective vegetative reproduction because of bud mutation can be used as a means of improving varieties.

It seems likely that the degeneration of varieties noted by the earlier horticulturalists may be due entirely to disease accumulation or to bad bud selection rather than to lack of sexual reproduction.

5. EXPERIMENTAL EVIDENCE FOR SENESCENCE

In the section above we have given observational evidence for senescent degeneration of plants continually propagated by asexual methods as well as observational and some experimental evidence that the degeneration is due to causes other than senescence. More recently some experimental evidence has appeared indicating senescence in various perennial plants.

Benedict (1915) claims that as a plant passes from youth to old age, reckoning its age from its origin from seed, areas of leaf tissue enclosed by the smallest branches of fibro-vascular bundles, "vein islets," become smaller. That is, the proportion of vascular tissue to active parenchyma tissue increases with age. Propagation by cuttings does not modify at all the venation of the leaf but propagation by seed is necessary for rejuvenation of the venation. Likewise, the photosynthetic and respiratory intensity of the leaves decreased with age as a result of the increased proportion of less active vascular tissue. Other changes in leaves that he considered probable with age were increase in number of stomata per area and decrease in imbibition power and decrease in size of stomata guard cells, palisade cells, and nuclei of the border parenchyma cells. The main part of Benedict's work was done on a wild grape, *Vitis vulpina*, and on other grapes but some attention was given to several varieties of peaches, apples, and plums, and to some other plants.

Ensign was unable to confirm Benedict's results and attributes the latter's errors to faulty technic. Ensign, unlike Benedict, used clearing agents to make all veins in the leaves visible. He also used much higher magnifications than the latter. He concludes that Benedict's methods failed to detect from 17 to 62 per cent of the smaller veins. Ensign (1919) first studied the seedlings from polyembryonic seeds of *Citrus grandis*. One of the seedlings from each seed he assumes to result from the sex act and therefore should show rejuvenation in the Benedict sense while the other seedling or seedlings from the same seed must be apogamous, formed without the sex act. He found no difference in vein islet size of the leaves of gamic and apogamic plants. Ensign (1921) later extended his studies to white oak, American planetree, two species of barberry, and *Vitis vulpina*, but found no relation between vein islet size of the leaves and age of the plant.

Ensign states that Dr. Heinicke found no relation between vein islet size of apple varieties and their age. A recent letter from Dr. Heinicke on this subject contains the following statements:

"The reference in Ensign's publication is to work done by myself in the department of Plant Physiology as a minor thesis. The study involved a good many varieties of apples which were grown in our collection at the University orchards.

"There is no evidence to indicate that the sizes of vein islets decreased with the age of the variety. We found some of the varieties that had been in existence for several hundred years to have much larger vein islets than those of more recent origin. Furthermore, the range in size of islets for seedlings which were but one year old was so great that we concluded that the size of the islets was as much a characteristic of the variety as color or quality of the fruit."

Levin (1929) studied the vein islet size of leaves of 9 species of *Barosma*, 5 species of *Cassia*, 2 species of *Erythroxylon*, and 4 species of *Digitalis*, all used as drugs or drug substitutes. He made all measurements midway between the midrib and leaf margin because the size was most nearly constant in this position and much smaller than the vein islet size near the margin or the midrib. He found the size of the vein islet sufficiently constant for use as a valuable specific character. The average vein islet size in leaves of *Barosma venusta* was more than four times that of *B. peglerae* and *B. scoparia* and from two to three times the size in several other species. This again raises the question whether vein islet size is not more a specific or varietal character than an indicator of plant age.

Tellefsen (1922), one of Benedict's students, using cuttings from black willow trees of various ages, confirmed the vein islet claims of Benedict. She also states that epidermal and cortical cells of roots of the cuttings seem to become smaller and the xylem and meristematic cells seem to become larger as the parent plants become older. Some doubt is thrown on Tellefsen's conclusions because she failed to clear the leaves for her vein islet studies. It is also questionable whether the slight difference she found in the cell size of the various root tissues is significant.

Finardi (1925), using the leaf clearing methods of DeVries, found in agreement with Benedict that the vein islet size of leaves decreased with the age of the plants. The degree of this change, however, varied very greatly with the species studied. In black walnut the vein islet area in leaves of one-year-old seedlings was more than six times that in 50-year-old trees. The same difference in age made a three-fold difference in the vein islet size of the leaves of the European beech. Six other perennial trees showed a decrease in the vein islet size with age but of considerable less magnitude than the walnut and beech. Finally in the Japanese varnish tree, *Sterculia platanifolia*, it was doubtful whether there was any difference in vein islet size of leaves from 2 and 40-year-old trees. In one set of measurements the vein islets were slightly larger from the 2-year-old trees and in a second set considerably smaller. Bergamaschi (1926), working with a grape (*Vitis vinifera*), confirms Tellefsen's conclusions in part on the cell size of tissues of roots of cuttings as affected by age.

In this paper attention has been given to all researches that bear on Benedict's conception of senescence in perennial plants because it is the only experimental evidence we have for age degeneration in such plants. There are some things about the character of the evidence favorable to the hypothesis that need critical consideration. In a leaf that is carrying on photosynthesis it is not only important to have chlorophyllous tissue to carry on the synthesis but it is also important to have conductive tissue for removing the synthate to other parts of the plant to prevent hindering of synthesis due to accumulation of the synthate. Just what is the size of vein islet and proximity of vascular strands that will insure maximum efficiency in photosynthesis?

Since Heinicke finds such a large difference in vein islet size of different varieties of fruits regardless of age of the variety and Levin finds similar differences between different species of the same genus and even between different regions of the same leaf, one must wonder whether Benedict is right in assuming such a strict relation between vein islet size and efficiency in the synthetic activity of the leaf. This brings us to the weakest point in Benedict's evidence, his studies of metabolism in the leaf. To obtain reliable results requires very carefully controlled experiments, because of the many variables that modify the rate of photosynthesis. Among these variables are light intensity, water content of the leaf, carbon dioxide concentration of the air, and finally the age of the leaf. We shall see the significance of the latter in a later section of this paper. Benedict ran very few experiments on photosynthesis and those that he did run lacked precision. What has been said about Benedict's photosynthetic studies applies in the main to his respiration studies.

In all the work with vein islet size the plants used were comparatively young. The oldest plant employed in any of the experiments was 100 years old (sycamore maple, Finardi, 1925) but mostly the plants were 50 years old or less. If in comparatively young plants there is such a great reduction in vein islet size, how long does this reduction continue with advancing age and does it really indicate age degeneration? There are plenty of plants that are several centuries old or that have been propagated vegetatively for centuries that could be used in such studies.

Benedict's hypothesis should not be considered too seriously until much reliable evidence has been accumulated involving the study of really old plants on which exact metabolic studies have been made. In the next section of this paper some very successful plants will be mentioned that are reproduced without involving at any time the sex act. It is possible that some perennials become senescent when propagated vegetatively continuously while others do not.

6. APOGAMOUS PLANTS

There seems to be irrefutable evidence that some plants do not become senescent or degenerate in absence of sexual reproduction. This is true of plants that reproduce exclusively apogamously (Sharp, 1934, p. 402; Schürhoff, 1926, p. 333; Chiarugi and Francini, 1930), that is, without fusion of male and female cells. Among the PTERIDO-PHYTES the following are known to reproduce apogamously only: *Marsilia drummondii*, *Athyrium filix-foemina* var. *clarissima*, and *Scolopendrium vulgare* var. *crispum-Drummondae*.

Many species of seed plants are known to produce only apogamous seeds. Billings (1937) has just reported in detail on *Isomeris arborea*, cytologically one of the simplest instances of apogamous seed production. In this plant all tissues have 17 chromosomes, probably the monoploid number. This is very different from the situation in plants that form seeds sexually. In such plants the egg and male cells have the monoploid number of chromosomes, the somatic cells twice this number, are diploid, due to the fusion of the egg and one male nucleus, and the endosperm cells have three times this number of chromosomes, i.e., are triploid, due to the fusion of the diploid nucleus of the embryo sac (formed by fusion of two polar nuclei) with the other male nucleus.

In *Isomeris arborea* no egg is formed and while the pollen tube enters the embryo sac its contents are not released into the sac but instead the contents of the tube become encased in a thick wall. The embryo of the seed develops from one of the monoploid endosperm cells in a purely vegetative way.

Besides this case the three authors mentioned in the second paragraph above mention 13 different genera and 8 different families of flowering plants, some species of which are known to produce only apogamous seeds. A complete study of all seed plants in this regard would no doubt multiply the list many fold. One of the more successful families of flowering plants, so far as natural competition is concerned, is the COMPOSITAE. Six of the thirteen genera that are known to include species producing strictly apogamous seeds belong to this family. Among apogamous COMPOSITAE are such persistent weeds as the common dandelion (*Taraxacum officinale*) and several species of *Hieracium*, or hawkweeds.

The existence of higher plants that reproduce exclusively apogamously is certainly fatal to the concept that every sort of higher plant must be regenerated from time to time by the sex act. It also raises the question whether the sex act is necessary to prevent age degeneration in plants that reproduce sexually.

7. AGEING IN TEMPORARY ORGANS OF PERENNIAL PLANTS

In the second section above we have considered the following question. Do the leaves of perennial plants by their structural and physiological characters indicate the age of the plants that produce them? However this may be, there is no doubt that temporary organs (leaves and fruits) of such plants show a definite life cycle with rather early appearance of signs of senescence finally resulting in death.

The rate of assimilation of leaves (Singh and Lal, 1935) shows a definite curve varying with age at least when optimum conditions for the process are maintained. In young leaves the rate is slow, rising to a maximum at maturity and then slowing down with ageing, and finally ceasing. Likewise there is a relation between respiratory intensity of leaves and their age. With ageing the respiratory intensity (Nicolas, 1918) of the leaf falls and finally ceases with death.

The chlorophyll and water content (Dastur and Buhariwalla, 1928) of leaves vary with age; the young leaves are low in these constituents, the mature leaves the highest, while the older leaves show a declining content. The leaves finally lose their chlorophyll and partially dry up before falling. In the late senescent stage of leaves (Schertz, 1921) not only does chlorophyll decompose but the chloroplasts themselves are partly disintegrated. All nitrogenous compounds including chlorophyll undergo partial decomposition and removal to other parts of the plant. While the chlorophyll is disappearing there seems to be an increase in the yellow pigments, carotin and xanthophyll.

Kidd (1934) has made a very thorough study of the stages of development of the fruit of the late fall apple. Figure 4 shows the developmental stages, the periods of the growing season during which the several developmental stages occur, and the intensity of respiration, fresh weight basis, for each stage.

The multiplication of cells all occurs during June and ends about three weeks after petal fall. At the end of this period the ordinary apple contains about one hundred million cells and is about the size of

a walnut.   The respiratory rate falls rapidly during this period to about
one-fifth the original rate.   The cells are filled with protoplasm and
only a few small vacuoles are present.   The concentration of sugars is
low and no starch is present.

The stage of cell enlargement extends over a period of three months
during which period the respiratory rate gradually falls.   Vacuoles
enlarge until they occupy about 80 per cent of cell space, also sugars,
mainly sucrose and fructose, rise from 1 to 9 per cent of the fresh weight.

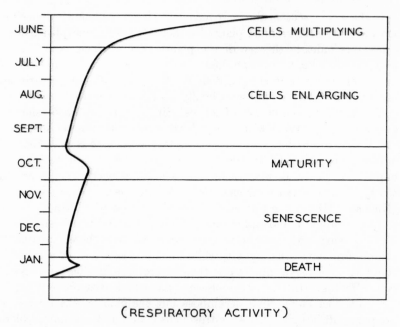

(RESPIRATORY ACTIVITY)

Fig. 4. Respiratory activity of the apple throughout its life.   Determinations
based on CO_2 produced per unit fresh weight.   (Reproduced by permission of
the author (Kidd 1934)).

Starch accumulates in the cytoplasm up to about the middle of this
period and then diminishes and disappears by the end of the period.
The cell walls reach their maximum thickness early in this period.

During October the apple reaches the stage of maturity which is
marked by a rather sudden rise in the rate of respiration.   This period
is also marked by the development of flavor, aroma, and color.

The senescent period is marked by a gradual functional as well as a
gradual cellular breakdown of the fruit.   Accompanying these changes

is a gradual fall in respiratory rate which shows a sudden rise just preceding the death of the fruit when respiration ceases.

8. AGEING OF SEEDS

Considerable attention has been given to the ageing of dormant organs in plants including seeds, spores, and pollen. These studies include life duration of these organs stored under various conditions and the internal changes involved in the gradual fall in vitality with duration of storage and the ultimate death. Much more attention has been given to seeds (Crocker, 1938) than to the other two; also the behavior of seeds is similar in most respects to that of spores and pollen. For these reasons a statement on seeds will suffice for all.

In nature and in ordinary storage the life span of seeds varies from several centuries (East Indian lotus) to a century and a half or more (certain hard coated legumes) down to a few days (willows, poplars, sugar cane, water or Indian rice, etc.). On the basis of their life span under optimum conditions Ewart divides seeds in three biological classes: (A) *microbiotic*, seeds whose life span does not exceed 3 years; (B) *mesobiotic*, whose life span ranges from 3 to 15 years; and (C) *macrobiotic*, whose life duration ranges from 15 to more than 100 years. As we shall see later, we do not have final information on the optimum storage conditions of many sorts of seeds. Indeed it is questionable whether we have it for any sort of seeds. Until we have such information, these terms do not have very definite meaning. As we learn better and better storage conditions for a given sort of seed it may jump from the microbiotic to the mesobiotic or even to the macrobiotic class. Some seeds will endure artificial desiccation considerably or far beyond the air-dry condition. Others will endure full atmospheric drying, while still others will endure little drying below the water content at time of shedding.

In seeds that will endure drying in the air or further desiccation, the best storage conditions for long retention of vitality are: maximum desiccation that the seeds will stand without injury; hermetically sealed storage in total absence of oxygen and at very low temperatures. In these conditions *Delphinium* seeds that in ordinary storage degenerate markedly in one year still have full vitality and vigor after eleven years of storage, with the experiment still running. In short, proper storage conditions lengthen the life of these seeds more than eleven-fold.

Methods have been developed for lengthening the life of short-lived seeds so they can be shipped to distant points or carried over until seeding time. Sugar cane seeds when thoroughly dry are placed in a suitable vessel with some calcium chloride. The air is then exhausted and replaced with carbon dioxide, the vessel sealed and stored at a low temperature. The seeds stored in this way can be shipped to sugar growing regions in any part of the world and grown months after they are harvested. Water or Indian rice seeds can be placed in water at the freezing point and carried over from fall harvest to spring sowing. Other methods have been developed for prolonging the life span of other short-lived seeds.

One of the best authentic records we have of various long-lived seeds is that furnished by Becquerel (1934). He had access to a batch of old seeds in a storage room in the National Museum of Paris. The time of collection of these seeds varied from 1819 to 1853. He ran germination tests on these seeds in 1906 and again in 1934. For the 1934 test Humbert and Metman furnished him about 20 seeds of *Cassia multijuga* Rich. which were collected in 1776. These seeds were all hard-coated so they demanded special treatment. The seeds were sterilized, the coats broken, and the seeds put to germinate in tubes under sterile conditions at 28°C. The seed stock was considered so precious that only ten of each sort were used for the test. In the *Cassia multijuga* only two seeds were used. Table I shows the results obtained for the 13 sorts of seeds showing germination in either the 1906 or the 1934 test. In the last column Becquerel estimates the probable life span of several of the seeds based on the data for the two tests.

All these seeds are LEGUMINOSAE except *Lavatera* (MALVA-CEAE), and *Stachys* (LABIATAE). The seeds of *Cassia multijuga* germinated after 158 years of storage. This exceeds the records of Robert Brown for *Nelumbium speciosum* from the British Museum, which were 150 years, also the records of Ewart for *Goodia lotifolia* and *Hovea heterophylla* which were 105 years, and still more the records of Turner for *Anthyllis vulneraria* and *Trifolium striatum* which were 90 years. Becquerel believes the long life span in all these seeds is made possible by impermeability of the coats which prevents any exchange of gases or water between the embryo and endosperm and the outside atmosphere, and by the high degree of desiccation and absence of oxygen in which the embryos exist within the hard coats. Hard seeds such as Becquerel studied have in themselves close approach to the several optimum conditions for storage as we defined them above. The hard coats seal the seeds individually instead of en masse, as one does with other seeds. This prevents exchange of water or gas with the outside air. According to Becquerel the water and oxygen content of hard seeds is low. This cares at least in part for proper drying and for storing in absence of oxygen. One optimum condition we mentioned above is lacking low temperature storage.

Perhaps the most interesting case known of long-lived seeds is that of East Indian lotus (*Nelumbo nucifera*) seeds of the water lily family. Ohga (1927) obtained a large quantity of these seeds from a naturally drained lake bed in Manchuria. These seeds must have been produced by the water lilies before the lake was drained for there is no other

TABLE 1

Becquerel's record of old seeds

Macrobiotic species	Date collected	Seeds growing in 1906	Seeds growing in 1934	Deter- mined long- evity	Probable long- evity
				years	*years*
Mimosa glomerata Forsk.....	1853	5 out of 10	5 out of 10	81	221
Melilotus lutea Gueld........	1851	3 out of 10	0 out of 10	55	
Astragalus Massiliensis Lam.	1848	0 out of 10	1 out of 10	86	100
Cytisus austriacus Linn......	1843	1 out of 10	0 out of 10	63	
Lavatera Pseudo-olbia Desf..	1842	2 out of 10	0 out of 10	64	
Dioclea Pauciflora Rusby....	1841	1 out of 10	2 out of 10	93	121
Ervum Lens Linn............	1841	1 out of 10	0 out of 10	65	
Trifolium arvense Linn......	1838	2 out of 10	0 out of 10	68	
Leucaena leucocephala Linn..	1835	2 out of 10	3 out of 10	99	155
Stachys nepétifolia Desf......	1829	1 out of 10	0 out of 10	77	
Cytisus biflorus L'Hérit......	1822	2 out of 10	0 out of 10	84	
Cassia bicapsularis Linn.....	1819	3 out of 10	4 out of 10	115	199
Cassia Multijuga Rich.......	1776		2 out of 2	158	

possible local source of the seeds. They were buried in the peat of the lake bed at a depth of five or six feet. Concerning the age of these seeds Ohga (1927, p. 1) says: "In one of these papers, the age was estimated (1) as more than 120 years from the size of the trunk of the willow trees which are still growing in the peat bed, (2) more than 200 years from the genealogy of Mr. U. Liu, the land owner, and (3) more than 400 years from the depth of the river bed which passes through the basin."

One immediately asks, How can seeds lie so long in moist soil without germinating or being destroyed? The answers are two: first, the seeds have hard coats which prevent water from entering the seeds, and second, under this condition the protoplasm of these seeds is very stable. The structure of the seed coat of new seeds is shown in figure 5B. The water resisting portions of the coat are the epidermis, *a*, and the outer portion of the palisade cells, *b*, down to the portion *m*, the so-called "light line." In the old buried seeds the epidermis layer was absent, also the outer portion of the palisade layer was partly eaten away, both probably due to the action of fungi and bacteria during the

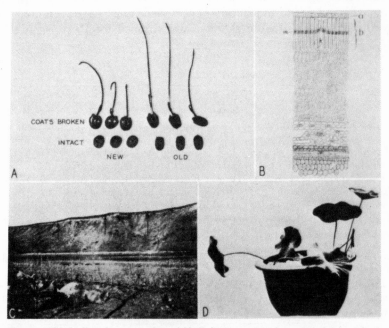

FIG. 5. Old Indian lotus seeds. (*A*) Relative rate of growth of freshly-harvested and old seed. (*B*) Structure of the seed coat showing water-resistant layers. (*C*) Location at which the seeds were found. Arrows indicate the soil layer. (*D*) A plant grown from one of the old seeds.

centuries in the soil. It is likely that in many of the seeds these resistant structures had been destroyed down to the "light line." Such seeds had of course germinated and the seedlings had perished due to deep burial and only those with the more resistant coats had remained intact. It is probable that a few seeds with less resistant coats had been germinating from time to time during the centuries. The structures that make the Indian lotus seed coats resistant to water are very similar to the structures that make most of the coats of the LEGUMI-

NOSAE seeds hard. The significance of hard coatedness in the longevity of legume seeds has been mentioned above.

It is interesting that these old lotus seeds not only gave 100 per cent germination, but they produced very vigorous seedlings. Figure 5A shows the relative rate of growth in freshly-harvested and old seeds when the coats were broken and the seeds were placed in water. Below the seedlings in each case are samples of freshly-harvested and old intact seeds. The difference in shape of the new and old seeds indicate that they may represent different strains of the species. This rather than age may account for the greater vigor of the old seeds. The arrows in figure 5C indicate the position in which the seeds were found in the escarpment formed by the eroding river, and figure 5D shows a plant grown from the old seeds.

Dr. Beal's buried weed seed experiment (Darlington, 1931) shows that various weed seeds (yellow dock, evening primrose, moth mullein, black mustard, and common smartweed) will lie in the ground for 50 years still dormant and capable of germinating. The experiments of the United States Department of Agriculture (Goss, 1924) show that seeds of many weeds as well as seeds of some cultivated plants (timothy, Kentucky blue grass, beet, several sorts of clovers, tobacco, and celery) remain dormant and alive for 20 years in natural soil conditions. Since in many cases a large percentage of these seeds still germinate, both experiments are planned to run well over a century with the hope of determining the maximum longevity of various seeds in natural soil conditions. Hard coats which prevent water absorption by the Indian lotus seeds have been mentioned as a factor contributing to their very great longevity in the soil. This cannot be called in as an explanation for the great longevity of some of the seeds mentioned in the two buried seed experiments above for timothy, tobacco, and several other seeds that live for a long time in the soil absorb water readily. The protoplasm of such seeds is apparently very stable in spite of high water content. Nature's trick of making seeds capable of remaining dormant and viable in the soil for long periods is one of her provisions for persistence of the species. While this is good for nature it is bad for the practical grower for it makes his fight against weeds, once his soil is well seeded down, a full life-time job. This delayed or distributed germination of seeds of wild plants is also an annoyance to practical growers when they put wild forms into cultivation.

What about the growth of mummy wheat? Every student of seed longevity will pronounce such a claim a pure fake. In real mummy wheat (Luthra, 1936) the grains are so nearly completely carbonized that they disintegrate into a black ash when they are placed in water. There is such a demand for mummy wheat by the tourists visiting the tombs that venders have found it profitable to satisfy this demand with modern wheat. If so-called mummy wheat has grown in recent years it is because new wheat was substituted for the real mummy wheat. Ewart (1908) speaks of the seeds of most cultivated plants, including wheat, as mesobiotic, i.e., having a life span of 3 to 15 years. There is no doubt, however, that Ewart did not realize the significance of "optimum storage conditions," in lengthening the life span of seeds, although he used the phrase in his definition. Percival (1921) found that grains of wheat, if dried and stored in tightly corked bottles, still gave 16 per cent germination after 25 years' storage and Dillman and Toole (1937) found that flax seed stored in the dry atmosphere of Mandan, North Dakota, still gave 58 per cent germination after 18 years of storage. In both of these experiments the moisture content of the seeds was low. If to this good storage condition vacuum storage and low temperature had been added, no doubt the life of these seeds would have been lengthened much more. It seems safe to say that under optimum conditions of storage, proper drying followed by vacuum storage at low temperature, the life of wheat grains and seeds of many other cultivated plants may be lengthened to 50 or even perhaps to 100 years. This is far, however, from 3000–6000 years required by mummy wheat and the latter was not stored under optimum conditions.

What are the changes within stored seeds that lead to their ageing— gradual degeneration and final death? Many explanations have been offered from time to time, such as degeneration of enzymes within the seeds, exhaustion of stored food, and denaturing of the proteins of the embryo. More recently it has been found that ageing, high temperature treatment, and X-ray treatment all seem to lead to the degeneration of seeds in the same way. All of these lead to dislocations in the mitotic mechanism of the cells of the embryo. These conditions bring about such changes as crossing over, fragmentation of chromosome with the fragments attaching to other chromosomes or being set free in the cytoplasm, similar dislocations of entire chromosomes, and finally production of polyploidy. Depending upon the intensity of application of the three degenerating factors mentioned above, the plants resulting from the treated seeds show greater and greater changes. Among the changes shown in plants grown from such seeds are: new forms of plants or mutants, slower germination and growth, partial or entire sterility, deformed leaves, and in extreme treatments death in the early seedling stage or failure to germinate at all.

9. SUMMARY

There is a great difference in the life span and life cycle of different sorts of plants growing in their natural habitats, also the life span and life cycle of most plants can be modified greatly by artificial cultural conditions. This makes it impossible to discuss the ageing of plants under a single concept.

Single-celled plants that reproduce continuously by cell division may be considered immortal.

Klebs was able to modify almost at will the life span and life cycle of various algae, fungi, ferns, and seed plants by modifying the growth conditions.

Some plants are monocarpic, that is, mature seeds but once and die. This is the nearest approach in the plant kingdom to the closed type of life cycle so common in the animal kingdom. Some monocarpic plants are annuals, some biennials, and still others perennials. By proper control of growth conditions, many annuals may have their lives indefinitely extended; biennials may be transformed to annuals or perennials; perennial monocarpic plants may have their usual life lengthened or shortened. In any case an individual monocarpic plant always dies after it matures seeds. Two explanations have been offered for the death of monocarpic plants after seed production: starvation due to exhaustion of foods in seed production and poisoning by substances formed during seed production. To date it is not known which or even whether either explanation is correct. Many perennial monocarpic plants reproduce vegetatively as well as from seeds; consequently the age of such plants, measured from the origin from seed, may be very great.

Many perennial plants produce seeds repeatedly without any evident injury to the plants. Some such plants attain ages as great as 4000 to 7000 years. Some plant scientists believe perennial plants become physiologically senescent in time and that reproduction from sexually formed seeds is necessary for physiological rejuvenation. Others hold the opposite view.

In horticulture as well as in nature many plants have been reproduced vegetatively for a very long time. Such reproduction does not furnish the so-called rejuvenating effect of sexual reproduction.

Some horticulturalists hold that varieties reproduced vegetatively soon degenerate and that the sex act is necessary for rejuvenation. There is no doubt that varieties of potatoes, raspberries, and many other plants do degenerate and that the rate of degeneration varies tremendously with the regions in which they are grown. The degeneration of many varieties of plants can be explained by the accumulation of virus diseases in them and the variation in rate of degeneration is a function of the proximity of sources of infection and abundance of insect carriers.

Since virus diseases are rarely transmitted through seeds, reproduction by seeds will rejuvenate plants degenerated by virus diseases. This fact, along with the fact that our knowledge of virus diseases has been developed mainly during the last two decades, explains why early horticulturalists mistook virus-degeneration for age-degeneration.

Bud mutations are fairly common among hybrid varieties. If a horticulturalist were not careful he might select inferior mutants for propagation and get an apparent degeneration of the variety. Horticulturalists are now making much use of bud mutants to obtain new and better varieties. The improvement in the latter case comes about through vegetative propagation without involving the so-called rejuvenating effect of the sex act. Vegetative reproduction due to bud mutations may lead to either degeneration or improvement of varieties.

Benedict claimed that as a plant passes from youth to old age, reckoning its age from its origin from seed, areas of leaf tissues enclosed by the smallest branches of fibro-vascular bundles, vein islets, become smaller. He also claimed that metabolic efficiency of the leaf fell with vein islet size. Some other investigators have confirmed Benedict's conclusions and found some other cytological or morphological evidence of age degeneration, but still other workers have criticized Benedict's technic and found no such reduction in vein islet size with age. The latter have claimed also that vein islet size of leaves is a varietal or specific character rather than an indicator of age. This is the only experimental evidence we have for physiological ageing in perennial plants as well as for the necessity of the sex act for rejuvenation; therefore the lack of agreement should be cleared up by further investigation.

Some fern-like plants reproduce only apogamously, that is, without fusion of male and female nuclei, and a number of seed plants produce only apogamous seeds. Some apogamous plants, like the dandelion, are very successful and persistent weeds. In strictly apogamous plants sexual reproduction certainly is not required for physiological rejuvenation.

Temporary organs of plants such as leaves and fruits show definite physiological and morphological life cycles ending in senescence and death. Seeds in dry storage gradually age and die. Optimum storage conditions lengthen the life span of seeds tremendously over the life span in ordinary storage conditions. The age degeneration of seeds is due to a gradual degeneration in the cell nuclei of the embryos which leads to dislocations in the chromosomes when the cells divide.

REFERENCES

BAILEY, L. H. 1927. The standard cyclopedia of horticulture. New York, Macmillan Co., 3 v.

BALDWIN, HENRY I., AND SHIRLEY, HARDY L. 1936. Forest seed control. J. Forestry, **34**, 653-663.

BECQUEREL, PAUL. 1934. La longévité des graines macrobiotiques. Compt. Rend. Acad. Sci. [Paris], **199**, 1662-1664.

BENECKE, W., AND JOST, L. 1923-24. Pflanzenphysiologie. 4. umgearb. Aufl. Jena: Gustav Fischer. 2 Bd.

BENEDICT, HARRIS M. 1915. Senile changes in leaves of *Vitis vulpina* L. and certain other plants. New York [Cornell] Agric. Exp. Sta. Mem., **7**, 275-370.

BERGAMASCHI, MARIA. 1926. Nuove richerche sui caratteri di senilita nelle piante. Atti Ist. Bot. Univ. Pavia, 115-145. (*Abstr. in* Biol. Abstr., 1929, **3**, 72, cit. 801.)

BILLINGS, FREDERICK H. 1937. Some new features in the reproductive cytology of angiosperms, illustrated by *Isomeris arborea* Nutt. New Phytol., **36**, 301-326.

BREGGER, J. T. 1933. Present status of mutation studies in deciduous fruit varieties. Proc. Amer. Soc. Hort. Sci., **29** (1932), 144-150.

BRIERLEY, PHILIP. 1933. Studies on mosaic and related diseases of dahlia. Contrib. Boyce Thompson Inst., **5**, 235-288.

BRYAN, BRUCE. 1934. Reading history from the diary of the trees. Amer. Forests, **40**, 10-14, 44-45.

BUSHNELL, JOHN. 1928. Do potato varieties degenerate in warm climates? Examples of vigorous potato clones in Ohio. J. Heredity, **19**, 132-134.

CHAMBERLAIN, CHARLES JOSEPH. 1932. The age and size of plants. Sci. Monthly, **35**, 481-491.

CHIARUGI, ALBERTO, AND FRANCINI, ELEONORA. 1930. Apomissia in "*Ochna serrulata*" Walp. Nuovo Giorn. Bot. Ital., **37**, 1-250.

CROCKER, WILLIAM. 1938. Life span of seeds. Bot. Review, **4**, 235-274.

DARLINGTON, H. T. 1931. The 50-year period for Dr. Beal's seed viability experiment. Amer. J. Bot., **18**, 262-265.

DASTUR, R. H., AND BUHARIWALLA, N. A. 1928. Chlorophyll from tropical plants and its quantitative determination by means of the spectograph. Ann. Bot., **42**, 949-964.

DILLMAN, A. C., AND TOOLE, E. H. 1937. Effect of age, condition, and temperature on the germination of flaxseed. J. Amer. Soc. Agron., **29**, 23-29.

DOUGLASS, A. E. 1919. Climatic cycles and tree-growth. A study of the annual rings of trees in relation to climate and solar activity. Carnegie Inst. of Washington. Publ., 289, 127 pp.

———— 1934. Tree growth and climatic cycles. Carnegie Inst. of Washington. Publ., 9, 1–15.

EASTWOOD, H. W. 1930. The propagation of banana plants. Agric. Gaz. New South Wales, 41, 713–724.

ENSIGN, M. R. 1919. Venation and senescence of polyembryonic citrus plants. Amer. J. Bot., 6, 311–329.

———— 1921. Area of vein-islets in leaves of certain plants as an age determinant. Amer. J. Bot., 8, 433–441.

EWART, ALFRED J. 1908. On the longevity of seeds. Proc. Roy. Soc. Victoria, 21(1), 1–210.

FINARDI, LUISA. 1925. Caratteri di senilita nelle piante. Atti Ist. Bot. Univ. Pavia, 3 Ser., 2, 305–333.

GARNER, W. W., AND ALLARD, H. A. 1920. Effects of the relative length of day and night and other factors of the environment on growth and reproduction in plants. J. Agric. Res., 18, 553–606.

———— 1923. Further studies in photoperiodism, the response of the plant to relative length of day and night. J. Agric. Res., 23, 871–920.

GLOCK, WALDO S. 1934. The language of tree rings. Carnegie Inst. of Washington. Publ., 9, 16-25.

GOSS, W. L. 1924. The vitality of buried seed. J. Agric. Res., 29, 349-362.

HARTMANN, MAX. 1921. Untersuchungen über die Morphologie und Physiologie des Formwechsels der Phytomonadinen (Volvocales). III Mitt. Die dauernd agame Zucht von *Eudorina elegans*, experimentelle Beiträge zum Befruchtungs- und Todproblem. Arch. Protistenk., 43, 223–286.

HITZER, KÄTHE. 1935. Die Bedingungen der Blütenbildung von *Stellaria media*. Flora, 129, 309–335.

KIDD, FRANKLIN. 1934. The respiration of fruits. Roy. Inst. Great Britain. Weekly Evening Meeting. Nov. 9, 33 pp.

KLEBS, GEORG. 1904. Über Probleme der Entwickelung. Biol. Centralbl., 24, 257–267, 289, 449, 481, 545, 601.

———— 1905. Über Variationen der Blüten. Jahrb. Wiss. Bot., 42, 155–32).

———— 1910. Alterations in the development and forms of plants as a result of environment. Proc. Roy. Soc. [Lond.] B., 82, 547–558.

KNIGHT, THOMAS ANDREW. 1795. Observations on the grafting of trees. Phil. Trans. Roy. Soc. London, 290–295.

———— 1810. On the parts of trees primarily impaired by age. Phil. Trans. Roy. Soc. London, 178-183.

KÜSTER, E. 1921. Botanische Betrachtungen über Alter und Tod. Abh. z. Theoret. Biologie, 10. (*Abstr. in* Bot. Centralbl., 1922, 143, 1.)

LEVIN, FREDERICK A. 1929. The taxonomic value of vein islet areas. Based upon a study of the genera *Barosma, Cassia, Erythroxylon* and *Digitalis*. Quart. J. Pharm. & Pharmacol., 2, 17–43.

LUTHRA, J. C. 1936. Ancient wheat and its viability. Current Science, 4, 489–490.

LYSSENKO, T. D. 1932. Iarovizatsiia sel'sko-khozialstvennykh rastenii. [Yarovization of agricultural plants.] Biull. Iarovizatsii, 1, 14-29.

McKay, M. B., and Warner, M. F. 1933. Historical sketch of tulip mosaic or breaking. The oldest known plant virus diseases. Nation. Hort. Mag., 12, 179-216.

Nicolas, G. 1918. Contribution a l'étude des variations de la respiration des végétaux avec l'age. Rev. Gén. Bot., 30, 209-225.

Ohga, I. 1927. On the age of the ancient fruit of the Indian lotus which is kept in the peat bed in South Manchuria. Bot. Mag. [Tokyo], 41, 1-6.

Percival, John. 1921. The wheat plant. London. Duckworth and Co., 463 pp.

Reinisch, E. F. A. Weakening effect of continual artificial reproduction. Flor. Exch., 70 (17), 96.

Schertz, F. M. 1921. A chemical and physiological study of mottling of leaves. Bot. Gaz., 71, 81-130.

Schürhoff, P. N. 1926. Die Zytologie der Blütenpflanzen. Stuttgart. Ferdinand Enke, 792 pp.

Shamel, A. D., and Pomeroy, C. S. 1932. Bud variation in apples. J. Heredity, 23, 173-180, 213-221.

——— 1937. Bud selection in citrus and other tree fruits. Calif. Citrogr., 23(1), 24, 26-28, (2), 78, 83-85.

Shamel, A. D., Pomeroy, C. S., and Harmon, F. N. 1932. Bud variation in peaches. U. S. Dept. Agric. Circ., 212, 22 pp.

Sharp, Lester W. 1934. Introduction to cytology. 3rd ed. New York. McGraw-Hill Book Co. 567 pp.

Singh, B. H., and Lal, K. N. 1935. Investigation of the effect of age on assimilation of leaves. Ann. Bot., 49, 291-307.

Sperlich, Adolf. 1919. Die Fähigkeit der Linienerhaltung (phyletische Potenz), ein auf die Nachkommenschaft von Saisonpflanzen mit festem Rhythmus ungleichmässig übergehender Faktor auf Grund von Untersuchungen über die Keimungsenergie, Rhythmik und Variabilität in reinen Linien von *Alectorolophus hirsutus* All. Sitzungsber. Akad. Wiss. Wien Math. Naturwiss. Kl. Abt. I., 128, 379-476.

Stout, A. B. 1921. Sterility and fertility in species of *Hemerocallis*. Torreya, 21, 57-62.

——— 1926. The capsules, seed, and seedlings of the tiger lily, *Lilium tigrinum*. Bull. Torrey Bot. Club, 53, 269-278.

Tellefsen, Marjorie A. 1922. The relation of age to size in certain root cells and in vein-islets of the leaves of *Salix nigra* Marsh. Am. J. Bot., 9, 121-139.

Thompson, H. C. 1934. Temperature as a factor affecting flowering of plants. Proc. Amer. Soc. Hort. Sci., 30(1933), 440-446.

Wallace, Raymond H. 1928. Histogenesis of intumescences in the apple induced by ethylene gas. Am. J. Bot., 15, 509-524.

Chapter 2

SENESCENCE AND DEATH IN PROTOZOA AND INVERTEBRATES

H. S. JENNINGS

Baltimore

1. PROBLEMS IN THE STUDY OF PROTOZOA

The questions which arise in the study of ageing and death in the Protozoa are mainly the following:

Does life in single cells involve decline, senescence, death? Does to live mean eventually to wear out, and to accumulate waste products that produce decline and death, even when it occurs in but a single cell?

Or is the life of single cells so carried on that wear is repaired as it occurs and waste products eliminated as they are produced, so that their life may continue without end? Are senescence and death phenomena that have taken origin only as organisms became multicellular and differentiated? Are they the consequence of division of labor, specialization, and interdependence among the cells of a multicellular organism, as many have held? What is the nature of the processes of repair that underlie the long-continued life of many unicellular organisms?

In view of the nature of the life cycle of the Protozoa, the age problem here has a two-fold bearing:

(1) The individual is a free cell, which performs all the fundamental operations of life. Does ageing play a rôle in the life of such a single individual?

(2) More important is the following. The single cellular individual as a rule does not as such die; instead it grows and divides into two individuals. This continues, so that chains of free individuals are produced, stretching for many cell generations. These are interrupted at long intervals by the union of two individuals in sexual reproduction. After this, the chain of free individuals continues. In relation to this, the question arises: Does the chain of successive living cells, through the processes of living, gradually become senescent in its later links, so that it declines and finally dies, unless something intervenes to save it?

These two aspects of living in free cells will be considered separately.

2. LIFE OF INDIVIDUAL PROTOZOAN

The single individual is produced by the division into two of an earlier individual. The parent has a typical differentiated structure, in many cases with typically arranged motor appendages (figure 6). The typical structure is necessarily altered and disordered by the division of the individual, so that the new individuals produced are not like the parent. But developmental processes occur by which the new individuals assume the same typical structure that was present in the parent. This development involves an extensive reorganization of the body. In cases in which the parent has complexly arranged appendages, these appendages are commonly absorbed and disappear during fission, while

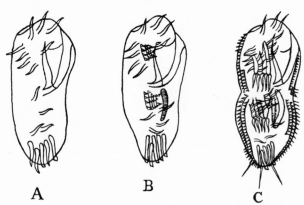

A   B   C

Fig. 6. Division with reorganization in the infusorian *Stylonychia*, after Wallengren (1901). (*A*) Parent before reproduction. (*B*) Appearance of two groups of small projections that are to form the appendages of the two offspring. (*C*) Division: the two groups of embryonic appendages are spreading out to take their final positions, while the old appendages have not yet disappeared.

at the same time many other bodily differentiations disappear. The typical structure and appendages are then developed anew in each of the new individuals. The details of this reorganization differ in different species; it appears to be less complete in species having a less highly differentiated structure.

This reorganization involves the nucleus of the cell, as well as the cell body. In the higher Protozoa,—the ciliate infusoria,—the nucleus is in two parts (originally derived from one). One is the very large macronucleus, the other the minute micronucleus (see fig. 7). It is the large macronucleus that participates in metabolism, growth and other activities of the cell, while the micronucleus is a reserve part, having little relation to the cellular processes except to maintain its own existence, and to produce new macronuclei.

At fission, both nuclei divide. During the process the macronucleus is in many cases known to be extensively reorganized. In some cases a portion of the macronucleus is eliminated and dissolved (fig. 8). In other cases a visible "reorganization zone" begins at a definite spot and traverses the entire nucleus, changing its structure (fig. 9). At the same time it seems probable, as has been suggested, that certain materials are eliminated, perhaps in a liquid condition.

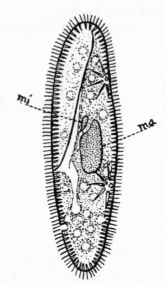

FIG. 7. The infusorian *Paramecium caudatum*, after Wenrich (1928), from Kalmus (1931), showing the large macronucleus (*ma*) and the small micronucleus [Stylonychia] (*mi*).

For accounts of such reorganization phenomena the following recent papers may be consulted: Kidder, 1933; Calkins, 1934; Kidder and Diller, 1934; Tittler, 1935; Summers, 1935. An excellent illustrated and detailed account of these and other matters relating to ageing and rejuvenescence in Protozoa will be found in Calkins' *Biology of the Protozoa* (2nd edition, 1933).

Thus after fission the newly produced individuals have been completely reorganized, both inwardly and outwardly; they are "young" as compared with the parent. Certain physiological changes as the individual recedes from youth have been revealed by studies of regeneration. But these are the reverse of what might at first be anticipated, revealing the peculiar nature of individual life in these organisms. Calkins (1911) found that in *Uronychia* there is no regeneration if parts are removed in "young" individuals immediately after fission, and very little if they are removed later during "adult" life. But if in "old" individuals that are getting ready to divide, parts are removed, they are fully regenerated. The end of the individual life is here not death, but division into two, and this is preceded by an increase of

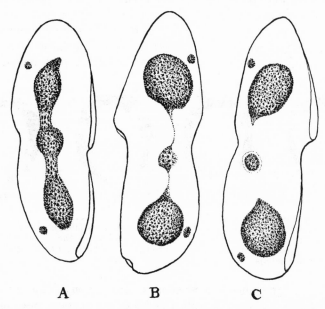

A   B   C

Fig. 8. Division of the macronucleus in *Ancistruma*, with extrusion of a central portion which is later absorbed and disappears. The small round bodies above and below are the micronuclei. After Kidder (1933).

growth energy instead of by senescence. However, such greater regenerative power just before division appears to be absent in some species (in *Spathidium*, according to Moore, 1924).

Under some unfavorable conditions the individual cell may undergo a reorganization without division. This occurs as a rule (but not exclusively) in connection with encystment. Conditions that induce encystment and reorganization are, in different cases, the following: mechanical injuries to the cell, drying, lack of food, increase of salt content in the water, the presence of excretion products, and the like.

The first step in such a reorganization is a dedifferentiation of the cytoplasmic structures. The conspicuous buccal groove disappears, the motor appendages are absorbed, and the cell takes a spherical form, appearing as an undifferentiated mass containing the nuclei. Usually this spherical mass secretes a wall about itself, becoming thus a cyst, which is resistant to drying and to other injurious conditions. De-differentiation in the large and complex unicellular form *Bursaria* is described in detail by Lund (1917).

Within the cyst thus formed there occurs in many cases a reorganization of the nuclear apparatus. In its most pronounced form, this includes the breaking up and dissolution of the macronucleus and its replacement by a portion of the micronucleus. The latter divides, one part enlarging to become a macronucleus, another part remaining in

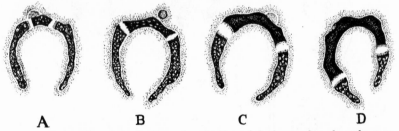

A   B   C   D

FIG. 9. Successive stages in the reorganization of the horse-shoe shaped macronucleus at division in *Aspidisca lynceus*, after Summers (1935). Before division two "reorganization bands" appear near the middle of the horse-shoe; these traverse the horse-shoe in each direction to its tips, inducing a thorough reorganization of the nucleus.

reserve as a micronucleus. Such a reorganization of the nucleus is known in many cases; it is called *endomixis*. In some cases no such pronounced nuclear reorganization occurs in the cyst. The detailed nuclear changes during encystment are in need of extensive study.

Under favorable conditions the undifferentiated cyst is awakened to active life. Redifferentiation occurs; the typical structures and appendages are again produced, the cell escapes from within the cyst wall and resumes its free existence. In cases in which before encystment the vitality was low, it is found that the reorganized individuals emerging from the cysts have a heightened vitality and reproductive power, as compared with the situation before encystment (Calkins, 1915; Beers, 1930). Encystment may occur at times when the vitality is high, being induced by unfavorable environmental conditions; in such cases encystment does not increase vitality.

The life of the individual cell as such is normally terminated by its division into two cells. Hartmann (1928) has shown that by repeatedly cutting off a part of the cell (in Ameba and Stentor) division may be suppressed. Individuals on which removal of a part is thus practiced at regular intervals may live indefinitely without division. Hartmann thus kept an individual Ameba alive for four months without division. It appears that cutting off a piece of the body induces reorganization, with the same effect as results from cell division.

3. AGEING OF PROTOZOA THROUGH MANY GENERATIONS

As shown in the foregoing section, reproduction by fission involves reorganization and development. The new individuals produced are physiologically young as compared with the parent individual.

But the question remains whether the rejuvenescence so produced fully restores the pristine condition. The chain of living cells extends for hundreds, thousands, of generations. Are the later members of the chain as physiologically young as the earlier members? Or do the later members become senescent and finally die, unless something intervenes to save them? And by what sort of intervention may they be saved?

To obtain factual answers to these questions an astonishing amount of labor has been expended. The present state of knowledge will be summed up in a series of numbered sections.

1. When the chains of living cells are kept under observation in the laboratory, so that their fate can be determined, as has been done with many species of Protozoa, it is found that as a rule, after some hundreds of generations they do decline. Fission and other life processes become slower, resistance decreases, functions are imperfectly performed. Varied structural changes occur. Frequently the protoplasm becomes opaque; the cell body is swollen, or in other cases wastes away. Structural differentiations become less marked; appendages may be lost. Nuclear abnormalities occur; at times the micronucleus disappears. The organisms give a picture of senescence, finally extending to death. Figure 10 shows three stages in these changes as observed by Maupas (1888).

The curve of declining vitality is well represented by the graph of daily fission rate, which for any given biotype appears to be a good measure of vitality. A typical graph is shown in figure 11. A large number of such graphs for different species, are given by Jennings 1929.

The period during which the animals continue to multiply, before declining to death, varies greatly. It usually includes some hundreds of generations. Such a declining curve of *Paramecium caudatum*, as studied by Calkins (1904) covered 659 days, during which there were 742 generations.

2. Such declining stocks are in some cases visibly rescued from death and restored to high vitality by the intervention of sexual reproduction,—the union of individuals in conjugation.

Whether sexual union does in fact result in rejuvenescence was long a subject of controversy. When conjugation occurs at periods when

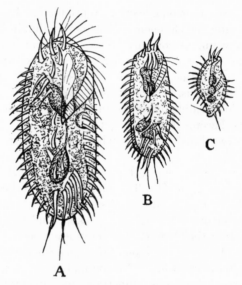

Fig. 10. Three successive stages (drawn to the same scale) in the decline and degeneration of *Stylonychia pustulata*, after Maupas (1888).

the vitality has not been lowered, it does not result in increased vitality. Moreover, conjugation has many other aspects; it results in producing new combinations of the genes; and it is a complex process, which may take place in an imperfect or abnormal way. In consequence, it often results in an actual lowering of vitality; it may even result in abnormality and death. It has now been fully demonstrated however that in certain species, if conjugation occurs at periods of lowered vitality, it results in increased vitality, in rejuvenescence. This was demonstrated by Calkins (1919) for *Uroleptus*, and by Woodruff and Spencer (1921) for *Spathidium*. After conjugation, in these cases, the lowered curve of vitality rises, the life processes proceed again rapidly and efficiently, and death is averted.

How sexual union produced this effect was long a mystery; it gave rise to mystical theories. The explanation now seems clear; it will be set forth in later paragraphs.

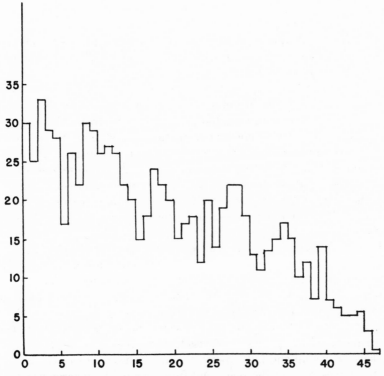

Fig. 11. Graph of the fission rate in successive ten-day periods in isolation cultures of *Pleurotricha lanceolata*, in the experiments of Baitsell (1914). The horizontal scale shows the number of successive 10-day periods, the vertical scale the number of fissions in each period. The fission rate declines (with many fluctuations) till the culture ends in death.

3. It has now been shown that there exist stocks or species of Protozoa which may continue indefinitely to reproduce by fission, without senescence or decline—the consecutive chain of cells continuing endlessly to multiply at a high level of vitality; and this without intervention of sexual union.

This was demonstrated by Woodruff (1926) in *Paramecium aurelia;*

the organisms were kept in uninterrupted vegetative multiplication for years, and for thousands of generations. It was similarly demonstrated for *Paramecium caudatum* by Metalnikov (1924), by Hartmann (1917) for *Eudorina*, by Belar (1924) for *Actinophrys*, and by other workers for other species of Protozoa.

Thus in these species the constitution of the organisms is such that the life processes can go on indefinitely. Regulatory processes, repair of wear and elimination of waste keep step with the other processes of life. One of the major questions appears to be answered by these observations. Senescence and death of the cell are not inevitable accompaniments or results of living.

4. But the deeper significance of these facts was brought into question by discovery of the nature of some of the regulatory processes which make possible this uninterrupted living. In the free cells that have been most studied in connection with these questions,—the ciliate infusoria—the nucleus, as before set forth, is in two parts. There is a large physiologically active macronucleus, and a minute reserve, the micronucleus. If the macronucleus is removed, life processes soon stop, but they may continue for generations in the absence of the micronucleus. If the major processes of living wear and use up the nuclear material, it is upon the macronucleus that this exhaustion must fall.

It was discovered by Woodruff and Erdmann (1914) that in *Paramecium aurelia* and *caudatum* there occur at intervals of many generations of active life a replacement of the entire active macronucleus from a part of the reserve micronucleus. This is the same process (endomixis) mentioned on an earlier page as occurring during encystment. But it was now found to occur in these species during active life, without interruption of the processes of vegetative reproduction. The macronucleus breaks up and fades away, the micronucleus divides and a part of it enlarges to take the place and functions of the macronucleus.

It has further been shown that this replacement of the worn macronucleus from the unworn micronucleus is effective in keeping up or restoring the vitality of the organism. If endomixis is omitted for long periods the organisms decline in vitality, resistance is decreased, and finally, if endomixis does not occur, they die. This was first observed by Woodruff (1917), and has been extensively confirmed in the laboratory of the writer. After endomixis has been long postponed, the fission rate falls, and the fall continues, becoming progressively greater the longer endomixis is held off, till death occurs (Jennings and Sonneborn, 1936). If after the fission rate has notably fallen, endomixis occurs, with its substitution of a new macronucleus for the old one, the fission rate in many cases is at once restored to the usual level, and the chain of cells lives far beyond the period at which it would have died. Normally in these species endomixis occurs before there has been a detectable fall in vitality, so that decline is entirely prevented. A delicate test gives evidence that in *Paramecium aurelia* the vitality is directly pɪ ˀportional to the recency of endomixis. This test is presented by the fact that the undergoing of the endomictic process is itself a severe ordeal, so that individuals of lowered vitality may die during or in consequence of it. The greater the period since the last endomixis, the greater the proportion of individuals that die at or after the occurrence of the next endomictic process (unpublished results of Pierson and Gelber).

The meaning of the occurrence of endomixis, with its renewal of vitality, appears to be as follows. An essential part of the cell, the nucleus, is indeed exhausted or poisoned in the process of living, so that life can be continued only by the substitution for this worn organ of a nucleus which has not partaken of the active life of the cell. In these species at least it appears to be this substitution of a reserve for a worn out part that makes it possible for life to keep indefinitely in progress. The necessary repair and elimination, it appears, are not carried out as part of the ordinary continuous physiological processes, but at intervals exhausted parts must be rejected and unexhausted parts substituted, such substitution occurring within the single cell itself. In place of the death of the entire cell there is the dissolution and replacement of the macronucleus.

This gave the clue to the restoration of lowered vitality by sexual union. In this process too the macronucleus breaks up and dissolves, and its place is taken by a part of the reserve. The substitution has the same effect in warding off senescence and renewing vitality, whether it occurs in connection with sexual reproduction or apart from it. In some of the Ciliata, beside the replacement of the macronucleus at sexual reunion, there is a visible reorganization of the entire cell. Appendages and other visible structures are lost and developed anew.

With these discoveries the balance seemed to incline again toward the inevitability of exhaustion through full active living, although reserve parts, it appears, can live unexhausted as a result of not participating in the major activities of life. One becomes inclined to suspect that the keeping in store of fresh unexhausted parts, whether they are entire cells as in higher organisms, or parts of cells as in these Protozoa, is the secret of continued life.

5. But another step in discovery brought again into question the general validity of such a conclusion. Certain stocks or species of Protozoa, it was found, can continue to live and multiply indefinitely, although in them there is no separation of the nucleus into active and reserve portions, and hence no replacement of the former by the latter. This is the case in Eudorina (Hartmann, 1921), and in Actinophyrys (Belar, 1924). Furthermore, in many species of ciliate infusoria, in which there is such a separation of active and reserve parts, there is no substitution of the reserve for the active part during the active life of the organisms, but only at encystment. Yet some of these species can live indefinitely in an active condition. And in certain species in which normally there exist macronucleus and micronucleus, at times stocks are found in which there is no separate micronucleus. Such a condition commonly occurs in the final stages of senescence, when the organisms are predestined to early death. But Dawson (1919) found a stock of Oxytricha hymenostoma in which the micronucleus was missing, yet vitality was high, and though vitality declined in isolation cultures, in mass cultures these infusoria lacking a micronucleus would live indefinitely.

Thus it appeared that in these species the substitution of a reserve for the active nucleus is not necessary. The balance seemed to swing again away from the conclusion that exhaustion and senescence are inevitable unless such substitution occurs.

But the last word on this matter has not been said. As set forth earlier, in the account of the life of the individual, at cell division parts of the active macronucleus are eliminated, in some species of infusoria. At division into two, a third piece of the nucleus is formed, and this is dissolved and disappears. In other cases, as already mentioned, a visible reorganization of the macronucleus occurs, which is not obviously accompanied by elimination of parts (unless the eliminated material is in liquid condition). Such phenomena are commonly interpreted as cases of elimination of exhausted portions of the nucleus, with presumably their replacement from reserve parts; or at least as processes of reorganization by which exhausted parts are renewed (see especially Calkins, 1934). They are of extreme interest, though it is much to be regretted that there appears no prospect of making an experimental test of the assumption that they actually result in a renewal of vitality.

All this leaves open the possibility that there are in all continuously living cells processes of substitution occurring on so minute a scale that they are difficult to detect or to test, and that this is the secret of the power of living indefinitely. Yet to conclude that these processes are so minute and so nearly continuous, is practically equivalent to the conclusion that the ordinary processes of life include repair and elimination so effective that life can continue indefinitely without exhaustion; to the conclusion that senescence and death are not in all free cells inevitable consequences of living,—though in some they are.

6. But another set of observations is important in relation to this matter of senescence. In the same species or stocks which under favorable conditions may live indefinitely without senescence there occurs under less favorable conditions a slow decline in vitality as generations pass. This is true both in those stocks in which substitution of unworn for worn parts is known to occur, and in those in which it is not. The effect of the unfavorable conditions cannot be perceived in one generation; often not in ten generations. But they apparently slow down repair and elimination, and after many, perhaps hundreds, of generations they produce senescence and final death. Decline in some of these stocks is checked and in large measure remedied by substitution of the reserve for the active nucleus, but in time even this fails; *Paramecium caudatum* and *Paramecium aurelia*, with their periodic endomixis, eventually under poor conditions become old and die.

Thus the cell constitution in many Protozoa is such that under certain conditions life may continue indefinitely; while under other conditions it may continue for a great number of generations, but eventually yields to senescence and death.

7. Finally, there exist also stocks in the Protozoa in which senescence and ultimate death are unavoidable, occurring under all conditions, including the best.

Such stocks are frequently produced, in Paramecium, at sexual reproduction. In the Protozoa, as in higher organisms, sexual reproduction is a process of producing many diverse genetic constitutions. Some of these genetic constitutions are such as may continue to live long, or even indefinitely, when the conditions are good. But others are of such a sort that the lines of descent to which they give origin may live for a number of generations, many or few, then they inevitably decline and die.

Many such short-lived stocks have been found to arise at conjugation in *Paramecium aurelia*; some of these are described by Jennings, Raffel, Lynch and Sonneborn (1932). Some of these stocks live for but a few generations after conjugation, producing a small number of descendants, which all die. Others continue to multiply for 10 to 40 generations or more, giving rise to a large population; but after a time all the members of the population decline and die. In some cases such a stock gives rise to a few lines that continue long, while the great majority of the lines are predestined to early death, as in the stock 11a, described in the paper just referred to.

Thus after a stock of Protozoa has gone through conjugation there is a great process of selective elimination occurring among their descendants. A considerable proportion of the descendants of diverse genetic constitution so produced cannot continue to live indefinitely; after a small or large number of generations they decline and die, leaving only the more vigorous lines of descent.

This occurrence of stocks that are predestined by their genetic constitution to decline and death after multiplying for a number of generations, is a matter not to be neglected in a consideration of senescence and death in free cells. Ageing and death from intrinsic causes is not foreign to organisms that are single cells, as is often asserted. Death from intrinsic causes by no means owes its first origin to the evolution of multicellular organisms. It is a widespread and abundant phenomenon in unicellular organisms.

Summarizing the relations of free living cells to senescence and death, as we have set them forth above, we find many gradations, many diversities of constitution. Some free cells are so constituted that they are predestined to decline and death after a number of generations. Some are so constituted that decline occurs, but this is checked or reversed by substitution of reserve parts for those that are exhausted; they can live indefinitely, but are dependent on this substitution. In some the constitution is such that life and multiplication can continue indefinitely without visible substitution of a reserve nucleus for an exhausted one; but whether this is due to the continued substitution, on a minute scale, of reserve parts for those that are outworn cannot now be positively stated. This perfected condition, in which living itself includes continuously the necessary processes of repair and elimination, is found in some free cells, but not in all.

(Many of the matters discussed in the foregoing pages will be found more fully described or discussed in the present author's *Genetics of the Protozoa* (1929), and in Calkins' *The Biology of the Protozoa* (1933)).

4. INVERTEBRATES CONTRASTED WITH PROTOZOA

The invertebrates of course present a wide variety of conditions as to length of life, senescence and death. The length of life varies from the few days of the male rotifer to the sixty-six or more years of the actinian (Ashworth and Annandale, 1904). A summary of the chief known facts as to length of life and related matters is given by Korschelt (1917), and many important relations touching them are investigated and discussed in the writings of Pearl (1922, 1928). The present discussion will deal in the main with matters that touch the questions raised in the foregoing section on Protozoa, together with certain additional relations for which the invertebrates furnish favorable material. There are many parallels in the relations of the two groups to senescence and death.

In the invertebrates, as in the Protozoa, we find extensive if not universal use of the device of keeping certain parts of the organism out of the main current of the life activities, forming a reserve, which is substituted at intervals for worn or senescent parts of the active organism. In the multicellular organisms these reserves are distinct cells, not mere reserve portions of cells, as in the Protozoa. These reserve cells have the capability of developing and of taking on all the activities of the organism. They are best known to us as germ cells, but many organisms have other reserve cells, known as embryonic or regenerative cells, which remain dormant, but can be roused to active life by appropriate conditions. They play a great rôle in vegetative reproduction and in regeneration.

Besides substitution of reserve cells for exhausted or injured active ones, there may occur, as in the Protozoa, dedifferentiation and reorganization of differentiated cells, which thereupon take on new functions and differentiations. Such reorganization takes place readily in the partially differentiated cells of early embryonic periods, so that the "prospective fate" of the cells is changed. It becomes infrequent as adult conditions are reached. Different groups of the invertebrates differ greatly as to the readiness with which the "prospective fate" of the cells can thus be changed. In general it may be said that the extent and distribution of such reorganization of differentiated cells is not fully worked out.

The reserve cells known as germ cells are commonly aroused to full activity by the processes of sexual union. But the many cases of parthenogenesis, natural or artificial, show that they, like the regenerative cells, may be awakened to full activity independently of sexual union.

In the invertebrates, as in the Protozoa, the cells which take an active part in the life of the individual are subject as a rule to decline, to senescence.   As we have seen in the Protozoa, such decline occurs in free cells as well as in those forming the differentiated multicellular body. In addition to the senescence of the individual cells, or in consequence of it, there is, as in the vertebrates, a general senescence of the entire body, culminating in death.

5. DETERMINATE AND INDETERMINATE GROWTH OF INVERTEBRATES

With relation to these matters there may be distinguished in the invertebrates certain different groups.   On the one hand there are those having determinate growth.   In these the body reaches a definite form and size, then ceases growing.   The period of growth is commonly followed by a definite period of maturity, then of age, followed by death. Examples of these are the insects, and the rotifers.   In another group growth is indeterminate; the form and size are not definitely fixed, and growth may continue for an indefinite period.   Marked examples of these are many sponges, and the branching hydroids.   Many invertebrates show mixed or intermediate conditions.   Examples of these are some of the free-living flatworms, in which the individuals have a definite form and size, yet may grow indefinitely by the budding off of new individuals.

Invertebrates with determinate growth.   In the most pronounced types of strictly determinate growth, as in the rotifers and the insects, embryonic or reserve cells may be lacking in adult life, except for the germ cells.   Such organisms are usually without the power of regenerating lost parts, and all the cells except the germ cell are subject to senescence and death.

In these organisms the individual life is commonly divided into definite limited periods, differing in their relation to development.   It will be worth while to note the characteristics of these in the rotifer as an example of strictly determinate development.

In the rotifer there is first a brief period of cell division, lasting but a few hours.   At this time are produced all the cells of the various bodily tissues.   According to some observers, the number of cells in each tissue is very sharply defined and limited, so that the exact number of cells in the body can be given; thus Martini (1912) gives the number of cells in the body of *Hydatina senta* as 959.   According to Shull (1918) there is some inconstancy in the number of cells in particular tissues, but the fact of definitely limited cell production remains.   The body is formed on a pattern in which the number of cells in each part is extremely constant.   Cell division occurs until the number of cells required for completing the pattern is supplied, then it ceases. At this time the cells are packed solidly together, and have not taken on their definitive forms, so that the individual is a minute nearly spherical mass of cells.

Upon the cessation of cell division, a period of growth and differentiation follows. Without increase in the number of cells, the various organs take on their adult forms, their cells differentiate, growth in size occurs, till the normal size and structure of the organisms are produced. Thereupon growth ceases. This period of growth lasts in the rotifers but a few hours.

Next follows a brief period of maturity, during which reproduction occurs. It lasts in most species but a few days, and is definitely limited, though it is not quite so uniform as the periods of cell division and of growth. The reproductive period varies in *Proales sordida* from 3 to 9 days (Jennings and Lynch, 1928).

Next follows a period of senescence, ending in death. The period of senescence is limited, like the others, though with a somewhat greater amount of variation. In *Proales sordida* it varies from 1 to 17 days. The total life in this animal falls within 23 days, divided as follows: cell division, one day; growth, one day; reproductive period 3 to 9 days; senescence 1 to 17 days.

As appears from the above, the different life periods, except possibly the last, are dedicated to certain definite functions, ceasing when those functions are accomplished, so that they are thereby sharply limited. The entire life proceeds upon a rather definite schedule, occupying but a few days. In many cases the organisms are so constituted that early decline and death forms one of their most definite characteristics. In the male of most rotifers there is no alimentary canal, so that life lasts but a few hours, and a similar situation occurs in other groups. Death at a particular time in the schedule appears as definite a characteristic of the species as form of body or limbs.

Such organisms have raised in certain minds the question whether in them senescence and death, like cell division, growth and reproduction. are not essentially functional; whether the time at which they occur has not become fixed by the same evolutionary processes that fix the color of eyes or form of limbs. Of this character was a famous theory of Weismann, holding that death at a certain period had been developed through natural selection, as an advantage to the species, rather than as an inevitable consequence of exhaustion through the wear and tear of living.

Invertebrates with indeterminate growth. In the invertebrates in which development is indeterminate, as in hydroids and some flatworms, life of the body appears to continue indefinitely, through continued branching, budding, or division. Yet the parts that are early formed and differentiated commonly become in time senescent and finally die. It is only the newly formed buds or branches that continue to live indefinitely,—through further budding or branching. A valuable detailed study of these phenomena in the flatworm Stenostomum is given by Sonneborn, 1930. In such organisms the senescence that occurs seems to be a true decline or "decay" resulting from wear or incomplete elimination of waste products.

In the formation of the "new" parts of the body, that continue to live, reserve or embryonic cells that have not taken part in the full life of the body are known to play a large rôle. When such embryonic cells are destroyed by radiation, new parts are not further produced; regeneration no longer occurs (Curtis, 1928). In some cases also dedifferentiation of differentiated cells plays a rôle; they take on anew the embryonic condition, later developing and differentiating anew. In many highly differentiated cells such restoration to the embryonic condition appears not possible. The extent to which dedifferentiation plays a rôle in these matters has not been fully elucidated.

6. GENETIC CONSTITUTION AND SENESCENCE

In any given species, particularly in those organisms having determinate growth, the length of life and the time of occurrence of senescence and death, depend (as in Protozoa) both on environmental conditions, and on the genetic constitution. Important investigations on both these aspects of the matter in invertebrates, we owe to Pearl and his co-workers (see Pearl, 1922, 1928, and Gonzalez, 1923). The rôle of genetic constitution in determining length of life they have demonstrated fully in the fruit fly, *Drosophila melanogaster*. Under given conditions, certain stocks, marked by visible structural characteristics, live much longer than others. Gonzalez (1923) found that while the normal "wild type" fruit fly lives on the average 39.5 days, a stock differing from this in having much reduced wings ("vestigial wings") has an average length of life of but 18.2 days. The vestigial stock differs from the wild type in but a single gene. Gonzalez shows also that changes in other single genes result in greatly altering the length of life. The average duration of life in days for a number of stocks differing in but a single gene (or in the case of "Quintuple" differing from the others in five genes) is given by Gonzalez (1923) as follows:

	days
Wild type	39.47
Black	40.68
Purple	25.54
Vestigial	18.22
Arc	26.81
Speck	42.66
Quintuple	10.88

As is well known, every gene (with seemingly a few exceptions) plays an essential rôle in the life and development of every cell of the body. It is not surprising therefore that changing single genes may so alter the cellular processes as to change the length of life.

When stocks differing in length of life are crossed, Pearl shows that in the descendants the length of life depends upon their genetic constitution. In the immediate offspring of the cross (F_1), the mean length of life is greater than in either parent stock, so that these offspring show "hybrid vigor." In a cross of a "type I" (mean life 44.2 days) with a "type IV" (mean life 14.1 days), the mean life in the immediate offspring was 51.5 days (Pearl 1922). In later generations of the descendants, groups with diverse lengths of life are formed, in proportions showing that inheritance of this character, like that of others, occurs in accordance with Mendelian laws.

In general it has been found that in Drosophila the mutated types tend to have a higher mortality rate, and a lower length of life than the unmutated or "wild" types,—almost any mutation in a gene tending to shorten life.

In invertebrates, as in man, there is much variation in the length of life among the individuals of a given species or race. If in a population the proportion of survivors is plotted at successive intervals, a curve of typical form is produced. Pearl brings out that in the invertebrates, so far as these matters have been studied, this survivorship or mortality curve is of the same form and type as in man. Pearl and Doering (1923) have illustrated this in detail for Drosophila and the rotifer, *Proales decipiens*, in comparison with man.

What are the causes of the variations in length of life, and the typical distribution of these variations shown in the survivorship curves? In a human population, both environmental and genetic factors are certainly involved, genetic differences among the individuals perhaps supplying the main cause of variation. In the rotifer, *Proales sordida* however, there is a similar mortality curve, although the individuals are all derived by uniparental reproduction from a single ancestor, so that genetic diversities based on varying distribution of the genes are not to be expected. The differences in duration of life possibly point to the existence of congenital diversities of a different type from those due to differences in distribution of genes; diversities hardly perceptible in other ways.

7. SUMMARY

Our present knowledge of ageing and death of protozoa and invertebrates indicates the importance of at least two factors.

The first of these is the substitution of reserve parts for those that become exhausted. Some protozoa are provided with both a large (macro) and a small (micro) nucleus. The latter functions as a reserve. In the invertebrates and in man a comparable intracellular reserve is not seen but there is an intraorganismal reserve of cells. These include the sex cells capable on union of producing another whole multicellular organism to take the place of the old one and of various relatively undifferentiated cells which by multiplication make good parts of the organism which may wear out. Among the latter are the reserves, being called upon as long as the individual lives, to produce new blood cells and epidermal cells of the skin.

The second is genetic or hereditary. There can be no doubt that in all animals from the single celled protozoa, through the invertebrates to man, the length of life is largely determined by inheritance. In fruit flies a single gene may make a great difference in length of life. In humans there are long and short lived families and further study will probably reveal the importance of genetic constitution as one factor in ageing.

REFERENCES

ASHWORTH, J. H., AND ANNANDALE, N. 1904. Observations on some aged specimens of Sagartia troglodytes, and on the duration of life in Coelenterates. Proc. Roy. Soc. Edinburgh, **25**, (pt. IV), 1–14.

BAITSELL, G. A. 1914. Experiments on the reproduction of the hypotrichous infusoria. II. A study of the so-called life cycle in Oxytricha fallax and Pleurotricha lanceolata. Jour. Exp. Zool., **16**, 211–235.

BEERS, C. D. 1930. Encystment and restoration in the ciliate Didinium nasutum. Jour. Exp. Zool., **56**, 193–208.

BELAR, K. 1924. Untersuchungen an Actinophrys sol Ehrenberg. II. Beiträge zur Physiologie des Formwechsels. Arch. f. Protistenkunde, **48**, 371–434.

CALKINS, G. N. 1904. Studies in the life history of Protozoa. IV. Death of the A series. Conclusions. Jour. Exp. Zool., 1, 423-464.

——— 1911. Regeneration and cell division in Uronychia. Jour. Exp. Zool., 10, 95-116.

——— 1915. Didinium nasutum. I. The life history. Jour. Exp. Zool., 19, 225-241.

——— 1919. Uroleptus mobilis, Engelm. II. Renewal of vitality through conjugation. Jour. Exp. Zool., 29, 121-156.

——— 1933. The Biology of the Protozoa. 2nd Ed., 667 pp., Philadelphia.

——— 1934. Factors controlling longevity in Protozoan protoplasm. Biol. Bull., 67, 410-431.

CURTIS, W. C. 1928. Old problems and a new technique. Science, 67, 141-149.

DAWSON, J. A. 1919. An experimental study of an amicronucleate Oxytricha. Jour. Exp. Zool., 29, 473-513.

GONZALEZ, B. M. 1923. Experimental studies on the duration of life. VIII. The influence upon duration of life of certain mutant genes of Drosophila melanogaster. Amer. Nat., 57, 289-325.

HARTMANN, M. 1917. Über die dauernde rein agame Züchtung von Eudorina elegans und ihre Bedeutung für das Befruchtungs- und Todproblem. Ber. d. preuss. Akad. d. Wiss., Phys.-Math. Klasse, 760-776.

——— 1921. Die dauernd agame Zucht von Eudorina elegans, experimentelle Beiträge zum Befruchtungs- und Todproblem. Arch. f. Protistenkunde, 43, 223-286.

——— 1928. Über experimentelle Unsterblichkeit von Protozoen-Individuen. Ersatz der Fortpflanzung von Amoeba proteus durch fortgesetzte Regenerationen. Zool. Jahrb., Abt. f. allg. Zool. u. Physiol., 45, 973-987.

JENNINGS, H. S. 1929. Genetics of the Protozoa. Bibliographia Genetica, 5, 105-330.

JENNINGS, H. S., AND LYNCH, R. S. 1928. Age, mortality, fertility, and individual diversities in the rotifer Proales sordida Gosse. I and II. Jour. Exp. Zool., 50, 345-407 and 51, 339-381.

———, RAFFEL, D., LYNCH, R. S., AND SONNEBORN, T. M. 1932. The diverse biotypes produced by conjugation within a clone of Paramecium aurelia. Jour. Exp. Zool., 62, 363-408.

———, AND SONNEBORN, T. M. 1936. Relation of endomixis to vitality in Paramecium aurelia. C. R. XIIe Congr. Internat. de Zool., Lisbon, 416-420.

KALMUS, H. 1931. Paramecium, das Pantoffeltierchen. Jena: 188 pp.

KIDDER, G. W. 1933. On the genus Ancistruma Strand (Ancistrum Maupas). I. Structure and division of A. mytili Quenn. and A. isseli Kahl. Biol. Bull., 64, 1-20.

———, AND DILLER, W. F. 1934. Observations on the binary fission of four species of common free-living ciliates, with special reference to the macronuclear chromatin. Biol. Bull., 67, 201-219.

KORSCHELT, E. 1917. Lebensdauer, Altern und Tod. Jena: 170 pp.

LUND, E. J. 1917. Reversibility of morphogenetic processes in Bursaria. Jour. Exp. Zool., 24, 1-33.

MARTINI, E. 1912. Studien über die Konstanz histologischer Elemente. III. Hydatina senta. Zeitschr. f. wiss. Zool., **102**, 425–645.

MAUPAS, E. 1888. Recherches expérimentales sur la multiplication des infusoires ciliés. Arch. de. Zool. Exp. et Gén. (2), **6**, 165–277.

METALNIKOV, S. 1924. Immortalité et rajeunessement dans la biologie moderne. 283 pp., Paris.

MOORE, E. LUCILE. 1924. Regeneration at various phases in the life-history of the infusorians Spathidium spathula and Blepharisma undulans. Jour. Exp. Zool., **39**, 249–316.

PEARL, R. 1922. The biology of death. 275 pp., Philadelphia and London.

———— 1928. The rate of living. 185 pp., New York.

———— and C. DOERING. 1923. A comparison of the mortality of certain lower organisms with that of man. Science, **57**, 209–212.

SHULL, A. F. 1918. Cell inconstancy in Hydatina senta. Jour. Morph. **30**, 455–464.

SONNEBORN, T. M. 1930. Genetic studies on Stenostomum incaudatum (nov. spec.). I. Jour. Exp. Zool., **57**, 57–108.

SUMMERS, F. M. 1935. The division and reorganization of the macronuclei of Aspidisca lynceus Müller, Diophrys appendiculata Stein, and Stylonychia pustulata Ehrbg. Arch. f. Protistenkunde, **85**, 173–208.

TITTLER, I. A. 1935. Division, encystment and endomixis in Urostyla grandis. La Cellule, **44**, 189–218.

WALLENGREN, H. 1901. Zur Kenntniss des Neubildungs- und Resorptionsprocesses bei der Theilung der hypotrichen Infusorien. Zool. Jahrb., **15**, 1–38.

WENRICH, D. H. 1928. Eight well-defined species of Paramecium (Protozoa, Ciliata). Trans. Amer. Micr. Soc., **47**, 275–282.

WOODRUFF, L. L. 1917. Rhythms and endomixis in various races of Paramecium aurelia. Biol. Bull. **33**, 51–56.

———— 1926. Eleven thousand generations of Paramecium. Quart. Jour. Biol., **1**, 436–438.

————, AND ERDMANN, R. 1914. A normal periodic reorganization process without cell fusion in Paramecium. Jour. Exp. Zool., **17**, 425–518.

————, AND SPENCER H. 1921. The survival value of conjugation in the life history of Spathidium spathula. Proc. Soc. Exp. Biol. and Med., **18**, 303–304.

Chapter 3

AGEING OF INSECTS

L. O. HOWARD

Washington, D. C.

The true insects—the Hexapods—of the great group Anthropoda, are extremely fugitive individuals, although they belong to an extremely old and rapidly increasing and expanding group. The individual is so fugitive, in fact, that it dies before it seems possible that it is old.

The insect class is of course enormous. It comprises the majority of living animals. And it is very old in the history of life on this globe. It has had millions of years in which gradually to evolve a type of creature fitted to absolutely all sorts of conditions. And this fit type has constantly been growing fitter, and increasing in its infinite number of variations, and in its enormous number of individuals. It is today increasing rapidly, and man is unwittingly assisting in this increase. Moreover, the rapidity of multiplication and shortness of life are, and have been, facts of prime importance in this remarkable evolution.

When we consider the enormous number of families, genera, and species involved, it is obvious that there must be infinite variations in structure to enable the classification that the taxonomists have made. But it is not so obvious that this prodigality of life should necessarily include such a variety of life habits and of life histories. However, an astonishing variety does exist. This is so great as to preclude, in many respects, the possibility of generalizations. So we cannot generalize satisfactorily about ageing of insects—there are such extremes and so many ways of living. In a very recent attempt to discuss "the ages of animals" in an admirable book entitled *The Living World* (Williams, 1937) all that the author has said of insects is: "Some insects live but a few hours or days. Most insects live but a single season, but there is a record of a buprestid beetle having lived for 37 years."

As a matter of fact, a very good and useful attempt at more or less of a generalization was made by Riley in 1893, when he took as the subject of his presidential address before the Entomological Society of Washington, "Longevity in Insects." He wrote with a very wide knowledge, and had as his assistant at the time, E. A. Schwarz, who had had wide experience and an enormous acquaintance with the literature. Therefore, it is fair to take this address (Riley, 1895) as

53

a very fair summary of our knowledge of the subject down to 1893. But down to that time entomological writings had been concerned mainly with matters of "taxonomy, life history, and behavior." Applied entomology was in its advanced beginning, and the general subject of physiology of insects was not only almost unknown to the entomologists, but also to the other group of general zoologists. (There was such a group then!) Down to the time of this paper of Riley's, no good general account of senescence in insects had been published in English, but there were many notes recording how this adult beetle, or moth, or some other insect, had been kept in confinement for so and so many months or years, and many pages might here be spent in detailing observations of this kind, but we must remember that these were the exceptions and not the rule, and that Riley's paper, taking up the insects order by order, really brings our knowledge down nearly to the beginning of the present century. From the temporary lives of the May flies, or "day flies" as they are sometimes called (Ephemeroptera) in the adult stage, down through the three years of the life of the May beetles in larval stage to the long life of the periodical cicada or "17-year locust," Riley has summarized it well, and has referred to the somewhat prolonged life of certain insects when deprived of sufficient food and moisture, certain insect parasites of birds, and mammals, (including the bed bug), and of certain beetle larvae feeding in trees which are cut down and made into furniture. He also calls especial attention to the variation in life with the social insects—the bees, wasps, ants and termites. He states of the honeybee that the queen is known to live at least three years, the drones only for the summer. The workers live from three to eight months. With the ants, he states that there is a great variation among the different forms, and refers to Lubbock's well known experiment of feeding a queen of one species in confinement for six and thirteen years. Of the termites, he says that the workers are for the most part limited to a year, the soldiers a little longer, and the queens "much longer."

So much for the old knowledge prior to 1893. The publication of Packard's text book of entomology in 1898 marked the first issue in the English language of a big competent work on the internal anatomy of insects, and to a certain extent of their physiology. He gives rather extensive cytological data, and prints a big bibliography (largely German) at the close of each chapter.

And then gradually came an interest in the physiology of insects— in the bringing together and digesting of the scattered, and not properly known, or considered, publications of earlier entomologists from the days of Newport down, and of the early general physiologists of the last century, who occasionally turned to insects to illustrate the especial subject on which they were working. When Wigglesworth (1934) wrote his *Insect Physiology* he had nearly 2,000 publications to study, and he lays the recent great interest in the physiology of insects to a new element—the applied entomologist—who has wanted to know more about the nutrition of insects, about the laws governing their responses to sensory stimuli, their reactions to parasites and climatic conditions, and to toxic sprays and gases.

Before the publication of Wigglesworth's book a most important work was going on. The Empire Marketing Board of the British Empire, had financed the preparation of an elaborate summary of the literature on "Insect Nutrition and Metabolism." This great task was assigned to the very competent B. P. Uvarov, of the British Museum of Natural History, and the result was astonishing. I am sure that no worker in any other field of entomology had any idea how much had been done, and how many papers had been written on these important subjects. Very fortunately this bibliography has been printed (Uvarov, 1928) with a careful summary by Uvarov himself of the papers, the whole covering 88 pages of the Transactions of the Royal Entomological Society of London. It was also issued as a separate, and is and will be of most valuable assistance to all present and future workers in this great field. The key as to just why insects die is probably locked up in this great summary.

Only a few years after the publication of this paper by Uvarov, there appeared a useful and informative paper by Hoskins and Craig (1935) entitled "Recent Progress in Insect Physiology" which gives an admirable account of the work done in the preceding five years. The authors had studied no less than 1200 papers and selected and cited 444 of them in a bibliographical list. In their text they carefully classified the investigations and summarized them. Here again we fail to find exact facts about the occurrence of a definite senescence, but there is here a combination of studies leading to a very greatly improved knowledge.

What a greatly increased activity these two last mentioned papers show, and what an advance over Riley's paper written in 1893.

1. BEES AND WASPS

We have only suggested that the life of the so-called social species of insects necessitates a somewhat longer life in certain individuals than is found in non-social or wild species. These, of course, comprise the bees, wasps, ants and termites, and so we shall give a reasonably up-to-date summary of each of these groups. I naturally wrote at once to Mr. J. I. Hambleton, Chief of the Bee Culture work, in the Bureau of Entomology and Plant Quarantine, for late facts on the honeybee. In his absence, his very competent assistant, Mr. W. J. Nolan, wrote me substantially as follows:

"As you know, the life span of the worker bee is governed largely by the intensity of its activity. During the busy summer season its average length of life is five or six weeks. The first half of this time is spent in duties within the hive, and the second half in field duties. The specific duties vary with the age of the bee. Under winter conditions, because of reduced activity, the worker lives not only through the winter but also long enough in the spring to be replaced by newly reared bees. In the *Journal of Agricultural Research* for May 1937, Dr. Haydak (page 792) reports having kept worker bees under experimental conditions in a greenhouse for 236 days.

"That the division of labor in the bee is a manifestation of the ageing of the worker physiologically is shown by the work of Rösch, Soudek, and others. For instance, the pharyngeal glands, the source of the secreted larval food, do not reach their maximum development until the worker has been active in the hive a few days. Consequently, newly emerged bees do not function as nurse bees. The pharyngeal glands begin to degenerate when the worker is about two weeks old or a few days before the time for taking up field duties. Likewise the wax glands seem to reach their maximum development during the period of hive duties. Although the ability of both sets of glands to secrete appears to become greatly reduced in old age, neither set degenerates so completely as to become altogether functionless. Therefore, old bees can act in a limited degree either as nurse bees or wax secretors if the normal age grouping in the colony becomes disturbed.

"On leaving the hive for the field the worker gradually wears out or 'ages' in various visible respects. Thus the worker's field duties lead to a fraying of the wings to such a degree that flight is no longer possible. The chitinous hair on the thorax and other parts of the worker wear off, leaving the creature shiny and perhaps less able to collect pollen.

"The worker thus does have a stage of old age somewhat comparable to that of humans. However, there is no social security provision for the worker when it reaches this stage. On the contrary, it is rushed from the hive as are deformed workers in earlier life or unproductive drones.

"Queens may live six or seven years. In advanced age their egg-laying activity becomes greatly reduced. They also show outward signs of old age. On reaching this stage the workers take matters in their own hands, or should we say tarsi or mandibles, and rear another queen to replace the failing one. Both old and young queens may be tolerated together for even a few weeks but the old queen usually soon disappears.

"As for the drone, too little is kown as to his old age or even his youth. They survive several weeks at least, and at last are chased from the hive as are old workers. The drone is not functionally mature until several days after emergence. The same may apply to the queen but this is not definitely known.

"Drone, worker, and queen, pass three days in the egg stage, and six days as unsealed larvae. Whereas the queen emerges seven days after sealing, the worker does not emerge for twelve days, while the drone remains sealed for fifteen days. This makes the total length of developmental period from egg to adult as follows: 16 days for the queen; 21 days for the worker; and 24 days for the drone."

As to the length of life of the adult worker whose senescence and expulsion from the hive are mentioned by Dr. Nolan in a preceding paragraph, it seems that Dr. C. C. Farrar, of the field laboratory at Laramie, Wyoming, has been doing some careful experimental work with especially marked bees, and Dr. Nolan informs me that he (Dr. Farrar) found in one colony from one to five bees in each of the following age groups: 320, 310, and 296 days of age, and that in another colony he found a like number of worker bees 307 days old.

We should refer at this point to Helen L. M. Pixell-Goodrich's important and careful paper (1920) on "Determination of Age in the Honeybee." Her summary is perhaps a good attempt to answer the question as to how and why workers die. She writes "It is important to be able [in the study of diseases] to eliminate bees dying of old age, and this cannot be done with certainty by observing outward symptoms. Moreover, the age of bees which normally work almost necessarily for about six weeks and then die, may be determined with some accuracy from the study of the brain cells. With advancing age the cytoplasm of these cells undergoes gradual reduction peripherally until in senescence only a vestige is left surrounding the nucleus." The author adds: "The condition of the head glands which do not appear to have been previously recorded gives some indication of age in normal healthy bees."

It should be added that as early as 1894 C. F. Hodge (1894) had written on changes in ganglion cells from birth to senile death; and that Smallwood and Phillips (1916) had written on the "nuclear size in the nerve cells of the bees during the life cycle."

Hodge's work seems especially suggestive. He cross-sectioned and studied the brains of young and old bees. The young ones were taken just as they issued from the brood cell, and the old ones were chosen by "age signs, and worn and frayed wings, abraded hairs, and general behavior, many bees no longer active but humped up in some corner." He showed that the brain dwindles greatly in size in the short worker life, that the protoplasm of the individual cells is all but absent in the old bees, and that the nucleus was greatly shriveled. Moreover, the cells grow lesser in number with age. As Hodge expressed it "As the work of life is being done the cells [brain] one by one are worn out. A stage is reached where only nerve cells remain to barely support processes requisite for life, no extra work being possible. Finally the number of cells fails and the functions of life must cease (either then or just before they are thrown out of the hive).

Smallwood and Phillips (1916) have criticized Prof. Hodge's results. They conclude, after describing much experimental work with the nerve cells of the honeybee, that "the changes in nuclear size cannot be explained as due to the effect of old age or fatigue."

No facts are known about the wild bees, the stingless bees of South America nor the not distantly related insects known as wasps (Vespidae). Only brief generalizations are possible. Among the so-called wild bees, the bumble bee (Bombidae) is a good example. There are underground colonies which are founded in the spring by comparatively few fertilized and overwintering females. They exist only for the season, and the life of the individuals, of whatever sex or caste, is less than a single year.

Much the same may be said of the social wasps, most of which make nests of paper. Like the bumble bees, and unlike the honeybees and the ants, their colonies have only a temporary existence. On the approach of winter the males and the workers usually die, and the fertile females crawl into protected places and pass the winter in a dormant state. At the opening of spring each surviving female founds a new colony.

Thus it seems that the social life of the wasps is rather primitive and that the life of the individual is fugitive. These statements are made after a careful reading of the delightful books of the Peckhams' (1905) and the Raus' (1918), but these fine books are by Americans and refer to American insects only. So the thought occurs—what can be said of the tropical social wasps of the genus Polybia that build numerous nests six feet long, and of the common South American form, that makes paper so thick that it resembles pasteboard? I do not know. Very possibly some of them live longer than our United States wasps.

2. ANTS

When we come to the ants we cannot do better than to consult that great book by William Morton Wheeler (Wheeler, 1913). Wheeler says on page 86, after stating that the embryos live from 19–22 days, the larvae from 24–29 days, and the pupae from 19–22 days, for the genus

Aphenogaster, "Although the development periods given above are immensely long for metabolic insects, the longevity of adult ants is still more remarkable. The male is supposed to be very short lived, and there can be little doubt that in most species it dies soon after the nuptial flight. Still Lubbock (1894) mentions males of *Myrmica ruginodis* which lived in an artificial nest from August 14 until the following April, and Janet (1894), page 40) kept males of *M. rubra* alive from October 12 until the beginning of April. The males undoubtedly live as long, or even longer, in many species of *Campnotus* and *Prenolepis*, whose sexual forms do not mate until the following spring. The longevity of workers is certainly much greater than that of males. Lubbock (1894, page 12) had *Formica cinerea* that lived nearly five years, workers of *F. sanguinea* that had lived at least five years, and some individuals of *F. fusca* and *Lasius niger* that attained an age of more than six years. That the workers of Myrmicinae are almost all quite as long lived, may be inferred from the fact that Miss Fields has kept those of *A. fulva* under observation for a period of three years, but even greater than the longevity of the workers is that of the female, as would be expected from the larger size and vigor of this caste. Janet (1904, pages 42–45) records the age of a female *Lasius alienus* as fully ten years, and Lubbock kept a female *F. fusca* alive from December 1874 until August 1888 "when she must have been nearly fifteen years old, and of course may have been more. She attained, therefore, by far the greatest age of any on record."

This quotation from Wheeler is already 27 years old. A great deal of work has been done with the ants since that time. Wheeler himself did much of it, but I cannot consult him, since he died last year. There is a small army of younger workers, however, who have been studying the ants since this great book quoted from was published, many of them having been inspired and led to the study of the group by the book itself, and they have found out naturally a good many things, in addition to having described many new species. One of these workers, Mr. M. R. Smith, at present working in Washington under the Bureau of Entomology and Plant Quarantine at the United States National Museum, tells me that the old idea of a single queen per colony of ants no longer holds. He states that the number of fertile queens per colony of ants varies according to the species. It is true that the so-called legionary ants of our southern States, and many others, have only a single queen; hence it is self-evident that the queen must live many years to establish such large and populous colonies as these ants have.

However, he himself has counted from 200 to 600 fertile queens in a nest of so-called "Argentine ants" (*Iridomyrmex humilis* Mayr). He tells me that nuptial flights of this species are rare events and that a given colony is increased by daughter queens (virgins) mating in the nest with their brothers and discarding their wings, joining their mother, or mothers, as the case may be, in the reproductive work of the colony. He also states that such a condition is no doubt true of *Tapinoma sessile* Say, a close relative of the Argentine ant, and he has found as many as several hundred queens in the nest of this ant. Under such a condition he states that there is an overlapping of the death of queens, and as the older queens die there are young queens constantly arising to replace them. Mr. Smith goes on further to say that the Texas leaf-cutting ant (*Atta texana* Buckley) is a species which builds very large and conspicuous nests. He has seen nests near Provencal, La., which have been known to be present in the same place for from 35–60 years. He thinks that there are many nests older than that, and tells me that only a half dozen or so fertile queens have been found in one of these nests. He is inclined to think that the queens of this ant must live much longer even than the queens of *Lasius* and *Formica* cited by Wheeler.

A posthumously published book by Wheeler (1937) deals with so-called "mosaics" and other anomalies among ants, and is based largely on the studies made by Dr. Neal Weber in Trinidad, Guiana and Venezuela, of a fungus-growing ant, *Acromyrmex octospinosus*, a colony of which contained many anomalous individuals. Research on these anomalies and Weber's extensive notes gave Wheeler new ideas on the origin of the castes and resulted in the publication of an erudite and important book. While it is true that it does not bear directly upon the age of the individual, it is nevertheless very suggestive as to possibilities.

3. TERMITES

The termites have been written about rather extensively, but there seems to be a lack of observed facts about the length of life of the individual. The length of life of the colony is much more often discussed. The old theory of Grassi, and other earlier workers, that new queens are especially manufactured from worker nymphs on the approaching death of old queens (who began fully winged and had had a nuptial flight) has been largely abandoned after the studies by numerous workers with very many forms. C. B. Thompson and T. E. Snyder (1919), in their extensive studies devoted principally to the question of

the phylogenetic origin of the different castes, have classified three reproductive castes: (1) with long wings, (2) with short wing pads and,
(3) entirely wingless, and have shown that the life of the colony may
be carried on for years without a nuptial flight, and they further show
that the second, and possibly the third, reproductive types produce
sterile workers and soldiers and their own fertile type. All this is
rather puzzling to one brought up on the old stories, and who is familiar
with much more recent semi-popular books by Maeterlinck (1930) and,
(more recently still) Marais (1937), but it is all scientifically true.

Dr. T. E. Snyder writes me (October 28, 1937) that the workers and
soldiers of our common native termite (genus *Reticulotermes*) only live
for one or two years. He thinks this is rather difficult to check, but
from data in his possession he would say that the life is "probably one
year with a two year maximum." As to the length of life of the individuals of the reproductive forms, Dr. Snyder is somewhat in doubt.
With the same *Reticulotermes*, he has kept reproductive forms of all
three types alive for at least six years in artificial colonies, and he tells
me of a colony of *Neotermes castaneus* from Florida that was kept for
many years by Odenbach of Ohio, who later passed it on for observation
to Alfred Emmerson. This colony, which contained no reproductive
forms of type one, but only of two and three, lived for over 25 years
with, it is believed, the same reproductive types. Dr. Snyder thinks
it quite possible that these were the same individuals but is not absolutely certain.

It seems to the more or less ignorant present writer that this sup-
position is very likely to be wrong, and that the individual life of these
females was probably considerably shorter than the 25 year period;
but Dr. Snyder knows the termites well and I do not.

At any rate this carries us back to Dr. Wheeler's comments on the
life of Sir John Lubbock's queen of the ant *Lasius alienus*, which I
quoted Wheeler as stating that she attained by far the greatest age of
any on record, for, if Dr. Snyder is correct Lubbock's female ant was
greatly outlived by the *Neotermes*. And that brings us back again to
the very modern statement quoted on an early page from Williams
(1937) in which he referred to "an authentic record of a buprestid
beetle having lived for 37 years."

4. BEETLES

Of course, Wheeler was writing only of ants when he made the statement about Lubbock's pet, not of insects in general. And the numerous

long lives are well summarized, although not mentioned individually in Riley's 1893 address. He (Riley) writes "There are many recorded cases of such prolongation of life in the Ptinidae and Cerambycidae when confined in dry wood made into furniture" and O. Nickerl (1889) has mentioned many instances of prolonged life in beetles of one family or another.

We should perhaps also mention here a later paper by A. Labitte (1916) on longevity of certain insects in captivity (translated). It refers only to beetles and only to the adult stage. It represents, however, long and earnest effort and shows that the Tenebrionidae lived the longest, the Stercorary beetles next, to be followed by the Hydrophyllids, the Carabids, the Cerambycids, Lucanids, Cetoniids and Melolonthids following in order. An interesting table of maximum longevity concludes the article, and in this table we note that he kept the adult of *Blaps gigas* alive for 5,349 days.

To go back to the Buprestidae, my esteemed and learned colleague, Dr. A. Böving, calls my attention to a comprehensive footnote in J. V. V. Boas' *Forst Zoologie* covering such cases, and from which Dr. Böving has kindly translated the following concerning a buprestid larva mentioned by Meinert (1889). Dr. Boving has verified the reference and translates from Boas as follows: "This larva 3 cm. long emerged in 1889 from the step of a staircase in the library in the University of Copenhagen. The step, made from foreign pine wood, was laid in 1860, and the larva, a foreign species, must therefore have been in the wood for at least 27 years because an 'infection' of later date must be regarded as completely out of the question." To this 27 year life in the library step must naturally be added the unknown length of life of the larva in the growing pine wood and in the cut lumber before it was made into the library step.

This carries this prolonged larval life to more than 27 years. What about the 37 year period for the buprestid larva mentioned by Williams in his generalization?

Dr. Williams himself states that he found this reference when he was working in the Library of the Linnean Society of London, but he cannot lay his hands on the exact reference. However, he informs me that it also occurs in Hammerton's *Wonders of Animal Life*. I looked it up there and found that the beetle was *Buprestis splendens* but again no exact reference was given. Further research, however, turned up a reference in Marsham (1810) which may be the case on which these statements have been founded. The species was the same and the length of the life was extensive. The writer also included references to even earlier publications on the longevity of insects.

Other cases involving Buprestidae have been recorded in the different entomological journals and transactions that involve more than 20 years of larval life in wooden furniture. In these cases absence of air and moisture and, where furniture is involved, the presence of a coat of varnish or paint make life very difficult, and we can only marvel at the survival of the insects.

And here is still another case that should be mentioned—this time of a Cerambycid larva. When C. J. Gahan was President of the Entomological Society of London, he showed a specimen and read a letter from F. G. Clemore (1918), stating that it came from a wooden pencil box that he had carried with him during extensive travels in India, Persia, Egypt, Arabia, and Russia for 25 years, possibly longer. I got on the track of this note through a letter from Dr. Walther Horn of Berlin-Dahlam; he mentioned it from memory and attributed it to Gahan.

We might mention also another frequently cited case (Waterhouse, 1895). Mr. Waterhouse exhibited before the May 1, 1895 meeting of the Entomological Society of London, a living Cerambycid larva found in a boot tree that had been in constant use by the owner for 14 years (the last seven in India). The specimen had been brought to the British Museum of Natural History in 1890 and placed in a block of beechwood in which it had lived ever since (five years). This is often referred to as a larval life of nearly 19 years.

The rather numerous published instances of the survival of wood-boring beetle larvae in furniture, or something of the sort, have always been considered as perfectly reliable, for in some cases the insect (when it could be identified) was entirely outside of its normal geographic range, as was the case of the buprestid in the library steps of the University of Copenhagen.

Dr. F. C. Craighead, head of the Forest Insects Investigations, of the Bureau of Entomology and Plant Quarantine, after telling me of a correspondent who once sent him a larva of the Cerambycidae, *Eburia quadripuncta*, that had been taken from a wooden bed that had been in use for 20 years, wrote me the following significant paragraph (letter of November 11, 1937). "I would like to comment on these observations by saying that it is not impossible for larvae of these insects to live for such a long period, but it is rather improbable   All the extensive rearing work that we have done in the past 25 years has never given a record of more than three to five years on the so-called dry wood-borers, or often called 'powder post borers'. Furthermore all these records are based on species which will lay their eggs on dry seasoned wood, although very few Cerambycidaes have this habit. The eggs are laid in a secretion and thus protected." He adds that certain Buprestidae, particularly the genus *Buprestis*, have similar habits of laying their eggs on dry wood and covering them with a secretion.

It is interesting to know that those old wonder tales (at least some of them) may be susceptible to an explanation differing from the one that has been accepted for so many years and that has found its way into so many books. I am taking the liberty of quoting from a letter by A. B. Champlain, a very well known student of the habits and development of insects, to Dr. Craighead, November 19, 1937. In reference to these instances of very long lives of beetle larvae in dry wood or furniture, Dr. Champlain writes: "I have seen articles or notes in reference to such occurrences, but as I was skeptical concerning such stories, did not take them seriously enough to remember the source."

Dr. Craighead sent me at the end of January a paragraph from a manuscript report by his agent F. P. Keen of Portland, Oregon. It reads as follows: *"Buprestis aurulenta* L. and *B. langi* Mann. Year after year requests come in concerning the emergence holes of these buprestid borers in Douglas fir flooring, siding and other parts of houses. While there are many records of remarkably retarded development of these beetles in seasoned wood products, it does not necessarily follow that all beetles that emerge from buildings have been in them since the time of their erection. It is quite probable that in the Douglas fir region eggs may be laid and one or more complete life cycles take place in buildings. Early in July 1937, *B. langi* emerged in numbers from a large Douglas fir timber that had been in use for eleven years on the municipal docks in Vancouver, Washington."

Janisch (1923), according to Dr. Horn, working with what we call "the drug store beetle," (*Sitodrepa panicea*) has surely made a contribution to what we may really term "the senescence" of insects. Both larvae and adults feed on grains and store drugs (even old pyrethrum powder and tobacco—it is sometimes called the "cigarette beetle"). In the adults the abdomens are much swollen, and in fact are not covered by the tergites and elytra. The existence of a large corpus adiposum (fat body) allows the adult to live without feeding. But this fat body gradually disappears and then begins the period of senescence, the abdomen becoming completely covered by the elytra and tergites.

The adults then feed and may try to mate, but if the females lay eggs these fail to hatch. This beginning of senescence is called by Janisch the critical age, and he thinks that the coming of this age (when the insect is comparatively innocuous) can be hastened by a very mild injection of CO_2 into the infested mills or other premises.

Dr. Janisch is a well known German scholar who has written much on the factors which aid or retard growth in the different stages of insects. For example, there is one in English (Janisch, 1932) which was read before the Royal Entomological Society of London, by B. P. Uvarov that has the suggestive and attractive title "The influence of Temperature on the Life History of Insects."

This will be the best place to insert an observation made by Dr. Horn himself, which he submitted in a letter dated September 7, 1937. Dr. Horn is the best authority in the world on the interesting "tiger beetles" (Cicindelidae). He has noticed numerous times, in studying the gigantic African specimens of the genus *Manticora*, that some of them had lost more or less of the bristles on all of their legs—on the femora, tibiae and tarsi—and that such specimens had in most cases very narrow legs. He considered rightly that these were old individuals whose chitin had become weaker and whose bristles had therefore fallen out, "in the same way as older people become thinner and are losing their hair."

Short notes from the time of Wheeler's (1913) summary about the ants were occasionally followed by notes on extended age with certain insects in the entomological journals and transactions. But they contained nothing significant to our present purpose, although many are of much interest and several of them accompanied hard and thorough study—notably Baumberger (1914). I will not here take the space to mention more of these articles, but they are all recorded in the bibliography kept in the library of the Bureau of Entomology and Plant Quarantine of the United States Department of Agriculture, where they may be consulted at any time. Collectively they will bring Riley (1893) in a way down to date.

5. DROSOPHILA FRUIT FLIES

Early in the present century something significant happened. The whole science of genetics sprang up. Zoologists and botanists entered the field and helped and developed it to an enormous extent, so that now the old fashioned zoologist and botanist are overshadowed just as the old fashioned "naturalist" has disappeared, and the mass trend is in this physiological direction. The significant and important thing from our point of view is that an insect was chosen for much of this important work—the minute "vinegar flies" or "fruit flies" of the genus *Drosophila*. These were chosen naturally for their ready handling in laboratory, and for their great rapidity in multiplication. There ensued necessarily a most intense study of these creatures, and out of this study we would expect important results bearing on the subject of age with insects, in addition to many other things of vastly greater importance that Morgan and his army of followers have ascertained and that have founded a great school.

One of the early workers in this field was Raymond Pearl, the great student of vital statistics and of most things relating to physical life and death. His first broad and general statement seems to be in his book *The Knowledge of Death* (Pearl, 1920) in which he gives the results of his long studies of *Drosophila* with significant plotting of the life curves under many conditions, from which he deduces that the effective magnitude of the specific longevity factor in each particular case is determined by heredity.

Then there followed a number of papers running through the next five years by Pearl and S. R. Parker (1921-2-3-4) entitled "Experimental Studies on the Duration of Life." With the results of all these fresh in his mind, Pearl wrote his very important book "The Rate of Living" (1928b). In the summary of his book (Chapter VIII) we find the statement that the life duration of *Drosophila* in days is almost identical with that of man in years, and again (on page 151) that the length of life depends inversely on the rate of living. "In short" he writes in another publication (Pearl, 1928a) "the faster an organism lives the sooner it dies."

A glance through the different biographical lists indicates a very considerable interest among modern biologists and geneticists in the subject of senescence and death, and Pearl's books, articles, and lectures have clearly inspired much of this activity. It has really been contemporaneous with his work. But, even though the creature mainly used for experiment was an insect, nothing has been shown that gives us much basis for any generalizations on the length of life of the individual, or indeed as to the real cause of senescence and death, except to show that there is much difference of opinion among modern biologists in this regard.

An East Indian worker, N. R. Dhar, of the Chemical Laboratory of Allahabad University has paid much attention to the subject, and one of his latest publications (Dhar, 1932) is well worth consulting, although he attempts to show in this, and other papers, that senescence is an inherent property of body cells.

One of the most interesting papers brought out by the *Drosophila* workers is by Stefan Kopeč (1928) who deals with the influence of intermittent starvation on the longevity of the adult stage of *Drosophila melganogaster*. In reading all these papers it becomes necessary for the average reader to hark back to Pearl's early conclusion that a day in the life of *Drosophila* means approximately a year in the life of a human being. An important contribution by Imms (1937) is recommended.

Mr. J. F. Yeager of the Bureau of Entomology and Plant Quarantine, called my attention to a short article by Tisek (1927) in which are summed up certain then recent publications on the pH contents of certain insects, and records his own work on *Dixippus*, showing that the pH content decreases with age and that therefore the Hysteressis of protoplasm in insects takes a course analogous to that of the vertebrata. In other words, it may be a causality of senility.

6. SUMMARY

Evidently insects are very numerous and varied. For ages they have been increasing and expanding, and that they are very short-lived and have practically no definite period of senescence. In this evolution many strange things have developed, like parthenogenesis, polyembryony and paedogenesis, which hasten the rapidity of multiplication. There is usually rapid feeding and very quick growth in the larval condition, and so soon as the imaginal stage is reached there is rapid reproduction and then death without old age and in many cases without further feeding. Exceptions to this occur in the fertilized females of the honeybees, the ants, and the termites, where continued feeding and reproduction may last for several years. The writer has attempted no generalizations as to the length of life of an individual insect owing to the remarkable degree of variation.

But the actual facts, so far as they are known, can easily be learned from any up-to-date and general treatise on entomology, and hence it is unnecessary to repeat them here. It is impossible for the authors of these general works to do more than point out, Order by Order, and in many groups, Family by Family, just what seems to be the normal life round and length of time that the different stages normally live. But to attempt to digest all that for this chapter would cover far too much space. Obviously what entomologists need is a series of very careful articles on the bionomics of every large group comparable to the remarkable paper of Balduf (1935), cited in the bibliography.

An attempt has been made to discuss briefly the social insects, since among them occur some of the few approximately long-lived insects, and since one form (the honeybee) has actually been practically a domestic animal for very many years and has been studied rather intensively.

Modern views, in some respects differing rather radically from those of the last century, are mentioned on two other groups of social insects—the ants and the termites.

Special emphasis has been placed (in certain general books) on the length of life of the larvae of certain wood-boring beetles (Cerambycidae and Buprestidae) in furniture and manufactured wooden articles, claiming that they have, under exceptional conditions, the longest term of life recorded among insects. The writer, therefore, has given the facts in several instances and has recorded the opinion that undoubtedly in some of them the generally accepted life period may be far too long, since the eggs may not have been laid originally in the growing tree, but upon lumber, or possibly lumber made up into one thing or another.

A statement is made as to the rapid advances made in the study of the physiology of insects during the present century, and a short estimate of this work, with references to the best summaries, is given. It is suggested that important facts leading to a knowledge of how and why senescence may be found in this mass of literature, but I have not been able to find many facts of significance to quote here.

There is a great mass of published observations on certain little two-winged flies (*Drosophila*) and the whole science of genetics has been greatly forwarded by these observations. Obviously the genus *Drosophila* was chosen on account of ease of handling and rapidity of multiplication, and a host of interesting facts has been learned as to life processes and the factors that alter or control them. Raymond Pearl and his associates have been leaders in this work and they have been able to make several important generalizations relative to life and death from their studies of these insects.[1]

[1] I am thankful to Dr. Walther Horn, of Berlin-Dahlam, Germany, and to Dr. C. H. Richardson, of Ames, Iowa, for references and information, and to the following workers in the Bureau of Entomology and Plant Quarantine for similar help:

Dr. F. C. Craighead, Dr. T. E. Snyder, Dr. W. J. Nolan, Dr. J. I. Hambleton, Dr. Adam Böving, and Miss Mabel Colcord, Librarian and her helpers. What would poor scientific men do without librarians? I am also indebted to Miss Laura Bennett for her intelligent clerical assistance.

REFERENCES

BALDUF, W. V. 1935. The bionomics of entomophagous Coleoptera. St. Louis (etc.), John S. Swift Co., inc. 220 pp.

BAUMBERGER, J. P. 1914. Studies in the longevity of insects. Ann. Ent. Soc. Am., 71, 323-353.

BOAS, J. E. V. 1923. Dansk forstzoologi. Ed. 2. Kobenhavn (etc.) Gyldendalske boghandel, 22, 761.

DHAR, N. R. 1932. Senescence, an inherent property of animal cells. Quart. Rev. Biol., 7, 68-76.

GONZALEZ, B. M. 1923. Experimental studies on the duration of life. VIII. The influence upon duration of life of certain mutant genes of Drosophila melanogaster. Am. Nat., 57, 289-325.

HAMMERTON, J. A. (Editor). 1930. Wonders of animal life by famous writers on natural history. London, Waverley Book Co. Ltd., 4, 1353-1800.

HODGE, C. F. 1894. Changes in the ganglion cells from birth to senile death; observations on man and honey-bee. J. Physiol., 17, 129.

HOSKINS, W. M., AND CRAIG, R. 1935. Recent progress in insect physiology. Physiol. Rev., 15, 525-596.

IMMS, A. D. 1937. Recent advances in entomology. Ed. 2. Philadelphia, P. Blakiston's Son & Co., Inc., 400 pp.

JANISCH, ERNST. 1923. Über Alterserscheinungen bei Insekten und ihre bekämpfungsphysiologische Bedeutung. Die Naturwissensch, 11, 929-931.

———— 1932. The influence of temperature on the life-history of insects. Tr. Ent. Soc. London, 80, 137-168.

KOBEE, STEFAN 1928. On the influence of intermittent starvation on the longevity of the imaginal stage of Drosophila melanogaster. Brit. J. Exper. Biol., 5, 204-211.

LABITTE, ALPHONSE 1916. Longévité de quelques insectes en captivité. Bull. Mus. d'Hist. Nat. Paris, 22, 105-113.

MAETERLINCK, MAURICE 1927. The life of the white ant; translated by Alfred Sutro. New York, Dodd, Mead & Co. Inc. 238 pp.

MARAIS, EUGENE 1937. The soul of the white ant . . . translated by Winifred DeKok. New York, Dodd, Mead & Co., 184 pp.

MARSHAM, THOMAS 1811. Some account of an insect of the genus Buprestis, taken alive out of wood composing a desk which had been made above twenty years. In a letter to Alexander MacLeay, Esq. F. R. S. and Sec. L. S. . . . Tr. Linn. Soc., London, 10, 399-403.

MEINERT, FR. 1887-1888. Om vore faunistiske fortegnelser. Ent. Meddelelser. 1, 151-164.

NICKERL, O. 1889. Carabus auronitens Fab. Ein Beitrag zur Kenntniss vom Lebensalter der Insecten. Ent. Zeitung, Stettin, 50, 155-162.

PEARL, RAYMOND 1922a. The biology of death, being a series of lectures delivered at the Lowell Institute in Boston in December, 1920. Philadelphia and London, J. B. Lippincott Co., 275 pp.

———— 1922b. Experimental studies on the duration of life. VI. A comparison of the laws of mortality in Drosophila and in man. Am. Nat., 56, 398-405.

PEARL, RAYMOND. 1925. The biology of population growth. New York, A. A. Knopf, Inc., 260 pp.

———— 1928a. Experiments on longevity. Quart. Rev. Biol. **3**, 391–407.

———— 1928b. The rate of living, being an account of some experimental studies on the biology of life duration. New York, Alfred A. Knopf, 185 pp.

PEARL, RAYMOND, MINER, J. R., AND PARKER, S. L. 1927. Experimental studies on the duration of life. XI. Density of population and life duration in Drosophila. Am. Nat., **61**, 289-318.

PEARL, RAYMOND, AND PARKER, S. L. 1921. Experimental studies on the duration of life. I. Introductory discussion of the duration of life in Drosophila. Am. Nat., **55**, 481–509.

———— 1922a. Experimental studies on the duration of life. II. Hereditary differences in duration of life in line-bred strains of Drosophila. Am. Nat., **56**, 174–187.

———— 1922b. Experimental studies on the duration of life. V. On the influence of certain environmental factors on duration of life in Drosophila. Am. Nat., **56**, 385–398.

———— 1924. Experimental studies on the duration of life. IX. New life tables for Drosophila. Am. Nat., **58**, 71–82.

PECKHAM, G. W., AND PECKHAM, E. G. 1898. On the instincts and habits of the solitary wasps. Madison, Wis., Pub. by the State, 245 pp.

———— 1905. Wasps, social and solitary. Boston and New York, Houghton, Mifflin and Co., 310 pp.

PIXELL-GOODRICH, H. L. M. 1920. Determination of age in honey-bees. Quart. J. Microscop. Sci., **64**, 191–206.

RAU, PHIL, AND RAU, NELLIE 1918. Wasp studies afield, with an introduction by William M. Wheeler. Princeton, Princeton University Press; London, Humphrey Milford, Oxford University Press, 372 pp.

RILEY, C. V. 1895. Longevity in insects. Proc. Ent. Soc. Wash., **31**, 108-125.

SMALLWOOD, W. M., AND PHILLIPS, R. L. 1916. The nuclear size in the nerve cells of bees during the life-cycle. J. Comp. Neur., **27**, 69-75.

THOMPSON, C. B., AND SNYDER, T. E. 1919. The question of the phylogenetic origin of termite castes. Biol. Bull., **36**, 115-132.

TISEK, MUDR. A. 1927. Beiträge zum Studium der Protoplasma-Hysteresis und der hysteretischen Vorgänge (zur Kausalität des Alterns). Archiv. f. Entw. d. Org., **112**, 255-257.

UVAROV, B. P. 1928. Insect nutrition and metabolism. A summary of the literature. Tr. Ent. Soc., London, **76**, 243-255.

WATERHOUSE, C. O. 1895. Longevity of larva of a longicorn beetle. Tr. Ent. Soc., London, Proc. 18.

WHEELER, W. M. 1913. Ants; their structure, development and behavior. New York, Columbia University Press, 663 pp.

———— 1937. Mosaics and other anomalies among ants. Cambridge, Mass., Harvard University Press, 95 pp.

WIGGLESWORTH, V. B. 1934. Insect physiology. London, Metheun & Co. Ltd., 134 pp.

WILLIAMS, S. H. 1937. The living world. New York, The Macmillan Co.. 704 pp.

CHAPTER 4

AGEING OF VERTEBRATES

T. WINGATE TODD

Cleveland

Aschoff (1937) speaks of physiological death as occurring commonly in animals but rarely in Man. It is perfectly true that there are many pathological processes, not in themselves lethal, which are to be found in the bodies of the old whether Man or Beast. Examples are dental caries, undue increase in subcutaneous or intra-abdominal fat, arthritis deformans, vertebral inflammation and arteriosclerosis. Their importance lies not in the fact that they are present but in the certainty that their presence gives of a metabolic aberration by which their presence has been rendered possible. They are all disabilities, it should be noted, occurring in what Carrel (1935) calls that closed system of tissues and plasma which, far earlier than the organs, reveals to us the fluctuations of physical well being.

The distinction between life span and duration of life has been very clearly defined by Pearl (1926) and is illustrated for Man in comparisons of mortality records obtained from observations on skeletons in several prehistoric and ancient populations (Todd, 1927).

Ray Lankester (1870) defined natural longevity in a species as the average age attained by the normal members living under the conditions to which they have been adapted by nature. Specific longevity, according to him, is the expectation of life at birth of a normal individual of the species. It is determined partly by constitution, partly by accidents, enemies and other external conditions to which the species is naturally subject. Potential longevity, on the other hand, is the age which may be attained by an individual which, by good fortune or artificial interference, has been removed from the hardships natural to its lot and placed in an environment relatively ideal.

Metchnikoff (1907) suggested that there is on the whole an inverse relation between the relative capacity of the large bowel and the duration of life, animals with a capacious large bowel being usually shorter lived in proportion to their size than those with a colon of small capacity. This explanation however will not hold on closer study. The Rodents, for example, have a relatively high viability compared with the Insectivores, despite their long and capacious colon. The high viability of Rodents however was pointed out by Chalmers Mitchell (1911) to be associated with the fact that they are a highly successful group with remarkable powers of adaptation to differences of environment. Observations in certain birds further emphasize this objection to Metchnikoff's theory. The theme will be more fully discussed in a forthcoming article from my laboratory (Todd, Todd and Todd).

In fishes reproductive power continues throughout life whereas mammals may continue to live for years after the power of reproduction has waned. We therefore have to consider in mammals two kinds of longevity, namely that which is significant for perpetuation of the species and that which is important only for the individual (Flower, 1935).

Doubt lies upon the genuine absence of lethal factors in those animals, autopsies upon which fail to show advanced definitive organic disease. The melancholia into which bears will fall is really a long continued malnutrition ultimately ending in refusal of food and inevitable death. Nostalgia, or homesickness, in deer and in opossums likewise results in death with no other postmortem character, as Fox (1937) points out, than atrophic change in the alimentary canal from prolonged fasting. External parasites occurring in animals kept in captivity in the country which is their regular habitat will result in a decline of health which ends in death without gross organic change. Indeed one of the chief reasons why animals transported for captivity into another climate are easier to maintain in health than those confined in the country of their origin is their freedom from their usual parasites (see also Leiper in Chalmers Mitchell, 1911, p. 544).

Chalmers Mitchell (1911) is inclined to explain the shorter viability of European animals in captivity as due less to parasites than to fear of Man which they have acquired in the wild state and carry over into captivity, thus bringing to them death by accident or, more frequently, by reaction of the mental state upon the physical health. Whatever the cause, some species of animals in captivity are a poor viability risk, others a good one (Flower, 1935). Death from sheer old age without any lethal condition whatever is considered possible in parrots by Fox (1937) who however finds in them a number of irreversible changes such as peripheral arteriosclerosis.

On the theme of minor malnutrition of long standing McCollum and Becker (1937) have recently made an important contribution. They point out that in 152 rats which died as the result of the lowering of one or more of the inorganic elements in the diet, 70 showed hypertrophy, abnormal color and marked pitting on the surface of the kidneys: in several there were watery cysts. The capsule however was always easily stripped from the organs. Animals of the same age on the breeding stock ration seldom show these anomalies and, if they do, never to the same extent. Kotsovsky (1935) has pointed out that for Man himself the mortality curve from forty years onward and the rate of mortality are expressions of the disturbance of physiological equilibrium. The greater number of diseases in advancing age is therefore but another expression of the basic biological problem of growing old.

Sherman and Campbell (1935) have noted that rate of growth and length of life vary independently of each other. Of animals of the same sex and same heredity on the same normal diet those which grow faster and those which grow more slowly have equal prospects of longevity. But that the average length of life, though not the life span (Pearl, 1926), can be modified to some extent has been illustrated both by these authors and by McCay and Crowell. Sherman and Campbell (see 1935) have recorded experiments in which an improvement by better quantitative adjustment of natural foods in a diet, already adequate to maintain normal nutrition and health for generation after generation, results in an increased rate and efficiency of growth, a higher level and longer period of adult vitality and an extension of the average duration of life. McCay and Crowell (1935) have also prolonged the average duration of life in rats by a diet, otherwise adequate for health, but restricted so as to diminish the rate of growth in the animals. Aschoff (1937) refers objectively to the constitutional changes of ageing in terms of connective tissue, cells, tissue fluid, changes in secretion and excretion and in pH of the entire tissue-plasma system of which mention has already been made.

The relation of family strain to longevity has been shown for Man to be by no means a matter of chance (Stoessiger, 1933). General health has been found to be strongly inherited in brothers and sisters (Pearson, 1904) and in parent and child (Pearson and Elderton, 1913). Yuan (1932) working in Pearl's laboratory has questioned the appropriateness of the statistical methods used by the Pearson school, but Pearl himself (1934) submits the hypothesis that the extremely long-lived among Mankind are differentiated from the general mass as not only the physically most fit of the race but as a group able to transmit to their offspring likewise a definite superiority. Pearl and Miner (1935) maintain that there is no universal "law" of mortality but that different species may differ in the age distribution of their dying just as characteristically as they differ in their mortality.

In a contribution of his own published in 1923, Geiser summarized the literature on the sex-linked differential mortality of fishes and demonstrated that, just as in Man, males show a lesser viability which cannot be due to deleterious influences in the environment but is merely the expression of a greater survival value in the females. Landauer and Landauer (1931) followed this by an investigation on the mortality of the domestic fowl. They conclude that there are no observations on record inconsistent with the assumption that there is a higher metabolic rate in males and offered this sexual difference in rate and stability of metabolism as a working hypothesis for the differential mortality in the two sexes. E. V. Allen (1934), in reviewing the relationship of sex to disease in Man, pointed out that, speaking comparatively, the price of maleness is weakness. MacArthur and Baillie (1932) in critically reviewing the subject, emphasize the inacceptability of the theory that greater mortality in males is due to the presence of one X chromosome since, in the common fowl, in pheasants and in twelve out of thirteen species of Lepidoptera, the males which are known or presumed to have two X chromosomes, are nevertheless shorter lived than the females. Allen (1933) gives an instructive table on the sex-linked difference in mortality among fishes and invertebrates culled from records by Geiser.

Setting on one side the sex-linked differences in viability and all questions of specific disease incidence, we may inquire into the probable life span of the vertebrates, a subject already considered by Chalmers Mitchell (1911) but to which the greatest contribution has been made by Major Stanley Flower whose long experience as director of the Giza Zoological Garden at Cairo gives his observations special authority.

Excellent records of the age of animals for comparison with those of Flower are to be found in the report of the Zoological Society of Philadelphia for 1937 (see Duetz, 1937).

1. FISHES

In fishes problems of longevity, rates of growth, age at spawning, life histories, migrations, influence of environment, influence of fisheries on a species and the composition of fish stocks illustrate the practical significance of age determination. As Flower (1935) remarks "In fact, from the cod-liver oil of Newfoundland and the caviare of Russia to the fighting-fish of Siam and the introduced trout of New Zealand, the commercial value of a fish may depend on a knowledge of its age."

The age of fishes is assessed by four different methods, namely, by size, scales, otoliths and marking. Age estimation by size is a most uncertain proceeding and it is impossible to tell the age by weight or length. Scales give a fair estimate of the rapid and periodical growth of young fish but the age of an old fish cannot be proved by this source of evidence. Otoliths may differ on right and left sides. They have been used as a check upon or a substitute for age determination by scales. But preservation in formalin, though not in alcohol, will render them useless for age determination within a month (Flower, 1935). The marking of fish seems to have been long in use for Flower (1935) mentions reviews by Van Oosten and by Nall recording the work of John Shaw, a headkeeper to the Duke of Buccleugh, who marked salmon in 1834 by cuts on their fins and in 1835 by copper wire. Fish marked with bright metal labels are apt to be short lived owing to their being mistaken for bait by other fish which swallow both label and label-bearer (Flower, 1935). There are species of Goby (Gobius), the entire life span of which is less than one year, in which all the adults of one generation die before the next generation grows up. The Ice-fish (Salanx) is also a short lived fish, dying within the year. At the opposite extreme is the European Sheat-fish (Silurus) of which one specimen is known to have lived sixty years. Eels, Sterlet (Acipenser) and Carp are also long lived fishes, all being capable of living fifty years. This is a very different story from that in popular currency on the viability of the Carp which, like the Pike, is supposed to attain an age of 150 years. There is however no reliable evidence that either fish has ever reached an age greater than that recorded in this chapter (see Flower, 1925a).

The Halibut (Hippoglossus) is known to live to thirty, perhaps forty years. Goldfish (Carassius) may live to thirty years, Plaice (Pleuronectes) twenty-five to thirty years, the Striped Bass (Roccus) to twenty-five years, Trout to about twenty years, Small mouthed Bass (Micropterus), Haddock and Cod (Gadus), Salmon and Pike to about fifteen years.

Regarding the life span of sharks and rays little is known. The latter live to twenty years at least and the Nursehound (Scytorhinus) is also known to live to twenty years. Of the Crossopterygii the African lung fish (Protopterus) has reached an age of eighteen years.

It is interesting to note that by determinations on scales and otoliths it has been possible to determine the age of fossil fish and, so far as our present knowledge goes, no specimens even from the earliest periods show any marked change in longevity from that which may be expected of modern fishes (Flower, 1935).

2. AMPHIBIA

The problem of duration of life in Amphibia is more difficult than that of other vertebrates owing to the changes which may or may not be passed through. The majority pass through three stages, namely, egg, tadpole and adult form. The egg stage lasts from thirty hours to twelve weeks. The tadpole stage, including both that of the quiescent clinging phase when it exists and the free swimming phase, lasts from two or three weeks to two or three years. In some species there is no tadpole stage but the animals commence independent existence as miniature replicas of the adult form. Some Amphibia become sexually mature and reproduce while still in the tadpole stage.

There is no evidence for great longevity in the Toad in which five years are required for the attainment of full growth nor is there justification for the stories of toads found in stones or buried in impossible places (see Flower, 1925b).

Of the limbless Amphibia or Coecilidae the longest lived specimen known is one which belonged to Professor J. P. Hill. This animal (Siphonops) had a known life of over nine years (Flower, 1925b).

The larger the species the longer is the potential span of life, but the longest life known is that of a specimen of Giant Salamander (Megalobatrachus) which attained fifty-five years (Flower, 1936). The Brown Toad (Bufo) has been known to live for thirty-six years, the Hellbender (Cryptobranchus) twenty-nine years, the Axolotl (Amblystoma tigrinum, larval form) twenty-five years but the Tiger Salamander (Amblystoma, adult form) only eleven years. The Spotted Salamander (Amblystoma maculatum), on the other hand, has been registered at eighteen years. The North American Bull Frog (Rana catesbaiana) has attained sixteen years, the Tree Frog (Hyla) perhaps twenty-two years. The American Toad (Bufo) reaches ten to fifteen years, the Mud Puppy (Necturus) and the Giant Toad (Bufo marinus) nine years. The Water Frog (Rana esculenta) and the Leopard Frog (Rana pipiens) reach only six years of life (Flower, 1936).

3. REPTILES

Reptiles have been stated to grow very slowly, to take many years to reach maturity and to live to a great age. But it has also been claimed that growth may be very rapid and that great size is not a proof of great age (Flower, 1925c). Of six Alligators kept in our laboratory four died after a few months but two have lived for thirteen years and are still living. The one has a large appetite and is half again as large and heavy as the other, the appetite of which is small. Both were of equal size at the beginning of the experiment and both are apparently in good health and still equally active. Neither however has grown at the rate recorded by McIlhenny (1934).

In some reptiles the eggs hatch the moment they are laid. In others such as the Tuatera (Sphenodon) thirteen months have been claimed to elapse between the laying and hatching of the egg (Flower, 1925c).

Toothlessness in crocodiles is not a sign of great age. Flower records one in the Giza Garden which became nearly toothless at about fifteen years of age. Wray had one in the garden of the Perak Museum which lost most of its teeth but grew a new set (Flower, 1925c). Our own alligators are fed on raw beef once in three weeks. Their teeth rapidly become yellow and repeatedly fall out, apparently irregularly, but are replaced in about three months.

Stories of the great age of tortoises are complicated by the facts that they are not slow growers, that age cannot be estimated by size and that scarred and rubbed shells depend, not on age, but on the nature of the environment and the number of tortoises which are kept together (Flower, 1925c). Several tales of great age in tortoises mostly belonging to Bishops have been analysed and largely discredited by Flower (1937).

The life of snakes in captivity is frequently terminated by simple refusal of food which is described by Flower (1937) as inanition of body and mind, or by infections of skin, mouth, intestines and lungs (Ratcliffe, 1937).

Flower's conclusions on the life spans of reptiles are given in this paper of 1937. Chameleons have not been kept in captivity more than two years and six months. Species of both lizards and snakes, not withstanding differences in bodily size, live to thirty years or even more. Crocodilians can certainly live more than fifty years. Tortoises live to ages greater than those of other vertebrates, the longest lived being a specimen of Marion's Tortoise (Testudo sumeirei) which attained 152, perhaps 200 years.

4. BIRDS

Whereas the eggs of some amphibians take as much as sixty-seven times as long to hatch as others do, the egg of the Ostrich is hatched in twice the time of the Hummingbird's egg. The variation in time required for hatching in the eggs of birds is so small that the eggs of the Albatross, Emu and Condor, which all take about fifty-five to sixty days, require only five to six times as long as the eggs of the Finches and Weaver birds (Flower, 1925d). The Buff-backed Heron of Egypt and the Wren of England hatch their eggs in fifteen to sixteen days. The eggs of the Pelican hatch in thirty-six to thirty-eight days, those of the Stormy Petrel, a very much smaller bird, in thirty-six to forty-two days. Likewise the eggs of the Raven, the Emerald Hummingbird and the Snipe all take nineteen to twenty-one days to hatch despite the difference in size of the adult birds.

After twenty-six years of study Flower (1925d) states that we do not yet know whether some families among birds are longer lived than others. The smaller Passeres, like the Finches and Weaver birds, and the smaller Gallinae, like the Partridges and domestic fowl, but particularly the Grouse (see Tobin, 1935), have the shortest lives in captivity. Large birds as a rule live longer than the smaller ones. Birds long in incubation do not live longer than those which hatch quickly. In general birds live longer than mammals but the longer a bird lives the harder it is to prove the facts of its individual longevity. So far as present evidence goes no bird has a specific longevity of thirty years but many birds have a potential longevity of more than thirty years.

The longest lives recorded by Flower (1925d) are those of the European Eagle-Owl (68 years), the African Bateleur Eagle (55 years), the Madagascan Larger Black Parrot (54 years), the South American Condor (52 years), the European Pelican (52 years) and the Australian Cockatoo (51 years).

Particular instances of longer life are however recorded like that mentioned by Gordon (1936) for the Golden Eagle which was shot in France in 1845. It had around its neck a collar of gold with the following inscription: Caucasus patria Fulgor nomen Badinski dominus, mihi est 1750. Major Flower does not refer to this bird even in his latest article (Flower, 1938) though he mentions a carrion crow which may have lived about a hundred years. He also speaks of a Griffon Vulture which was in captivity in Vienna in 1706. When Prince Eugène built his menagerie at Belvedere in 1716 he transferred the bird there and Fitzinger was satisfied that it was the same bird which died in 1824 at an age of 117 years. Professor Antonius however warned Major Flower that it may have been an "understudy" which died in 1824 carrying on the glory and the glamour of Prince Eugène's famous bird.

5. MAMMALS

The potential life of most mammals is naturally controlled by the state of the teeth: when these wear away or fall out starvation or attack quickly closes the record. Certain mammals however are rendered independent by peculiarities of their structure. The Water Vole has "persistently growing" cheek teeth but we have no idea of what would happen to these teeth in real old age (see Todd, Todd and Todd) for, in other genera of Microtinae (Voles and Lemmings), the cheek teeth are known to be limited in growth, closing their pulp cavities and cement spaces below, developing roots and wearing out in old age (Hinton, 1926). This is what happens in course of time to the teeth of the horse so that an animal of thirty years shows very definite completed roots for each tooth. The incisors of all Rodentia have persistent pulps. These teeth are apt to break and, in malnutrition, loosen in their sockets and may be shed, in which case difficulties of occlusion and even death rapidly follow.

Some animals, like some of the Whales, swallow their prey whole regardless of teeth.

In the Duckbilled Platypus the teeth are succeeded by horny plates on the gums: these perform the shell-crushing function indefinitely.

A few mammals use the tongue in place of teeth to procure food or force it down the throat. These are all the anteaters, the Whalebone Whale and certain bats.

Information on the gestation periods of mammals can be got from the Appendix to Jennison's popular little book (1927) but there is no relationship between length of gestation and duration of life.

Concerning very few mammals is there any convincing evidence on which to base an estimate of life span: these few are the domesticated Cat and Dog, oxen, sheep, goats and horses, the Hippopotamus, the Giraffe, the Lion and the Kangaroo. Despite thousands of years of domestication the life spans of cats and dogs are not prolonged beyond those of their wild "unimproved" relations. Dogs may live thirteen to seventeen years but there are records of one living twenty-two and another thirty-four years. Cats have about the same life span. One animal has been proved to live twenty-one years; higher records are claimed for others. The oldest horse on record is a Manchester Canal horse which died in 1822 at sixty-two years. For sheep the record of potential viability is that of an Egyptian Four-horned Ram living at Giza until it was between fifteen and sixteen years old. A goat which belonged to the Rifle Brigade lived to nearly seventeen years: wild goats have been known to live from nineteen to twenty-two years. Oxen usually live twelve to fifteen years but examples of the American Bison have attained thirty-three years. The Giraffe, like the Camel, may live to thirty years, the Hippopotamus to more than forty. The extreme of life has been reached in the Kangaroo at seventeen years, in leopards and tigers at about twenty and in lions at nearly thirty years.

There are mammals with a life of five years or less, namely Insectivores and insectivorous Bats. The small Rodents live six to seven years. Most mammals however have a life span of between fifteen and twenty-five years. A few reach thirty or more years, namely bears, seals, whales, horses, rhinoceros, tapirs, hippopotamus and baboons. Probably the life-time of the giant anthropoids, the Gorilla, Chimpanzee and Orang considerably exceeds thirty years but I hazard this suggestion on the basis of the very great and unique material in the Hamann Museum, my experience of the time taken by non-lethal irreversible changes, such as arthritis, to develop and my knowledge of the period required in the Chimpanzee for full adult development.

The only mammals known to exceed fifty years of age are the Asiatic Elephant, the Horse and Man.

6. SUMMARY

With this rapid survey of the potential longevity as shown in specimens of all types of vertebrates of proved age we must conclude our record of Ageing in Vertebrates. With few exceptions among mammals, birds, reptiles and perhaps fishes, fifty years is the probable limit of vertebrate life. The majority, no matter what their size, reach the extreme of survival at between twenty-five and thirty years. From that downwards to approximately fifteen years there is a range of life into which most of the Vertebrata would fall. A few, the smaller as a rule, do not reach more than five to seven years and occasional examples, like the Goby and Ice Fish, reach the end of their potential life within the year.

REFERENCES

ALLEN, E. V. 1933. The difference in mortality of animals by sexes. Proc. Staff Meet., Mayo Clin., **8**, 755–757.

ALLEN, E. V. 1934. The relationship of sex to disease. Ann. Int. Med., **7**, 1000-1012.

ASCHOFF, L. 1937. Zur normalen und pathologischen Anatomie des Greisenalters. Med. Klin., **33**, 1-3.

CARREL, A. 1935. Man the unknown. New York: Harpers, 346 pp.

DUETZ, G. H. 1937. Exhibition periods of animals still living in the Garden compared with the maxima of those that have died in Philadelphia and elsewhere. Rep. Penrose Research Laboratory, Zool. Soc., Phila., 31-40.

FLOWER, S. S. 1925a. Contributions to our knowledge of the duration of life in vertebrate animals. I. Fishes. Proc. Zool. Soc., London, 247-268.

———— 1925b. II. Batrachians. *Ibid.*, 269-289.

———— 1925c. III. Reptiles. *Ibid.*, 911-981.

———— 1925d. IV. Birds. *Ibid.*, 1365-1422.

———— 1931. V. Mammals. *Ibid.*, 145-234.

———— 1935. Further notes on the duration of life in animals. I. Fishes: as determined by otolith and scale-readings and direct observations on living individuals. Proc. Zool. Soc., London, 265-304.

———— 1936. II. Amphibians. *Ibid.*, 369-394.

———— 1937. III. Reptiles. *Ibid.*, **107**, 1-39.

———— 1938. IV. Birds. *Ibid.*, ser. A, **108**, 195-235.

FOX, H. 1937. Personal communication.

GEISER, S. W. 1923. Evidences of a differential death rate of the sexes among animals. Am. Midland Naturalist, **8**, 153-163.

GORDON, S. 1936. Rare birds in the Highlands. Manchester Guard. Weekly, **35**, 515.

HINTON, M. A. C. 1926. Monograph of the Voles and Lemmings (Microtinae). London: British Museum, 488 pp.

JENNISON, G. 1927. Natural history animals. London: Black, 337 pp.

KOTSOVSKY, D. Z. 1935. Allgemeine Symptome des Alters. Biol. generalis, **11**, 87-106.

LANDAUER, W., AND LANDAUER, A. B. 1931. Chick mortality and sex-ratio in the domestic fowl. Am. Naturalist, **65**, 492-501.

LANKESTER, R. 1870. On comparative longevity in man and the lower animals. London: Macmillan, 135 pp.

MacARTHUR, J. W., AND BAILLIE, W. H. T. 1932. Sex differences in mortality in Abraxas-type species. Quart. Rev. Biol., **7**, 312-325.

McCAY, C. M., AND CROWELL, M. F. 1935. Effect of retarded growth upon length of life span and upon ultimate body size. J. Nutrition, **10**, 63-79.

McCOLLUM, E. V., AND BECKER, J. E. 1937. The inorganic elements in the nutrition of the rat. Science, **86**, 477.

McILHENNY, E. A. 1934. Notes on the incubation and growth of alligators. Ann Arbor: Copeia, 80-88.

METCHNIKOFF, E. 1912. The prolongation of life, English translation, ed. by P. Chalmers Mitchell. London: Putnam, 343 pp.

MITCHELL, P. C. 1911. On longevity and relative viability in mammals and birds. Proc. Zool. Soc., London, 425-548.

PEARL, R. 1926. Span of life and average duration of life. Natural Hist., **26**, 26-30.

PEARL, R., AND MINER, J. R. 1935. Experimental studies on the duration of life. XIV. The comparative mortality of certain lower organisms. Quart. Rev. Biol., **10**, 60–79.

PEARSON, K. 1904. On the inheritance of the mental and moral characters in Man, and its comparison with the inheritance of physical characters. Biometrika, **3**, 131–190.

PEARSON, K., AND ELDERTON, E. M. 1913. On the hereditary character of general health. Biometrika, **9**, 320–329.

RATCLIFFE, H. L. 1937. Reptiles. Rep. Penrose Research Laboratory, Zool. Soc., Phila., 30–31.

SHERMAN, H. C., AND CAMPBELL, H. L. 1935. Rate of growth and length of life. Proc. Nat. Acad. Sc., **21**, 235–239.

STOESSIGER, B. 1933. On the inheritance of duration of life and cause of death. Ann. Eugenics, **5**, 105–167.

TOBIN, V. E. 1935. Known high figures of life in menagerie specimens. Rep. Penrose Research Laboratory, Zool. Soc., Phila., 22–27.

TODD, T. W. 1927. Skeletal records of mortality. Scient. Monthly, **24**, 481–496.

TODD, T. W., TODD, A. W., AND TODD, D. P. Epiphysial union in mammals with especial reference to Rodentia. (In press).

YUAN, I. C. 1932. A critique of certain earlier work on the inheritance of duration of life in Man. Quart. Rev. Biol., **7**, 77–83.

CHAPTER 5

HUMAN CULTURAL LEVELS

CLARK WISSLER
New York

The ultimate objective in this book is an understanding of old age in man. When human material is reported upon, observations are usually limited to contemporary whites. But the contemporary white is a subdivision of mankind, whereas the task assigned this chapter of the book is to explore the human fauna for differential age changes. The contemporary human fauna is usually divided into three main divisions or subspecies, the Caucasoid, Mongoloid, and Negroid. It is natural to ask if age changes are strictly parallel in these three forms of man. Again, it is possible to set up time levels in the evolution of these subdivisions of man, but until more skeletal material is available, no data on sequential skeletal changes in old age are to be expected. Finally, it is customary to group mankind according to certain types of culture which, in turn, fall into chronological levels. Another matter of interest here is the social significance of old age, an approach to which can be made by noting the varying social practices and institutions which are based upon age distinctions.

Our method is necessarily comparative. We are to compare the various classes of individuals resulting from the application of the foregoing systems of classification. The point of departure, or the standard of comparison, is usually the contemporary white.

Since one field of exploration is among the recognized biological classes of human beings, a statement as to the distribution of the human fauna may be useful. The geography of the world as of 1600 A.D. shows the three great divisions of mankind segregated, the Caucasoid in the middle, the Mongoloid on one side, the Negroid on the other. But taking a different view of the phenomenon, we see a few large organized populations practicing writing and many small populations innocent of this art. This is one of the most convenient culture distinctions, the literate and the non-literate. Non-literate peoples function in small, inbreeding groups, but between these groups there is crossing in varying frequencies. New groups are forming by division and by the combination of remnants of declining groups. Obviously, all populations were formerly on the non-literate level.

83

ANTHROPOMETRY OF OLD AGE

Growth in size and proportion has been investigated by measurement. Many interesting and unsuspected features of growth have been discovered in this way, but in most cases it is assumed that once man grew up, no normal changes occurred. Yet eventually some age differences in the mature came to notice, which, if not growth phenomena, simulate them. Age changes in the human skeleton are discussed in Chapter 11 so we are limited to a review of the data for the living.

Ideal data for such study would be yearly measurements upon the same individuals from birth to death. Such are not available in numbers sufficient to be significant. However, we can follow the time-honored method of measuring individuals at random and then classifying them by age. Either method presents limits to interpretation. The literature of the subject reveals that changes in adult stature were recognized more than a century ago. Later, some observations were recorded for the dimensions of the head. A review of this literature was published by Hrdlicka in 1936, revealing that the data, as usually compiled, disregard all changes after the age of fifty or sixty as pathological. Consequently, there is little information available respecting bodily change in form and size in what may be termed old age.

In America, Hrdlicka (1925) and Goldstein (1936) sought to establish the average age for maximum size among whites. The number of individuals for each age was not large so the differences were tabulated in three age groups, 0–27, 28–50, 51+. Differences appeared in all the measurements made and were consistent with the results of other observers. Hrdlicka compiled similar tables for American Indians, using estimated ages. In the main, the results are similar to those for whites. However, the large age differences used in these tabulations tend to obscure trends in age changes.

Sullivan and Wissler (1927) published a study of Hawaiian (Polynesian) adults. The ages of these individuals were checked against official registration records and so have a high reliability. This publication presents age distributions for nine measurements and eight indices. See table 2.

The following is a brief summary:

Stature: The tallest males are 36 to 40 years old, after that age the decline is regular to the 76–80 age group. Females are tallest in the 31–35 age group, from this point on they decline, but to a less degree than males.

Head length: Males show a regular increase in length of head even in the 76–80 class; females of the 46–50 class show the longest heads, after which there is a decrease.

TABLE 2

Anthropometric age differences among Hawaiian males

(Wissler, 1927, p. 438)

Age	Stature	Head length	Head width	Minimum frontal	Face width	Face height	Nose height	Nose width
6–10	133.3	173.3	147.2	103.1	124.1	105.9	45.9	35.0
11–15	147.3	178.5	149.9	105.6	129.9	112.4	48.7	37.1
16–20	162.2	183.6	153.4	107.9	136.8	119.3	52.1	39.9
21–25	168.0	186.3	156.5	108.1	140.8	123.4	54.1	41.4
26–30	169.9	185.7	157.9	107.8	143.0	125.3	55.1	42.4
31–35	170.1	185.9	158.6	107.5	144.3	125.9	55.7	42.7
36–40	171.1	187.4	158.6	108.1	145.6	126.3	55.9	43.5
41–45	170.0	188.3	158.2	108.0	145.7	125.4	55.7	43.9
46–50	168.9	188.8	157.5	107.7	145.3	125.1	55.5	43.8
51–55	167.9	188.6	157.2	107.3	145.7	125.6	56.3	44.2
56–60	167.2	189.1	157.2	106.7	145.6	126.5	56.8	44.4
61–65	167.2	188.8	157.4	106.4	145.7	127.5	57.8	44.8
66–70	167.1	189.7	157.0	105.7	146.0	128.4	59.0	45.1
71–75	165.2	190.7	156.6	104.1	144.5	129.2	60.2	44.8
76–80	163.5	192.2	155.8	102.6	143.1	131.1	61.3	44.5

Age	Cephalic index	Fronto-parietal index	Cephalo-facial index	Zygo-matico-frontal index	Zygo-matico-gonial index	Facial index	Nasal index	Ear index
6–10	84.7	70.1	84.3	83.1	77.2	85.3	76.1	56.3
11–15	83.7	70.5	86.5	81.5	76.9	86.3	76.1	55.0
16–20	83.0	70.2	89.0	78.9	76.5	87.1	76.9	52.9
21–25	83.7	69.1	90.0	76.8	76.1	87.6	77.5	52.0
26–30	84.8	68.3	90.7	75.3	76.2	87.7	77.8	52.0
31–35	85.3	68.0	91.0	74.4	76.4	87.3	78.0	52.0
36–40	84.7	68.1	91.7	74.2	77.0	86.8	78.6	52.0
41–45	84.0	68.2	92.2	73.9	77.3	86.1	79.2	51.2
46–50	83.4	68.3	92.3	74.1	77.6	86.1	79.3	51.3
51–55	83.5	68.1	92.5	73.6	77.5	86.5	79.0	51.2
56–60	83.2	67.9	92.5	73.4	76.8	87.1	78.7	51.1
61–65	83.5	67.7	92.6	72.0	76.7	87.5	78.1	51.1
66–70	83.1	67.1	93.2	72.3	76.3	87.8	77.3	50.3
71–75	82.5	66.8	92.5	71.9	76.3	89.6	75.3	49.7
76–80	81.5	66.9	92.0	71.6	75.7	91.6	73.4	48.9

Head width: Males of class 36–40 reach the maximum, decline then sets in; females practically duplicate the curve.

Minimum frontal: Class 21–25 males and females reach the maximum, after which decline is continuous.

Face width: Class 66–70 for males presents the maximum, with little change between 36 and 70, then falls; females rise to class 51–55 and then decline.

Face height: The general tendency is for both sexes to increase throughout; for 36 to 60 with males and to 65 with females a kind of plateau appears.

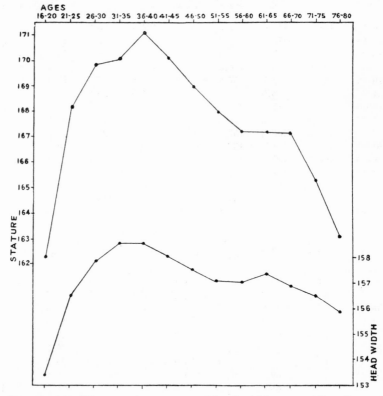

Fig. 12. Age differences in stature and head width among Hawaiian males (Wissler, 1927).

Nose height: Both sexes increase; however, for 31 to 50, males, and 36 to 55, females, there is a plateau.

Nose width: Both sexes increase.

Some measurements and indices for males are given in the accompanying tables from which the trends can be determined. The graphs (figs. 12 and 13), present two types of age trends. Naturally, in all studies of this kind the number of individuals measured is small; for the Hawaiians between the age classes of 16–20 and 61–65 the maximum number for the four-year groups was 113, the minimum, 48. Yet the consistent trends in the average measurements for the age groups increase the probability that the observed differences are real.

These measurements of Hawaiians show the same kind of age trends as were suggested in the more grossly tabulated data of other anthropometric investigators. The increments in size appear small when

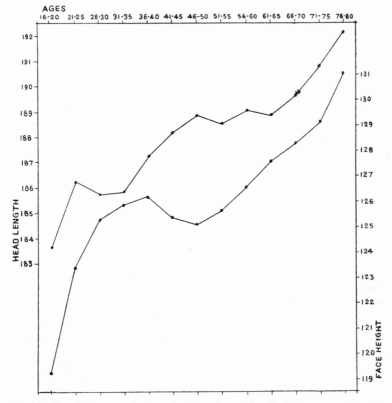

FIG. 13. Age differences in length of head and face height among Hawaiian males (Wissler, 1927).

compared with the increments for the years 0 to 20, but the consistency in trend, shown throughout the data, certifies to the reality of these age changes.

Unfortunately, we have no data upon the same individuals throughout adult life. Selection and internal changes in successive generations could distort the picture but since measurements upon the same children throughout the growing period show the same type of growth curve as results when age classes are used, there is reason to assume that the same similarity will hold between results obtained by comparing contemporary old age classes as would result from repeated measurements upon the same individuals.

In the literature available, we note that similar changes are indicated among Hawaiians, U. S. Indians, and American whites, suggesting that the phenomena are common to *Homo sapiens*, though eventually some small group differences may be discovered. Similar sex differences appear in all.

In conclusion, bodily changes in size and proportion have been recorded, suggesting age trends similar to those observed in performance tests. The comparison made between Polynesians (Hawaiians), whites, and Indians suggests that in the main the observed age changes are common to all mankind, but until these researches extend beyond the exploratory period, nothing positive can be stated. All we can say is that changes take place which are susceptible of study by anthropometric methods.

2. LENGTH OF LIFE

The life span and average length of life for the white race are considered in another part of this volume. Our point of view is comparative, so with the accepted white standards in mind, we turn to non-literate peoples. The observations of explorers are contradictory, for some remark that many old people are to be seen among the non-literate, whereas others are equally positive that few reach the age of fifty. The more critical observations of anthropologists favor the latter. However, non-literates do not keep track of their ages by years. For good data, then, we turn to non-literates in transition, as Indians upon reservations, Australian Blacks, Polynesians, etc. The official data for Indians in Canada seem the most reliable, but even here age data are not available until about 1890. Our problem, then, is whether the onset of age changes is earlier, or proceeds faster, among the non-literate, as represented by American Indians. If variation in age-at-death is largely a social phenomenon, then a study of reservation Indians should show differences from United States and Canadian whites, because these Indians are still culture hybrids.

Clements (1931) demonstrated that the age-at-death frequency profile for some United States Indians differed markedly from the white profile on the one hand, and from that for the American Negro on the other. (See also Krogman, 1935; Wissler, 1936d; and Powdermaker, 1931.) One might assume these differences to be inherent in the biology of the Caucasoid, Negroid and Mongoloid divisions of man, respectively. However, the profiles for Indians, Whites, and Negroes differ widely among themselves when treated as tribes and local groups, the suggested correlation being with social differences rather than with those in anatomy and physiological function (Wissler, 1936d).

3. AGE PROFILE

Data for age-at-death are wanting among most non-literates, but age profiles among certain living Canadian Indian tribes are available. In 1805 a fur trading company made a census of the Indian tribes in territory now falling within the provinces of Alberta and Saskatchewan, Canada (Wissler, 1936c). The data were as follows:

	Men	Women	Children
Actual	4,823	13,632	45,906
Per 1,000	74	212	714

The term children seems to include all the unmarried young people. Naturally, ages were not kept accurately by such wild Indians, but the data available suggest that the term children includes on the average females under sixteen and males under twenty. This would exaggerate the excess of women. Even so, the large number of minors is surprising, but since there are similar counts for other Indian tribes, the data cannot be dismissed as absurd. For many years the Canadian Indian Agencies have kept vital statistics (Wissler, 1936c) and for a band of Indians under Carlton Agency still living mainly by hunting, we note the following ratios per thousand:

	Men	Women	Minors	Population
1904	177	212	611	165
1929	187	244	569	296

There are other bands of Indians under this agency less dependent upon hunting, so combining their population statistics, we have the following:

	Men	Women	Minors	Population
1909	212	258	530	969
1929	206	258	536	1,287

The data for each successive year show the trend expressed by the above sample years.   Further, all bands enjoy the many safeguards to life which a civilized government is able to give.   Yet the differences between 1805 and 1904 are not astonishing.   There are more men in 1904 but still an excess of women notwithstanding accurate age data. The full data suggest that in 1904 the hazards to men in hunting were still high, and that in 1805 the additional hazards of inter-tribal wars would account for the still smaller number of men surviving.

When all the data available are considered, we get the following tentative picture of non-literate tribal populations.   The birth rate is about the physiological maximum, 42 and upwards per thousand of the population; the death rate is high, approximating 40 per thousand (Wissler, 1936c; Aberle, 1931; Powdermaker, 1931).   Minors will greatly exceed adults, in many cases the ratio will approximate two minors to one adult.   However, adult males are in the minority, the ratio varying from one man to three women in extreme cases, to two men to three women in others.   Where selective infanticide is practiced on a large scale, an excess of males may result, as formerly among certain Eskimo tribes, but the prevailing expectation would be an excess of adult females.   The chances for old age are smaller than among literate peoples.   On the other hand, there is reason to expect that a few non-literates will live as long as among the literates.   The mode of life will be the chief determinant.

In literate populations, the life span is assumed to be about 100 years. This cannot be demonstrated empirically.   What can be determined is the average length of life based upon the age profile of the population in a given year.   If adequate observations were made upon non-literate groups, as Bushmen in Africa; Blacks in Australia; Indians in the Upper Amazon; etc., we might come to a satisfactory conclusion as to whether the life-span is the same for all divisions of *Homo sapiens*. What we do know of other bodily functions suggests that the life-span will differ but slightly, if at all, as between primitive non-literate and civilized groups, regardless of race.

There may be small sex differences, but when travelers say that non-literate women age rapidly because of their hard life, they may be deceived by differences in customs.   In the culture of the white observer, many devices are known to conceal the marks of old age.   Traddition seems to bias us to associate unkemptness with age.   Yet the question remains unanswered as to whether observable and measurable ageing processes have differential tempos in mankind at large.

4. BIOLOGICAL AND SOCIAL IMPLICATIONS

A tribe or village among hunting non-literates rarely has a population of more than 1000. In terms of the 1805 census for Indians, the aged, as we conceive the term, would be relatively few; of the 74 adult Indian males in a population of 1000, at most but 2 or 3 would exceed 65 years; of the 212 women perhaps 6 to 10. In 1900 the registered reservation Indians in Alberta and Saskatchewan, Canada, including some of the tribes covered in the 1805 census, revealed 18 males and 28 females per thousand of the population as over 65 years of age; total population 12,789. In 1934, the ratio had risen to 24 and 31 respectively, which compares favorably with the surrounding white population.

Turning to social functions, anthropologists tell us that such tribes are largely man-controlled, even though males are in the minority. In our typical tribe the 74 males would rule. Upon the basis of age distribution for modern Indians (Wissler, 1936), we hazard the following hypothetical age grouping:

Ages	1805 Males	1904 Males	1805 and 1904 Females
21–40	45	108	129
41–64	26	62	74
65+	3	7	9

The 45 younger males of 1805 would constitute the chief hunters and the lines of offense and defense. The 29 older men would control the tribe because of superior knowledge and experience; they, with about 80 older women, carry the culture, conserve it and guarantee its continuity. Further study of the situation might reveal other social and economic implications. Even these estimated adult ratios should correct the impression that in hunting societies the men do nothing, since the 45 younger adults (21–40) will kill most of the game needed to feed 1000 persons.

In 1904 there were no wars and no occasion to defend the camp, the chief job being to hunt for food and furs; 108 men carried most of this burden. White influences had raised the standard of living so that the output per man should have been about the same as in 1805. The 41–64 age group of men will spend a lot of time in conducting rituals, making sacrifices, doctoring, etc., but these functions are considered necessary in every such culture. Further, the universality of male domination, even where their numbers are relatively small, suggests something fundamental.

Male dominance is less variable than sex divisions of labor, for while woman is the feeder and preparer of food, her other occupations are of secondary importance (Buxton, 1924; Lowie, 1920). Men do the hunting among tribes to whom that is the chief support. Women do some agriculture when that is secondary in food production, but when it becomes primary, usually the men make it their own task. In ritualistic activities, man plays the primary rôle, woman the secondary one.

Turning to the biological consequences of excess ratios for women, there is no reason to believe that the birth rate will fall below the physiological maximum. As a breeding group in 1805 the number of males might be somewhat larger than 74, including all sexually mature boys; the number of females, on the other hand, might be about 180. The expectation would be about one breeding male to two females. The more aggressive males would dominate. Such a situation should make for a more homogeneous type; if so, tribal types would be accentuated, the tribe being an in-breeding group.

5. AGE DIFFERENCES AS RECOGNIZED IN NON-LITERATE SOCIETIES

The intent under this head is to test the assumed functional importance of age limitations by reviewing the recognition given them in non-literate societies. Human beings under every form of society reflect, rationalize, and formulate procedures for social practice. Responses may be spontaneous as in defense reactions, but a human can reflect upon his responses to the end that a formula for future action is realized. For example, the rationalization of property rights may have been influenced by the universal reaction to the attempts of another to seize an object one holds and values. As a further suggestion lactation is believed to set off responses which underlie attachment to offspring and this in turn may set off the responses which everywhere lead woman to assume the rôle of the feeder and the cook. Again, no tribe of humans is likely to escape spontaneous classification by sex, but once sex is recognized as a line of cleavage, secondary and irrelevant distinctions will be formalized and institutionalized, for example, divisions of work, differences in dress, etc. Almost equally obvious everywhere are certain progressive cycles in life, as birth, death, childhood, maturity, old age, etc. Menstruation sharply demarks three successive age periods in the life span of females. Corresponding changes in the male are less obvious but still recognizable and usually accentuated by artificial procedures, like circumcision, tattooing, knocking out teeth, etc. Again we see on every hand evidences that age differences in physical and mental capacity for technological and ceremonial pursuits, are not only recognized but institutionalized.

We should expect to find, then, that most societies, in one way or another and to varying degrees, have formulated concepts concerning age values and have set up patterns of procedure in accordance with the spirit of the place and the time. It would be easy to show that the biological and social functionings of society present many provocative situations, spontaneously resolveable into concepts of age change. In addition to those we have just cited is the measuring of one's age by his fellows. Even the most primitive man knows that certain persons were child companions; that certain others have always been older, etc. All through life he tends to associate automatically with those of his age class, not because he ever heard of a calendar, but because they have so many capabilities in common, the same limitations to experience, etc. No matter what the social pattern, there will be a spontaneous grouping by age. This is not the place to cite the history of the calendar, but the most primitive calendars known are year-counts set down in picture-writing and kept by a specific person; if they endure beyond the death of the recorder, it is because they are taken up and continued for a time by another individual who associates the calendar with his own life. But until a society becomes literate the individual has no way of recording his age except by age classes, or in relative terms. Yet we see that the recognition of age is none the less real.

6. AGE CLASSES

Now and then we find non-literate tribal groups giving formal recognition to the tendency among males to form pairs and larger units of chums and comrades. One form in which this tendency appears is known technically as "age societies." Among the Plains Indians of North America such organizations were once conspicuous. Taking the Blackfoot tribes as an example, we note a series of ten societies, arranged in sequence, so that normally males entered the lowest society and progressed step by step, as in the grades of a school. Every four years the members of each society moved to the next higher. The average age in the initial society was eighteen years, ranging from fourteen to twenty-two (Lowie, 1916; Webster, 1908).

A member entering at eighteen would reach the last grade at fifty-four and at fifty-eight would normally be a "has been." One result of this system is a group of organized contemporaries who go along together through life. The total population of one Blackfoot group in 1870 was estimated at 2,500; adult males 480, females 720. Of the 480 adult males, roughly, fifteen to twenty should survive to graduate from the last society; for the first society about one hundred males should be available. However, the number taken in was not fixed, our informants considered forty members a maximum. It would thus be a selected group. Death would thin the ranks rapidly, but gaps could be filled from the same age rank. The last rank never boasted many members. In the aggregate the total society membership would constitute a majority of existing males over 35. What we see, then, are organized groups of men, approximately equal in age, but in combination covering the active period of adult life. These societies had leaders and subordinate officers and all were subject to ritual sanctions and taboos.

We are told that when the chief executive of the political group assigned duties, he called upon the leaders of one or more of these societies. The classification by age was a distinct advantage. Thus, the traditional assignments to the lower age societies were to patrol the outskirts of the camp both day and night, to guard the horse-herds, etc.; to the intermediate societies were delegated scouting duty, police duty, the main line of defense and offense, and the control of buffalo hunting. The two or three higher ranks were advisers and councilors, formally called upon in emergencies.

So an executive officer taking note of the task to be assigned, would choose the age rank supposedly best qualified by strength, discipline, and experience. The social practicality of this arrangement is obvious.

Finally, we learn that from two to four elderly men were taken into the lower societies to. see that the rituals and taboos were properly observed. Similarly in the upper societies two to four young men were added to run errands, attend to the fires, etc. Again, to the lower societies an elderly woman or two were added, apparently as a symbol of a much needed mother.

In some other parts of the world the society membership does not change, but at regular intervals of three to five years a society is made up of adolescents who are members for life. The result is about the same, a series of age classes for males.

The literature of social science contains many long and learned discussions of such age classes in primitive societies, how they came to be and what they signify (Lowie, 1920). We need not consider these problems here. It is sufficient to note these methods of tagging males according to age, and the existence of well formulated concepts as to the average competence of men at each age level.

7. REGIMENTATION

The organizing of society for public work, defense, etc., is by no means modern, but becomes conspicuous when a population rises above the non-literate culture level. Thus, in the Inca Empire of pre-Columbian Peru we find an all-embracing age classification of the entire male population (Means, 1931). Peru, under the Inca, was a kind of socialistic state, food and raw materials were produced by regimentation and issued from public ware-houses. Our present interest is with the age-classes of which there were ten. The number is obviously arbitrary and one of convenience.

Age classes for males in Peru

1. Baby in arms	1
2. Able to stand	2– 3
3. Under six	4– 6
4. Bread receiver	6– 8
5. Boy playing	8–16
6. Coca picker	16–20
7. Worker	20–25
8. Head of family and tax payer	25–50
9. Half old	50–60
10. Old man sleeping	60+

We note that men over fifty ceased to be tax payers and were left to their own devices and after the age of sixty their privilege was to sleep. Some work was demanded of boys over eight years of age, special tasks assigned to those sixteen to twenty and real labor exacted in the period twenty to twenty-five. Further, this seems to have been the age rank from which most of the soldiers were recruited.

In all the examples so far noted, women seem exempt from regimentation and minute age classification. Four age classes seem to be the rule; girls, maidens, married women, old women. When women are drafted for special service in the arts and in religious work, the tendency is to require celibacy. The amount of labor exacted of women in some societies is looked upon as excessive, yet in all schemes of regimentation it is chiefly men who are involved. Seemingly woman is regarded as the feeder and the bearer of children. Everywhere the child-bearing function appears as a stumbling block in the way of political and economic sex equality.

8. CONCEPT OF GENERATION LEVELS

We turn now to a more complicated social phenomena, in part comprehended under the head of relationship systems (Wissler, 1929). These are systems for the classification of relatives in a population The following generation levels are usually observed:

(3) Great grand parents
(2) Grand parents
(1) Older brothers and sisters
(0) Self
(1) Younger brothers and sisters
(2) Children
(3) Grand children
(4) Great grand children

Some societies do not bother with younger and older brothers and sisters, and in such cases our scheme would be shortened by placing self, brothers and sisters in a single category. However, taking the scheme as it stands, the tendency is to classify all members of the community according to these age levels; thus, mother's and father's sisters may be given the same designation as mother, and all women in the same social group of the same generation level may be included. In our own society we extend the term cousin not quite consistently as to the generation level, but the idea is there. The subject is complicated because there is great variation in applying such classifications, nor can it be said that all groups recognize the same fundamental scheme. Among the concepts in common are those which recognize the sequences of parent and child and the extension of these terms to contemporaries. Among peoples lacking calendar systems and methods of writing, ages are remembered in such relative terms as elder brother, child, parent, etc. With this as a measuring device, most of the population in a group can be roughly classified by associating with each individual a name for his generation or age level.

This brief survey shows that age differences have an important place in all culture levels. They are probably recognized, formalized and institutionalized because their biological realities forced such recognition. We fail to see how even a tribe of non-literates could carry on without such recognition. Some of the concepts as to age limitations may have been based upon poor data, at times they may have been matters of magic, but everywhere social experience is clever in pointing to correct solutions. We assume the purpose of this volume is to stimulate the search for more reliable data as to yearly differences in function and capacity. Presumably such data could be used in contemporary culture for the same purpose as in non-literate societies. In short, every culture assigns the individual tasks selected according to formal standards of age capacity. This is reflected in the universality of age classification.

9. ATTITUDE TOWARD THE AGED

Old age in social practice is a relative term. In contemporary life seventy or seventy-five usually comes to mind when the term is used, but in societies where the average length of life is much shorter, forty years might be looked upon as old age. Any system of universal old age pensions must eventually adjust its age qualifications to what the individual is capable of doing at each age level.

Non-literate peoples everywhere seem to recognize the onset of incompetence as a sign of old age. All seem to recognize an obligation to their aged, but the formulations of this obligation vary widely.

Thus, the Witoto in South America; Polar Eskimo in Greenland, Tasmanian in Australia; et al., abandoned the aged, infirm, and the sick; These are itinerant peoples, but the equally itinerant Arunta in Australia, show great respect for their aged and care for them solicitously. Other examples of respect for old age are to be found among the Hottentots, Iroquois, Haida, Ainu, Semang, etc. In southwestern United States, the Hopi, and to some extent the other Pueblos seem to ignore old age, each individual struggling along to the very end. In parts of Siberia the old were "mercifully" executed. This suggests that among the peoples of the world attitude toward the aged ranges from the execution of the aged, through indifference, to extreme care.

All people recognize that age gives increased experience and knowledge, often comprehended under the term wisdom. The rationalization of this leads in some societies to the veneraton of the aged, the acceptance of advanced age as the symbol of wisdom, etc. Perhaps as an outgrowth of this, or its antithesis, is the relaxation of social discipline among the aged, relief from responsibilities, and even the waiving of taboos. For example, among the Aztecs of Mexico, to become intoxicated was a capital crime, but the old of both sexes could be drunk whenever they chose. Perhaps this was the Aztec method of rewarding the righteous. Again among many peoples, women past the child-bearing age are free to speak and joke with strange men of any age, whereas the opposite extreme is enforced against younger women.

Yet, whatever the attitude toward the very old, the adult males of

40 to 60 and upward dominate in tribal societies. They have the self confidence and knowledge needed to maintain the group; they know how to control the younger people, they maintain the relentless momentum of the living culture. In the main, it is an old man's world. This may be why the old are considered conservative; it is up to them to conserve culture by disciplining and conditioning young people. The memories of the aged are the guarantee that the culture will have the continuity upon which its very existence depends.

10. SUMMARY

That a human being grows up, matures, and declines is accepted as a truism. Anthropometry shows that this is true of stature but not always for other bodily dimensions. Hence, we need further research by the methods of anthropometry. Once age changes are known for the whole life span, some correlations with internal organs and functions may be attempted. Anthropometry has achieved nothing positive for the comparison of human groups; we can form no satisfactory hypotheses as to whether the bodies of all peoples and under all environments, age in the same way and at the same time.

Respecting the duration of life, some comparative concepts can be formulated. Increasing numbers of old people are observable in contemporary populations. Sedentary peaceful cultures favor long life and populations in which the sexes approach equality in number. On the other hand, hunting and war-like non-literate peoples show an excess of women, due to the higher death rates among adult males. The causes for these differences seem to be social; that is, when two populations follow the same mode of life, their age profiles should tend toward identity. This may mean that the span of life is a constant for the human fauna as a whole.

We sought evidence for the assumption that biological age changes determined the individual's place in the culture of his group. We find that all societies have formulated concepts of age capacity and treated the individual accordingly. Since no society ignores age changes, it seems safe to assume that they are deeply enmeshed in every form and state of culture. Their social significance is fundamental.

Turning to the old age problem, we find it necessary to recognize the relativity of the term when comparing culture groups. Though all take note of old age and the group's responsibility to do something about it, the solutions to the problem seem to exhaust the possibilities. The relative number of aged among the non-literate is small, which may account in part for the diversity of solutions. In large political societies the old cannot be disposed of so easily and are accorded treatment which seems to us more humane.

As in other contemporary social problems the need is for factual guidance. First of all, more information as to the annual change in capacity for work, leadership, and judgment. The problems are for the most part specific and complex. If society demands that the person of sixty do his part, it should check the validity of its traditional assumptions as to the proper culture load for such an individual.

REFERENCES

ABERLE, SOPHIA B. DE 1931. Frequency of pregnancies and birth interval among Pueblo Indians. Am. J. Phys. Anthrop., 16, 63-80.

BUXTON, L. H. D. 1924. Primitive labour. London: Methuen & Co., Ltd., VIII, 272 pp.

CLEMENTS, FORREST 1931. Racial differences in mortality and morbidity. Human Biology, 3, 397-419.

GOLDSTEIN, MARCUS S. 1936. Changes in dimensions and form of the face and head with age. Am. J. Phys. Anthrop., 22, 37-89.

HRDLIČKA, ALES 1925. The old Americans. Baltimore: The Williams & Wilkins Company, XIII, 433 pp.

——— 1936. Growth during adult life. Proc. Am. Philos. Soc., 76, 847-897.

KROGMAN, W. M. 1935. Vital data on the population of the Seminole Indians of Florida and Oklahoma. Human Biology, 7, 335-349.

LOWIE, ROBERT H. 1916. Plains Indian Age-Societies: Historical and comparative summary. Anthropological Papers Am. Mus. Nat. Hist., 11, 877-992.

——— 1920. Primitive Society, New York: Boni and Liveright. 463 pp.

MEANS, PHILIP AINSWORTH 1931. Ancient civilizations of the Andes. New York: Charles Scribner's Sons. XVIII, 586 pp.

POWDERMAKER, HORTENSE 1931. Vital statistics of New Ireland (Bismarck Archipelago) as revealed in geneologies. Human Biology, 3, 351-375.

SULLIVAN, LOUIS R., AND WISSLER, CLARK 1927. Observations on Hawaiian somatology. Mem. Bernice P. Bishop Museum, 9, 3-341.

WEBSTER, H. 1908. Primitive secret societies. New York: The Macmillan Co., XIII, 227 pp.

WISSLER, CLARK 1927. Age changes in anthropological characters in childhood and adult life. Proc. Am. Philos. Soc., 66, 431-438.

——— 1929. An introduction to social anthropology. New York: Henry Holt & Co., X, 392 pp.

——— 1936a. The excess of females among the Cree Indians. Proc. Nat. Acad. Sci., 22, 151-153.

——— 1936b. The effect of civilization upon the length of life of the American Indian. Scientific Monthly, 43, 5-13.

——— 1936c. Changes in population profiles among the Northern Plains Indians. Anthropological Papers Am. Mus. of Nat. Hist., 36, 1-67.

——— 1936d. Distribution of deaths among American Indians. Human Biology, 8, 223-231.

CHAPTER 6

LONGEVITY IN RETROSPECT AND IN PROSPECT

LOUIS I. DUBLIN

New York

The term "life span" is loosely used. In the popular mind, it connotes with equal frequency the limit of duration of the individual human life and the average length of life of a group of persons. I shall attempt, in this chapter, to consider broadly the ideas that are behind each of these points of view with regard to human longevity.

1. LIFE SPAN

The "life span," properly conceived, is the limit beyond which human life does not extend even in the most favorable circumstances. When we examine into this limit, we find ourselves almost at once in a sphere of vagueness and conjecture. There is no evidence of some definite age at which all human life must necessarily cease. It is difficult, as a matter of fact to find a body of authentic data with regard to the length of life of persons in the advanced ages. Until fairly recently, birth registration was practiced in a relatively few countries and even in these such registration was not always complete. And so if we find persons who claim to be 150 and more years old in various semi-civilized and rural populations, we may be neither surprised nor impressed with the reliability of such claims. It is significant that claims for extreme old age are frequent in just such backward places where one would hardly expect great longevity.

On the other hand, in more advanced countries where correct recording of age is possible, it is an extremely rare occurrence to find persons who are more than 100 years old. There are, of course, a few individual instances which are very striking. The most quoted example is that of Christen Jacobsen Drakenberg, the Dane, who was supposedly born on November 18, 1626, and died on October 9, 1772, thus living 146 years. Authentic centenarians do exist, but they are very few in number and they pass out of the picture rapidly. We are thus led to the conclusion that in current times the century mark is, for all practical purposes, the limit of the human life span.

Despite our lack of authenticated data, there is no reason to believe that the life span of the human race, indefinite as it is, has varied appreciably within historical times. The extraordinary life spans referred to in Genesis are obviously mythical and need not concern us here. For some reason, homo sapiens very rarely has the ability to pass the mark of 100 years of life, a fact which may seem strange to some who have grown accustomed to the incessant boast of our increasing longevity. For these people it becomes necessary to distinguish clearly between two fundamentally different concepts, namely, the life span, which has already been defined, and the mean length of life, which is the average number of years lived by all persons born at a given period. The second of these concepts leads us at once to a brief description of the life table, a most useful statistical tool, by means of which we can follow quantitatively and accurately the effect of the ageing process on a population traced from birth to death.

2. LIFE TABLE

The life table, such as that shown by way of example on page 102, is really a simple document to understand when stripped of its technicalities. The basis of the life table is a series of figures showing the death rates for each age of life (see, for example, column 4 of table 3) as derived from our national mortality reports and census volumes, which contain, respectively, the numbers of deaths and the population classified by age. It is characteristic of the column of death rates in a life table that, once the hazardous first year of life is passed, the figures drop rapidly to a minimum at about age ten. From here on, the figures increase slowly to the fifth decade of life, during which the effects of the ageing process become very noticeable in the death rates. Thereafter the death rates increase with accelerating rapidity.

The survivorship column of the life table (column 2) is easily derived from the column of death rates. Thus, in our example, we start with 100,000 newly born white male babies who experienced, according to the figure opposite age zero in column 4, a death rate of 60.86 per 1,000. Among these 100,000 babies there were, therefore, 6,086 deaths (column 3) in the first year of life, leaving 93,914 to reach their first birthday. Since the death rate at age one was 9.88 per 1,000 living at that age, among 93,914 persons there were

$$93,914 \times \frac{9.88}{1,000} = 928$$

deaths. The number living to attain age 2 is thus 93,914 − 928 = 92,986. This procedure is continued to the end of the life table. It

TABLE 3

Life table for white males in the United States,* 1929 to 1931

1	2	3	4	5	1	2	3	4	5
	Of 100,000 Born alive		Rate of mortality per 1,000	Complete expectation of life or mean after-lifetime; average number of years lived after age x per person surviving to exact age x		Of 100,000 Born alive		Rate of mortality per 1,000	Complete expectation of life or mean after-lifetime; average number of years lived after age x per person surviving to exact age x
Age	Number surviving to exact age x	Number dying between ages x and $x+1$	Number dying between ages x and $x+1$ among 1,000 living at age x		Age	Number surviving to exact age x	Number dying between ages x and $x+1$	Number dying between ages x and $x+1$ among 1,000 living at age x	
x	l_x	d_x	$1,000q_x$	$\overset{\circ}{e}_x$	x	l_x	d_x	$1,000q_x$	$\overset{\circ}{e}_x$
0	100,000	6,086	60.86	59.31	30	85,944	354	4.12	37.57
1	93,914	928	9.88	62.12	31	85,590	365	4.26	36.72
2	92,986	496	5.33	61.74	32	85,225	377	4.42	35.88
3	92,490	345	3.73	61.06	33	84,848	391	4.61	35.04
4	92,145	276	3.00	60.29	34	84,457	408	4.83	34.20
5	91,869	231	2.51	59.47	35	84,049	426	5.07	33.36
6	91,638	200	2.18	58.62	36	83,623	447	5.35	32.53
7	91,438	176	1.92	57.75	37	83,176	471	5.66	31.70
8	91,262	151	1.66	56.86	38	82,705	496	6.00	30.88
9	91,111	138	1.51	55.95	39	82,209	524	6.38	30.06
10	90,973	132	1.45	55.03	40	81,685	555	6.79	29.25
11	90,841	134	1.47	54.11	41	81,130	587	7.23	28.45
12	90,707	142	1.56	53.19	42	80,543	619	7.69	27.65
13	90,565	155	1.71	52.27	43	79,924	654	8.18	26.86
14	90,410	171	1.89	51.36	44	79,270	690	8.70	26.08
15	90,239	190	2.10	50.46	45	78,580	727	9.25	25.30
16	90,049	210	2.33	49.56	46	77,853	767	9.85	24.53
17	89,839	229	2.55	48.68	47	77,086	808	10.48	23.77
18	89,610	247	2.76	47.80	48	76,278	852	11.17	23.02
19	89,363	264	2.95	46.93	49	75,426	898	11.91	22.27
20	89,099	278	3.12	46.07	50	74,528	948	12.72	21.54
21	88,821	290	3.27	45.21	51	73,580	1,001	13.61	20.81
22	88,531	301	3.40	44.36	52	72,579	1,060	14.60	20.09
23	88,230	309	3.50	43.51	53	71,519	1,122	15.69	19.38
24	87,921	316	3.59	42.66	54	70,397	1,189	16.89	18.68
25	87,605	321	3.66	41.81	55	69,208	1,259	18.19	17.99
26	87,284	326	3.73	40.96	56	67,949	1,332	19.60	17.32
27	86,958	331	3.81	40.12	57	66,617	1,406	21.11	16.65
28	86,627	338	3.90	39.27	58	65,211	1,482	22.72	16.00
29	86,289	345	4.00	38.42	59	63,729	1,559	24.46	15.36

* Exclusive of Texas and South Dakota.

TABLE 3—*Concluded*

1	2	3	4	5	1	2	3	4	5
	Of 100,000 Born alive		Rate of mortality per 1,000	Complete expectation of life or mean after-lifetime; average number of years lived after age x per person surviving to exact age x		Of 100,000 Born alive		Rate of mortality per 1,000	Complete expectation of life or mean after-lifetime; average number of years lived after age x per person surviving to exact age x
Age	Number surviving to exact age x	Number dying between ages x and $x+1$	Number dying between ages x and $x+1$ among 1,000 living at age x		Age	Number surviving to exact age x	Number dying between ages x and $x+1$	Number dying between ages x and $x+1$ among 1,000 living at age x	
x	l_x	d_x	$1{,}000 q_x$	$\overset{\circ}{e}_x$	x	l_x	d_x	$1{,}000 q_x$	$\overset{\circ}{e}_x$
60	62,170	1,638	26.35	14.73	80	17,339	2,226	128.38	5.27
61	60,532	1,720	28.41	14.12	81	15,113	2,093	138.52	4.97
62	58,812	1,803	30.65	13.52	82	13,020	1,941	149.05	4.69
63	57,009	1,888	33.11	12.93	83	11,079	1,772	159.92	4.43
64	55,121	1,973	35.79	12.35	84	9,307	1,594	171.23	4.18
65	53,148	2,057	38.70	11.79	85	7,713	1,412	183.11	3.94
66	51,091	2,139	41.86	11.25	86	6,301	1,233	195.66	3.71
67	48,952	2,217	45.28	10.72	87	5,068	1,059	209.03	3.49
68	46,735	2,289	48.97	10.20	88	4,009	895	223.33	3.27
69	44,446	2,355	52.98	9.70	89	3,114	743	238.66	3.07
70	42,091	2,413	57.33	9.22	90	2,371	605	255.13	2.88
71	39,678	2,463	62.08	8.75	91	1,766	482	272.84	2.69
72	37,215	2,503	67.25	8.29	92	1,284	375	291.89	2.52
73	34,712	2,531	72.90	7.86	93	909	284	312.38	2.35
74	32,181	2,544	79.05	7.43	94	625	209	334.41	2.18
75	29,637	2,541	85.75	7.03	95	416	149	358.09	2.03
76	27,096	2,521	93.04	6.64	96	267	102	383.50	1.88
77	24,575	2,481	100.96	6.27	97	165	68	410.77	1.75
78	22,094	2,420	109.53	5.92	98	97	43	439.98	1.61
79	19,674	2,335	118.69	5.59	99	54	25	471.24	1.49
					100	29	15	504.65	1.37
					101	14	8	540.32	1.26
					102	6	3	578.33	1.16
					103	3	2	618.80	1.06
					104	1	1	661.82	

will be noted that in the process of computing the survivorship column, we obtained, incidentally, the third column of the life table, which shows how many, out of the 100,000 born alive, die in each age of life. Let it be assumed, for the sake of simplicity, that each person lives, on the average, one half year in the age of his death; for example, that each of the 6,086 who died in the first year of life lived, on the average, one half year; that each of the 928 dying in the second year of life lived one and one half years, etc., to the oldest age shown in the table. Altogether, the 100,000 live born babies lived a total of

$$6086 \times \tfrac{1}{2} + 928 \times 1\tfrac{1}{2} + 496 \times 2\tfrac{1}{2} + 345 \times 3\tfrac{1}{2} + \text{etc.} =$$
$$5{,}930{,}771 \text{ years of life}$$

Each of the 100,000 newly-born babies lived, therefore, 5,930,771 ÷ 100,000, or 59.31 years of life on the average. This figure, 59.31 years, is commonly known as the mean length of life or expectation of life at birth. The expectation of life at any age may be conceived in a like manner. Thus, of the 89,099 persons alive at age twenty, 278 died after living one half year in that age, 290 died $1\tfrac{1}{2}$ years after attaining age 20, etc. The total number of years lived by the 89,099 in the remainder of their lifetime is thus

$$278 \times \tfrac{1}{2} + 290 \times 1\tfrac{1}{2} + 301 \times 2\tfrac{1}{2} + \text{etc.} = 4{,}104{,}772 \text{ years of life}$$

The expectation of life at age 20 is therefore

$$4{,}104{,}772 \div 89{,}099 = 46.07 \text{ years}$$

It is to be noted that the life table shows what would be the number of survivors to successive ages, what would be the number of deaths at successive ages, and what the expectation of life would be *if the death rates at each age remained constant as of the calendar year or period for which it is constructed.* With this understanding, let us examine what the life tables constructed for the past have to tell us.

3. HISTORICAL RETROSPECT OF LONGEVITY

Investigators working with data obtained from inscriptions on Roman tombstones have estimated that the mean length of life in antiquity may have been on a level with that of such places as India today, say somewhere between 20 and 30 years. There is some evidence that in the more healthy places the mean length of life may have been as high as 35 years, but this figure is rather doubtful. From this era we must pass to the end of the seventeenth century for our next indication of the mean length of life. In 1693, Halley, a noted English astronomer, published the results of his investigation of mortality in the City of Breslau during the period 1687–1691. Although the life table produced by him can not be accepted as typical of that period, the resulting mean length of life, 33.5 years, does not indicate any marked advance over the crude estimates for antiquity.

An extended series of life tables for Sweden, beginning with 1755 and reaching up to 1930, enables us to follow the progress of longevity in a typically Western country which has taken advantage of modern public health practices. The earliest life table, that for the years 1755–1776, showed a mean length of life of 34.5 years, not far from what Halley found for the City of Breslau. The next life table, reflecting conditions during 1816–1840, had a mean length of life of 41.5 years, an advance of 7 years over the previous table. Tables constructed for successive decennia beginning with 1861 show a steady progress in expectation of life from 44.6 years to 57.0 years for the period 1911–1920; in the next decade, the 60 year mark was passed with a figure of 61.8 years for the first quinquennium and 62.3 years for the second. The course of the expectation of life in the remaining Scandinavian countries, Holland, and England has been much the same as that just outlined. For us, in this chapter, a particular interest attaches to the situation in the United States.

The first American life table, known as Wigglesworth's Table, was crudely constructed for the year 1789 from data gathered in several towns in New Hampshire and Massachusetts. The mean length of life was found to be 35.5 years, a figure corresponding to that for Sweden of about the same time. Progress for some time thereafter was slow; according to a life table for Massachusetts in 1850, our longevity had advanced to only 40 years by the middle of the nineteenth century.

Shortly before the turn of the century came what may be called the era of discovery of the basic facts with regard to the control of environment, causation of disease, and that series of practical administrative measures which have since been crystallized in the modern public health movement. As this program developed, the expectation of life at birth responded rapidly and definitely so that each new set of tables showed a corresponding increase in the expectation of life. By 1900, the expectation in the United States had jumped to about 50 years; by 1920, to 55 years and by 1930, to a little over 60 years. The rapidly improving longevity witnessed so far during this century presents some characteristics that call for special consideration.

4. LONGEVITY CONSIDERED WITH REGARD TO AGE

Analysis of available data indicates that the constant gain in longevity which we have noted has been largely concentrated in the earlier years

TABLE 4

Expectation of life and mortality rate per 1,000 among white males and white females in the United States. Original death registration states in 1901, 1910, 1919–1920, 1929–1931, for the decennial ages of life

Sex and calendar period	Age									
	0	10	20	30	40	50	60	70	80	90
Expectation of life, years										
White males										
1901	48.23	50.59	42.19	34.88	27.74	20.76	14.35	9.03	5.10	2.85
1910	50.23	51.32	42.71	34.87	27.43	20.39	13.98	8.83	5.09	2.99
1919–1920	54.05	52.82	44.29	36.47	28.85	21.37	14.62	9.09	5.19	2.75
1929–1931	58.84	54.50	45.50	36.88	28.48	20.83	14.24	8.93	5.09	2.75
White females										
1901	51.08	52.15	43.77	36.42	29.17	21.89	15.23	9.59	5.50	3.02
1910	53.62	53.57	44.88	36.96	29.26	21.74	14 92	9.38	5.35	3.C0
1919–1920	56.41	53.82	45.16	37.61	29.95	22.26	15 29	9.59	5.57	3.11
1929–1931	62.37	57.14	47.98	39.33	30.78	22.70	15 51	9.69	5.55	3.12
Mortality rate per 1,000										
White males										
1901	133.45	2.74	5.94	7.99	10.60	15.37	28.59	58.94	133.53	262.78
1910	123.26	2.38	4.89	6.60	10.22	15.53	30.75	62.14	135.75	255.17
1919–1920	92.43	2.27	4.59	6.47	8.44	13.02	26.48	59.00	129.63	253.60
1929–1931	61.22	1.54	2.94	3.87	6.93	13.95	29.04	60.60	133.07	270.00
White females										
1901	110.61	2.46	5.54	7.72	9.31	13.37	25.06	53.69	121.15	245.32
1910	102.26	2.06	4.20	6.03	8.03	12.59	25.83	56.63	125.79	247.59
1919–1920	73.61	1.91	4.64	6.84	7.32	11.77	23.64	54.74	119.88	240.40
1929–1931	48.38	1.16	2.61	3.55	5.32	10.43	22.88	51.80	120.25	239.56

Source: L. I. Dublin and A. J. Lotka, "Length of Life—A Study of the Life Table." (Ronald Press, 1936), p. 68.

of life. For example, we see, in table 4, that among white males in the original death registration states of our country,[1] the expectation of life at birth increased from 48.23 years in 1901 to 58.84 years in the

[1] The original death registration states included all of New England, New York, New Jersey, Indiana, Michigan and Washington, D. C. For sake of comparability, the table was confined to data of this constant area.

period 1929–1931, a gain of 10.61 years. At age 40, the corresponding gain was only 0.74 years; at higher ages the differences are negligible. Although greater gains in expectation of life are observed among the females, the situation is, fundamentally, much the same. In England and a few other countries, conditions in this regard are somewhat better, but even in these instances, the gains after age 40 are small.

We are inevitably led to the conclusion that the greater part of the gains in the expectation of life at birth may be attributed to the control of infant mortality, to the practical elimination of certain diseases of childhood, and to the curtailment of conditions once considered typical of adolescence and early maturity. Altogether our progress with the diseases of late maturity and old age has not been of any consequence. To date, we have not been able to stretch the life span. We observe savings only at those ages where lives were heretofore unnecessarily shortened by the impact of fortuitous factors like the bacterial diseases, many of which are coming under control. The viewpoint thus established naturally leads us to inquire further. What causes of death are typical in the "ageing process" and at what ages do they first become noticeable? What are the chances of dying from any of the causes typical of old age? How many years of life may be added, on the average, if it were possible in some way as yet unknown to eliminate any of these causes?

5. VARIATION IN CAUSES OF DEATH WITH AGE

Aside from the predominance of the congenital conditions as a cause of death in early infancy, deaths at ages under 40 are largely of infectious or accidental origin. Beginning with age 40, however, the cardiovascular-renal[2] diseases, typical of the ageing process, assume rapidly increasing importance. According to the data shown in table 5, which relate to white persons in the general population, more than one quarter of all the deaths in the age group 40 to 49 years arise from the degenerative conditions included within this category. The proportion of deaths from the cardiovascular-renal diseases thereafter mounts until in the age group 80 to 89 years it accounts for two thirds of all deaths. Cancer, also, first becomes an important item at age 40. Among females between the ages 40 to 59, this cause takes about one fifth of all deaths; among males between ages 50 to 69, about one eighth of all deaths arise from cancer. Accidents, an important factor in mortality during youth and early maturity, are of importance again in old age.

[2] The cardiovascular-renal diseases include, principally, the chronic diseases of the heart, chronic nephritis, cerebral hemorrhage, and paralysis without specified cause, diseases of the arteries, and angina pectoris.

Influenza and pneumonia as causes of death present a situation some-what parallel to that for accidents. These diseases are, in fact, im-portant factors of mortality at all ages of life. At ages under 20, about one seventh of all deaths arise from influenza and pneumonia; among males in the age group 40 to 49 years, their toll is almost one tenth of

TABLE 5

Per cent distribution of deaths from specified diseases or conditions. United States death registration states* in 1930

Disease or condition	Age group							
	0-19	20-39	40-49	50-59	60-69	70-79	80-89	90-99
White males								
All causes	100.0	100.0	100.0	100.0	100.0	100.0	100.0	100.0
Cardiovascular-renal dis-eases	2.4	11.5	25.9	40.3	52.4	61.8	66.0	62.4
Cancer	0.5	3.0	7.7	12.0	13.4	11.4	7.1	4.5
Accidents	11.3	25.0	14.3	8.8	5.6	3.9	4.1	5.1
Influenza and pneumonia	14.9	8.9	9.5	7.5	6.3	6.2	7.3	8.0
Tuberculosis	2.7	17.6	11.4	6.4	3.2	1.5	0.6	0.2
Diabetes	0.3	0.8	1.0	1.8	2.3	1.9	1.0	0.4
All other causes	67.9	33.2	30.2	23.2	16.8	13.3	13.9	19.4
White females								
All causes	100.0	100.0	100.0	100.0	100.0	100.0	100.0	100.0
Cardiovascular-renal dis-eases	3.2	13.1	28.4	39.6	51.5	61.3	64.3	61.3
Cancer	0.6	6.9	20.4	22.4	17.5	12.5	7.5	4.3
Accidents	6.4	5.1	3.6	3.2	3.1	3.9	6.0	8.0
Influenza and pneumonia	15.5	6.7	6.6	6.0	6.5	7.1	8.1	8.4
Tuberculosis	4.8	21.1	7.9	4.1	2.3	1.4	0.6	0.2
Diabetes	0.5	0.9	2.1	4.4	5.2	3.0	1.2	0.3
Puerperal state	1.2	15.3	2.3	†				
All other causes	67.8	30.9	28.7	20.3	13.9	10.8	12.3	17.5

* As constituted in 1920.
† Less than 0.05.

the total, while among females it is appreciably less. Although tuber-culosis is a sizable item during ages 40 to 49, taking one ninth of all deaths among males, it decreases in proportion to the total with ad-vancing age. Diabetes is of particular importance among females in the higher ranges of life.

With a continuance of mortality conditions prevailing in 1930, practically 50 per cent of all children born will eventually die of some cardiovascular-renal disease (see table 6). The chances of dying from this category of conditions increase thereafter with advancing age and reach 60 per cent by age 60. For females, the chances of dying from cancer are appreciably greater than for males; at birth, the figures are 12 per cent and 9 per cent respectively. The chances of dying from

TABLE 6

Chances per 1,000 of eventually dying from specified diseases or conditions. United States death registration states,* in 1930

Disease or condition	Age						
	0	10	20	30	40	50	60
White males							
Cardiovascular-renal diseases....	453.1	496.4	504.9	520.1	539.4	566.1	598.5
Cancer........................	90.1	98.6	100.3	103.3	106.5	109.3	107.1
Accidents.....................	79.4	80.8	75.6	67.2	60.3	52.4	45.3
Influenza and pneumonia........	79.5	71.3	71.0	70.7	69.4	67.0	65.5
Tuberculosis..................	42.7	45.3	44.6	39.6	33.0	25.3	17.5
Diabetes......................	14.8	16.1	16.2	16.5	16.9	17.5	17.4
All other causes...............	240.4	191.5	187.4	182.6	174.5	162.4	148.7
White females							
Cardiovascular-renal diseases....	478.8	515.2	521.5	535.1	551.1	570.1	595.8
Cancer........................	121.6	130.8	132.6	136.0	137.3	132.5	119.0
Accidents.....................	45.5	44.9	43.8	43.3	43.3	43.8	45.5
Influenza and pneumonia........	78.1	70.9	70.6	70.9	70.9	71.2	72.8
Tuberculosis..................	35.3	36.5	34.2	26.6	21.0	16.9	13.4
Diabetes......................	26.8	28.8	29.0	29.6	30.4	31.1	29.1
Puerperal state...............	12.1	13.0	12.2	7.0	1.5		
All other causes...............	201.8	159.9	156.1	151.5	144.5	134.4	124.4

* As constituted in 1920.

cancer become a maximum at age 40, where they are practically 14 per cent for females and 11 per cent for males. Among males, the chances of eventual death from some accidental cause are markedly greater than among females at all ages of life. Influenza and pneumonia shows no partiality between the sexes until age 50, where the chances of death from this combination of causes become greater for the female. Throughout life, the white male has a greater risk of eventual death from tuberculosis than the white female; even at age 50, the figure for white males is as high as 2.5 per cent. Practically 3 per cent of all females will eventually die of diabetes; for males the chances are about half that for the females.

The question is often raised as to the increase in the mean length of life which would result from the elimination of any one particular cause of death. The answer is of some importance, for it indicates in a forceful manner, the directions in which efforts must be led to achieve the most substantial results in prolonging human life. We find, for example, that if there had been no deaths from the cardiovascular-renal diseases in the general population as constituted in 1930, 7.2 years would have been added to the average length of life for white males and 7.5 years for white females. These figures have only academic interest, however. It is quite impossible to expect the complete elimination of the cardiovascular-renal diseases, for the processes of degeneration are inevitable. On the other hand, the figures do show that we have, in these diseases, the greatest room for increasing the average length of life. If it were possible to eliminate cancer as a cause of death the average white male life would be extended 1.1 years at birth and the average white female life 1.8 years. Although the progress in the fight against tuberculosis has already been marked, the average length of life would be extended 1.1 years by its complete eradication. Deaths from accident have become an important factor in our mortality picture; by their complete elimination, the white male would gain 2.1 years in average length of life at birth, the white females, 0.8 years or close to 10 months. The presence of diabetes as a cause of death curtails the average length of life by 0.2 years and by 0.4 years, respectively, among white males and females.

6. HYPOTHETICAL LIFE TABLE

One may speculate a bit also on the possibilities of further life extension in the future. We have just seen that in the field of the cardiovascular-renal diseases, cancer, and tuberculosis there is an appreciable margin within which human longevity may be extended. These margins for improvement, together with a more intensive application of our present knowledge concerning the communicable diseases of childhood and early adult life may make it possible to stretch the expectation of life to a maximum of 75 years. However, our record of what has been accomplished and of where we have so far failed, and our knowledge of what may be accomplished by a more widespread appreciation of the available public health facilities indicate that a mean length of life of 70 years is possible in the immediate future.   This figure, which is not

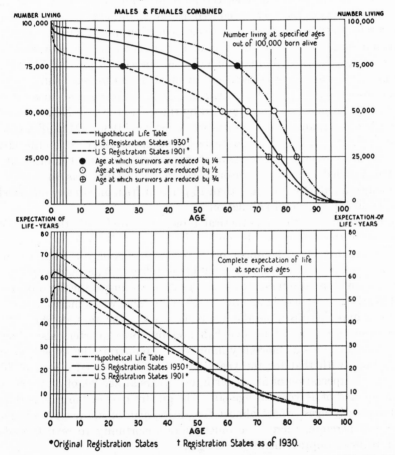

COMPARISON OF SURVIVORS AND OF COMPLETE EXPECTATION OF LIFE

Life Tables for U.S. Registration States, 1901* *and* 1930†
and Hypothetical Life Table.

FIG. 14. Comparison of survivors and of complete expectation of life (Dublin and Lotka, 1936).

far removed from an expectation of life of 67.88 years observed among females in New Zealand during 1931, is obtained from a hypothetical life table constructed upon the following assumptions as to improvement in mortality. In the first place, it was assumed that a mortality rate of 25 per 1,000 may before long be attained in the first year of life, instead of a value of about 50 which now prevails. In New Zealand, they had already reached the low figure of 25.5 per 1,000 for females in 1931. At age one, there was assumed a reduction of 10 per cent from the mortality observed among New Zealand females in 1931. For each succeeding age after age one, the mortality rates for females in New Zealand during 1931 were reduced by an additional quarter of one per cent, until at age 21 a 15 per cent reduction was obtained. It was then assumed that this reduction of 15 per cent from the mortality of the table considered is attainable for all succeeding ages to 74, after which the reduction was decreased by one per cent for each subsequent age until it was only 10 per cent at age 79. For ages 80 to 88, the hypothetical mortalities are guided by those observed for New Zealand females, 1931, and United States white females, 1930. Mortalities for the remaining ages of life were based on those observed in the last mentioned life table. The assumptions as to improvement in mortality here outlined are not unreasonable. In no instance has there been assumed a reduction of more than 15 per cent from an already observed mortality in a general population.

The results of the hypothetical table, compared with those of life tables for the general population in 1901 and in 1930 are shown graphically in figure 14. The upper panel portrays strikingly the savings in lives made possible by improvement in mortality. Whereas one quarter of the children born failed to attain age 25 according to the life table for 1901, the corresponding age by the 1930 life table was almost 50 years; in our hypothetical table the age is 63 years. The ages at which the survivors are reduced by one half and by three quarters also show marked advances as mortality improves. Comparing the hypothetical life table with that for the year 1930, there is observed a gain of 10 years in expectation of life at birth, of 7 years at age 20, of $5\frac{1}{2}$ years at age 40, and of $3\frac{1}{4}$ years at age 60. The greater part of the gain is thus at the early ages, where almost the entire span of life lies ahead and where, therefore, there is so much more opportunity to reap the advantages of improvements at all ages.

7. LONGEVITY AND POPULATION STRUCTURE

The consequences of the changing picture of mortality and longevity are many. In this chapter, we need be concerned only with those which flow from the inescapable fact that we are becoming a nation of elders.

As more lives are saved from premature death, larger numbers will survive to a ripe old age. This is a fundamental concept that will continue to operate as long as our public health practices move to higher levels. Another factor in this ageing process of primary importance is the steady and rapidly declining birth rate so characteristic of the period since the World War. Although no official figures exist prior to 1915, it is estimated that the birth rate in the United States in 1900 was approximately 30 per 1,000; by 1915, it had fallen to 25 and at the present time it is not much over 16 per 1,000. It is significant that the 1930 census revealed, for the first time in our national history,

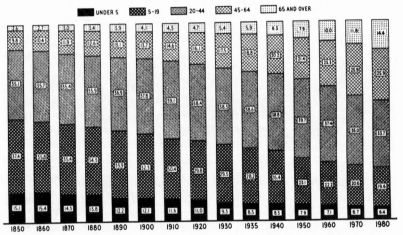

FIG. 15. Present distribution of total population by age

two noteworthy findings: one, that we had fewer children under age five than at the census previously taken; two, that there were actually fewer children under age five than in the next older age group, five to nine years. By careful analysis of recent trends in fertility and mortality, we learn that our present annual excess of births over deaths arises solely from a large concentration of population at the reproductive ages of life—ages which also experience low mortality. Actually, the present generation is not reproducing itself. With a continuation of current tendencies in fertility and mortality, the proportion of the population at the younger ages will continue to decline, and the proportion at the older ages will increase.   Immigration, once a factor of great importance in this regard seems destined to a minor rôle in our future population picture.

This suggests that we trace briefly the changes in the age composition of the American population since 1850.   We see in figure 15, that in 1850 over a half, or 52.5 per cent, of the total population was under 20 years of age.   At each subsequent census this percentage declined; by 1900 it was 44.4 per cent; the 1930 census gave the figure as 38.8 per cent, and according to a recent estimate for 1935, it dropped further to 36.7 per cent.   Even more interesting are the figures showing the proportionate increase among those 65 years of age and over during the same period.   In 1850, they formed only 2.6 per cent of the total; fifty years later, they formed 4.1 per cent; in 1930, the figure rose to 5.4 per cent; and for 1935, the estimate is 5.9 per cent.

The effects of these changes in the age structure of our population will take place so gradually that, on the whole, we will hardly be aware of them.   But when we look back little more than a generation, we can see that changes have come; and when we project present trends into the future we cannot avoid the conclusion that these changes will loom large in the life of the individual and the community of which he is a part.   Thus, it is estimated that by 1980, those at ages 65 years and over will constitute 14.4 per cent of the total population.

Although it is impossible to trace all the sequences propagated by these alterations in our age composition, mention may be made of some of the effects upon our political, economic, and social life.   Obviously, men in industry will meet the changing demands of an ageing population by adjusting their programs of production and distribution accordingly. With a marked slackening in population growth, expansion of manufacturing facilities may proceed at a slower rate than in the past; replacement of existing equipment will become a more important source of business.   What effect the altered age composition of the population will have upon the general standard of living cannot be judged by itself, for the future pace of economic progress introduces uncertainties into the situation.   However, there is to be considered the possibility that standards of living may fall, for a population with an increasing proportion of elders will make heavier the burden among those in the productive ages, whose labor will have to provide, more than before, to support the aged.   Our recently enacted social security program has made this situation more concrete.   Persons in industry are being taxed directly to provide for their own old age; indirectly, they are being taxed to provide benefits for the indigent aged as well.

Perhaps the most important single effect of such changes in our population structure as we have discussed will be in the mental outlook of the nation. Conservatism may become much more characteristic of our thinking than it is today. The ever-growing number of older people will play a larger part in determining the policy of the country. There may be expected fewer radical departures from accustomed ways, and suggestions for new forms in all phases of life will probably be met with increasing resistance. With a greater proportion of accumulated wisdom in the nation, there will perhaps be a stronger tendency to curtail waste, to utilize the natural resources for the public good, and to guide more intelligently the channels of production and distribution. More attention will probably be given to the advantages of concerted action against the daily risks of life. Our experiences in social insurance, and those of other countries, will presumably be carefully studied for possible improvements and extensions. Another accompaniment of the change in population structure is the disturbance in the sex ratio. A larger part of the older survivors will be women, since female mortality in adult life, and especially at the older ages, is considerably lower than that among males. But it is difficult and even dangerous to say what effects this shift in ratio will produce.

Whether there will be more or fewer annual deaths in the future than there are now will depend, to a large extent, on the total numbers of our population and on the trend of our death rates, besides the age structure of our population. It is inevitable, however, that, with an increasing concentration of population in the older ages of life where the death rates are highest and in the absence of any marked reduction in mortality at those ages, our country will experience a greater death rate per head of total population than that with which it is now favored. Conditions of morbidity and mortality associated with old age will become more frequent, relative to the total population, than is now the case. With a larger proportion of deaths and of cases of morbidity coming from the higher ages of life, the cardiovascular-renal conditions, cancer, diabetes, the pneumonias, influenza and certain types of accidents will become relatively more common. In fact, a very large part of the increase that we have already experienced in the mortality from such conditions as heart disease and the other degenerative diseases, as well as from cancer and diabetes, may be attributed to the shift in the age distribution of the population within the last half-century. This phenomenon will undoubtedly become more accented.

Under the régime of an ageing population, the conditions of morbidity and mortality typical of old age may receive the attention to which they have long been entitled, but have not always received. Closer study will probably be given to the part played by the infectious diseases in hastening the degenerative processes associated with old age. Recently acquired knowledge of the relations that exist between endocrine disorders and the ageing process is now regarded as only the initial development in a field of research that promises much. Inheritance of longevity will perhaps be studied more intensively; search will be made for other factors that may affect the ageing process.

An environment which concentrates on the problems of old age cannot help but affect the individual. As his social and economic relations shift, he may be expected to show greater concern in his own prospects for longevity. The possibilities for postponing old age and for mitigating its effects have always found willing ears; the audience will grow more attentive. Individual differences in longevity will be noted more carefully and discussed in the light of the various factors bearing on the chances of attaining a ripe old age.

8. LONGEVITY AND THE INDIVIDUAL[3]

There are many factors that bear upon an individual's prospects for a long life. One that will probably remain outside human control is the heritage of longevity bequeathed by the family, for studies that have been conducted on the subject indicate that this characteristic is a hereditary trait. However, gains in average longevity since the beginning of the century have been greater than the differences observed between the best and poorest classifications by parental longevity. The average individual can, therefore, more than overcome biological discrimination by personal and collective action toward the intelligent control of environment, although he cannot altogether avoid the consequences of the qualities that are born with him.

It is now fairly well established that a direct relation exists between social-economic status and mortality. The prospects for a long life are best in the most favored classes and poorest in the unskilled laboring classes. Many industrial workers are exposed to a wide variety of specific occupational hazards although both legislation and invention are used to minimize the dangers involved. The individual who, at the outset of his career, has freedom of choice in profession or occupation,

---

[3] The subject of this discussion is treated in detail in "Length of Life—A Study of the Life Table," by Louis I. Dublin and Alfred J. Lotka (Ronald Press, 1936); see particularly Chapters 4, 7, 8, 9 and 10.

is indeed in a fortunate situation so far as influencing his own longevity is concerned.

The average length of life has also been found to vary with geographic locality.   Those individuals who live in the prairie states of the midwest, and those living in the northwest, have, on the average, the best longevity in the country, while those who live along the Atlantic seaboard have relatively inferior longevity.   However, these variations in longevity may be influenced by occupational characteristics of the different areas; the midwest is predominantly rural, while the east is essentially industrial.   Another factor to be considered in this connection is that public health activities in the past have been largely concentrated in urban areas.   Thus, the individual's chances for a long life are affected by the locality he lives in, besides the work he does.

There is now an abundance of evidence to show that the married generally experience lower death rates than either the single or widowed. The exception is found among young married women who are exposed, in large numbers, to the risks of childbirth.   Such differentials in mortality by marital status may be expected, for marriage is essentially a selective process into which only the more physically fit of the single and widowed enter.   That it also confers benefits of various kinds, which directly or indirectly are conducive to longer life, can hardly be questioned.

An individual's personal history of physical or mental ailments has a very significant bearing upon his prospects for a long life.   Insurance investigations have shown that a history of certain impairments is often associated with mortality in excess of normal.   Many of the illnesses to which the individual falls a victim during the course of his lifetime leave indelible marks that affect his longevity.   Abnormalities of build, such as marked overweight or underweight, also involve some degree of curtailment in longevity.

The factors indicated in the preceding paragraphs are obviously but a few of the more important items which affect the length of life of the individual.   Perhaps more important than any of these factors are the steps that the individual may take on his own behalf to correct or control the hardships of his environment.   Evidence of value is accumulating that through the practice of better personal hygiene and by means of a well ordered existence, the average man may add many years to his expectation of life.   The possibilities along these lines have never been fully explored.   There are many instances of greatly improved physical condition and of enhanced longevity through the practice of personal hygiene. Professor Irving Fisher has made much of this type of evidence and has predicted an extraordinary increase in the life span as a real possibility for man in the future. Time alone will determine the accuracy of his judgment. In any case, the individual certainly can take advantage of current medical skill to a greater degree than in the past, not only during periods of illness but also to forestall serious developments through periodic health examinations. Among other steps the individual may take on his own behalf are to make his home in a more desirable locality and to avoid unhealthful occupations. However, in taking these steps, he is benefited from the collective efforts made in the past to promote human longevity. They indicate clearly what may be accomplished when this practice becomes more general among large numbers of individuals.

9. SUMMARY

By some inexorable law, still to be discovered and clarified, nature has allotted to man a life span of about one hundred years. But very few lives complete this span. Some are so malformed at the beginning of their existence that they cannot continue to live; others inherit limitations on account of constitutional weaknesses. The great majority of newly created lives, which are prepared to live through an existence that terminates only by physical degeneration, are constantly exposed to adverse influences in their environment that threaten either to destroy their existence or to accelerate the degenerative processes. It is within the powers of man, with his natural gift for controlling the forces of his environment, to mitigate or remove these adverse influences. The individual may accomplish much for himself in this direction by accommodating his routine so as to follow sound rules of personal hygiene and by showing an intelligent interest in current public health activities. Acting collectively with his fellow-men either through governmental or private bodies, he has at his disposal vast resources that may be used to meet and overcome difficulties affecting the public health. By such individual and collective efforts, it should be possible to extend the average length of life to a maximum of about 75 years.

REFERENCES

CARREL, A. 1937. The problem of the prolongation of life. Proc. of the Association of Life Insurance Presidents. New York, p. 154.
DORN, H. F. 1937. The increase in average length of life. U. S. Public Health Reports, Dec. 5, p. 1776.

DUBLIN, L. I. 1928. Health and wealth. New York: Harpers, Chapts. VII and XV.

DUBLIN, L. I., AND LOTKA, A. J. 1936. Length of life—A study of the life table. New York: Ronald Press.

GUMBEL, E. J. 1937. La Durée Extrême de la Vie Humaine. Paris.

PEARL, R., AND PEARL, R. DEW. 1934. The ancestry of the long-lived. Baltimore: Johns Hopkins Press.

STEFFENSEN, J. F. 1930. Some recent researches in the theory of statistics and actuarial science. Cambridge Press, pp. 5 and 6.

YOUNG, T. E. 1905. Centenarians and the duration of the human race. London.

CHAPTER 7

CARDIOVASCULAR SYSTEM AND BLOOD

ALFRED COHN

New York

1. NORMAL AND ABNORMAL COMPARED

Ageing is either disease or not disease. On first approach, the notion that growth and death, observable in all living organisms are intercurrent or accidental occurrences seems to do too great violence to the belief, now uncritically and generally adopted, that the processes of nature are orderly. If the conclusion were ultimately reached that ageing is an orderly natural process, a technique needs to be devised to show what is meant by orderly; what in short is natural and for that reason, normal. A decision has not been made less difficult by discovering to how great an extent, as Stockard (1937) has pointed out, behavior is under the dominance of mechanisms which seem controllable. The view may be held, however, that behavior has been a *usual* thing always, obviously, modifiable. To possess the means of modification does not mean that they will be employed or that it is profitable to employ them. If it were, the search for what is basic, unmodifiable, behavior would be sought much as is the basal metabolic rate. The concern would then center about the fate of the basic organism. This chain of notions anticipates though a situation which is, as yet, scarcely upon us.

In discussing the ageing of the cardiovascular system there is a special problem because the features which presumably constitute the evidences for ageing may also be, and often are, regarded as indications of disease. How to decide what is usual, or normal; and what is unusual, atypical, pathological or abnormal depends in this, as it does in many other situations, upon what is habitual, what is conspicuously familiar. The difficulty consists in defining in what manner such conceptions are formulated. Obviously, the notion "health" is central in this discussion. But the notion "health" is itself obscure. It depends on preconceptions based on rough experience and secondarily on an estimate of functions amenable to measurement. Height, weight, acuity of vision, the blood pressure, the pulse rate, the basal metabolic rate, the cardiac output (W. H. Lewis, Jr., 1938) represent such measurements.

The persons included in the groups to be measured are themselves selected as a result of judgments representing first rough approximations as to their conformity to the notion "health." Some notion of health becomes then the basis of selection of the individuals of whom measurements are to be made illustrating the state of special functions. But the precise states of special functions, even when assembled, synthesized, some would say, do not constitute the state "health" of an individual. Measurements of value have not, obviously, been developed to estimate all the essential functions which taken together constitute the physiology of a person. Of the tissues, organs and systems of the animal body, not one falls as yet in a category of which it can be said that the measurements available taken together describe that structure. This point is not made to document a defect. Contrariwise—that defect cannot, in all probability, be made good and if it could, would not suffice to produce a description that could be designated "health."

Meanwhile it is important to develop the notion "normal." Of normal it must become possible to say, normal in respect to what? Normal is not a measurement nor a conception which, like the decalogue, is something given. Reflection will disclose the fact that it exists, not in a Platonic, but in an Aristotelian sense. It results from experience on the part of a critical observer. He knows, for example, when, in a street travelled by fast-going traffic, it is safe to cross. For that kind of inference, no formal arithmetic is necessary. Where numbers can be used, entrance into what is called scientific method has begun. The measurement of the blood pressure may serve as example. At a given age persons of one sex, said to be healthy, are measured. At first, weight, height, and psychological state seem irrelevant considerations. They turn out to be important if the measurements are too scattered. Resort is then made to taking the pressures under what are called basal conditions—when all the obvious external disturbances are eliminated. When these precautions and reservations are regarded, averages are found for large numbers of persons, from which the figures of individuals differ by amounts taken to be not significant. What is accepted is a number, which has been obtained after several sortings— the criteria being race, "health," sex, age, state (e.g., basal), weight, height, social habits,—and perhaps others equally important. It has been found often enough, that attention to such matters is required, so that an average shall have characteristics in respect to a total experience, that will make that average credible. Without that the notion "normal" is meaningless. But since this choice of conditions is arbitrary, it is permissible to choose others provided, of course, they serve a use. Conditions not basal run the risk of yielding averages from which too many measurements will differ by significant amounts. But where an average is obtained which seems valid in that, in a distribution curve, a large fraction of cases falls in a narrow region, a "normal" figure for that function is deemed to have been obtained. Abnormal is a measurement which in relatively rare instances falls far away from usual experience. Persons who yield such measurements are of one of two classes— either abnormal or exhibiting a physiology peculiar to themselves. How to decide in which class to place them requires further analysis. The primary sorting may have been inadequate—persistent severe headache, or dizziness, or liability to fatigue may have been overlooked. In that case, a measurement discloses an error in the first rough sorting. Actually, this is the manner in which cases of so-called arterial hypertension are not infrequently discovered.

Reference has been made to a number of criteria according to which classes are made, at first arbitrarily perhaps, but later, if necessary, to arrive at necessary refinements. Sex, age, weight, height, are such criteria. When the effort is made to take these four into account, by decades or half-decades of age, the measurements yield averages from which the deviations are small. The average points at succeeding decades represent smooth curves. In so far as smooth curves tell consistent stories, success has attended the effort to find whether investigation has been undertaken of a process of which it can be said that the measurement represents a function which is normal. In that case, systematic changes consistent with a variable like age are obtained when measurements of individuals, not part of the group serving in the original experience, fall within proper distance of the descriptive curve.

This search for what is normal has been a laborious process. It will be recognized though that this procedure is actually the one which is habitually followed. It seems, now, to be the method of choice, having been generally adopted as the one by which successful prediction of the situation of a case can be made. Chance, lack of classification, has given way to order, to law.

The description of growth may be called the physiology of a long continuous process. Customary physiology has been descriptive of behavior at a selected time only—of young males. The description of ageing requires however more extended attention. The facts at each age are required so that it may be known whether occurrences, certainly some occurrences, at age 70 are normal. Abnormal in comparison with normal at 21, may not be abnormal, but normal at age 70. Making these distinctions has long been overdue. There is scarcely a province in the description of form or of function but that such information is required. When it is available, what is to be anticipated statistically, within the framework of the system of sorting that has been under discussion, will be recognized as normal. Wide deviations, either in quantity or in quality, will be regarded as abnormal. If sclerosis of an artery is to be anticipated at 70, its discovery at that age cannot be regarded as pathological. Its presence is normal for 70. When the view is adopted that these statements are correct, a new insight into the description of growth will have been attained. The description of growth becomes then the description of usual anticipated changes in structure and of usual anticipated changes in behavior. Growth in this sense is not a phenomenon limited to the development of bulk alone. It comprises what are customary changes with age. What constitutes these changes and what may be the mechanisms which underlie them, it is unnecessary, perhaps impossible, to define now. Whether they take place and can be recognized is what is essential.

In any discussion of ageing these two conceptions—"normal" and "growth"—are involved and a comprehension of them is of first-rate importance. When occurrences affecting the cardiovascular system are to be viewed in the light of these ideas, the fact that human disability so often accompanies changes in them, whether these are to be anticipated, as has been suggested and are therefore normal, or are accidental and not anticipated and therefore abnormal, renders inescapable, appraisal of the meaning of these changes. They have, perhaps uncritically, been regarded as evidence of disease, of being pathological. The definition of "disease" becomes therefore also a matter requiring attention. Attempts at definition have been legion. A review of them is not now desirable. Nor is it adequate to regard disease merely as the reverse of health in the light in which health has just been discussed. If health, or that synthesis of behavior we call health, is what is to be anticipated, disease clearly is accident. If, in a given person, the presence of certain bacteria occasion infection here, of the tonsils, joints, or heart, elsewhere on this planet that same association may not at all have this consequence. Diseases apparently are conditioned, among other factors, by time and place. Of many disabilities, whether they are diseases in this sense, there need be no doubt. Tuberculosis of the lungs or rheumatic fever, or typhoid fever are such disabilities.

But the disabilities incident to age belong in a different category. Geography may exert no influence on their occurrence. Their presence may occasion quite as much discomfort but—they may be inescapable. The idea disease carries with it, in our day, is the idea of cause. It may be cause operating in a favoring environment, but a single factor is nevertheless regarded as precipitating an ailment. There may be more than one named "cause"—symbiotic ones for example. Or if it is in a different realm, the disturbing factor may consist in too much or too little activity on the part of an organ or a tissue—the thyroid gland or the pancreas or the pituitary gland or the liver, a consequence of faulty "anlage" or of injury acquired within or without an organism. Whatever its nature, it is the unbalanced state of one's physiology which occasions the new appearance.

But in the disabilities which attend growth or senescence the situation is different. What has been called the togetherness of the organism provides, in time, for complex, reciprocal interactions which very gradually and very subtly alter the appearance and behavior of a person or an animal to such an extent, that to assign to any substance or mechanism, leadership in the process appears to present insuperable difficulty. But that view too has had advocates and the effort to find such substances has engaged the energies of distinguished men.

The separation of ailments incident to growth or ageing from those occasioned by "disease" is, as this discussion is designed to emphasize, difficult. Success in the effort has far reaching consequences. It matters whether an ailment is a response to a "cause"; removal of the cause disposes of the problem—at least in a narrow sense. The situation changes though when no cause can be assigned, when what we recognize, perhaps incorrectly, as among inexorable natural occurrences, precludes the possibility of preventive action. And the natural difference between these processes is decisive in the search for remedies. In processes of simple causation, believed to be reversible, cures may be sought justifiably—agents designed to neutralize or to inhibit the continuance of the process. But in processes which are irreversible, to attempt to bring about disappearance seems inappropriate; relief, amelioration, lessening of the effect, may represent the limits of possible action. In this view, the approach to therapeutics varies in the two types of affection, and the difference may have far-reaching results.

2. POINTS OF VIEW

In describing the state of knowledge of the cardiovascular system even in that relatively small section which touches on the matter of ageing alone, the literature is sufficiently abundant to render undesirable specific references to more than a small number of published researches. Those of which mention will be made are illustrative of the phenomena observable in the course of ageing. A description of the changes in the circulatory system should include both morphological and physiological matters, and should discuss from these two aspects, events taking place in the heart, the great vessels, the smaller vessels, and the blood itself. Concerning the blood, I am indebted for the information to be presented to Doctor Karl Landsteiner, Member of the Rockefeller Institute for Medical Research.

The evidence that can be submitted for the general point of view to be presented is two-fold—structural and functional, or anatomical and physiological. In both respects, the changes which take place with time should exhibit orderly progression. The average measurement of a function at a given period should form, with other averages similarly obtained, a curve which describes the anticipated course of events. Cases to be regarded as normal are those which do not deviate significantly from the curve. Those which do, are presumably pathological. The matter is perhaps not so simple as this numerical form of description suggests. It suffices in such matters as the blood pressure, where the state of this phenomenon is determining for the entire status of a person. But when, in a situation, there are elements which are not measurable or which cannot now be understood in measurable terms, the existence of a pathological state must be regarded as having a qualitative basis. To what extent less well defined ailments can be expected ultimately to be described quantitatively can, of course, merely be surmised. There are several situations: (1) There are those, like arterial hypertension, in which it may suffice to know the level of the blood pressure and its course. The collateral phenomena may conceivably depend on this one, though this is by no means certain. A similar case is the clearance of urea by the kidneys as a measure of renal function, the level of this being regarded as indicative of the presence of Bright's disease and fluctuations in level, of the course of that disease. (2) Then there are those, as in typhoid fever, in which there is no single measurable function suitable for giving an insight into its presence or the course of events. The temperature is not such a measurement nor is the presence of typhoid bacilli. (3) And finally there are those, as in senile dementia or insanity, in which there is no agreement that a measurement of any kind is possible.

These are the various forms under which diseases may be recognized—quantitative or partly quantitative or wholly qualitative. The deviations are from averages when numerical description is possible, or from familiar appearances only, when qualitative.

If the process of ageing can be shown to conform to orderly evolution or to the orderly evolution of certain forms and functions, the view which is taken in this description may be regarded as justified. This chapter is written where this is possible from this point of view.

3. HEART

Initially the heart occupies a position in the chest more nearly central than it does in advanced life. Its position is moreover erect in comparison with the situation later when it assumes a more horizontal position. Its bulk increases with years. Reliance has long been placed on the painstaking measurements of Müller (1883) in establishing curves of the growth of the heart. His results have been confirmed with modifications (Herrmann and Wilson, 1921–22; Lewis, 1913–14) a number of times. In making estimates of normal size and weight, factors apart from the mere weight of the heart should be taken into account. Among such factors are sex, stature, state of nutrition, occupation practised by the individual, type of individual (roughly, race). These factors may be assumed to influence the form of curves and attention to them may tend to limit the wide scatter often found in distributions. There are important relations between growth of the heart and that of the body as a whole, for the heart continues to grow after the body has ceased to do so, the ratio of heart weight to body weight decreases gradually through this period. Similar phenomena have been observed in other animals (fowl and rabbits) (Ehrich and Cohn, 1931). Subpericardial fat tends to increase along the grooves of the coronary vessels, especially in the auriculo-ventricular groove at the base of the right auricle. Its amount becomes sufficient so that in securing weights, it has become customary first to remove these accumulations. There is a tendency for the pericardium to become opaque, especially over the surface of the base of the right ventricle.

The *valves* undergo continuous change. Their softness and pliability are gradually lost so that later their structure tends to become rigid and their leaflets are less nicely approximated. These changes result from increase in fibrous tissue, from changes in the quality of elastic tissue, from the deposition of fats, and from the formation of calcium deposits. It is uncommon in older persons to fail to find deformity of these structures in varying degrees. The valves of the left side of the heart, the mitral and aortic, are far more severely involved in these processes than those of the right, the tricuspid and pulmonary. On the left side the degree of deformity may in fact be very advanced. Certain of these changes appear to be reversible. Lipoid is deposited, for example, in the aortic flap of the mitral valve very early sometimes in the first year. Later it disappears. The occasion for this change may be sought in diet and the changes in diet.

Changes take place also in the endocardium, the fibrous quality of that of the left auricle increasing so that it becomes a substantial membrane. It is not infrequent that the endocardium of the left ventricle covering the septum, being in any case a complicated structure (Nagayo, 1909), exhibits increasing thickness. That at the apices of the papillary muscles, even in the absence of older attacks of inflammation, tends to be thick.

The *striated muscle* fibers which constitute the essential bulk of the heart undergo important alterations. So far as is now known (Karsner, Saphir and Todd, 1925) the number of fibers undergoes no change. At first, individual cells form the substance of the muscle. Later these become modified, coalesce, and form the well-known syncytium. In very young hearts, cross striation is not as conspicuous as it comes later to be. In advanced age, about the nuclei, striation begins again to disappear. It is as if the spaces which become vacated, do so to accommodate the developing pigment. About the time of birth intercalated discs make their appearance. These exhibit a simple structure at first, but later undergo increasing complexity, being arranged in very irregular steps, their direction being not always uniform but changing one or more times as they traverse a fiber from side to side. The significance of these phenomena is still unknown. There is a tendency on the part of the fibers in older bodies to become fragmented and to do so, some observers have thought, at the location of the intercalated discs. But it is still uncertain whether that is correct. It seems likely though that the tendency to fragmentation increases with years. The view has been entertained (Warthin, 1925) that regeneration is possible after injuries like diphtheria, but the evidence is not conclusive. The size of individual fibers increases, undoubtedly, during the earlier decades, but declines again later. The impression is gained that late in life the discs are less tall, but a judgment of this is not simple because alterations take place during fixation and because an effect is exerted on their state in consequence of rigor mortis. Mention has already been made of the probability that in growth hyperplasia of muscle elements does not take place. *Pigment*, lipochrome in nature, begins to be laid down at the poles of nuclei in the earlier decades, increasing continuously in amount afterward. Older hearts, exhibit this appearance to which the term brown atrophy is applied, as a result of decrease in the concentration of water,[1] a part perhaps of the general process of desiccation which takes place with time; and an increase in the amount of the pigment to which reference has already been made.

The *nuclei*, centrally placed within fibers look vesicular at first and are contained within smooth nuclear membranes. But the nuclei increase much in size, become complex in structure, irregular in outline, appear something like cumulus clouds, and take on more dye than in youth.

Aside from its appearance in the aorta, the belief is entertained (Miller and Perkins, 1927) that the amount of *elastic tissue* found in cardiac muscle varies so much with age and is so characteristic that, in normal hearts, it may be possible to arrive at an estimate of age in terms of the amount present. The auricles exhibit this phenomenon more than the ventricles.

The *coronary arteries* undergo changes but not all of them in a uniform manner. The *ramus descendens arterior* matures earliest. Change in the *ramus descendens posterior* can in fact lag five to ten years. Nor in any branch does advance take place uniformly. The process is accelerated in certain locations as, for example, at a point about a centimeter from its origin in the *ramus descendens anterior*, where calcification and ultimately constriction and thrombosis develop. Various views have been entertained to account for the changes. One set of changes characteristic of ageing takes place in the intima (Ehrich, de la Chapelle, and Cohn, 1931). In this view the internal elastic lamella splits early in life, the intima undergoing continuous change until finally it gives the appearance of being quite disorganized. The process is one in which progressing alteration in elastic tissue and ground substance occur along with the deposition of cholesterol, and calcium in the form of droplets. Under what influence these occurrences take place is so far unknown. A somewhat different view is taken by Winternitz (1938) who thinks there is evidence to show that underlying all changes are numerous small haemorrhages on the basis of which subsequent occurrences develop. The precise mechanism accountable for the continuous alterations, so easily observable, it is of prime importance to learn. So far the results of experimental arteriosclerosis

---

[1] The view that desiccation is characteristic of growth is developed by O. Glaser, Biological Reviews, 1938, **13**, 20–58.

in rabbits (Anitschow, 1933; Leary, 1934) have yielded insufficient information concerning occurrences in human beings, although undoubtedly much can be learned from this method. The assumption that the two processes are identical is widely made. Leary thinks the evidence for this view is strong. Further studies of the metabolism of the sterols and of the function of hormones, will no doubt yield valuable additional information on these crucial phenomena. It does not go without saying that a mechanism, responsible for the course of events in a tissue or an organ, as in the heart, is identical with that operating elsewhere, as in the brain or in the kidneys.

In a series of diagrammatic drawings Sappington and Cook (1936) have shown in a striking fashion how, from birth to 84 years, the coronary arteries, in the same individual, are subject to intimal and medial changes to a far greater degree than are the radial arteries. The radial arteries are, in fact, relatively little affected, less, in their opinion than in that of Thayer and Fabyan (1907). Indeed, the radial arteries at 65 years have not developed further than the coronary arteries at 20 years. The coronary arteries, on the other hand, very rarely exhibit medial calcification (Mönckeberg) resembling in this regard, elastic and not muscular arteries. In comparison with the renal arteries they show greater change but less than the splenic.

It was thought by Gross (1921) that after birth and with the development of the heart, especially in the early years, anaemia of the walls of the right ventricle takes place, relative to that of the left, due to decrease in the number of arteries to be observed. If the arteries of a size at about the limit of visibility are actually counted, it appears that this inference can scarcely be drawn (Ehrich, de la Chapelle, and Cohn, 1931). The number of such arteries bears a relation to the weight of the ventricles. Taking the increase in weight of the two ventricles into account, the blood supply to both increases, that to the left twice as much as that to the right, an expression of the relative weight of the two. Later in life when there is decrease in the weight of the heart, the blood supply, that is to say the number of arteries, seems again to diminish, an appearance which now affects especially the left ventricle.

It seems unlikely that the number of arteries in the heart increases during life. The increased demand for blood is met by increase in the diameter of those arteries which are just visible, macroscopically, to the extent of about two-and-a-half times. At its maximum, the heart muscle has increased about twenty times its weight at birth, the total area of the arteries only 6 or 7 times. But if the square (that is, the area of the cross sections of the arteries) is raised to the cube (the volume of the muscle) the correspondence in dimensions becomes clearer (Ehrich, de la Chapelle, and Cohn, 1931).

The *rate* of the heart beat is, as is well known, a function of age. Beginning at birth there is progressive slow decline during the first decade. At the third decade the rate reaches a plateau and declines again slightly after the fifth. This statement applies to Western European and to the White races in America. A somewhat different curve shows the rate to decline from birth (130 to 140) to about 25 years (70), and then gradually to mount to a level of nearly 80 at 95 years (Bramwell, 1937). In general similar statements can no doubt be made in the case of other races, but the facts are not available. Undoubtedly stature is a factor which enters into the result. In general, the rate of metabolism of smaller animals being higher than that of larger ones, it should be expected that the cardiac rates of smaller, slighter human beings are more rapid.

The *rhythm* of the heart tends in younger persons to be regular. Even in severe diseases, disturbances in rhythm are relatively infrequent among affected persons. These statements are unfortunately not facts—but estimates. As time progresses there is marked tendency for abnormalities in rhythm to multiply. A distinction should be made between abnormalities which occur incident to diseases of the heart and those which occur when, in other respects, the heart is believed to be sound. Such abnormalities as *heart block*, except in a relatively few cases of congenital origin, occur, it is perhaps not too much to say, exclusively as the result of lesions acquired during life—as results of syphilis, arteriosclerosis, or other abnormalities. Apart from obvious, easily detectable, structural changes, irregular action has a tendency with age increasingly to take place—*premature contractions* are not infrequent, nor are attacks of brief or even of longer periods of *fibrillation* of the auricles.

The ventricles, it appears, give rise more frequently to premature contractions than the auricles. Their frequency varies a great deal. For some persons they occasion discomfort, others are wholly unaware of their occurrence. Of what these irregularities are a sign, it is impossible to say, now. The rhythm of the heart results from many factors—specific, that is to say, differentiated, systems of muscles; the nervous system, sympathetic and parasympathetic nerves, extra and intracardiac ganglia; hormones, metabolites; a very complex situation the significance of each part not yet adequately unraveled. And yet there are collateral phenomena which contribute to establishing the fact that with age subtle changes occur that facilitate irregular action of the heart. Patients suffering from lobar pneumonia, for example, are sometimes seized with auricular fibrillation, but those who are so taken are almost exclusively older persons, the more frequently, the older the persons.

Another indirect indication that the function of cardiac muscle changes with age is found in the experience of patients suffering from hyperthyroidism (Ernstene, 1938). In them, auricular fibrillation is more common after age 45 years, whether the irregularity is transient or permanent, before or after operation.

In recent years methods have become available (Grollman, 1932; Henderson and Haggard, 1925; Field, Bock, Gildea and Lathrop, 1924; Burwell and Robinson, 1924) for measuring the amounts of blood which are discharged from the ventricles of the heart per minute and, of course, per beat. These methods have been carefully utilized in the study of older men from 40 to 90 years (Lewis, 1938). Under so-called basal conditions, in trained men, no significant change in output has been observed. That this should be the fact is perhaps surprising. The output of the heart appears, however, to be a response to the body's needs. Under basal conditions the amount is not reduced to a minimum but it is, nevertheless, small enough so that more can be expelled, perhaps much more, than is then (under basal conditions) required. But this state does not explain the whole situation for under basal conditions the basal metabolic rate declines with progressive ageing (see Lewis, 1938, Table 1). A clue it was thought may be found in the arterio-venous oxygen difference which declines 3.2 per cent. The consumption of oxygen declines meanwhile, 9.3 per cent. The decline in oxygen utilization (A-V oxygen difference) does not therefore tell the whole story.

The effort has been made meanwhile to ascertain what the facts are when, with very slight exercise like elevating one foot, work may be expected to increase the cardiac output. These studies are still in progress but appear not to be fruitful when the cardiac output rises more than 10 liters. Indeed it rises to this level on very slight exercise so that an answer under these circumstances is not yet available.

Aside from the actual work which hearts do—a difficult measurement in human beings with the means now available—an insight into the amount of oxygen they consume can be gained. This measurement cannot be made now in human beings. In animals it is also difficult to measure, but in them an answer can be obtained by experiment. Such experiments have been undertaken. Heart-lung preparations were made of thoroughbred wire haired female fox-terriers of known age (Cohn and Steele, 1932). The ages of the dogs varied between 3 months and 13 years—approximately their life span. It was found that as the animals grew older their hearts, per gram of heart muscle, consumed less oxygen to a significant degree, even when correction was made for disturbing factors, such as that larger hearts consume less oxygen per unit of weight and that the consumption of oxygen per gram of heart increases with rate or decreases with the slower rates of older hearts. But when, as has just been said, these corrections are made, the decrease in consumption of oxygen with age remains significant. The decreasing ability to consume oxygen suggests essential changes in the constitution of muscle with time. This change in capability is not indicative of the mechanism within the muscle which is involved, but suggests what substances constituting these mechanisms must be. Advancing knowledge of the substances, the proteins, the carbohydrate and respiratory catalysts may be expected with time to unravel certain of these problems. Protein, for example, constitutes a very large percentage (19 per cent, Mirsky, personal communication) of the substance of muscle and, there begins to be reason to believe, partakes, perhaps basically, in the act of contraction. It will be the task of research in the future to discover what this substance is, the factors which condition its work, the changes in that substance and in these conditions which are modified with time so that decrease in energy which is so obvious may be "explained." Both protein and its environment—organic and inorganic substances take part, no doubt, in this behavior. What is true of cardiac muscle from this point of view is true also of substances which are found in the vascular system and in the blood.

About alterations with age in the *innervation of the heart* little is known. A few have been brought to light and these concern the autonomic nerves distributed to the heart. However simple the appearance of this influence, the nature of the mechanism has so far escaped analysis. As age advances, Gilbert (1923) has found that pressure on the vagus nerves, now known to be pressure not on the nerves but on the carotid sinus, has a greater effect with advancing years—the rate of the heart is more and more slowed, and the rate of conduction of impulses from auricles to ventricles is more and more prolonged. A collateral phenomenon was described by Crawford (1923). His observations likewise concern the vagus nerves, in his study by way of bringing about release of their influence as inhibitors of the rate of the heart beat. He found that when atropine is injected the increase in rate is greatest in the young and that its effect decreases with advancing age. The release (increase in rate) is maximal between 20 and 30 years. Afterward the effect is somewhat less at first but after 50 the increase becomes slight. How these two phenomena are related is not now clear—pressure on the carotid sinus with consequences to the functioning of a reflex, and action on terminals in the muscle of the vagus nerves. In the former case, the effect is apparently wrought in a way different from that in the latter.

The carotid sinus seems to become more sensitive to pressure, and the neuro-muscular junction less capable of being influenced. If the sensitiveness of the junction has changed, and its influence has been completely removed, the muscle, now uncontrolled, appears to be less capable of developing rapid rates. Presumably the intrinsic rhythm of the muscle has become slower. That is a result which points to fundamental changes in essential systems within the muscle reminiscent of its declining ability to utilize oxygen.

Evidence that changes of a profound nature take place is observable in *electrocardiograms*. Systematic studies of the phenomena are still too few to permit general statements. Whether resulting merely from alteration already referred to in the position of the heart from vertical to horizontal, or from further changes in balance of muscle between right and left ventricles, the direction of potential of the action current shifts, its direction becoming more horizontal, as if the hand of a clock changed from a position at 30 to one at 20 minutes. Other changes occur. There is a tendency for the voltage, that is to say the height of the curves, to decline; there is a tendency for the second ventricular complex (the T-wave) to become inverted especially when the current is derived from the left arm and the left leg (Lead III); there is a tendency for the first ventricular complex (the Q-R-S waves) to become intricate; there is lengthening of the interval between auricular and ventricular waves, representative of slowing of conduction between auricles and ventricles. No more is possible than to state these facts— their meaning still is obscure. Of especial interest is lengthening of the Q-R-S waves just mentioned. The assumption is that the passage of the stimulus to contraction is obliged to proceed in ways more devious because of disruption in normal pathways, resulting in electrical patterns less simple and in duration more prolonged than in youth. The mechanism in older persons which necessitates this change is still obscure though evidence is available that lesions have occurred in the conduction system.

4. ARTERIES

The arterial system cannot be regarded as a system having either uniform structure or uniform functions. The lack of uniformity is characteristic not only of arteries of different sizes but also of arteries of the same size. To make this statement is no doubt to outrun available information. Yet there is reason to think this description suggests matter of importance. There seem to be arteries not only of greater vulnerability but also arteries the alterations in which, though slighter, differ nevertheless. It is much too early in the history of researches of this nature to entertain ideas concerning the bases of difference, but the opportunities for difference are numerous, in the intima and in the media, in the sense that these regions may be sites for continuous reorganization of ground substance and elastic tissue, of fatty materials (sterols), of calcium, and no doubt of other elements not yet identified and of mechanisms not yet understood.

The difference in gross function among arteries has become well known—the difference between arteries which serve as reservoirs, and passages which are predominantly elastic and those of muscular quality. The aorta, as the type of the elastic variety, presents evidence for ageing beginning at its very root. As it issues from the heart, it undergoes well defined changes (Gross and Silverman, 1937). The junction is a complicated arrangement consisting of root, wedge and annulus. At birth these structures are devoid of capillaries but as early as the middle of the first decade they begin to appear and, in the wedge, take on sinusoidal appearance. The annulus becomes hyalinized and receives lipoid material. In its further length changes in its elasticity have been studied by a variety of methods (Wilens, 1937; Steele, 1937). The results point to a loss of elasticity with age though, as has been pointed out (Benninghof, 1930), there is no actual loss, but perhaps even an increase in amount, of elastic tissue. Its form changes though, as does its tinctorial properties. A study of elasticity in its various aspects and as a property of various structures in the body would be a rewarding undertaking.

It is important to recognize that the arteries in the same individual which branch from the abdominal aorta—the coeliac axis and the splenic artery, for example, undergo changes much more conspicuous than those in arteries to the extremities such as the femoral or the brachial, and their branches.   This reference is naturally not to arteries the subject of diseases—as thrombo-angiitis obliterans or syphilis. The arteries of the heart and those of the brain undergo changes distinctly more numerous and more far-reaching than do those to the kidneys or the lungs or the liver.   For these differences, reasons deserve to be sought.   But it is perhaps not incorrect to assume that processes of profound importance are at play which account for what can be observed so easily.   Whether these processes are different, and whether they depend on the organs which they serve or on local mechanical requirements or on matters intrinsic to the arteries themselves, is not known now.   But matters of indifference they certainly are not.[2]

The alterations in vessels of unequal size are very different in ap-

[2] Winternitz, Thomas, and LeCompte end their recent volume (The Biology of Arteriosclerosis, Springfield, Ill., Thomas, 1938, 142 pp.) with these sentences: "The cause of arteriosclerosis is probably not to be found in a single factor.   The pleomorphism of the process, its characteristic irregularity of distribution and rate of development are sufficient evidence of this.   But surely an approach to the problem which is based on recognition of the artery as a vascular or potentially vascular organ, and therefore subject to the same pathological processes to which other tissues are subject, may prove more fruitful than one in which the lesions are regarded as primarily 'degenerative' or as the inevitable concomitants of age."

The phrases "single factor," "characteristic irregularity of distribution and rate of development," in connection with the histogensis of arteriosclerosis are very happy phrases.   Obviously, in respect to the last sentence there can be complete agreement in regarding an "artery as a vascular or potentially vascular organ."   But whether there is anything in this statement antithetical to the view that such lesions, arteriosclerotic ones, are "primarily 'degenerative' or . . . the inevitable concomitants of age" is doubtful.   The intention is, I suppose, to suggest that there is.   What the word "degenerative" means is a matter of definition, one which it is unnecessary now to formulate.   It may, and should be, suggested though, that when lesions are described the "causes" of which cannot be assigned because unknown, growth, as being a phrase which includes in its meaning "the inevitable concomitants of age," cannot be dismissed as one of them.   If emphasis is placed on arteriosclerosis as a process, a case for its "pathological" nature is not won by insinuating that ageing is not also a process. Both are, without doubt.   Would it be remarkable if arteriosclerosis should turn out to be only a single aspect, no matter how important and essential, of ageing? Evidence to support the second phrase quoted is supplied by the course of events in different branches of the coronary arteries.   One wonders whether in the last sentence it *follows* that because an artery is a vascular organ, it becomes subject to the same pathological processes to which other tissues are subject.   Nor is it obvious why an "approach" to solving the problem of arteriosclerosis is likely "surely" to be more "fruitful" if arteries are recognized as being vascular organs than if they (the lesions) are "primarily 'degenerative' or . . . the inevitable concomitants of age."   May not the inevitable concomitants of age be vascular change?

pearance, irrespective of whether initially these differences originate in the same injury. The plaques in the aorta, the scars in the splenic artery, the miliary aneurisms in the cerebral arteries, intimal hyperplasia in many locations, the annular narrowing in the coronary arteries are all striking lesions and all, at least superficially, different. How they originate, through what intermediate phases they pass, and to what disability each ultimately leads, deserves thoroughgoing study. Specifically what kinds of alteration take place and where in the vessel walls are they located?

There seems to be general agreement that small cerebral arteries differ in structure from arteries elsewhere of the same size (Baker, 1937). The *elastica interna* is thicker, it takes on the stain irregularly; and the media possesses less elastic tissue and muscle but a great deal more collagen. With advance in age the *elastica interna* is split already in the third decade and takes up the dye in a uniform manner. The media exhibits decreasing amounts of elastic tissue and muscle early in life; there is complete fibrosis here before collagen appears elsewhere, collagen having become hyalinized. Red blood cells break through the walls of the vessels and sometimes form rings of red blood cells around them; finally, calcification takes place as an independent process without concomitant hyalin or fibrotic change.

Apart from the small vessels of the cortex, the basal arteries show conspicuous changes with age. They occur earlier than in the cortical ones and are more extensive. Here hyalinization is frequent and calcification is found. The entire process is already advanced at the fourth decade.

There was a time when the term arteriosclerosis sufficed to designate the state of the arteries—sclerosis meaning hard. The split which takes place in the *elastica interna*, the further alterations in the intima which becomes progressively thickened and disorganized or perhaps reorganized chiefly through increase in connective tissue, the deposition of calcium constitute what are regarded as the chief lesions that occur. Aschoff attempted, about 20 years ago, to distinguish between the hardening process and a process in which the metabolism of fatty substances, the sterols, notably cholesterol, is involved. In recent years changes in the arteries have been described chiefly from the viewpoint of this metabolic process. Experiments have been undertaken to analyze this phenomenon. Much is now known of the results of experiments especially in rabbits to which cholesterol has been given with their food (Anitschkow, 1933).

It is unnecessary to trace the changes which occur in all the smaller arteries. It will suffice to describe those in a single branch of the left coronary artery—the *ramus descendens anterior*. The first change which takes place occurs in new-born children; the *lamina elastica interna* is split. The "elastic muscular layer" is formed. This layer lies between the *lamina elastica interna* and the inner limiting lamella. Inward from this, the hyperplastic layer develops and may be perceived as early as the first decade. It is characterized by hyperplastic elastic tissue in the more outward part and by connective tissue in the more inward. The two are not always easily distinguishable. When the inner limiting lamella is much split, the limits of this layer can scarcely be recognized. In this case the inner portion of the intima is spoken of as the "diffuse layer." How to distinguish these structures, when this is possible, has been described by Jores (1903). Now there are striking differences in the rate of development of these changes even among branches of the coronary arteries. In the *ramus descendens anterior*, the internal elastic lamina is split in places in the new-born. But this phenomenon does not take place in the posterior descending ramus until the first decade. The hyperplastic layer appears in the anterior descending ramus in the first decade, but in the posterior descending ramus not until the third. And again, in the anterior descending ramus, beading is detected in the first decade and calcification in the third, though in the posterior descending ramus, neither was observed until the seventh decade (Ehrich, de la Chapelle, and Cohn, 1931; Wolkoff, 1923, 1929; Bork, 1926).

Arteries of practically the same size, although they undergo similar changes, do so, in the same organ, at very different rates. The meaning of this difference is quite unknown. But in any formulation of the meaning of the development of arterio- or athero-sclerotic changes, the peculiarity should be seriously taken into account. If the difference is attributed to difference in function, structure in some way, genetically, has responded to the demands placed upon it. In the clinic the observation is frequently made that structure is not equal to demand. It is, for example, common to find the *ramus descendens anterior* the site of important lesions, resulting in serious disability of the heart—often in death. But it is this ramus which exhibits the highest differentiation, presumably in response to its need. Did it not so respond, accidents might not befall it. But the assumption is, nevertheless, the changes result from stress. Whether the response is a source of increased strength or of weakness, is not yet understood.

The deposition of cholesterol and of calcium in the walls of the vessels, where this takes place, and the mechanism of its occurrence is by no means solved (Anitschkow, 1933).   More is known about this process in animals used for experiment, especially in rabbits, than in human beings.   If, as is urged, this occurrence depends on diet, or on environment in a larger sense, the fact remains that, in the same subject, arteries differ—even when they are of the same size in the same organ, as the heart.   Of possible factors, environment (diet), structure, function (stress), internal environment (hormones), it is obvious that structure differs with locality—presumably a response to stress.   And the difference in structure suggests a different need in order to respond to stress on the part of the structure in that locality.

An important consequence of the change in structure of arteries is a change in their behavior in response to the movement of the pulse (pressure) wave.   The rate at which the *pulse wave* travels along arterial walls can be expressed as a function of age.   This phenomenon has been investigated several times (Friberger, 1912; Bramwell, Hill, and McSwiney, 1923; Hallock, 1934; Wezler, 1935; Steele, 1937) always with the same result.   The waves travel with increasing celerity with advance in years.   Bramwell was able, for example, to draw a smooth curve descriptive of the facts he observed.   At 5 years the rate was 5.2 meters per second; at 20 years, 6.2 meters; at 40, 7.2; and at 60, 8.0.

It has long been thought, it seems incorrectly, that the levels of the *blood pressures* change consistently and continuously with age (Faber and James; 1921; Alvarez, 1923; Burlage, 1922; MacWilliam, 1925). They are relatively low in childhood but rise sharply during the second decade and continue to do so through the ninth decade (80 to 89 years). There are differences between males and females, the level being lower in women.   The technique of taking blood pressures has varied.   The custom has been general to make readings either directly after periods of exercise or after a short period of rest.   It is doubtful whether a given method can be regarded as correct; each has value for the purpose for which it is employed.   For purposes of comparison to make readings after a night's rest, in what are called basal conditions, has advantages. This method has been employed a number of times (Lewis, 1938; Addis, 1922; Blankenhorn and Campbell, 1925; Brooks and Carroll, 1912), notably in men between 40 and 89 years by Lewis.   It now appears that the average systolic pressure at 40 to 44 years is 116 mm. Hg.   It rises gradually until age 60 to 64 (124 mm. Hg); then rises sharply between 65 to 69 (134 mm. Hg).   At 85 to 89 it is 158 mm. Hg.

The average diastolic pressure varies within narrow limits only, between 75 and 85 mm. Hg. Under these circumstances the pulse pressure reflects predominantly the changes in the systolic levels.

There are changes also in venous pressure (Hooker, 1916). It rises between ages 5 and 85 years from 83 to 267 mm. of water. The point has been made, however, that these measurements are obtained with subjects in the sitting position. When the position is prone, no difference referable to age is said to be observable (Castellotti, 1923; Eyster and Middleton, 1924; Eyster, 1926).

The *internal secretions*, especially of the pituitary gland and of the adrenals are known to exert important influences on the state of the walls of the arteries and probably also of the capillaries and veins. What is not known but what can easily be surmised is that as the arteries change so do the secretory glands. But what the changes are and how they affect the behavior of the arteries has not been investigated. The fact should be taken into account that all arteries, presumably in younger persons, are not affected identically by chemical or pharmacal agents. The reaction of the coronary arteries to adrenalin, for example, is different from that of other arteries. But the analysis here again is not simple for the integrated action upon arteries involves the effect of drugs upon the nerves which innervate them. That their response changes with time, or may do so, has already been described in discussing the action of the vagus nerves and of atropine upon them.

5. CAPILLARIES

What the fate of the capillaries is in the course of life is a matter of very great concern. There is little that can be asserted unequivocally. The progressive decrease in the number of glomeruli, the result apparently of influences at work upon the capillary tufts is familiar. The decrease is systematic, beginning very early in life (Moore, 1931). The assumption is that their disappearance is a normal phenomenon. There are no other familiar obvious situations in which a parallel course of events can be traced. That the existence of capillaries need not necessarily be jeopardized at older ages is evidenced by the fact that wounds heal and that tumors grow during advanced years. The phenomenon which Krogh (1929) and others have observed, that all capillaries are not open all the time and so need not be missed, is scarcely relevant for were they completely shut, tissues would die without the chance for adequate nutrition or respiration.

Atrophy of organs or tissues would it seems likely exert an influence upon the numbers of capillaries.   The actual counting of cells or fibers or capillaries is a laborious undertaking which has occasionally been attempted.   But evidence on this relation is not available.   The skin offers a suitable object of study.   Wrinkling obviously takes place, but the mechanism of shrinking, whether accompanied by involution and disappearance of capillaries or whether by change in elastic and constituent tissue requires still to be learned.

Like the arteries there is reason to think that capillaries exhibit different structure in different parts of the body.   The size of the cells differs in arteries, capillaries and veins.   The permeability of capillaries is said to decrease with age though there is as yet no literature on this point.   There is a property or the loss of a property in capillaries which makes possible appearances in the aged not observable in youth as, for example, their dilatation in exposed portions of the skin of the nose.

The rôle which the capillaries play is, of course, of very first importance in respiration and nutrition.   It would be desirable to know better what part they take in those changes in the appearances of the body which become so obvious with the passage of time.   In the heart muscle, changes in structure of the muscle are apparent, but in other tissues comparable or correlative ones are not.   It is not necessary that these should be visible—a change in elasticity may not be.   Elastic tissue itself may lose its elasticity without loss of its distinctive staining reaction, a phenomenon familiar in the ageing of the aorta.   But to what extent all tissues do so, including the capillaries, is not yet understood.   It is not to be inferred that it is to this one property that all changes in form and function are to be referred.   To suggest a possible one, such as this, is all that is intended.   It would, in another direction, be a matter of great interest to learn through the use of isotopes, as Schoenheimer is doing, whether cells permeable to substances at one age lose that ability later or whether the reverse situation as to age obtains—gain rather than loss.   But of this also one can be certain, in different tissues and organs, the capillaries obviously permit the passage of substances not necessary elsewhere.   Three possibilities exist—either that capillaries can permit the passage of every relevant substance but depending on their location do not do so; or that, in relation to the needs of cells, capillary endothelium possesses a requisite degree of adaptability; or that all capillaries are identical and leave the matter of selection to the tissues which they serve.   With the differences in structure which are apparent, and with the differences in function which can be inferred, it appears possible to conclude that these differences enter into those situations which are recognized as phases of the ageing process.

Now endothelial cells differ a great deal in size, in the first place. Those forming the lymphatics are the largest. Next come those in the veins, then those in the capillaries, and finally those in the arteries. Nor are endothelial cells of the same thickness. In the lymph nodes, they are cuboidal in the veins.[3] Endothelial cells are not, furthermore, uniform. There are those of the liver, the Kupffer cells; second, those of the spleen; third, those of the bone marrow; fourth, those of the lymph nodes. These endothelia differ principally, it seems, in the degree to which they can act as phagocytes. The term reticulo-endothelial tissue has been used to designate two types of cells, first, free cells in the connective tissue, the phagocytic mononuclear cells; and second, the four specific endothelial cells just enumerated. What the fate of capillaries is, is obscure. That those in the glomeruli of the kidney atrophy had become hyaline is known. That they do so in the continuous fashion so that the numbers disappearing with age form a smooth curve has been shown (Moore, 1931). Their fate in the skin has also been studied. The view has been expressed (Wetzel and Zotterman, 1936) that the number of capillaries in certain regions as at the hand "show no appreciable change after growth ceases." But when the figures given are plotted there appears to be a distinct fall in the number with age. But too few cases have been examined, and these perhaps with inadequate methods, to be able to speak with assurance of the facts.

The point has been made that, even if capillaries disappear with age the ratio of capillaries to tissue remains unchanged because, with the going of the capillaries, the tissue must also be expected to have gone (Weiss and Frazier, 1930). But there is no evidence here that the capillaries actually atrophy. The skin, meanwhile, quite obviously has shrunk. In any case the number of capillaries in small groups was less (30 per sq. mm.) in arteriosclerotic persons than in normal ones (35 sq. mm.) or in persons with arterial hypertension (35 sq. mm). If there were value on this analysis, the fact that the average is less in arteriosclerotic subjects could be taken to mean that the capillaries disappear faster than the surrounding tissues.

6. BLOOD[4]

There are few studies which illustrate variation in the activity of of antibodies at different periods of life. Two cases can be distinguished

[3] I am indebted to Doctor Florence R. Sabin for these statements.

[4] These notes have very kindly been put at my disposal by Doctor Karl Landsteiner, Member, the Rockefeller Institute for Medical Research.

which differ possibly in principle—so-called natural antibodies and those which result from artificial immunization.

Natural antibodies, those found in the serum of men and animals and which are not due to antecedent diseases, have given rise to various views concerning their origin. More particularly, a discussion has arisen whether bacterial antibodies are always called into existence as a result of contact on the part of the body with bacteria; in this case they are in principle identical with antibodies arising through the process of immunization. The other possibility is that natural antibodies arise as the result of physiological processes.

The answer to this question is that neither explanation is exclusively valid. Certain investigations have shown that antibodies against pathogenic bacteria and viruses are demonstrable in a population only when an opportunity has occurred either to acquire a disease or to pass through an unnoticed infection with a corresponding bacterium. Among such investigations that of Hughes and Sawyer (1932) on antibodies against the virus of Yellow Fever may be mentioned. They found such antibodies only in regions in which the disease occurs. On the other hand, there is an instance in which undoubtedly the occurrence of antibodies must be regarded as a physiological phenomenon. This is the case with the inherited isoagglutinins in human beings, having a constitutional origin.

The age-curves describing changes in the content of antibodies can, in both the cases mentioned, have different significance. With those antibodies which are occasioned by external influence there is the increasing opportunity with age, for exposure to infectious agents. This factor plays no rôle in cases where antibodies have a physiological origin.

On the subject of human isoagglutinins and on the presumably related agglutinins and haemolysins of human serum for the blood of animals, a number of papers have been published which describe differences with age. Schiff and Mendlovicz (1926) and Thomsen and Kettel (1929) made determinations of the titer of isoantibodies which are presented in table 7 (see also fig. 16). These data and Thomsen's curve show that the titer of agglutinins begins to rise in infancy and reaches its maximum between the ages of 5 and 10 years, after which it begins to fall and reaches a low level in old age. It may be recalled incidentally that the degree of agglutinability of red blood cells remains unchanged even in extreme old age.

The other antibodies mentioned, the agglutinins and lysins in human serum have been examined in like manner (Friedberger, et al., 1929) and yield curves quite similar to those of the isoagglutinins. Another example in this category is the report of Blake in which the titer of pneumococcus agglutinins (not type specific) decreased with age. This observation is reported in a review by Baumgartner (1933–34).[5]

In connection with the results reported, investigations on the development of antibodies, at various ages, upon active immunization should be mentioned. These studies concern principally the increase in antibody formation during the period of adolescence. Investigations pointing to a decrease in antibody formation in old age were reported by

TABLE 7

Averages of the 4 agglutinins in given age groups

(Thomsen and Kettel)

	Age group												
	½–1	1–2	2–5	5–10	10–20	20–30	30–40	40–50	50–60	60–70	70–80	80–90	90–100
O α	27	130	287	386	332	291	246	179	174	118	149	81	38
O β	17	69	124	162	139	105	76	53	46	37	42	28	38
A β	18	55	99	214	176	156	81	56	66	44	51	33	40
B α	31	142	295	350	269	224	234	245	127	124	131	116	35

Five additional cases of individuals 100 years of age

Type	Sex	Age	α	β
O	♀	100	32	1
O	♀	102	4	4
O	♀	101	8	8
O	♂	100	4	1
A	♀	102		32

Thomsen (1917) who observed lessened susceptibility in old guinea pigs in anaphylactic experiments. Besides, Baumgartner (1934) found evidence that older animals, after immunization, yielded, possibly antibodies of lower titer and less avidity than younger ones. The differences were too slight however to be significant and the animals were not old enough ("over two years old") to permit a decisive conclusion in respect to the problem under discussion.

In the light of the results mentioned with normal antibodies one

---

[5] In this report the literature of immune reactions according to age is very fully discussed.

might well expect the production of antibodies to be diminished in older immunized animals. Systematic investigations on this subject, however, have not been undertaken. Were there a positive result it would be natural to surmise, in the case of diminution of antibody formation in old age, that the fault lay in an insufficiency of the reticulo-endothelial system, for to this system is commonly attributed the chief rôle in the development of antibodies. It would be desirable, there-

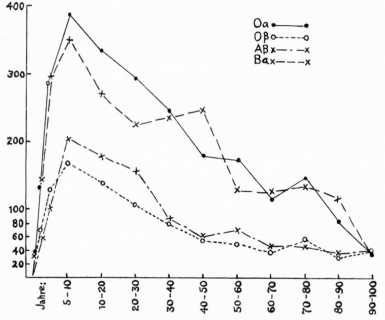

FIG. 16. Curves describing titer of agglutinines at different ages (Thomsen and Kettel).

fore, to institute investigations of the capability of this system in advanced age.

The claims of serological differences in human beings and in animals of different ages put forth by Picado (1929, 1930) would be very remarkable, if they should turn out to be correct. Rabbits were immunized (1) with the serum of children, and (2) with that of old individuals. The precipitins were then studied. The immune sera reacted more intensely on those sera with which the animals were immunized. Young rabbits immunized with sera of older ones were said to develop isoprecipitins which gave reactions with the serum of old but not of young animals. Friedberger and Gurwitz (1931) were unable, however, to repeat this experiment.[6]

Nattan-Larrier and Grimard-Richard (1932) and other authors believe that fully grown animals can be made sensitive to foetal serum. But even in the event that such an effect were observable, it would have a meaning for other questions than the problem of changes in blood in old age.

7. SUMMARY

Enough has been said to suggest that the organs of the circulation and their functions change with time. The question to which these remarks have attempted to answer is "Do they *age?*" Whether they do depends upon the view which is taken on the nature and the value of this kind of evidence. The position is taken that the evidence depends for its credibility on a combination of common sense and statistical inference, aided perhaps by the use of examples not particularly obvious. From this point of view, the belief that ageing takes place is founded on ground sufficiently firm. The evidence is varied and the account of it indicates the many directions in which it can be amplified. That amplification is desirable emerges from noticing how fragmentary the evidence actually is. Significant beginnings have been made, however, sufficient to justify the tentative position which has been adopted.

REFERENCES

ADDIS, T. 1922. Blood pressure and pulse rate levels. First paper: The levels under basal and daytime conditions. Arch. Int. Med., **29**, 539-553.

ALVAREZ, W. C. 1923. Blood pressure in 15,000 university freshmen. Arch. Int. Med., **32**, 17-30.

ANITSCHKOW, N. 1933. Experimental arteriosclerosis in animals. Arteriosclerosis, edited by E. V. Cowdry, New York, The Macmillan Co., 617 pp. (Chapter 10.)

BAKER, A. B. 1937. Structure of the small cerebral arteries and their changes with age. Am. J. Path., **13**, 453-462.

BAUMGARTNER, L. 1933-34. Relationship of age to immunological reactions. Yale J. Biol. & Med., **6**, 403-434.

———— 1934. Age and antibody production; qualitative changes in antisera associated with age. J. Immunology, **27**, 407-416.

---

[6] Picado contends that serum from older individuals coagulates at lower temperatures than that of older animals, the serum of very old individuals coagulating at 55-56°. He also states that the serum of children is less toxic for rabbits than that of older persons.

BENNINGHOF, A. 1930. Blutgefässe und Herz. Hdb. d. mikros. Anat. d. Mensch. **6,** 1–232. (Wilhelm v. Möllendorf. Springer, Berlin.)

BLANKENHORN, M. A., AND CAMPBELL, H. E. 1925. The effect of sleep on blood pressure. Am. J. Physiol., **74,** 115–120.

BORK, K. 1926. Über Kranzadersklerose. 1926. Virchow's Arch., **262,** 646–657.

BRAMWELL, C. 1937. (Lumleian Lecture) Arterial pulse in health and disease. I. The pulse. II. The pulse wave. Lancet, **2,** 239–247, 301–305, 366–371.

BRAMWELL, J. C., HILL, A. V., AND McSWINEY, B. A. 1923. The velocity of the pulse wave in man in relation to age as measured by the hot-wire sphymograph. Heart, **10,** 233–235.

BROOKS, H., AND CARROLL, J. H. 1912. A clinical study of the effects of sleep and rest on blood pressure. Arch. Int. Med., **10,** 97–102.

BURLAGE, S. R. 1922. Blood pressures and heart rates in girls during adolescence. A preliminary study of 1700 cases. Proc. Soc. Exp. Biol. and Med., **19,** 247–248.

BURWELL, C. S., AND ROBINSON, G. C. 1924. A method for the determination of the amount of oxygen and cargon dioxide in the mixed venous blood of man. J. Clin. Invest., **1,** 47–63.

CASTELLOTTI, FR. 1923 Contributo allo studio clinica della pression venosa. Mallattio del cuore e die Vas., **7,** 69, 277, 317.

COHN, A. E., AND STEELE, J. M. 1932. Studies on the effect of the output of blood from the heart. 1. The effect on the output of the dog's heart in heart-lung preparations. J. Clin. Invest., **11,** 871–895.

CRAWFORD, J. H. 1923. The influence of the vagus on the heart rate. J. Pharm. & Exper. Therap., **22,** 1–19.

EHRICH, W., AND COHN, A. E. 1931. Anatomical Ontogeny. A. Fowl. C. Rabbit. 1. A study of the nuclei of the heart. Am. J. Anat., **49,** 209–240.

EHRICH, W., DE LA CHAPELLE, C., AND COHN, A. E. 1931. Anatomical Ontogeny. B. Man. 1. A study of the coronary arteries. Am. J. Anat., **49,** 241–282.

ERNSTENE, A. CARLTON. 1938. The cardio-vascular complications of hyperthyroidism. Am. J. Med. Sci., **195,** 248–256.

EYSTER, J. A. E., AND MIDDLETON, W. S. 1924. Clinical studies on venous pressure. Arch. Int. Med., **34,** 228–242.

EYSTER, J. A. E. 1926. Venous pressure and its clinical applications. Physiol. Rev., **6,** 281–315.

FABER, H. K., AND JAMES, C. A. 1921. The range and distribution of blood pressure in normal children. Am. J. Dis. Child., **22,** 7–28.

FIELD, H., BOCK, A. V., GILDEA, E. F., AND LATHROP, F. L. 1924. The rate of the circulation of the blood in normal resting individuals. J. Clin. Invest., **1,** 65–85.

FRIBERGER, R. 1912. Über die Pulswellengeschwindigkeit bei Arterien mit fühlbarer Wandverdickung. Deutsch. Arch. f. klin. Med., **107,** 281–295.

FRIEDBERGER, E., BOCK, G., UND FÜRSTENHEIM, A. 1929. Zur Normalantikörperkurve des Menschen durch die verschiedenen Lebensalter und ihre Bedeatung für die Erklärung der Hautteste (Schick, Dick). Ztschr. f. Immunitätsforsch. u. exper. Therap., **64,** 294–319.

FRIEDBERGER, E., UND GURWITZ, I. 1931. Vergleichende Versuche über das antikörperbildende Vermögen von älteren und jüngeren Antigenen; nebst einem Anhang: "Ueber Alters-Isoantikörper." Ztschr. f. Immunitätsforsch. u. exper. Therap., **71**, 453–458.

GILBERT, N. C. 1923. The increase of certain vagal effects with increased age. Arch. Int. Med., **31**, 423–432.

GROLLMAN, A. 1932. The cardiac output of man in health and disease. Springfield, Ill.: Thomas. 325 pp.

GROSS, L. 1921. The blood supply of the heart. New York. Hoeber, 171 pp.

GROSS, L., AND SILVERMAN, G. 1937. The commissural lesion in rheumatic fever. Am. J. Path., **13**, 389–404.

HALLOCK, P. 1934. Arterial elasticity in man in relation to age as evaluated by the pulse wave velocity method. Arch. Int. Med., **54**, 770–798.

HENDERSON, Y., AND HAGGARD, H. W. 1927. The validity of the ethyl iodide method for measuring the circulation. Am. J. Physiol., **82**, 497–503.

HERRMANN, G. R., AND WILSON, F. N. 1921-22. Ventricular hypertrophy. A comparison of electrocardiographic and post-mortem observations. Heart, **9**, 91–147.

HOOKER, D. R. 1916. The influence of age upon the venous blood pressure in man. Am. J. Physiol., **40**, 43–48.

HUGHES, T. P., AND SAWYER, W. A. 1932. Significance of immunity tests in epidemiology as illustrated in yellow fever. J. A. M. A., **99**, 978–982.

JORES, L. 1903. Wesen und Entwicklung der Arteriosklerose. Wiesbaden; Bergmann. 172 pp.

KARSNER, H. T., SAPHIR, O., AND TODD, T. W. 1925. The state of the cardiac muscle in hypertrophy and atrophy. Am. J. Path., **1**, 351–371.

KROGH, A. 1929. The anatomy and physiology of capillaries. New Haven. Yale Univ. Press. 422 pp.

LEARY, T. 1934. Experimental atherosclerosis in the rabbit compared with human (coronary) atherosclerosis. Arch. Path., **17**, 453–492.

LEWIS, T. 1913-14. Observations upon ventricular hypertrophy, with especial reference to preponderance of one or other chamber. Heart, **5**, 367–402.

LEWIS, W. H., JR. 1938. Changes with age in the cardiac output in adult men. Am. J. Physiol., **121**, 517–527.

MACWILLIAM, J. A. 1925. Blood pressures in man under normal and pathological conditions. Physiol. Rev., **5**, 303–335.

MILLER, A. M., AND PERKINS, O. C. 1927. Elastic tissue of the heart in advancing age. Am. J. Anat., **39**, 205–217.

MOORE, R. A. 1931. The total number of glomeruli in the normal human kidney. Anat. Rec., **48**, 153–168.

MÜLLER, W. 1883. Die Massenverhältnisse des menschlichen Herzens. Hamburg & Leipzig. Voss. 220 pp.

NAGAYO, M. 1909. Zur normalen und pathologischen Histologie des Endocardium parietale. Beitr. z. path. Anat. u. allg. Path., **45**, 283–305.

NATTAN-LARRIER, L., AND GRIMARD-RICHARD, L. 1932. Action du sérum de foetus sur les animaux adultes de la même espéce. Compt. rend. Soc. de biol., **110**, 510–513.

PICADO, T. C. 1929. Propriétés antigeniques différentes des sérums d'animaux jeunes et des sérums d'animaux agés. Compt. rend. Soc. de biol., **102**, 631–633.

——— 1930. Effets des injections de sérum homologue sur la taille et la croissance des animaux. Ann. de l'Inst. Past., **44**, 584–603.

SAPPINGTON, S. W., AND COOK, H. S. 1936. Radial artery change in comparison with those of coronary and other arteries. Am. J. Med. Sci., **192**, 822–839.

SCHIFF, F., MENDLOVICZ, L. 1926. Quantitative researches on isoagglutinins with special reference to leukemia. Ztschr. f. Immunitatsforsch. u. exper. Therap., **48**, 1–22.

STEELE, J. M. 1937. Interpretation of arterial elasticity from measurements of pulse wave velocities. Amer. Heart Jour., **14**, 452–465.

STOCKARD, C. R. The interaction of the endocrine and the nervous system. 1. Mechanisms operating the body as a unit. (Joseph Collins Lecture, Dec. 2, 1937) (not yet published).

THAYER, W. S., AND FABYAN, M. 1907. Studies on arteriosclerosis, with special reference to the radial artery. Am. J. Med. Sci., **134**, 811–829.

THOMSEN, O. 1917. Studien über die Ananaphylaxie (Antianaphylaxie). Ztschr. f. Immunitätsforsch. u. exper. Therap., **26**, 213–257.

THOMSEN, O., UND KETTEL, K. 1929. Die Stärke der menschlichen Isoagglutinine und entsprechenden Blutkörperchenrezeptoren in verschiedenen Lebensaltern. Ztschr. f. Immunitätsforsh. u. exper. Therap., **63**, 67–93.

WARTHIN, A. S. 1924. The myocardial lesions of diphtheria. J. Infect. Dis., **35**, 32–66.

WEISS, S., AND FRAZIER, W. R. 1930. The density of the surface capillary bed of the forearm in health, in arterial hypertension, and in arteriosclerosis. Am. Heart J., **5**, 511–518.

WETZEL, N. C., AND ZOTTERMAN, Y. 1926. On difference in the vascular coloration of various regions of the normal human skin. Heart, **13**, 357–369.

WEZLER, K. 1935. Abhängigkeit der Arterienelastizität vom Alter und dem Zustand der Wandmuskulatur. Ztschr. f. Kreislaufforsch., **27**, 721–745.

WILENS, S. J. 1937. The post mortem elasticity of the adult human aorta. Its relation to age and to the distribution of internal atheromas. Am. J. Path., **13**, 811–834.

WINTERNITZ, M. C., THOMAS, R. M., AND LE COMPTE, P. M. 1938. The biology of arteriosclerosis. Springfield, Ill.: Thomas. 142 pp.

WOLKOFF, K. 1923. Über die histologische Struktur der Coronararterien des menschlichen Herzens. Virchow's Arch. f. Path., **241**, 42–58.

——— 1929. Über die Atherosclerose der Coronararterien des Herzens. Beitr. z. path. Anat. u. z. allg. Path., **82**, 555–596.

CHAPTER 8

LYMPHATIC TISSUE

EDWARD B. KRUMBHAAR

Philadelphia

The lymphatic system is one of the best examples of the generalization that various tissues of the human body do not age alike or at the same age periods, any more than they die at the same instant after death of the individual. Of its various components, it is well known, for instance, that thymic involution begins about the age of puberty and proceeds rapidly in adults to an advanced stage; tonsillar involution is marked in the 4th and 6th decades, though lymphatic elements persist throughout life; while lymph nodes and the spleen remain fairly rich in lymphatic tissue in adults with gradual atrophy in old age. Details of these morphologic changes must constitute the major part of this chapter, as unfortunately essential knowledge of the function of the lymphatic system lags far behind knowledge of its structure. That it is an important part of the defense mechanism of the body can be inferred from its morphological changes in many diseases. Just how it acts in these diseases and how its actions are modified at different ages, are important questions, which, as will be seen later, cannot yet be answered in any satisfactory way.

In the present chapter consideration of the lymphatic tissue will include those widespread tissue aggregations of lymphocytes found in liver, kidney, thyroid, skin, etc; the lymph follicles of the digestive and respiratory tracts, and the more complicated lymph nodes, tonsils, thymus and spleen. This of course necessitates brief treatment of those elements of the reticulo-endothelial system that are found in lymphatic tissue as well as of lymphocytes. Not only has this system become increasingly well established since the concept was first proposed by Aschoff in 1913; but also it is in the lymphatic tissue in general that the cells of this system are chiefly found. The lymphatic channels are not considered here, as their problems are more closely related to those of the blood vessels, which are treated in Chapter 7. As will be seen later, the scavenging function (ingestion of foreign particles), one of the chief functions ascribed to lymphatic tissue, is a characteristic of the reticulo-endothelial system, but not of lymphocytes. Here also

149

it is assumed, though by no means proven as yet, that the blood monocytes are functioning reticulum, or special endothelial, cells that have
wandered into the blood stream.

"Lymphatic tissue" is here regarded as a system widespread throughout the body, which in its most characteristic form is made up of more
or less encapsulated masses of lymphocytes alternating with a system
of pulp and sinuses. In the meshes of the pulp and to a lesser extent
in the sinuses are reticulum cells, while the sinuses are lined by special
endothelial cells. Aschoff's distinction between "lymphatic," in the
narrower sense, and "lymphoid," i.e., that the latter does not possess
the typical follicular, pulp and sinus structure, will occasionally be
used in this presentation, though in a wider sense "lymphatic" must
serve for the whole system as well. The term "lymphocytic tissue"
will be used to refer to that part of the lymphatic tissue that consists
predominantly of lymphocytes. The term "lympho-epithelial" is properly applied to some of the tissues discussed in this chapter—tonsils,
appendix, intestinal follicles, thymus. Omitting the significance of the
type of reticulum involved therein, an item that has provoked considerable discussion, it is here regarded merely as tissue in which lymphatic
and epithelial tissue are in close contact, with differences in function
from ordinary lymphatic tissue.

The lymphatic tissue taken as a unit—and excluding the frequently
included bone marrow—may be one of the largest "organs" in the body.
Insurmountable difficulties prevent presentation of any accurate figures
as to its weight; but B. K. Wiseman, who has spent much time attempting to estimate this point, believes (personal communication) that it
amounts to more tissue than is contained in the liver, for instance, the
largest single organ in the body.

1. DISTRIBUTION AND FUNCTION OF LYMPHATIC TISSUE

Before considering how the lymphatic tissue varies with increasing
age, a brief summary of its structure in various parts of the body must
be presented.

In the typical lymph node the afferent channels penetrate the capsule
into the marginal sinus and connect with a plexus of sinuses which are
gathered together into the efferent sinus, which leaves the node at the
hilus with the artery and vein. These sinuses are only partly lined
with endothelium; otherwise are unlined channels in the reticulum,
and often contain in their lumina a sparse reticulum whose cells show
the same ability to phagocyte and to become free wandering cells as

do those of other parts of the system. The sinuses normally contain lymph with a few lymphocytes and the variously named "monocytes." Between the sinuses is the reticular syncytium containing masses of lymphocytes, condensed especially in the outer zones into follicles. These are dense homogeneous masses (called secondary follicles by Stohr) of small and medium sized lymphocytes, with a thin skeleton of reticulum and sparse reticulum cells. They often contain pale centers, made up of large pleomorphic cells with vesicular nuclei to which various names and functions are still given. To Flemming (1885) sometimes both pale centers and dark outer zones were apparently "germ centers" (i.e., sites of new lymphocyte formation) or "secondary follicles," though at other times only the pale centers were regarded as germ centers. More recently the pale centers have been called "reaction centers" (Hellman, 1919a) or "defence foci" (Wetzel, 1928) in recognition of their reticulum cell component and marked ability to phagocyte débris.[1] This point of view, in which formation of new lymphocytes goes on throughout the lymphocyte mass, is supported by the appearance of younger as well as older lymphocytes in the outer zone of the follicle, occasional mitoses in these regions and also by the absence of pale centers in fetal life and in leukemia when lymphocyto-poiesis is very active and by their prominence when reactive or degenerative phenomena would be expected. The great difficulty in distinguishing lymphoblasts from monoblasts in "pale centers" will be readily conceded by most students of the subject, and it may well be that "pale centers" are sometimes due to young lymphocytes as well as to young reticulo-endothelial cells.

The *hemolymph nodes*—rare in humans—are like other lymph nodes except that their sinuses are normally filled with blood.

The *spleen* is in some respects like a large hemolymph node. Its chief lymphocytic content is in the Malpighian follicles, collections of lymphocytes about an eccentric "central" artery, which also have "pale centers," that react as do those of lymph nodes. Lymphocytes

[1] Sometimes darker staining, i.e., more concentrated, "solid centers," are found, which are undoubtedly lymphocytic and may well represent increased lymphopoietic activity. Recent suggestions are to regard solid follicles as primary; those with pale centers (whether lymphocytopoietic, reactional or transitional) as secondary; and those budding from secondary follicles as "pseudo secondary" or tertiary. The terminology of "primary" and "secondary" nodule has remained in such confusion since Flemming's ambiguous statements, confused by varying usage of later investigators, that such noncommittal terms as "pale" and "solid" centers have their advantages.

occur to a lesser extent in the periarterial lymphatic sheath as it emerges from the trabeculi and in moderate numbers throughout the red pulp; cells of the reticulo-endothelial system are found lining the sinuses, in the meshes of the red pulp, in the pale centers of the follicles, and to a less extent in their outer zones.   In 10 healthy men whose blood lymphocytes averaged 36 per cent and monocytes 6.7 per cent, Schilling (1928) found, in differential counts of the spleen pulp, averages of 3.4 per cent young lymphocytes; 85.3 per cent adult lymphocytes and 1.8 per cent monocytes.

Noduli lymphatici is a term here used to designate simple lymph tissue, such as Ranvier's "tâches laiteuses" of the omentum.   As shown by Marchand, in their early stages, these tâches are encapsulated collections of the phagocytic monocytes already mentioned.   It is only later that in the periphery of these cell groups of lymphocytes appear, producing a picture roughly analogous to the lymph follicle with its pale staining, large celled center.   These structures are very labile, tending to succumb to fat cell infiltration, but reverting to the original structure on demand.   While usually assembled near omental blood vessles, they may occur quite independently of them.

Even simpler units are those small collections of lymphocytes found in many parts of the body; e.g., subpleural, pericardial, peritoneal, peribronchial, perivascular, etc.   These also can come and go with considerable freedom.   They do not appear to be organized, but are merely more or less unorganized collections of cells.   Of similar nature are the submucosal collections in the genito-urinary and especially in the gastro-intestinal tract.

More permanent and more organized are the nodules of the intestinal tract, whether occurring as solitary follicles in the small and large intestine, or as the aggregations known as Peyer's patches in the small intestine, or the more or less confluent nodules of the vermiform appendix.   Such nodules may occur anywheres from a position buried beneath the mucosa to projecting above it into the lumen.   They all may contain pale centers, about which the same uncertainty maintains as in other regions.

Lymphocyte and monocyte.   The adult lymphocyte is the familiar, small (about 7μ), round cell, composed of a round, dense, deeply staining nucleus and a very small amount of almost transparent, slightly basophilic cytoplasm.   One or two nucleoli are demonstrable with supravital stains and frequently a few cytoplasmic azurophile granules with Romanowsky stains.   The lymphocyte is motile, progressing not much more slowly than a granulocyte and in a different manner. It has never been seen to phagocytize. Bunting (1921) estimated that some three billion lymphocytes enter the blood stream from lymphocytopoietic centers daily. Many escape through the blood capillaries into the tissues but may reënter the circulation by way of the lymphatics (Drinker and Field, 1933). Their ultimate fate is obscure. Presumably those in the circulation die and are disposed of as are other blood cells, but undoubtedly many leave the body by way of the alimentary tract. The number of lymphocytes in the peripheral blood may be more or less increased physiologically (as by an infant's crying spell) and in many disease conditions with or without corresponding increase in the lymphatic tissues (mumps, whooping cough, syphilis, tuberculosis, thyrotoxicosis, etc.). They are enormously increased in typical lymphatic leukemia, which is generally regarded as a neoplasm of the lymphocyte.

The *monocyte*, the other important cell of lymphoid tissue, has borne many names in the 50 years of its history. Macrophage, clasmatocyte, adventitial cells, resting wandering cells, histiocytes, reticulum and endothelial cells of Aschoff's system, the "large mononuclear and transitional cells" of the blood, all are now more or less generally accepted as indicating cells that lie in the reticulum or line the sinuses of lymphoid tissue as well as in connective tissue, serous membranes and certain special capillaries. They will be referred to in this chapter as monocytes. They constitute in the blood stream normally about 4 to 8 per cent of the total leukocytes, and are increased in late stages of a number of infections. In the tissues they vary greatly in appearance, from flat, inconspicuous cells to large, rounded or stellate structures, perhaps filled with phagocytized material (depending on their location and their functional, resting or active, state). In lymphatic tissue they occur in many abnormal conditions in large numbers greatly outnumbering the lymphocytic elements. This fact greatly complicates evaluation of normal ageing of lymphatic structures as seen post mortem. Actively ameboid, these cells are assumed to enter the blood stream with ease. Here they appear as large, spherical cells, 12 to 20μ in size. Their cytoplasm is more granular than that of the lymphocyte and the oval or slightly indented nucleus has a more finely woven reticulum. With vital stains such as neutral red and Janus green, they show red staining rosettes near the nucleus or vacuoles indicating phagocytosis and green staining mitochondria.

Very little indeed is definitely known about the function of the obviously important lymphocyte. Though lymphocytes are found constantly in characteristic positions in such common, important lesions as the tubercle and the gumma, their rôle there is unknown and has been even blithely dismissed as a mechanical walling off. Their increase in the blood stream in many diseases is vaguely connected with resistance to infection, while to the considerable lymphatic tissue through the body is ascribed the function of producing lymphocytes. To be sure, other possible functions have been investigated. Bergel (1919–1926) claimed to have found lymphocytes rich in lipase which became useful when the cells were attracted to bacteria with fatty envelopes or in connection with fat metabolism. This suggests a convenient use for the follicles in the intestinal tract, as do Settle's (1920) and Lefholz's (1923) report of the increase of lymphatic tissue in the body following a high caloric diet, especially if rich in fats. The fat found in mesenteric lymph nodes after a fat diet is conspicuously in the sinuses, either free or contained in monocytes. Fukuchi, also, found in the centrifugate of lymph serum considerable lipase that presumably comes from lymphocytes. He also (p. 171) found catalase in lymphocytes, though in smaller amounts than in the plasma. The number of lymphocytes in the blood stream and about lesions has been correlated with immunity to transplantable tumors and tuberculous infection by Murphy and his colleagues (1919); but unfortunately many of the studies in these fields have either been refuted or not sufficiently confirmed, or the results attributed to other cell units. Lymphocytes apparently also increase in number both in the blood stream and in the tissues on diets rich in fat or carbohydrate and are said to contain a carbohydrase.

Monocytes, with their outstanding power of ingestion and digestion of foreign material, may be inferred to possess proteases, are known to contain oxydases and very probably furnish the lipase that Bergel attributed to lymphocytes.

Some connection between lymphatic tissue and immunity is on a somewhat firmer basis. Toxins have long been known to be diminished by passage through lymph nodes, and thoracic duct lymph or lymph node extracts have been found potent in inhibiting bacteria growth and function (chemical filter). Also recently McMaster (1935) has definitely shown that after intracutaneous injection of bacterial antigen, specific agglutinins are formed within the lymph nodes. It has been more or less assumed that the protective substances come from the reticulo-endothelial elements (monocytes), because of their abundance in these tissues and their well known phagocytic function; but recent evidence points more toward the lymphocyte as the source. Ehrich (1934), for instance, found that while large doses of antigen produce many histiocytes and but little free antibody, smaller doses give more antibodies with but few histiocytes and many cells regarded as lymphocytes. Rich also (1936) has demonstrated with vital and motion picture studies of tissue cultures from the large cells that accumulate in spleen and lymph nodes in acute infections that these cells definitely belong to the lymphocytic and not the reticulo-endothelial series. As the same reaction occurs with non-bacterial foreign protein, it is suggested that the lymphocyte may be concerned with the handling of foreign protein in the tissues. In many inflammations, the monocytes and lymphocytes can roughly be regarded as second and third lines of cellular defense, of which the granulocytes are the first. The sinuses of lymphatic tissue, also, appear to act as filters mechanically, both to bacteria and to other foreign bodies (Drinker, et al, 1933).

It is obvious from even the above short explanation that little can yet be said about changes in the functioning of lymphatic tissue associated with the ageing process, except as inferred from the structural changes to be described. There is ground for hope, however, that more precise knowledge of function may ere long permit some evaluation of the effect of ageing on function.

2. AGEING OF LYMPHOCYTE AND MONOCYTE

The young lymphocyte, the lymphoblast, is a larger cell than the adult with more cytoplasm that is more basophilic. The ovoid nucleus is vesicular, with granular chromatin which in fixed preparations form a loose network. In Romanowsky stains of cells in the blood stream the nucleus is paler staining; the nucleoli more prominent than in the adult cell. The life duration of the lymphocyte is not established. In the tissues, there seems to be no good way of estimating its length of life, though it can multiply there with great rapidity; it apparently does not multiply in the circulation. Once in the circulation, according to Bunting's (1921) experiments, it probably lasts little more than 24 hours, migrating into the mucous membranes and into the lumen, especially of the gastro-intestinal tract. We do not know, however, how many are destroyed in the spleen and lymph nodes, nor do changes in form of the adult cell betray individual senescence or approaching death while the cells are circulating.

At birth, the lymphocytes constitute about 20 to 30 per cent of the total of 12,000 to 20,000 leucocytes in the peripheral blood. However, they quickly increase both relatively and absolutely, so that in the first few weeks they amount to from 50 to 75 per cent (marked variations with different observers), or 7,000 to 9,000 per cubic millimeter (Thursfield, 1929). Thereafter, they gradually decrease in number till they reach the adult normal level of 16 to 2400 per cubic millimeter, or from 21 to 35 per cent (Schilling). The lymphocytes in the blood become about equal to the granulocytic series in number at about the age of 4 or 5 years. Osgood (1935) gives distinctly higher normal percentages for young adults (15 to 19 years, mean of 41.9 per cent; 26–30 years, 37.8 per cent). They do not show any such increase in the blood in later adult life, as has been found in the case of some of the lymphatic tissues.

The monocyte in its youngest stage is practically indistinguishable from young lymphoblasts and myeloblasts. It gradually assumes a more granular, less basophilic cytoplasm, and the nucleus has more finely divided chromatin, less prominent nuclei, finally become deeply indented. Little may be said of the normal duration of life of this cell also. It is thought to be able to slip in and out of the blood stream with ease and to exist, perhaps for relatively long periods, in the tissues in a resting stage. Once called into strenuous phagocytic activity its existence may be quickly terminated.

The monocyte percentage in the peripheral blood is not known to vary regularly at different ages. Constituting normally about 4 to 8 per cent of the leucocytes in the adult, it has been reported by different authors in early life at various normal levels, varying from 0.16 to 12 per cent. In older life, Dobrovici (1904) found an average of 20 per cent lymphocytes and 5.4 monocytes in 11 persons from 67 to 81; Étienne and Perrin, (1909) 24.8 and 5.7 per cent respectively in 27 persons over 80. The ability of both lymphocyte and monocyte to appear in increased numbers in the blood stream under appropriate stimuli seems to persist throughout life with little if any impairment.

3. AGEING OF LYMPH NODES AND NODULES

Lymphatic tissue, being very sensitive to environmental influences, waxes and wanes throughout life on slight provocation. This and its widespread distribution in countless small units render it practically impossible to make any quantitative estimation of the effects of normal ageing on the tissue as a whole. Not only does existing tissue easily become hyperplastic, but it is even probable that new lymphatic structures may be formed. The large numbers of lymph nodes that are found in a given area in certain diseases strongly suggest this. Counts of the number of lymph nodes in the human body, therefore, become of little value. Sappey's (1874) figures of 600 to 700 for the whole body are unquestionably too few; Hellman (1921), for instance, in mesenteries made transparent found from 200 to 500 nodes, and the total number in the adult body is probably well in the thousands. Lymph nodes are said to occur in the fetus first in a primary group of axillary, inguinal, cervical and retroperitoneal chains; and in a later secondary group that includes epitrochlear, popliteal, intramesenteric and para-aortic.

Study of lymph nodes at different age periods leaves still unanswered the question as to when they attain maximum size. From Bichat to Bartels some have maintained that their greatest size is reached during childhood; for others this applies only to the maximum relative size (Sukiennikow, 1903); while Gundobin (1906) maintains that this is reached during infancy, and still others believe that their growth and involution parallel that of the body as a whole (Grossmann, 1896). The general view, however, is that maximum size is reached about the time of puberty and that regression begins shortly after. This view is undoubtedly influenced by analogy with lymphoid tissue elsewhere in the body and with the hypothesis that it is concerned with defensive mechanisms during adolescence and that it regresses when the body has acquired a resistance to noxa of various kinds. Needless to say this is pure hypothesis and not in accord with many clinical facts. An important point to be emphasized, at any rate, is that *the normal lymph node undoubtedly retains throughout life a marked ability to proliferate lymphocytes and reticulo-endothelial cells in response to infection.*

In other mammals, also, the lymph nodes are accepted as larger in younger than in older life (Ellenberger and Baum, 1915). In Hellman's (1914) excellent study of 100 rabbits in 12 different age groups, selected with the best possible attention toward permitting valid comparisons, it appeared that the mass of lymph nodes increased up to the age of 5 months (i.e., time of puberty) then grew smaller. Cervical and popliteal nodes, however, had a second growth period, with final regression only after 12 months. In old rabbits (averaging $3\frac{1}{2}$ years) the lymph nodes were reduced to about one-half their maximum size. In other words, in material where normality was beyond question, and far above that attainable in human material, *the lymph nodes grew quicker, reached their maximum sooner and began to regress earlier than did the rest of the body tissues.*

Histologic Appearance at Different Ages. At birth, the characteristic

structure of the lymph node is already present; only the secondary
nodules are lacking, to appear about the third month after birth—
between the second to sixth, according to different authorities.   I have
found one solid center (fig. 17A) in a lymph node of an infant of 41 hours;
while Ehrich (1929b) has observed a secondary nodule (pale centre)
in a stillborn whose mother had pneumonia (fig. 17B).   The lymphocytic

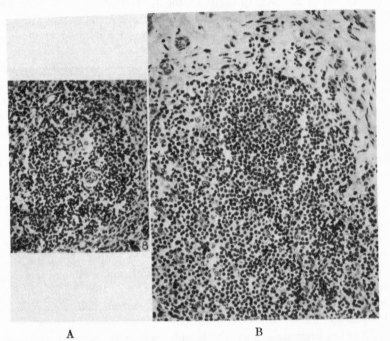

A   B

Fig. 17. A. Beginning reticular increase (*a*) in center of follicle, from a spleen
of a 34 cm. fetus from a mother suffering from pneumonia (Ehrich, 1929d).
   B. A "solid center" from a lymph node of a 74-hour-old infant dying of a
birth injury (U. of Pa., 1931–925) (× 260).

mass in the average is greatest in youth, though individual nodes in
older life may show an unexplained mass greater than this average.
   The generally accepted picture is that the parenchyma gradually
atrophies with age, to be replaced partly by connective tissue and
partly by fat, which starts at the hilus and progresses inward.   This
may become so extreme that the node consists almost entirely of fat.
The cortex is earliest affected by the atrophy: the lymphocytes diminish
in number, the cortex narrows, pale centers are rare.   The medullary
cords then elongate and become narrow; the network of the reticulum

becomes more compact with fewer reticulum cells both in and outside of the sinuses, and more and more space is occupied by delicate fibrous tissue. The coarser fibrous tissue of trabeculae and about blood vessels also contributes to the fibrosis. However, it is generally recognized that the lymph node can react to inflammation or enlarge in leukemia at any age. Marked sclerosis of a node, with hyalinization, calcification or even bone formation may be always ascribed to some pathologic process such as tuberculosis, and may be found at any age.

Different groups of lymph nodes are said to age differently: thus fatty infiltration is said to occur especially early and prominently in the axillary and inguinal nodes (Rössle, 1923), while the mesenteric

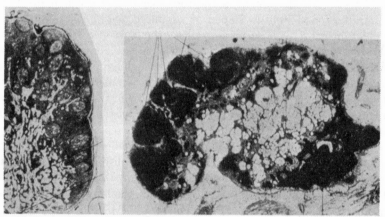

FIG. 18. A. Part of cross section of a fully developed human lymph node (from Hellman, 1930).
B. Senile human lymph node showing fatty infiltration (from Hellman, 1930).

nodes remain relatively unchanged (Zacharow, 1891). Though my own observations are handicapped by their basis on material mostly drawn from pathologic sources, I have the impression that the earlier involutionary changes due to age have been overemphasized, that most nodes go on at least to 60 years with but little atrophy, and that both lymphocytic and reticulo-endothelial elements can become hyperplastic on demand at any age, unless too badly damaged previously by some pathologic process. Lymphatic leukemia, probably a kind of neoplasm of the lymphocyte, may occur at any age; in fact in Curschmann's (1935) recent series twice as many cases started after the age of 50 than before. Lymphatic tissue disappears rapidly during starvation or wasting illnesses, and as this is always more or less a factor to be reckoned with in autopsy material, normal human lymph nodes are especially hard to acquire. Material removed for surgical biopsy is of course seldom normal.

Especially do these limitations apply to the pale centers (secondary nodules), which may often represent reaction to noxa. In normal animal material, however, as in the more questionable human material, they appear to be most numerous, largest and most prominent in younger life, though constantly absent at birth. Hille (1908) found them at a maximum in cattle and dogs at the end of one year; in horses at 2 years, but in swine well developed even in the aged. In the follicles of the rabbit tonsil, Hellman found that while they were best developed at 10 months, as in the corresponding age of humans, they were often found well developed at advanced ages. Positive findings in older life cause little surprise to those who look upon the pale centers mainly as reaction centers; though the larger amounts in younger animals might be taken as an indication of a high lymphoblastic content. A very approximate gauge of the changes in lymphatic tissue function at various age periods has been attempted on the basis of clinical findings. Thus it is widely accepted that resistance to tuberculous infection is but slight in the first year of life, increases toward puberty, reaching a maximum about that period, with an increased susceptibility to tuberculosis, typhoid, small pox, Hodgkin's disease and so on from puberty to the age of 30. This is inversely proportional to the amount of lymphoid tissue found at these ages, while the later decrease in susceptibility has a suggestive correlation with the increase in lymphatic tissue in late adult life referred to in several places in this chapter. W. S. Miller (1924–1925), however, does not find that lymphatic tissue in the lung decreases with age in the generally accepted way.

The *lymphoid nodules* of the mucosa of the gastro-intestinal tract by and large follow a similar course to that of the lymph nodes in general. They are largest and most numerous in younger life, when their "germinal centers" are most prominent. West (1924), who followed the histologic changes in cecal lymph nodules of 18 rats and 6 cats (4 and 2 of which, respectively, were known to be of great age), found that this tissue normally regresses with age almost to the point of complete obliteration. He found the regression to be correlated with the physiological rather than the chronological age of the individual and that it could be overcome by irritating factors. Thus in presence of intestinal parasites, the cecum might maintain abundant lymphoid tissue to advanced age. The regressive process appears to be initiated by decreased formation of lymphocytes, so that the nodules shrink, the pale centers are inconspicuous or absent, eventually many disappear and are replaced by connective tissue.

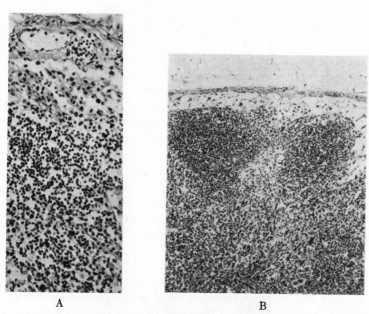

A   B

FIG. 19. A. Human mesenteric lymph node (white male, 73 years) showing sparsity of lymphocytes in the follicles and increase of reticulum. Death from peritonitis (U. of Pa., 1930-712) (× 140).

B. Human retroperitoneal lymph node (white male, 76 years), showing some fibrosis, but also persistence of cortical follicles. Death from acute cystitis (U. of Pa., 1931-910) (× 72).

4. AGEING OF APPENDIX, TONSILS AND WALDEYER'S RING

Lymphoid tissue appears in the human appendix early in fetal life, first near the cecum and last near the tip. The secondary nodules appear, as elsewhere, about the fourth month, and the lymphoid tissue continues to an early maximum. According to some (see Muthmann, 1913), regression starts in childhood, according to others (Berry and Lack, 1906; Corner, E., 1913) later in life—a difference of opinion that is very probably due to the use of diseased as well as normal material. According to the latest study (Bernardo-Comel, 1937), the maximum amount of lymphoid tissue is attained from 13 to 17 years and maintained to the 20th year. In the ensuing slow and steady regression, the pale centers diminish in size (question of less frequent stimulus to

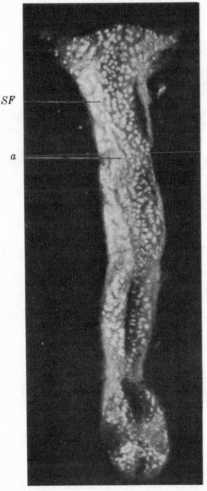

FIG. 20. Opened appendix from a young boy; cleared in acetic acid to show lymph nodules. *SF* = solitary follicle. At "*a*" a row of follicles occurs (from Hellman, 1930).

reaction ?) and the amount of lymphoid tissue decreases, beginning at the tip. In the 7th decade—the last examined—the lymphoid tissue was much reduced, consisting of isolated elements, with very few pale centers, near the proximal end. C. Stefanelli (1936) found normally no lymphoid follicles after the age of 75 or even earlier as a rule, though in cases of "subinvolution," he states that the appendix can be rich in lymphoid tissue at any age.

In 1884 the celebrated German anatomist, Waldeyer, described the ring of lymphatic tissue about the pharynx which has since gone by the name of Waldeyer's Ring. It is composed not only of the palatine (faucial), pharyngeal (so-called "adenoids"), tubal (about Eustachian tubes) and lingual tonsils, but also of an unusually rich distribution of lymphocytic tissue through the mucosa of the region. The importance of these structures, at a site where they are exposed to a maximum insult from external influences, though their mode of action and significance to the organism is still far from clear, is indicated by the fact that their homologues are found in practically all mammals, and many lower forms (they are especially prominent in birds). The practical importance of enlarged tonsils and adenoids in younger life is only too well known to parents and nose and throat specialists, even though the "tonsil problem" is still far from solved. Their form and function must be considered in some detail as a necessary prelude to the changes of ageing.

These structures are to be regarded as modified lymph nodes, similar to accumulations found elsewhere in the gastro-intestinal tract. The modifications consist in the lack of afferent lymphatic vessels (i.e., they are not ordinary lymphoid stations in a lymphatic chain) and of peripheral sinuses and in their close application to epithelial lined crypts. Out-wandered lymphocytes can always be found in the epithelial layers or in the crypts (salivary corpuscles), and these together with polymorphonuclears and plasma cells are greatly increased during inflammation. The out-wandered lymphocytes are most numerous at the age of puberty, after which they gradually diminish in number, only a few being found in aged persons (Wessel, 1933).

In the palatine tonsils, the tubular or branched crypts (10-20) are especially well developed. Beneath their several layers of stratified epithelium in the tunica propria and its extensions is the lymphoid tissue, containing indefinite masses of lymphocytic tissue, interspersed with numerous secondary nodules that behave in general like secondary nodules elsewhere. The rather distinct capsule (submucous layer) is pierced by an efferent vessel, carrying lymph to the jugular chain of lymphatics.

The pharyngeal tonsil ("adenoids") is a similar, though smaller, structure on the median dorsal wall of the pharynx. When enlarged in disease, it may obstruct the posterior nares, just as the tubal tonsils may obstruct the Eustachian tubes. The lingual tonsil is a collection of follicles on the back of the tongue, each consisting of an epithelial lined pit (through which lymphocytes wander to become salivary corpuscles) and lymphoid tissue, often containing several secondary nodules.

The function of the various tonsils, in spite of the vast amount of study given to the subject is still far from clear. Sciclunoff (1933) in a recent Sammelreferat considers 8 possible theories, only to reject most, such as the ancient theory of lubrication. A possible internal secretion he regards as debatable but definitely unproven, the evidence pro and con such items as growth stimulation being more than usually contradictory. Special functions such as producing reducing agents or effects on carbohydrate or lipoid metabolism may also safely be disregarded till more convincing evidence becomes available. The relation of the ring to immunity, or its existence as a series of protective organs, would best be regarded as part of the general function of lymphoid tissue in an unusually strategic position.

As a working hypothesis, only partially supported by evidence, let us assume that the chief function of Waldeyer's ring is to protect the body and especially the respiratory and digestive tracts from external noxa. Small numbers of bacteria, then, would be satisfactorily handled by the normal tonsil in the crypts or even when penetrating or carried into epithelium or lymphoid tissue. Larger numbers, on the other hand, might not be overcome, short of marked tissue reactions and fever or even suppuration or systemic infection. Such attacks inevitably would leave structural scars in the tonsils, which with accompanying lymphoid hyperplasia, might both permanently increase their size and decrease their efficiency. Frequent repetitions of the process or a state of chronic infection and reaction would produce obviously distorted organs that are more harmful than useful to the owner. Removal of such tonsils is obviously indicated, though it is not necessarily an unmixed blessing. An increase in the number of postoperative throat infections, however, often shows that the damaged organs were still exerting some protective action. Size alone is no indication of harmfulness, as the amount of lymphoid tissue is notoriously variable throughout the human body; and we have the disturbing factors both of individually variable normal size and of size changes due to ubiquitous minor disease changes to complicate any consideration of structural changes in these tissues due to age. Minor but frequent insults are so common here under modern conditions of life that it is impossible to say what constitutes undamaged material in the human. Grave (1934), for instance, found more or less wide signs of irritation in apparently normal tissue. Yet it is only recently that bacteria have been definitely demonstrated in the crypts of supposedly normal tonsils.

The concept of the "normal" palatine tonsil is made still more difficult by Eigler's (1935) observation that the structure of the tonsils can be not a little influenced by the type of feeding, considerable depletion of lymphocytes being obtainable on certain diets. Relying, however, on the definition of "normal" given by the Editor to be used in this book, some definite results of the changes that accompany ageing may be presented. First, the statement sometimes heard that normal palatine tonsils should disappear in the 3rd decade is definitely incorrect. Careful studies from autopsied cases dying from varied causes (less open to fallacious deductions due to the presence of disease than is operative material) show that the tonsils remain throughout life and some think remain at their fullest development until well after puberty (Kniaschetsky, 1899; Kayser, 1899; Hodenpyl, 1891; Mathies, 1935; Hieronymus, 1933, *literature*). Another group (Hett, 1913; Hett and Butterfield, 1909–1910; Dietrich, 1926; Hellman, 1927; Schönberger, 1928, etc.) believes that the tonsils are largest in children and that the involution of age sets in shortly after—from about 12 to 16 years. Hett and Butterfield found that atrophy of the deeper parts began as early as the fith year.

Kniatchetsky (1899) states that the tonsils of a yearling are $3\frac{1}{2}$ times as large as at birth; at 5 years, $3\frac{1}{2}$ times as large as at 1; and at 20 years, $3\frac{1}{2}$ times as large as at 5 (i.e., a greater development than that of the body as a whole). Mathies finds a strong development long past puberty and marked involution only in old age.

In Hieronimus' (1933) careful study of tonsils from 100 cases autopsied in miscellaneous diseases, the size of the palatine tonsils at different ages was found to be as in the accompanying chart. After a rapid rise to an average maximum size about the 12th year (maximum area of cross section 2.7 sq. cm.), the plateau is maintained until the first regression to about 1.8 sq. cm. between 35 and 40 years, and a second decline beginning at 70. Up to 2 years of age, all the tonsils measured less than 1 sq. cm. From then on they varied up to the 7th decade between 1 and 3 sq. cm., and after 60 years, from 0.4 to 2.7. Of the three cases with an area of over 4 sq. cm., one was 7 years old, one 13 years and one 36 years.

Histologically, the loss of tonsillar size is accompanied by an increase of the fibrous connective tissue and a greater tendency to fibrosis and hyalinosis of the arterioles with decrease in the calibre of the arteriole lumen.   The behavior of the secondary nodules in tonsillar tissue has been extensively studied, but mostly in respect to their general lymphoid significance (see earlier).   They usually make their appearance, as else-where, a few months after birth (Pol, 1923, 3rd to 12th month; Barnes, 1923, by the 6th month; Kniaschetsky, 1899, 6th month) and reach their highest development about the age of puberty.   As one who be-

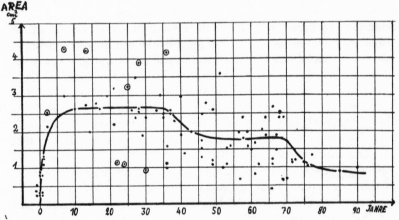

Fig. 21. Size of palatine tonsils at different ages (area of maximum cross section) (from Hieronimus, 1933).

lieves in the importance of their protective function would expect, however, their first appearance is by no means constant, and varies greatly, depending on the need for reaction by the tissues of the given individual.   In the involution periods, the secondary nodules show fewer lymphocytes, with an increase of reticulo-endothelial cells, hyaline and other kinds of amorphous pink-staining material.

The pharyngeal tonsils have not been as extensively studied quantitatively in man as have the palatine.   It is generally accepted, however, that they are largest in children, according to Kayser (1899) between 5 and 11, to Symington (1910) between 6 and 7 years.   Todd (1936) has shown that growth of the pharyngeal tonsils can be objectively and accurately measured with standardized roentgenograms.   He finds that they develop at about 12 months, increase in size to 3 years, usually to remain stationary till adolescence, after which they gradually regress. Most authors place the beginning of involution about the age of puberty (Kilian, 1898, in the second decade), with occasional cases

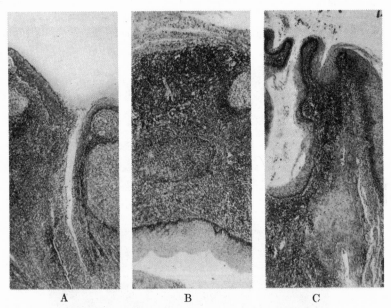

A B C

FIG. 22. A. Part of human palatine tonsil (male, 31 years), showing nodules with pale centers beneath the squamous epithelium which lines the crypt. Note the out-wandered lymphocytes at the mouth of the crypt (U. of Pa. Histol. Class Set No. 78) (× 37).

B. Part of a human palatine tonsil (female, 78 years), which though small has retained considerable lymphoid tissue, with follicles and pale centers. At the bottom is a cleft lined on both sides with normal squamous epithelium. Death from chronic valvular disease and congestive heart failure (P. G. H. 35,047) (× 37).

C. Part of a small involuted remnant of human palatine tonsil (female, 74 years), showing a cleft lined with a thin layer of epithelium and sparse lymphoid tissue beneath. To the right, is buccal mucosa with dense fibrous tissue between it and the tonsillar cleft. Death from cardio renal disease. One cannot, of course, eliminate the possibility in such cases that the changes may be the result of previous disease (P. G. H. 35,061) (× 37).

of involution beginning in the 3rd and 4th decade. They suffer a more marked involution (loss of lymphocytes) than the palatine tonsils. In older life the region may appear as sparse lymphoid aggregations scattered over the mucous membrane (Megevand, 1887) or perhaps with persistence of a median cleft.

The lingual tonsil is said to develop relatively late. Its structure is first clearly demonstrable about the age of puberty, according to Swain (1886) and Kayser (1899); while Wilson (1906) states that it has reached full development at the age of 12. In the same way, the involutionary changes of age are said to be delayed longer than in the other tonsillar tissues.

In general, then, Waldeyer's ring may be said to reach its highest

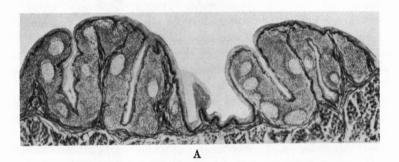

A

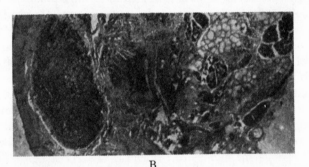

B

FIG. 23. A. The human lingual tonsil, showing slightly over-developed nodules (12 years) (from Barnes, 1923).
B. Involuted adult human lingual tonsil, showing loss of crypts and pale centres, and decrease of lymphatic tissue (from Cambrelin, 1937).

development about the age of puberty, to regress slowly thereafter, with more abrupt falls in the palatine tonsils in the 4th and 6th decades. Schönberger found peaks in the development of Waldeyer's ring at the 4th and 10th years.

It will be seen from the above that the significance of the changing structure of the tonsils at different ages is still obscure. If we subscribe to the views that they are essentially lymphoid in nature and therefore chiefly concerned with resistance to disease, then, without invoking pure teleology, we may infer that the need for such resisting tissue is greatest at puberty and young adult life. The efficient response of the tonsils to infection at any age and the fewer local infections in older life would indicate that the two involutionary periods in the 4th and 7th decades represent lessened need more than an obligatory atrophy of old age. Though the frequency of infected tonsils in the young does not preclude such cases from consideration here, one must recognize that ideal freedom from tonsillar infection would most probably produce a different life morphology for these elusive structures. Until adequate studies can be made, however, on populations conspicuously free from tonsillar infections of all grades—a condition that is not known to exist in civilized countries—we must content ourselves with the kind of evidence given above.

5. AGEING OF SPLEEN

In any attempt to follow behavior of lymphatic tissue at different ages, one would naturally turn to the spleen as the place where a considerable amount of such tissue occurs (in the Malpighian follicles) in a form utilizable for study.

It is pertinent to recall here a few details of spleen structure. It is made up chiefly of sinuses and red pulp—that contain a large depot of the important cells of the reticulo-endothelial system and a variety of other cells, including lymphocytes—and the white pulp, or Malpighian follicles that correspond to the follicles of the lymph nodes. The spleen is subject to great variations of size from contraction of the muscle fibers in capsule and trabeculae (reservoir function) as well as from depletion or congestion of the pulp in other ways. The branches of the splenic artery in the trabeculae send out branches into the pulp when a lumen of 0.2 mm. is reached. Beside the usual coats, these arteries have many lymphocytes in their outer walls (Weidenreich's *Lymphscheiden* or lymphatic sheaths); in fact, the cylindrical Malpighian follicles may be regarded in a way as a further development of this arrangement. Both sheaths and follicles are subject to rapid changes in volume under various circumstances, such as inflammatory stimuli on the one hand, or cachectic or still other depleting states on the other hand. It is obvious that it is impossible to take lymph-sheaths and the lymphocytes scattered diffusely through the pulp into account in any quantitative estimate of splenic lymphoid tissue. The Malpighian follicle, as is well known, contains an eccentric "central artery," surrounded by lymphocytes in such condensation that the follicle is easily recognized grossly and microscopically. However, in many cases—just as in lymph nodes and solitary follicles—the spleen follicle contains a round or oval pale area in the center (secondary nodule). Unfortunately also the margin of the Malpighian follicle is by no means sharp. Often an outer or "Randzone" of less concentrated lymphocytes merges almost imperceptibly into the surrounding pulp, thus further complicating attempts to measure lymphocytic areas of Malpighian follicles.

There have been many studies bearing on the amount of lymphocytic tissue in the spleen ever since Kölliker (1847) established the fact that the Malpighian follicles were composed of lymphatic tissue. Among early figures given by Hellman (1926) are Hessling's (1842) that the lymphatic tissue occupied about one-fifth to one-sixth the total volume of the spleen; Gray's (1854) of from one-sixth to one-eighth to one-fourth to one-fifth; Kölliker's that it constituted one-fifth to one-sixth the volume of the red pulp. More recently Groll (1919) found in healthy young soldiers that the lymphatic tissue of the spleen was best developed in his youngest group (19 and 20 years), and least well developed in those over 41. The excellent quality of this material, however, is considerably offset by his inability on field service to have done more than estimate the size of the follicles macroscopically!

By far the most valuable in this field is Hellman's (1925-1926) analysis of 100 cases, divided into 11 age groups, of persons dying sudden, violent deaths and proving at autopsy to have no noteworthy lesions of the spleen. This is truly admirable material, all of the cases dying within 12 hours of the injury, most of them instantaneously, and all but one within 3 hours, all studied grossly and microscopically and by the same person. They present a striking curve of quick increase of lymphocytic tissue in the Malpighian follicles from birth to an average of about 11 per cent in the first year of life, rising to a maximum of 18 per cent in the 18th year, with a sharp drop to 13.6 per cent at 25, remaining level till 45, then another drop to below 5 per cent in the oldest case studied (84 years). One hundred cases, however, is a very small number when distributed over 11 groups, especially as the individual "scatter" was great. There were, for instance, 12 cases below one year and 20 below 6, leaving an average of 10 cases for the other age groups and only 5 cases over 50 years of age. It should also be noted that the figures given represent percentages only and must be taken in connection with the total spleen weights in order to arrive at the actual amount of lymphatic tissue in the spleen at a given age.

Furthermore, they represent only the size of the Malpighian follicles, the outer edge of which is often open to considerable interpretation and they include the intrafollicular vessels and all pale centers, which many now believe not to be made up of cells of the lymphocytic series. Though the short interval between injury and death precludes changes secondary to wasting, sepsis, and so on, the considerable splenic pulp

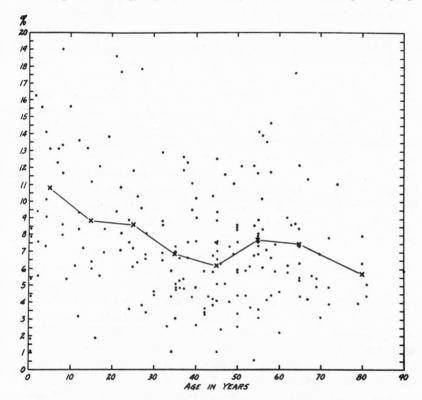

Fig. 24. Percentage of "net" lymphatic tissue in the Malpighian follicles of 200 spleens in cases of violent death. These percentages differ slightly from those given in the text which are based on 300 spleens that eventually became available.

change that results quickly after shock or hemorrhage cannot be excluded and remains a variable affecting the percentage that cannot be accounted for. We (Hwang, Lippincott and Krumbhaar, 1938) have, therefore, made a similar study, even though our series is also open to some of the above objections, hoping that larger numbers, especially in the older groups, will throw further light on the subject.

We have selected material, like Hellman, from persons dying violent deaths of various kinds, shortly after the violence occurred, and excluded those known either before death or at autopsy to have any recognizable disease.   The percentage of lymphocytic tissue was obtained by projecting microscopic fields under standard conditions (20 fields were found to be the minimum satisfactory number), outlining the Malpighian follicles and also their non-lymphocytic areas on paper and measuring these with a planimeter.   Thus it was possible to get figures for the percentage area of splenic tissue occupied by the Malpighian follicles as a whole (i.e., including pale centers and blood vessels); for the follicles excluding these features, and for the number of follicles encountered. On account of the greater sharpness of the end-point at the inner edge of the outer marginal zone, it was decided not to include this zone in the measurement.   This probably is the chief reason for our percentages being considerably smaller than Hellman's.   Our method also permits only a relative value for the figures obtained; but in any case they could not represent the true lymphocytic content of the spleen, as the lymph-sheath and the lymphocytes diffused through the red pulp have been included by neither Hellman or us for obvious reasons.   For technical reasons a microscopic slide from only one part of the spleen was used; but Hellman has demonstrated that the Malpighian follicles appear to be distributed equally throughout the spleen.   With the spleen and body weights known, it is then possible to get an approximate figure for the weight of the lymphocytic tissue in the spleen and also its ratio to the body weight at different ages.   For analysis of these last two sets of values, which did not produce much of additional value, the reader is referred to the original reports.   We have analyzed 300 cases of violent deaths distributed in 9 age groups from birth to 70 years and over. All the adult groups up to 70 years contain 29 or more cases each and there are 95 cases analyzed over 50 years of age, as compared with 5 cases over 50 in Hellman's study.   The chart shows that the individual "scatter" of lymphatic tissue percentage was as great as in Hellman's cases; a fact that is difficult to interpret other than on the basis of the unhelpful "individual idiosyncrasy."   Disturbing factors, such as diminution in size of the red pulp due to shock or severe hemorrhage, or its increase in early sepsis, could not be shown to be of moment.   The mean curve shows, that as in Hellman's series, the percentage of lymphatic tissue is low in the first year (4.5 per cent), though the number of Malpighian corpuscles is then at a maximum (5.6 per field).   The maximum percentage is reached in the first decade (10.8 per cent)— again as in Hellman's series—with 4.3 follicles per field.   Whereas his fell steadily throughout life, our curve dropped sharply to 7.7 per cent in the 11 to 30 age groups, tending to fall gradually in the next two age groups. After a slight rise in the two age groups from 50 to 70 years, it falls in the last group (comprising all cases over 70) to 5.8 per cent. When studied statistically in terms of the standard error and regression coefficient, it is found: (1) That the peak at the 1 to 10 year period is significantly higher than the level of the period on either side. (2) If the groups from 11 years on are considered, the regression coefficient shows that the line is not significantly different from horizontal, though it does have a slightly downward trend. (3) If the regression line is considered in three parts (i.e., from 11 to 50 years, from 41 to 70 years, and from 70 years on), three limbs result. The first of these is significantly downward, the second significantly upward and the third significantly downward. We have already seen, that Hieronymus found maintenance of tonsillar tissue between the regressions that occurred in the 5th and 8th decades and that the cervical and popliteal lymph nodes in Hellman's normal rabbits had a second growth period at a similar age. Aschoff (1926) also accepts the statement frequently made in the literature that there is an increase of human lymphoid tissue late in life, so that it is more abundant in those over 60 years than in earlier adult life. Should we, then, reserve as (*a possibility that there is a real increase of lymphoid tissue in late middle life and that it may be associated with increased resistance to various infectious processes?*)

Another line of study yielding information of indirect value for our main theme and one that has been extensively followed is the total weight of the human spleen at different ages. As this figure is influenced by a large number of variables, other than age (kind of human material, cause of death, histological condition, methods used in preparing tissue, etc.), it is not surprising that wide variations are reported by different investigators, and that even the average weight given for the spleen varies from 115 grams (Schridde) to 250-300 grams (Hyrtl, 1846). Vierordt (1893) gives 298 male and 305 female spleen weights divided into 36 groups between birth and 25 years. The weights (combined for both sexes) rise from 10.7 grams at birth to a maximum of 168.3 grams at 25 years, the most marked rise occurring about the age of 15, with the males' spleens (after the first 2 years) weighing slightly more than the females'.

Lubarsch (1926) has tabulated spleen weights for both sexes in 11 groups between birth and 40 years. There were 484 females and 541 males (total 1025), selected from the Charité Hospital, cases that showed no noteworthy splenic changes.   Starting at 9.5 grams as the spleen weight at birth for both sexes, the weights increased, with no significant differences between sexes, to 77 grams for the 10-15 age group, 121 grams at 15-20, 144 grams at 20-30, and 144 grams for 30 to 40.   He regards 150 grams as a good average weight for the adult spleen.   In 569 males and 233 females (total 802), selected in the same way by Rössle and Roulet (1932), somewhat similar figures were obtained.   Starting with weights of 11.2 and 10.2 grams at birth, the

TABLE 8

Data on the lymphatic tissue of Malpighian follicles in 300 cases of violent death

Group	Age	Number of cases	Net percentage	2SE	Gross	Weight of follicular lymphatic tissue	Ratio $\frac{\text{Follicular lymphatic tissue weight}}{\text{Body weight}}$	Number of Malpighian follicles	2SE
	years				*per cent*	*grams*			
1	Up to 1	7	4.5 ± 2.0		4.8	0.36	0.00019	5.6 ± 0.62	
2	1–10	22	10.8 ± 1.8		12.1	6.7	0.00030	4.2 ± 0.44	
3	11–20	18	7.7 ± 1.6		8.6	10.6	0.00019	3.5 ± 0.44	
4	21–30	36	7.7 ± 1.2		8.4	10.6	0.00016	3.2 ± 0.24	
5	31–40	54	6.7 ± 0.8		7.1	8.5	0.00014	3.3 ± 0.34	
6	41–50	68	6.3 ± 0.6		6.8	9.0	0.00012	3.0 ± 0.22	
7	51–60	53	7.0 ± 1.0		7.5	9.2	0.00013	3.3 ± 0.42	
8	61–70	29	7.3 ± 1.0		7.8	8.9	0.00014	3.9 ± 0.54	
9	Over 70	13	5.8 ± 1.2		6.3	5.7	0.00010	2.8 ± 0.54	

weights rise steadily to a maximum for males of 169.1 grams in the 3rd decade and for females of 153.7 in the 4th decade.   From then on, the spleen weights decrease with increasing age, averaging about 112 grams in the 7th decade, and about 103 grams for all persons over 70.   Two over 90 years of age averaged 65 grams.   Though the authors state that they found no "durchgehenden" difference between the sexes, their figures show greater weights for the male, as high as 25 per cent, in all but 6 of the 30 age groups studied.   Neugarten (1921), in Schridde's material, on the other hand, found an average weight for males in the 25 to 40 age group of 113.3 grams as compared to 140.0 grams for females. However, Moon (1928) and Ahronheim (1937), like ourselves, found slightly but consistently smaller figures for the female than the male spleens. Pearl and Bacon (1921-1924) found that the spleen increased in weight up to the 35 year period, after which it progressively declined. They computed from Oppenheimer's (1889) accidental deaths that at 25 years the male spleen averaged 164.8

TABLE 9

Spleen weights at different ages (combined "disease" and violent deaths)

Age	2000 "Disease" deaths			2000 Violent deaths			Total 4000		
	Number	Mean	2SE	Number	Mean	2Se	Number	Mean	2SE
years									
Up to 1	137	17.9 ± 2.2		19	12 ± 3.2		156	17.2 ± 2.0	
1–5	44	52 ± 8.2		71	58 ± 4.4		115	55 ± 4.4	
6-10	16	106 ± 30		73	78 ± 7.2		89	83 ± 8.2	
11–15	37	146 ± 30		57	107 ± 12.4		94	125 ± 14.4	
16–20	73	192.5 ± 23		111	154 ± 12.2		184	170 ± 12.0	
21–25	107	190 ± 16		163	148 ± 8.6		270	165 ± 7.6	
26–30	96	165 ± 5		214	136 ± 9.2		310	148 ± 7.6	
31–35	101	171 ± 17		191	146 ± 9.8		292	155 ± 8.8	
36–40	151	164 ± 13.2		209	135 ± 9.2		360	147 ± 7.8	
41–45	156	168 ± 14.4		175	139 ± 9.8		331	153 ± 8.6	
46–50	191	164 ± 11.8		164	129 ± 9.2		355	148 ± 7.8	
51–55	184	169 ± 12.8		142	137 ± 10.6		326	155 ± 8.8	
56–60	183	166 ± 14.6		142	135 ± 10.4		325	153 ± 9.6	
61–65	175	170 ± 16		102	135 ± 13.4		277	158 ± 11.4	
66–70	136	156 ± 13		89	113 ± 12.4		225	139 ± 9.6	
71–75	109	143 ± 13.8		43	107 ± 11.6		152	133 ± 10.2	
76–80	60	125 ± 14.8		24	116 ± 17.4		84	122 ± 11.6	
Over 80	44	116 ± 19.4		11	71 ± 13.2		55	107 ± 16.6	

grams, the female 160.7 grams. In Moon's 2000 cases (at the Philadelphia General Hospital before 1928) above 18 years of age, the spleen weight decreased progressively in each of the 8 decades studied.

In view of these differences, it seemed desirable to review our own material, (Krumbhaar and Lippincott, 1938) on a similar basis to that of Lubarsch and Rössle and Roulet, i.e., analyzing our routine autopsy material but omitting those cases that at autopsy or during histologic examination showed any considerable splenic lesions, such as leukemias, neoplasms, Hodgkin's disease, amyloidosis, and other

causes of splenomegaly.   All ages from birth to 95 years were included
in 18 semi-decades.   The body weight, presumably having an influence
on spleen weight, was compared where available.   Furthermore, recognizing that death from disease must necessarily affect the weight of the
spleen, we have attempted also to classify the 2000 cases into arbitrarily
erected disease types that might be regarded as having similar effects
on spleen weight.   We found 868 cases in this series where there had
been made a histological study of the spleen, which have been classified

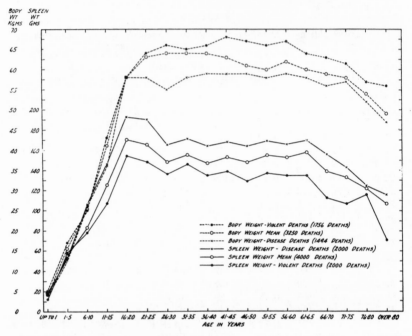

FIG. 25. Means of spleen weights and body weights in 2000 disease and 2000
violent deaths and combined.

according to the condition of the spleen.   In these ways it was hoped
that variations of the spleen weight curve might be illuminated.   The
well known fact that the spleen post mortem weighs less than it does
in vivo was a disturbing factor that had to be accepted.

The results (shown graphically in the uppermost and fourth curves
of figure 25) gave distinctly higher weights in this series than in the
German studies.   Also the maximum weight was reached earlier.   Statistical analysis showed that the 16-20 and 21-25 age groups had signifi-

cantly heavier spleens than any other group. The lower weight level of the 26-30 age group was maintained with but little change to the 65th year, after which there occurred a sharp and statistically significant loss of weight. Comparison with body weights shows that these had nothing to do with the peak from 16 to 25, though they are presumably a factor in the final decline. Analysis of the causes of death brings out that death from respiratory diseases were more prevalent in the 16-20 and 21-25 age groups; and, as would be expected, arteriosclerosis in the older age groups. It will be shown later, however, that the respiratory diseases could not be the only factors concerned in the younger groups; while arteriosclerosis in the old group is an important factor, though just how important it is impossible to say. In passing it may be stated that analysis of the cases classified by sex and color, showed that the female spleens were distinctly lighter than those of the males; and that spleens of negros were lighter than those of whites; but these had no important bearing on the data given above. The average weight for all adult spleens (16 years or over) was 150.7 grams; for spleens between the years of 16 and 70, 154.2 grams; for all 4000 spleens, 140.7 grams. Analysis of the histological appearance of the 868 spleens shows that 75 per cent were given diagnoses that should be accompanied by a tendency toward increased weight, even though such terms as "Congestion" are variably used in routine descriptions and though the cases would not have been included if the changes had been marked. Only 2.5 per cent were listed as atrophic. These figures, then, indicate that the splenic weights in this series of "disease" deaths tend to be above normal.

In order further to eliminate the disturbing disease factor, a series of spleen weights of persons dying *violent deaths* has been assembled from the records of and with the aid of the Medical Examiner's offices in Manhattan, Jamaica, L. I., and Boston, and the Coroner's physicians of Philadelphia. The only previous studies of this kind that we have knowledge of are the 100 cases of Hellman's, previously referred to. In Hellman's (1926) series, the spleens at birth weighed on the average 8.0 grams; at 1 year, 52.0 grams; from 2 to 5, 50.8 grams; from 6 to 10, 78.3 grams; from 11 to 15, 108.3 grams; from 16 to 20, 135.5 grams; from 21 to 30, 145.0 grams; from 31 to 40, 139.0 grams; from 41 to 50, 163.9 grams, and over 50, 114.7 grams. This surprising difference from the "disease" curves, with a maximum spleen weight in the 41 to 50 age group, would be of greater significance if based on more cases; but where only one group has more than 20 cases and 5 of the 11 has fewer than 10, with a marked "scatter" (from 45 to 250 grams, for instance, in the 12 cases of the 41 to 45 group) the figures must be regarded as chiefly suggestive.

In the 2000 cases that we have collected, it was of course not always possible to ascertain the time of death after the violence. Also there were included 342 cases where hemorrhage and shock was sufficient to be included in the cause of death, and 193 cases where some sepsis was noted. Separate analyses showed that whereas the hemorrhage and shock cases had spleens that averaged a few grams below the general average, the sepsis spleens averaged somewhat heavier. The fact that these tended to counterbalance each other, together with the certainty that these same factors were present in an unknown number of other cases, though unrecorded, made it seem reasonable not to exclude them. We have also, like Hellman, included certain acute poisonings, such as carbon monoxide, and acute (but not chronic) alcoholism, though these too may have affected the spleen weight. It is also recognized that these victims of violence may have coincidentally been sufferers from disease, though wherever the spleen was recognized as abnormal, or coincidental disease elicited, the spleen was discarded. The influence of nutrition—the spleen being smaller in the emaciated and Malpighian follicles apparently larger after meals (Hessling, 1842; Toldt, 1888)—has also had to be disregarded. While the spleens in this series, therefore, may not be regarded as "supposedly normal," they should be accepted as closer to normal than the "disease" series, and it should be recognized that truly normal human spleens are practically impossible to obtain. For many of the marked individual variations of spleen weight encountered no explanation was forthcoming. Thus a male white, aged 45, weighing 135 pounds, who committed suicide with cyanide, had a spleen which was reported as normal but weighed 400 grams; a Jewess of 32, weighing 150 pounds, was strangled—her "normal" spleen was found to weigh 415 grams. At the other extreme, an apparently normal Chinese of 40, weighing 124 pounds, was drowned and his spleen weighed only 20 grams. Such examples are too numerous to be attributable to error or oversight. This great individual variation is strikingly brought out in the accompanying spot chart (fig. 26); so that even when full allowance is made for the possible inclusion of undetected abnormalities, the normal spleen must be recognized as one of the organs in the human body most variable in size and weight.

Graphs of the means obtained for the spleen weights in the 2000 disease deaths and the 2000 violent deaths showed a remarkable parallelism, with the "disease" spleens probably averaging too high and the "violent" spleens too low. A grand total of the 4000 cases was therefore plotted, appearing in the chart as the middle line of the spleen and body weight curves. We believe that this comes nearer to the true normal of the human spleen than either of the other curves. It shows the same

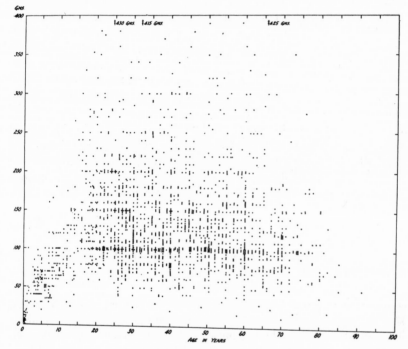

FIG. 26. Spleen weights in 2000 violent deaths, showing individual "Scatter"

peak of spleen weights in the 16–20 and 21–25 age groups, which is still significantly (more than twice the standard error) higher than weights in other age groups. As this peak occurs in the violent death series, where the factor of respiratory disease occurring in the disease series could not be operative, it must be regarded as due to the innate growth habit of the spleen. The plateau that extends from the 26–30 to the 61–65 year group is shown by the regression coefficient to be theoretically horizontal (i.e., the chances proved to be better than 1:1 that the trend was that of a level line). From 65 years on the slope is definitely and significantly down, though the body weights also are less in these groups.

Study of the ratio of spleen weight to body weight in the 4000 cases shows that it is highest and significantly above the others in the earliest age group (0.0042). From then on the slope of the ratio is slightly though not significantly down (from 0.0035 to 0.0022), except for a plateau in the groups between 51 and 65 years (0.0026), where the ratio is significantly higher than those of age groups on either side. This indirect indication of a possible increase of the body's lymphoid tissue about this period of life has already been commented upon. The ratio of spleen weight to body weight in all ages in the 4000 cases averaged 0.0027. Others have found similar results: the percentage of the spleen weight in the body weight having been found highest from 2 to 7 years (0.32–0.39 per cent), falling to 0.25 per cent at 25.

The oldest spleen of our series weighed 80 grams and showed both fibrosis and a considerable amount of lymphocytic tissue. It came from a negress of 95, who weighed but 72 pounds. She was a senile dement, suffering from hypertension, an enlarged heart, pipe stem radial arteries, etc., who gradually got weaker and died, with pulmonary congestion given as the chief cause of death. The spleen appeared markedly fibrotic with a wrinkled capsule, but also showed a surprising amount of lymphocytic tissue in the loosely constructed Malpighian follicles (no secondary nodules) and in the lymph sheaths. The next to oldest spleen was from a recluse of 90 years who killed herself with illuminating gas. Autopsy showed general arteriosclerosis and fibrosis of organs, including the spleen, which weighed 85 grams. Nevertheless the Malpighian follicles seemed but little decreased in size or number as compared with younger adult spleens. None contained secondary nodules. Their net area (i.e., excluding non-lymphocytic tissue such as vessels and reticulo-endothelial cells) constituted 5.95 per cent of the total and 3.1 follicles were encountered per standard field (see figure 24). This is just above the average percentage for the spleens of those over 70. The fibrosis of the red pulp and a slight thickening of capsule and trabeculae alone suggested an aged spleen under the microscope. Thus, while both these spleens support the general opinion that *fibrosis, arteriosclerosis and atrophy (low weight) are the rule in the aged, they also indicate that lymphocytic tissue may persist in considerable amounts even in extreme old age.*

We may sum up this study of the "normal" spleen's weight and lymphatic tissue per cent in general terms as follows: *the spleen appears to grow parallel with the growth of the body during childhood, but reaches its maximum weight (170 grams) earlier (i.e., in the 16–20 age group as opposed to 26–40 years for the body weight). From the ages of 26 to 65, its absolute weight remains approximately unchanged; though, compared with the average body weight, the spleen weight falls slightly, except for the 51 to 65 age group where it rises significantly. After 65, both spleen and*

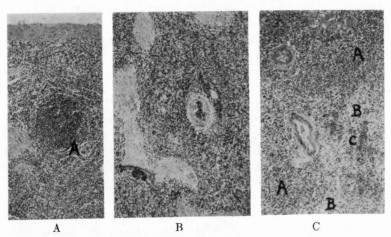

A   B   C

Fig. 27. A. Spleen (child of 7), showing a follicle with a "solid center" near the capsule. Note the eccentric "central artery" (A) in the looser outer margin of the follicle. Death from traumatic rupture of liver (Phila. Morgue, 1937. No. 1927) (× 72).

B. Spleen (weight, 90 gms., from a white female of 81), showing a sparsity of lymphocytes in the follicle, and numerous prominent trabeculae. The wall of the central artery is sclerosed. The fine fibrosis of follicle and pulp barely distinguishable at this magnification, has been lost in the half tone. Death from shock following multiple crushes and fractures (Phila. Morgue, 1937, No. 2334) (× 72).

C. Spleen (weight, 85 gms., from a white female of 90), showing persistence of considerable lymphatic tissue (A), with fibrosis of pulp (B), and areas of congestion (C). The "central arteries" have markedly hyalinized walls. Death from carbon monoxide poisoning (U. of Pa., 1933–1079) (× 72).

body weight fall steadily, the spleen weight more than the body weight, so that in the very old weights less than 100 grams are frequent.

The lymphocytic tissue in the Malpighian follicles, low at birth, quickly rises to a maximum percentage early in the first decade. It then drops, most sharply in the second decade, till the age of 50, when there is a distinct increase lasting till about 65. Thereafter it falls again eventually to reach a percentage similar to that of early infancy.

In both spleen weight and lymphatic per cent figures, we have found, as have others, a marked individual "scatter," which apparently should be regarded as one of the innate characteristics of the organ.

6. ANATOMICAL SIGNS OF AGEING OF THYMUS

Accepting Hammar's (1926) view of the thymus as an epithelial organ infiltrated with true lymphocytes (of mesodermic, not epithelial, origin),[2] its changing form at different age periods must be considered in this chapter. On account of its important probable endocrine relations to growth, however, and possible other endocrine functions, its functional significance at different ages is discussed by Carlson in Chapter 14. The thymus is here regarded as a combination of epithelial and lymphocytic tissue, by the action of which in unknown ways materials important for the body are constructed. That it may partake of some of the ordinary functions of lymphatic tissue, however, is indicated by its increase in lymphatic content after the injection of Staphylococcus toxin (Ehrich, 1929d). On the other hand, Young and Turnbull (1931) believe that "In so far as the product of the length, breadth and depth measurements. . .can be considered to give an approximation to the actual volume of the individual lymphatic structures, and in so far as selected glands and Peyer's patches can be considered in any way representative of the amounts of lymphoid tissue in different sites, there would appear to be no significant association between the weight of the thymus and the size of any of the other lymphoid structures with the possible exception of the lingual tonsils."

Starting in the fetus as an epithelial outgrowth from the third pharyngeal pouches, the thymic anlage sends out tubular projections (the lumina of which are soon lost) and irregular branches which, when surrounded by infiltrated true lymphocytes (thymocytes), form loose lobes, subdivided by connective tissue septa into lobules. These thymocytes are densest in the dark staining cortex of the lobule, merging into the paler medulla which contains reticulum and Hassall's corpuscles but few lymphocytes. The secondary nodules, peripheral and perifollicular lymph sinuses and the afferent lymphatics of ordinary lymph nodes do not exist in the thymus. Interlobular lymphatics, on the other hand, are recognized by von Ebner (1902) and Hammar, (1936) as draining upward, out and back in the human body to adjacent lymph nodes

---

[2] The earlier view of Stöhr and others that the small thymus cells were modified epithelium has recently been given some support by Popoff's (1927) tissue culture studies, but has not been generally accepted.

(Severeanu, 1909). The striking thymic (Hassall's) corpuscles of the medulla begin to appear as sparse, small, rounded bodies about the fifth fetal month. They are regarded by most authorities as degenerated entodermal epithelium, though some regard them as active constituents of the thymus, others as connective tissue masses, others as thickened blood vessel walls. Injection preparations, however, show that they are not connected with the vascular system. The concentric arrangement, with central obliteration of nuclei and frequent hyaline, fatty or calcifying changes, give an appearance similar to the "epithelial pearl" of carcinoma.

The changes in the thymus at different ages have been carefully studied by a number of authors; but especially by Hammar, of Upsala, who in the past 30 years has devoted many articles and 3 considerable volumes (1926, 1929, 1936) to his own work on this organ and a critical survey of the literature. His report will be largely followed in this presentation.

From the accompanying table, adapted from Hammar (1936), based on 345 cases, it appears that the human thymus grows rapidly through fetal life, weighing about 15 grams (range, 7.3 to 25.5 grams) at birth. Increase of absolute weight continues to a maximum at the 6th to 10th years, with a slow regression in weight after the 16–20 age group. These figures represent somewhat heavier weights than those usually given, but are substantiated by Löwenthal's (1932) series of 114 military cases between the ages of 16 and 50 with even higher figures: 16–20 years, average 22.5 grams (range 7–65 grams); 21–25 years, average 21.6 grams (7–52 grams); 26–30 years, 16.7 grams (5–30); 31–35 years, 25.7 grams (15–34); 36–40 years, 18.9 grams (4–37); 41–50 years, 22.5 grams (10–32). One is at once struck by the great variability in supposedly normal adults. In an analysis of 234 stillborns and 1891 postnatal deaths, Miss Boyd (1932) determined that "This analysis has again demonstrated that while the mean thymus weight in normal persons is about 2 grams more than the median, both increase rapidly in the first months of life, double their birth size by 2 years and triple it by 11 years; then both decrease slowly to about birth size in senility. This general progression holds for data from the United States, Germany, France, Sweden and England." Bremer (1936) says that the thymus at birth weighs from 5 to 15 grams, grows rapidly till the second year, then more slowly till puberty. It then begins to involute but persists through life.

This atrophy especially affects the cortex, which is at its maximum at 3½ years. At puberty it has only lost 6 per cent of its volume, while in the 15–20 age group, it has lost 44 per cent, as against 19 per cent of the medulla, and at 60 retains only 4 per cent of its maximum. The connective tissue of the thymus begins to increase even in utero; it increases much more rapidly in the post-puberty period and reaches its absolute maximum in the 4th decade—twice the pubertal value. In Edith Boyd's series of 207 cases of death from accidental causes within

TABLE 10

Mean weights of the thymus and its chief components at different ages.

(345 normal cases)

(Adapted from Hammar)

Age	Thymus (whole)	Paren-chyma	Cortex	Medulla	Ratio Cortex / Medulla	Connec-tive tissue
	grams	*grams*	*grams*	*grams*		
3rd fetal month	0.00122	0.00064	0.00042	0.00005	8.3	0.00058
4th fetal month	0.0409	0.0204	0.0139	0.0065	2.1	0.0205
5th fetal month	0.237	0.145	0.095	0.050	1.9	0.092
6th fetal month	0.846	0.550	0.386	0.164	2.4	0.287
7th fetal month	2.30	1.79	1.33	0.46	2.9	0.51
8th fetal month	4.79	3.79	2.81	0.98	2.9	1.00
9th fetal month	6.19	5.06	3.72	1.34	2.8	1.13
10th fetal month	11.67	9.23	6.98	2.25	3.1	2.44
Newborn	15.15	11.92	8.73	3.19	2.7	3.02
1–5 years	25.68	19.82	14.48	5.34	2.7	5.16
6–10 years	29.42	21.88	13.90	7.98	1.7	6.76
11–15 years	29.41	20.97	13.08	7.98	1.7	7.88
16–20 years	26.24	13.85	7.34	6.51	1.1	11.20
21–25 years	21.05	10.05	5.24	4.81	1.1	10.22
26–30 years	19.54	5.89	2.97	2.92	1.0	12.19
31–35 years	20.17	4.86	2.50	2.36	1.1	14.68
36–45 years	19.03	3.79	1.96	1.83	1.1	15.07
46–55 years	17.32	1.23	0.68	0.47	1.4	14.90
56–65 years	14.30	1.36	0.62	0.68	0.9	12.88
66–90 years	14.06	1.02	0.62	0.34	2.0	11.25

24 hours of injury, the cortex likewise began to involute at 4 years, while the medulla, with its Hassall's corpuscles, began, like the whole thymus, to involute at puberty, and the connective tissue and fat content continued to increase until old age.

The ratio of cortex to medulla was found by Hammar to be 2.7 at birth, 1.7 at puberty, and about 1 after puberty. This differs from Gedda's (1921) findings in rabbits, where the ratios for these periods

were 5, 3.7 to 4.5, and 3.9 to 7.2, respectively. These figures offer an
interesting correlation with the lymphocytes of the blood and suggest

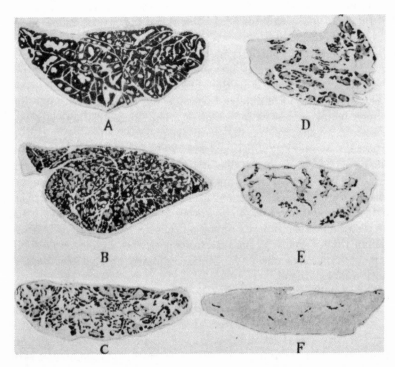

FIG. 28. Histology of thymuses at various ages showing age involution (from
Hammar, 1926).
  A. Male infant, died during delivery. Thymus weighed 15.64 grams. The
darker portion is parenchyma (82 per cent); the lighter portion is connective tissue.
  B. A healthy boy of 6 years, drowned. Thymus weighed 28.0 grams; parenchyma, 71 per cent.
  C. A man of 20, dying of hydrochloric acid poisoning. Thymus weighed
20.5 grams; parenchyma, 49 per cent.
  D. A man of 25, suicide by gun shot wound. Thymus weighed 24 grams;
parenchyma, 32.6 per cent.
  E. A man of 48, carbon monoxide poisoning. Thymus weighed 15 grams;
parenchyma, 12.4 per cent.
  F. A man of 90, hanged. Thymus weighed 20 grams; parenchyma, 0.7 per
cent. These selections from a large series of thymus glands, to illustrate progressive loss of parenchyma, should not obscure the fact that individual variations are so great that in single cases an older gland might have relatively more
parenchyma than a younger one.

again the possibility that the thymus lymphocytes are not unconnected
with somatic lymphocytic activities.
  Under the microscope the abundant lymphoid picture of early child-

hood—lobules rich in lymphocytes and placed close together with narrow interlobular trabeculae—is but little changed up to the age of puberty. In the post-pubertal period the interstitial tissue rapidly thickens, with infiltration of more and more fat between and into the lobules, so that by the 5th decade the connective tissue has reached twice its pubertal value. The cortex still contains more lymphocytes than the medulla; but the difference becomes less marked as age advances, the cortex appearing as darker areas in the narrowed medullary strands. There is great individual variation, so that some old thymuses resemble those of much younger persons (effect of reactive processes?) and vice versa (accidental involution, i.e., due to external causes).

Hassall's corpuscles, which in the fetus are first seen as a few small rounded bodies 12 to 20μ in diameter), increase rapidly in number and size, some reaching a maximum of 800 micra in the post-pubertal period. They gradually regress in size, so that from the 7th decade none surpass 300μ and the large corpuscles appear only rarely. Hammar also calls attention to an involutionary thickening of the walls of small thymic veins, though he recognizes that similar changes may occur in hyperthyroidism, congenital syphilis, or the accidental involution of childhood.

Cytologically, the lymphocytes are the cells chiefly diminished in the involution of ageing. Schridde (1911) stated that the eosinophiles (mostly myelocytes) disappeared at the beginning of age involution, except in cases of (the now somewhat discredited) Status Thymico Lymphaticus; Hammar has conceded a diminution of eosinophiles rather than a total disappearance. With the cellular atrophy of increasing age, the reticulo-endothelial cells of the medulla, as well as the connective tissue fibrocytes, are increased, relatively more than absolutely.

Study of the weight of the human thymus in different races and regions shows that weight differences exist; although, in view of such important complicating variables as differing diets, diseases, and endocrine ratios, they cannot be attributed with any assurance to race or locality alone. Castaldi (1923), for instance, found that the thymus was heavier in Skandinavians and Germans than in Latins and Russians; i.e., heavier in linear types of man than in lateral. Shellspear (1924) found in an autopsy study of 102 Chinese between 12 and 70 years of age (including 8 cases of violent death) that 46 thymuses weighed over 35 grams and were relatively rich in parenchyma for their age. Oppenheim (1925), however, could not confirm such findings in 100 Shanghai autopsies. In 119 Jewish children, Bratton (1926) found that the thymus was somewhat heavier, both absolutely and in relation to body weight, than in British children. In the Burmese goitre district, Ruskoff (1933) reported that in 841 new born children, the thymus sometimes weighed as little as 2 and 4 grams; the average weight in the first hours was 12.1 grams—a low figure but well within the range of Hammar's findings.

Weights lower than Hammar's average normals, also were found in thymuses of 141 Japanese (Ohmura, 1928) and 338 Filipinos (Nañagas, 1933):

Ohmura—141 Japanese		Nañagas—338 Filipinos	
Age	Weight	Age	Weight
	grams		grams
Newborn	12.0	2 days-2 months	5.6
1- 5 years	11.9	1½-13 months	4.8
6–10 years	31.9	3½-18 months	7.3
10–20 years	22.2	9 –36 months	6.2
21–25 years	15.7	1½- 4 years	9.3
26–35 years	17.0	3 – 7 years	13.5
36–45 years	11.7	5 – 7 years	11.7*
		7 – 8 years	10.0
		8 –11 years	31.0
		12 –15 years	19.4
		13 –15 years	17.8

* Few cases.

In the case of the Filipinos, however, poor nutrition appears to have been responsible for many of the low figures, and the ratio to body weight is not given.

From such incomplete data, with results differing from Hammar's own figures so inconclusively, it is obviously as yet impossible to draw definite conclusions as to racial or geographical differences in thymus weight.

In most diseases, the thymus loses weight as part of the general expression of malnutrition; and loses it rapidly, as one would expect in a member of the lymphatic family. This limitation of the value of published figures must always be borne in mind. Only in lymphatic leukemias, neoplasms of the thymus, status thymico-lymphaticus and exophthalmic goitre is an increase instead of a loss of weight known to occur; the age-weight thymus curve that includes these diseases will, of course, be correspondingly affected. One disposes unsatisfactorily

of the thymic enlargement in exophthalmic goitre by assuming an endocrine relationship.   Doubts continue to be cast on the very existence
of status thymico-lymphaticus; many now maintaining that the large
thymus, when it is large, is only so because the sudden death has not
given inanition a chance to reduce its weight and that so-called normals
based on the results of routine autopsies are really subnormal as the
result of the lymphatic atrophy consequent on disease.

The ageing changes of the thymus in other animals has received such
detailed attention that some findings are included here to illustrate the
results of comparative studies, even though the other units of the
lymphatic system have not been thus systematically treated in this
chapter.   In 80 *rabbits* of known age Söderlund and Backman (1909)
found that, as in man, the thymus lost weight with age, in spite of fatty
infiltration, chiefly by the organ getting thinner; but also that there was
great individual variation.   After the age of two the cortex is practically
indistinguishable from the medulla.   Hassall's corpuscles increase in
size and number up to puberty (Syk, 1909).   Then they decrease, at
first rapidly, then slowly; but at the age of two they are still large and
more numerous than at birth.   In an interesting comparison of sexual
maturity, thymus involution and per cent of lymphocytes in the blood
of 2 rabbit litters, Lindberg (1910) found that the appearance of spermatozoa and occurrence of pregnancy coincided with the maximum
number of the blood lymphocytes and beginning of thymic involution
(5 months).   In *rats*, the thymus grows to a maximum weight at 70
days (Jackson, 1913; and Watanabe, 1929 a, b, 1930), to 82 (Donaldson, 1924) or 85 days (Hatai, 1914), which corresponds to the time of
quick increase of gonads.   At 400 days, according to Donaldson, the
thymus only weighs 14 per cent of its maximum.   Relative to body
weight, the thymus weighs 0.15 per cent at birth; 0.25 per cent at 7
days and 0.38 per cent (the maximum relative weight) at 20 days
(Jackson).   Watanabe places the rat's attainment of maximum relative
weight of the thymus at 4 weeks.   As in man, the thymus persists,
with slowly increasing atrophy, throughout life.   Only Hammett
(1926) found a second rise of thymus weight in rats after the post-
pubertal regression.

As in man, also, the atrophy of older life chiefly involves the cortex,
where lymphocytes are replaced by fat and connective tissue.   Cell
collections resembling Hassall's corpuscles appear in the cortex, while
the medulla becomes gland-like or even cystic and Hassall's corpuscles
disappear.   According to Kinusaga (1930), the average weight of the

rat's thymus at birth is 0.01 grams; at 60 days 0.47 grams; at 70 days 0.52 grams, after which the weight falls. He found that at birth, the medulla constitutes 29 per cent of the gland; at 7 days, 15 per cent; at 14 days, 17 per cent; at 21 days, 19 per cent; at 53 days, 21 per cent; at 70 days, 25 per cent; at 90 days, 28 per cent; and at 240 days, 30 per cent.

In the 90-day *mouse* Masui and Tamura (1925–26) found a distinct sex difference, the non-pregnant female thymus averaging 0.038 grams, the male 0.021 grams. In the *guinea pig*, the thymus apparently reaches its maximum when a body weight of between 200 and 300 grams is reached (Paton, 1926). Jolley and Lieure (1929) found that involution began at $2\frac{1}{2}$ months, when the first sperm made it appearance. In the *horse*, as in other mammals, the thymus can be found at any age. Involution, here also, starts in the cortex with lymphoid atrophy and connective tissue increase (Shimpei, 1921). Involution of the medulla begins with increase in size and number of Hassall's corpuscles and with fat infiltration. Eosinophiles which in the fetus are found only in the medullary centers, are later more diffusely placed and often degenerated. In 462 *goats*, Schirber (1930) found a heavier thymus in females than in males—30.5 grams at birth; 35.5 grams at 3 years, falling to the average of 5.4 grams at 5 to 11 years. The thymus of male goats weighed 23.4 grams at birth; 23.0 grams at 3 years, and 11.9 grams at 5 years.

In a study of 110 *pigs* of known ages, Waschinsky (1925) found a maximum weight at 6 months—the age of beginning sexual maturity. In this species, the male appears to have a heavier thymus than the female. Hessdorfer (1925) found the maximum weight at 5 months, with one-half of maximum weight at 14 months, and one-sixth at 21 months. In *cattle* the thymus increases in weight for 7 to 8 weeks after birth; at 8 to 12 months it is in full regression (Krupski, 1924). In *dogs*, involution begins at 2 to 3 months, according to Ellenberger and Baum (1915); in the second year, according to Hammar (1936).

In *birds*, thymus involution appears to begin relatively late. In *hens* Hammar found it to be almost the same size at all ages studied, though in older birds the cortex gradually became thinner and developed epithelial-lined lumina. Even at 7 to 12 years, when the cortex was represented only by occasional small spots, the medulla remained well developed. Others, however, have found an involutionary regression in birds (Salkind, 1915), beginning at 3 (Riddle and Frey, 1924–1925) or 6 months (Latimer, 1925). In *doves*, Riddle and Frey found that the female thymus equalled the male thymus before involution; but was smaller after involution.

In *frogs* of 50 grams or over, Hammar (1936) found mucoid areas and cysts; the former never were found in frogs under 40 grams, though the cysts occurred as far down the age scale as in frogs of 2 grams. Histological signs of age were thinning of the cortex, with increased pigment and increased perivascular connective tissue.

In *fishes*, also, thymus involution appears to begin coincident with the arrival of sexual maturity (Hammar). Histologically, in older life, lymphocytes are fewer throughout the parenchyma, but especially in the cortex. Glandular and mucoid masses appear with increase of pigment, and the perivascular connective tissue becomes thickened and even hyaline. Deansley (1927), on the other hand, observing involution of the trout thymus at 2 years, could find no connection of involution with sex maturity. In Lophius budagassa, Picchio (1933) found that the histological distinction of cortex and medulla disappeared with age and that cavities of considerable size appeared.

Thus, though different species and classes naturally show individual differences, in general it appears that *the thymus begins to regress at or before sexual maturity, but can be found at any age. The regression affects first and chiefly the cortex.* There are sex differences, sometimes changed by involution; in mammals the female thymuses tend to be heavier; in birds, the post-pubertal male thymus. Though the involution of age bears some structural similarities to artificial or accidental involution, it is less modifiable by treatment, and unlike some of the other types appears to be irreversible.

7. SUMMARY

The various lymphatic tissues of the human body develop rapidly in early life and tend to begin involution earlier than body tissues in general, though there are, as would be expected, marked differences in various individuals and in the various units concerned. Lymph nodes and lymphatic nodules probably reach their maximum normal size in adolescence, and regress but slowly in adult life; tonsils appear to be at a maximum size at puberty with regression periods in adult life (4th and 8th decades). The spleen reaches its maximum weight in young adults but maintains a slightly lower plateau till the 7th decade, after which it loses weight. Its percentage of lymphatic tissue is at a maximum in the first decade, with a subsequent diminution throughout life, except for an increase about the years 50 and 65. The thymus begins to regress at or before puberty, with steady, marked loss of parenchyma. Lymphatic tissue, however, is present in all these organs, even the thymus, at all ages. Why the various lymphatic tissues undergo involution, or wasting, at different periods of the life span, is as yet unknown. To measure the involution quantitatively is extraordinarily difficult, but progress has been made with the thymus and the spleen.

Extravascular lymphatic tissue cells (lymphocytes and monocytes) are found in the tissues both diffusely and in aggregations. They live in special tissue fluid environments—the composition of the lymph closely approximating that of the tissue fluid of the region drained— and these environments are shielded from the homeostatically regulated blood stream (Chapter 23) by a layer of vascular endothelium. These tissue fluids are sluggish as compared with the circulating blood and therefore their composition has more opportunity to be modified by the various tissues and cells lying within, or limiting, them. The diversity which is to be expected in the relations of cell and fluid through the body (Chapter 24) may not be without influence on the lymphatic cells by promoting differences in rate of involution in different regions. As the circulation becomes impaired in old age, one would look for reflected changes in the lymph nodes of the aged; we cannot yet, however, evaluate the importance of this factor in the involutions of the ageing process.

The kind and degree of exposure to external stimuli need be considered as another modifying factor in the ageing of these tissues; but again we can do more than speculate about their influence at different ages. The lymphatic tissue of the lymph nodes and spleen remains fairly well developed at ages when the tonsils have regressed, and tonsils are "exposed" constantly. Furthermore, any lymphatic tissue may undergo "accidental involution" at any age after exposure that damages the parenchyma; yet, as we have seen, spontaneous involution (i.e., of ageing) occurs at considerably different periods in the various tissues.

Lymphatic tissue is an important part of the defense of the body, both against inanimate particles and living invaders. The lymphatic streams are essentially avenues of absorption of both harmful and nutritive material from the tissue fluids throughout most of the body and from the gastro-intestinal tract. Yet most people live and die without serious handicap from the failure of this tissue to function properly. In Dublin and Lotka's (1937) Metropolitan Life Insurance Company's figures, for example, a combination of diseases of the thymus spleen, pharynx, tonsils and lymphatic system, and of leukemias (all kinds) and Hodgkin's disease, were found to total 7.4 deaths per 100,000, as compared, for instance, with 116.6 deaths per 100,000 in the case of a single disease, tuberculosis. Appropriate, including disease, stimuli seem to be able indefinitely to delay the beginning of involution, or may even induce new formation of cell elements and new activity after involution has occurred. Such delay of involution and new formation very probably constitute important, though as yet imperfectly understood, factors in the structural condition of the lymphatic tissue and the individual's resistance to disease.

Thus the lymphatic system may be regarded as occupying a very probably central position in the phenomena of ageing. Until much more is known, however, of the function of these units and of lymphatic tissue in general, little can be said as to the significance of the morphologic changes outlined in this chapter.

REFERENCES

AHRONHEIM, J. H. 1937. The size of the spleen and the liver-spleen ratio. A statistical study based on 1000 autopsies. Arch. Path., 23, 33–52.

ASCHOFF, LUDWIG 1926. Die Lymphatischen Organe. Med. Klin., 22, Beihefte, 1–22.

BARNES, H. A. 1923. The tonsils, faucial, lingual, and pharyngeal. St. Louis: The C. V. Mosby Co., 217 pp.

BERGEL, S. 1926. Zur Morphologie und Funktion der Lymphocyten. Arch. f. Exper. Zellf., 3, 23–31.

BERNARDO-COMEL, M. C. 1937. Il tessuto linfoide dell' appendice umana nelle varie eta della vita. (Abstr. in Omnia Med., 15, p. 407) (Inst. Anat. d. l'Univ. R. di Milano).

BERRY, R. J. A., AND LACK, L. A. H. 1906. The vermiform appendix of man and the structural changes therein coincident with age. J. Anat. and Physiol., 40, 247–256.

BOYD, E. 1932. The weight of the thymus gland in health and disease. Am. J. Dis. Child., 43, 1162–1214.

BRATTON, A. B. 1926. The normal weight of the human thymus. J. Path. and Bact., 28, 609–620.

BREMER, J. L. 1936. A Textbook of Histology, Philadelphia: P. Blakiston's Sons & Co. Inc., 580 pp.

CAMBRELIN, G. 1937. L'Amygdale linguale, Paris: Masson et Cie, 147 pp.

CASTALDI, L. 1923. Applicazioni biometrici e statistiche di pesi timici, con determinazione del grado di influenza del timo sull'accrescimento corporeo del'uomo. Monit. zool., 34, 136–156.

CORNER, E. 1913. The function of the appendix and the origin of appendicitis. Brit. Med. J., 15, 325–327.

CURSCHMANN, HANS 1935. Zur Morbidität der Leukämien, insbesondere auch im höheren Alter. Deut. Med. Wchnschr., 61, 285–288.

DEANSLEY, R. 1927. Structure and development of the thymus in fish. Quart. J. Micr. Sci., **71**, 113-145.

DIETRICH, A. 1926. Rachen und Tonsillen. In Henke-Lubarsch Handb. d. Spez. Path. Anat. u. Hist., **IV**/1, pp. 1-75. Berlin: Springer.

DOBROVICI, A. 1904. Les leucocytes du sang chez les vieillard. Compt. rend. Soc. de biol., **56**, 970-972.

DONALDSON, H. H. 1915. The Rat. Data and reference tables for the Albino Rat (Mus norwegicus albinus) and the Norway rat (Mus norvegicus) Mem. Wistar Inst., No. 6, 1st ed. Philadelphia: [no publisher], 278 pp.

DRINKER, C. K., AND FIELD, M. E. 1933. The Lymphatics, Lymph and Tissue Fluid. Baltimore: The Williams & Wilkins Company, 254 pp.

DUBLIN, L. I., AND LOTKA, A. J. 1937. Twenty-five Years of Health Progress. New York: Metropolitan Life Insurance Co., 611 pp.

VON EBNER, V. 1902. Von der Thymus. In Kölliker's Handb. d. Gewebelehre, 6th ed., p 328-340. Leipsic: Engelmann.

EHRICH, W. 1929. (a) Studies of the lymphatic tissue, I. The Anatomy of the secondary nodules and some remarks on the lymphatic and lymphoid tissue. Am. J. Anat., **43**, 347-383; (b) II. The first appearance of the secondary nodules in the embryology of the lymphatic tissue, Ibid, **43**, 384-401; (c) Experimental study of the relation of the lymphatic tissue to the number of lymphocytes in the blood in subcutaneous infection with staphylococci. J. Exp. Med., **49**, 347-360; (d) Experimental studies on the effect of intravenous injection of killed staphylococci on the hehavior of lymphocytic tissue, thymus and the vascular connective tissue, Ibid., **49**, 361-385.

EHRICH, W., AND VOIGT, W. 1934. Ueber die Reaktion des Gefässbindegewebsapparates auf intravenöse Staphylokokken-Injectionen. Ziegler's Beitr., **93**, 348-370.

EIGLER, G. 1935. Die Funktion des lymphatischen Rachenringes. Arch. f. Ohren., Nasen u Kehlkopfh., **140**, 1-62.

ELLENBERGER, W., AND BAUM, H. 1915. In Handb. d. vergleich. Anat. d. Haustiere, Berlin: Hirschwald, 1047 pp.

ÉTIENNE, G., AND PERRIN, M. 1908. Les leucocytes chez un vieillard bien portant. Compt. rend. Soc. de biol., **65**, 250-252.

FUKUCHI, K. 1935-36. Ueber die Lipase (Butyrase) in Lymphozyten. Arb. a d. Anat. Inst. (Kyoto), Ser. D., No. 5, p. 76-78.

GEDDA, E. 1921. Zur Altersanatomie der Kaninchenthymus, Uppsala lak. för., **26**(IX), 1-27.

GRAVE, H. 1934. Die Reizzustände der Tonsillen und ihre Bedeutung. Rostock: Dissertation.

GRAY, H. 1854. On the structure and use of the spleen. London.: J. W. Parker & Son, 380 pp.

GROLL, H. 1919. Die "Hyperplasie" des lymphatischen Apparates bei Kriegsteilnehmern. Münch. med. Wchnschr., **66**, 833-835.

GROSSMAN, F. 1896. Ueber die axillaren Lymphdrüsen. Berlin: Dissertation.

GUNDOBIN, N. 1906. Die Lymphdrüsen. Jahrb. f. Kinderheilk., **64**, 528-539.

HAMMAR, J. AUG. 1926. Die Menschenthymus. In Gesundheit und Krankheit. Vol. 1, Das normale Organ. Leipzic: Akademische Verlagsgesellschaft,

570 pp. [Vol. 2, 1929, Ibid. "Das Organ unter anormalen Körperverhältnissen" is also a valuable reference on the thymus].

HAMMAR 1936. Die normal-morphologische Thymusforschung im letzten Vierteljahrhundert. Leipzig: Barth, 453 pp.

HAMMMETT, F. S. 1926. Studies in the thyroid apparatus, XXXVII. The rôle of the thyroid apparatus in the growth of the thymus. Endocrinology, 10, 370-384.

HATAI, S. 1914. On the weight of the thymus gland of the albino rat (Mus norvegicus albinus) according to age. Am. J. Anat., 1, 16, 251-257.

HELLMAN, T. 1914. Die normale Menge des lymphoiden Gewebes beim Kaninchen in verschiedenen postfetalen Altern. Uppsala lak. för. Suppl. 1-408.

———— 1919. Studien über das lymphoide Gewebe, 3, Die Bedeutung der sekundärfollikel. Uppsala lak. för., 24, 283-316.

———— 1921. Die Bedeutung der Sekundärfollikel. Beitr. z. path. Anat., 68, 333-363.

———— 1926. Die Altersanatomie der menschlichen Milz. Ztschr. f. Konstitutionslehre, 12, 270-415.

———— 1927. Der lymphatische Rachenring. In Moellendorf's Handb. d. mikrosk. Anat. V/1, 245-289. Berlin: Springer.

———— 1930. Lymphgefasse, Lymphknötchen und Lymphknoten, Ibid, VI/1, p. 233-396.

HESSDÖRFER, E. 1925. Ein Beitrag zur Anatomie und Rückbildung des Thymus beim Schweine. Berlin: Dissertation Veter.

HESSLING 1842. Untersuchungen über die weissen Körperchen der menschlichen Milz. Regensburg: F. Pufter, 20 pp.

HETT, G. S. 1913. The anatomy and comparative anatomy of the palatine tonsils and its rôle in the economy of man. Brit. Med. J., 2, 743-745.

HETT, G. S., AND BUTTERFIELD, H. G. 1909-10. The anatomy of the palatine tonsils. J. Anat. and Physiol., 44, 35-55.

HIERONIMUS, W. 1933. Die Grösse der Gaumentonsillen in den verschiedenen Lebensaltern. Rostock: Dissertation.

HILLE, H. R. 1908. Untersuchungen über des Vorkommen der Keimzentren in den Lymphknoten von Rind, Schwein, Pferd und Hund und über den Einfluss des Lebensalters auf die Keimzentren. Leipzig: Dissertation.

HODENPYL, E. 1891. The anatomy and physiology of the faucial tonsils with reference to the absorption of infectious material. Internat. J. Med. Sci., 101, 257-274.

HWANG, M. L., LIPPINCOTT, S. W., AND KRUMBHAAR, E. B. 1933. To be published, Am. J. Path.

HYRTL, J. 1846. Lehrbuch der Anatomie des Menschen. Prague: F. Ehrlich, 718 pp.

JACKSON, C. M. 1913. Postnatal growth and variability of the body and the various organs and systems in the albino rat. Am. J. Anat., 15, 1-68.

JOLLY, J., AND LIEURE, C. 1929. Sur l'involution du thymus. Compt. rend. Soc. de biol., 102, 762-764.

KAYSER, R. 1899. Die Krankheiten des lymphatischen Rachenringes. In Heymann's Handb. d. Laryngol. u Rhinol., II, 487-495. Wien: A. Hölder.

KILIAN, J. 1897-1898. Entwicklungsgeschichte, anatomische und klinische Untersuchungen über Mandelbucht und Gaumentonsillen. Arch. f. Laryng. u Rhinol., **7**, 167-203.

KINUSAGA, S. 1930. Functions of the cortex and medulla of the thymus, especially in their relation to the sexual glands. Keijo J. Med. **1** (From Hammar, 1936, as cited in Ber. wiss. Biol., **15**, 458, 1930).

KNIASCHETSKY, 1899. Ueber die Tonsillen der Kinder. St. Petersburg: Dissertation.

KÖLLIKER, A. 1849. Ueber den Bau und die Verrichtungen der Milz. Mitth. d. Naturf. ges. in Zurich, **1**, 120-125.

KRUMBHAAR, E. B., AND LIPPINCOTT, S. W. 1939. To be published, Am. J. Med. Sci.

KRUPSKI, 1924. Ueber die akzidentelle Involution der Thymusdrüse beim Kalb. Schweiz. Arch. f. Tierheilk., **66**, 14-21.

LATIMER, H. B. 1925. The relative postnatal growth of the systems and organs of the chicken. Anat. Rec., **31**, 233-253.

LEFHOLZ, R. 1923. The effects of diets varying in caloric value and in relative amounts of fat, sugar and protein, upon the growth of lymphoid tissue in kittens. Am. J. Anat., **32**, 1-36.

LINDBERG, G. 1910. Zur Kenntnis der Alterskurve der weissen Blutkörperchen des Kaninchens. Fol. Haemat., **9**, 64-80.

LÖWENTHAL, K. 1932. (a) Thymus. In Handb. innere Sekr. Max Hirsch, Editor. I, 709-866. Leipzig: Kabitzsch. (b) Die Lipoidablagerung bei der akzidentellen Involution der Erwachsenen, Virch. Arch., **283**, 448-457.

LUBARSCH, O. 1926. Pathologische Anatomie der Milz. In Henke and Lubarsch's Handb. d. Spez. Path. Anat. u. Hist., Berlin: Springer, pp. 373-774.

McMASTER, P. D., AND HUDACK, S. S. 1935. Formation of agglutinins within lymph nodes. J. Exp. Med., **61**, 783-805.

MASUI, K., AND TAMURA, Y. 1925-26. The effect of gonadectomy on the weight of the kidney, thymus and spleen of mice. Brit. J. Exper. Biol., **3**, 207-223.

MATHIES, W. 1935. Ueber die Entwicklung des Waldeyerschen Rachenrings. Beitr. z. path. Anat. u. z. Allg. Path., **94**, 389-403.

MEGEVAND, J. A. 1887. Contribution à l'étude anato-morphologique des maladies de la voute de pharynx. Geneva: Thesis.

MILLER, W. S. 1924-25. The pulmonary lymphatic tissue in old age. Am. Rev. Tuberc., **9**, 519-552.

MOON, V. H. 1928. Racial variation in size of spleen. A comparison. Arch. Path., **5**, 1040-1043.

MURPHY, J. B. 1919. Effect of dry heat on blood count in animals. J. Exp. Med., **29**, 1-24. Also pp. 25, 31 and following.

MUTHMANN, E. 1913. Beiträge zur vergleichenden Anatomie des Blinddarms und der lymphoiden Organe des Darmkanales bei Säugetieren und Vögeln. Anat. Hefte, **48**, H. 144, 65-114.

NAÑAGAS, J. C. 1933. Contributions to the study of the internal secreting glands in Filipinos. I. Topography and size of the thymus. Philipp. J. Sci., **51**, 281-322.

NEUGARTEN, L. 1921. Ueber das Gewicht der Milz bei gesunden Erwachsenen. Anat. Anz., **54** (11), 229-235.

OHMURA, T. 1928. Experimentelle Studien über die Thymusdrüse. II. Zustand während der Schwangerschaft und nach der Entbindung. Jibiinko ka, **1** (quoted in Hammar, 1936).

OPPENHEIM, F. 1925. Ueber die Häufigkeit einzelner Befunde bei 100 in Shanghai ausgeführten Chinesensektionen. Tungchi. Med. Monatschr., **1**, 1-33.

OPPENHEIMER, C. 1889. Ueber die Wachstumverhältnisse des Körpers und der Organe. Ztschr. f. Biol., **25**, 328-343.

OSGOOD, E. E. 1935. Normal hematologic standards. Arch. Int. Med., **56**, 849-863.

PATON, D. N. 1926. The relationship of the thymus and testes to growth. Edinb. Med. J., **33**, 351-356.

PEARL, R., AND BACON, A. L. 1924. Biometrical studies in pathology. III. The absolute weight of the heart and spleen in tuberculous persons. Johns Hopkins Hosp. Repts., **21** (V), 297-377.

PICCHIO, T. S. 1933. Ricerche sul timo di lophius budegassa Spin. e sulle sue modificazione nell' adulto. Arch. Ital. Anat., **31**, 549-568.

POL, R. 1923. Zur Funktionsfrage der lymphadenoiden Organe, insbesondere der Tonsillen. Verh. deut. path. Ges., **19**, 286-289.

POPOFF, N. W. 1927. The histogenesis of the thymus as shown by tissue cultures. Arch. exp. Zellf., **4**, 395-418.

RICH, A. 1936. Inflammation in Resistance to Infection. Arch. Path., **22**, 228-254.

RIDDLE, O., AND FREY, P. 1924-25. The growth and age involution of the thymus in male and female pigeons. Am. J. Physiol., **71**, 413-429.

RÖSSLE, R. 1923. Wachstum und Altern. Ergeb., Path., **20**, 369-569.

RÖSSLE, R., AND ROULET, F. 1932. Mass und Zahl in der Pathologie. Berlin: Springer, 144 pp.

RUSKOFF, P. R. 1933. Das Thymusgewicht bei Neugeborenen. Bern: Dissertation; also

———— 1934. Virch. Arch., **293**, 113-128.

SALKIND, J. 1915. Contribution histologique à la biologie comparée du thymus. Arch. Zool. exper., **55**, 81-322.

SAPPEY, C. 1873-74. Traité d'anatomie descriptive. Paris: Delahaye, **4**, 803 pp.

SCHILLING, V. 1928. Physiologie der blutbildenden Organe. In A. Bethe et al's Handb. d. nor. und pathol. Physiol. Berlin: Springer, **VI/2**, pp. 730-894.

SCHIRBER, A. 1930. Ein Beitrag zur Anatomie und Rückbildung des Thymus bei der Ziege. Berlin: Veter. Dissertation.

SCHÖNBERGER, M. 1928. Die Grösse der Gaumentonsillen im Kindesalter. Ztschr. f. Kinderheilk., **39**, 367-371.

SCHRIDDE, H. 1911. Die Bedeutung der eosinophil-gekörnten Blutzellen im menschlichen Thymus. Münch. med. Wchnschr., **58**, 2593-2596.

———— 1923. Die blutbereitenden Organe. In L. Aschoff's Pathologische Anatomie, 6th ed., **10**, 400 pp. Jena: Fischer.

Sciclunoff, N. 1933. Die Funktion der Tonsillen. Ein Sammelreferat. Rostock: Dissertation.

Severeanu, G. 1909. Die Lymphagefässe der Thymus. Arch. Anat. and Physiol. pp. 93-98. Anat. Abt.

Shellshear, J. L. 1924. The thymus gland in the Chinese. Caduceus, J. HongKong Med. Sch., **3**, 58-67.

Shimpei, E. 1921. Ueber die Involution der Thymusdrüse der Pferdes. Japan. J. Med. Sci., **1** (quoted by Hammar, 1936).

Söderlund, G., and Backman, A. 1909. Studien über die Thymusinvolution. Die Altersveränderungen der Thymusdrüse beim Kaninchen. Arch. mikr. Anat., **73**, 699-725.

Stefanelli, C. 1936. L'Appendicite acuta nei soggetti de eta nel vecchio. Policlinico, Sez Chir., **43**, 644-651.

Sukiennikow, W. 1903. Topographische Anatomie der bronchialen und trachealen lymphdrüsen. Berlin: Dissertation.

Swain, H. L. 1886. Die Balgdrüsen am Zungengrunde und deren Hypertrophie. Deut. Arch. f. klin. Med., **39**, 504-530.

Syk, I. 1909. Ueber Altersveränderungen in der Anzahl der Hassallschen Körper nebst einem Beitrag zum Studium der Mengenverhältnisse der Mitosen in der Kaninchenthymus. Anat. Anz., **34**, 560-567.

Symington, J. 1910. The pharyngeal tonsil. Brit. Med. J., **1**, 1147-1148.

Thursfield, H. 1929. Diseases of the Haemopoietic and Lymphatic Systems. In Garrod's Diseases of Children. London: Ed. Arnold & Co. 1106 pp.

Todd, T. W. 1936. Integral growth of the face, I. The nasal area. Internat. J. Orthodontia and Oral Surg., **22**, 321-332.

Toldt, C. 1888. Lehrbuch der Gewebelehre, 3rd ed. Stuttgart: Enke, 708 pp.

Vierordt, H. 1893. Daten und Tabellen. Jena: Fischer, 400 pp.

Waschinsky, G. 1925. Ueber den Thymus des Schweine. Berlin: Veter. Dissertation.

Watanabe, T. 1929. Thymusstudien I. Die Altersveränderungen des Thy-musgewichtes und ihre Beziehung zum Wachstum des Körpergewichte und der Geschlechtsdrüsen, Trans. Japan. Path. Soc., **17**, 332-340; also Ibid., **18**, 286-289; and Ibid., **20**, 257-262, 1930.

Wessel, O. 1933. Die Lymphozytendurchwanderung durch das Epithelium der Tonsillen. Rostock: Dissertation.

West, L. S. 1928. Observations on the lymphatic nodule, particularly with reference to histological changes encountered in senescence. Anat. Rec., **28**, 349-366.

Wetzel, G. 1928. Die Blutbildenden Organe. In Peter et al's Handb. d. Anat. des Kindes. I/1, 140-189. München: Bergmann.

Wilson, J. G. 1906. Some anatomic and physiological considerations of the faucial tonsil. J. Am. Med. Assn., **46**, 1591-1595.

Young, M., and Turnbull, H. M. 1931. An analysis of the data collected by the Status Lymphaticus Investigation Committee. J. Path and Bact., **34**, 213-258.

Zacharow, J. 1891. Zur Frage über die Veränderungen der Lymphdrüsen im Greisenalter. St. Petersburg: Dissertation.

CHAPTER 9

DIGESTIVE SYSTEM

A. C. IVY
Chicago

A question of prime importance to the ageing person is the likelihood of death from disease of this system. Although mortality statistics are not conveniently grouped so as to answer such a question accurately, the following rough comparisons are possible. Death in persons above 45 years of age is about as frequent from all diseases of the digestive system (7.0 per cent) as from chronic nephritis, slightly more frequent than from cerebral hemorrhage and paralysis, and about one-third as frequent as death from diseases of the heart. This relatively high rating of the diseases of the digestive system as a cause of death is due principally to the fact that cancer of the digestive organs is so prevalent. Cancer of the stomach, liver, gallbladder and bile ducts comprise almost one-third of the total of all forms of cancer. Two and six-tenths (2.6) per cent of all deaths are due to cancer of the stomach, liver and biliary passages. In addition, 13.6 per cent of all forms of cancer arise from the peritoneum, intestine, colon and rectum, and comprise 1.1 per cent of total deaths (Dublin and Lotka, 1937). To this should be added cancer of the buccal cavity (3.1 per cent of all forms of cancer and 0.25 per cent of deaths from all causes), and also of the pancreas. Thus, at least one-half of all forms of cancer which cause death arise in the organs or tissues of the digestive system, and account for more than one-half of the deaths due to diseases of the digestive system in persons above 45 years of age.

Some important sex differences exist. Cancer of the buccal cavity is six or seven times more frequent in males. Cancer of the stomach in males causes more than twice as many deaths as cancer of any other organ, and ranks second only to the uterus in females. According to Ewing (1931), cancer of the gallbladder affects four women to one man. This accounts for the higher incidence (about 22 per cent) of deaths from cancer of the liver and biliary passage in women, as is revealed by mortality statistics which do not separate deaths due to cancer of the liver and of the biliary passages (Dublin and Lotka, 1937).

Hepatic diseases rank next to cancer of the digestive organs as a cause of death in persons above 45 years; they account for about 1.6 per cent of deaths. Cirrhosis of the liver heads the list (about 0.9 per cent) and causes death in males about twice as frequently as in females. The death rate from biliary calculi (0.33 per cent) is about the same as the total from the other hepatic diseases (0.38 per cent), cancer and cirrhosis being excluded, and causes death about three times more frequently in females than in males (Dublin and Lotka, 1937).

Ulcer of the stomach and duodenum as a cause of death in the mature adult ranks third in importance among the diseases of the digestive system. Ulcer of the stomach causes death more frequently than ulcer of the duodenum, although the latter occurs more frequently. Both types of ulcer occur more frequently in males and cause more deaths in males. Deaths from these diseases do not become numerically important until after the age of 35, after which they increase up to the age of 75 (Dublin and Lotka, 1937).

Other fatal conditions due to disturbances of the digestive system that increase with age are intestinal obstruction, diverticulitis of the colon, and pernicious anemia. Hernia, one of the causes of intestinal obstruction, increases with age. Diseases of the pancreatic acinar tissue other than cancer rarely cause death. Deaths from diarrhea and enteritis, which occur for the most part in the years under 5, show an increase above the age of 55, indicating that the aged are susceptible and easily exhausted (Dublin and Lotka, 1937).

It will become evident from the discussion to follow that death from disturbances of the digestive organs is more frequently due to a disease not directly related to a wearing out or ageing process per se. Or, most elderly persons die with a digestive system, when not locally altered by cancer or by a toxic or an infectious process, that is capable of functioning beyond the ordinary life span. This will be demonstrated by an analysis of the available evidence pertaining to the development, maturity and involution of the functional activities of the digestive organs. In such an analysis it is necessary to attempt to distinguish between the functional and structural changes due to ageing per se and to disease. In fact, the chief purpose of this chapter is to summarize what is known concerning the functional and structural changes due to ageing.

1. SALIVARY GLANDS

1. *Anatomy.*

Data on the growth of the submaxillary gland have been provided for the rat by Donaldson (1924), but the effect of age has not been determined. In the human, Scammon (1923) has found that the salivary glands increase about three times in weight during the first three months, and about five times during the first two years after birth. The connective tissue and ducts are relatively more plentiful than the parenchyma in the salivary glands of the infant than in those of the adult. The glands do not become histologically typical of those of the adult until the end of the second year. According to Warthin (1929), the salivary glands of the aged are atrophied, but decisive evidence is not available. Goodpasture (1918), who studied the histology of the submaxillary gland in fifty old stray dogs, found degenerative changes which occurred most uniformly in the cells lining the intermediate ducts. These cells are considered to be the chief contributors of water to the saliva by Stormont (1928). Their degeneration in the aged may explain the observed reduction in the volume of saliva secreted by the aged.

Hamperl (1931, 1933) has reported that numerous large cells with acidophilic granules in their cytoplasm and pyknotic nuclei may be found in the salivary glands of elderly people. He has termed these cells "onkocytes." Up to the age of 30 years, these cells are found only in occasional cases, whereas after the age of 70 years, they are invariably present in considerable numbers. Although Steinhardt (1933) was unable to recognize "onkocytes" in his cases, Hamperl (1937) has reaffirmed their existence. Their physiological significance is highly speculative.

2. *Salivary secretion.*

Ptyalin is present in the mixed saliva of newborn and even of prematurely born infants. Its concentration increases during the first year, at the end of which it usually reaches the concentration found in young adults (Nicory, 1922; Mayer, 1929; Cocchi, 1924).

The only data available, which renders a comparison of the salivary secretion of young and old adults possible, is that obtained by Meyer and his collaborators (1937). Their essential experimental data are shown in table 11. In the aged, the concentration of ptyalin and the volume output of saliva on chewing "diabetic gum" are less, and the specific gravity of the saliva is slightly greater than in the young adult. The ptyalin concentration in the basal and stimulated secretion among the different individuals in the older group did not vary appreciably; greater variations between individuals occurred in the younger group. The basal secretion of ptyalin was quite constant in the individuals of both groups. A remarkable constancy of the ptyalin concentration of the stimulated saliva was observed in the individuals in the older group. Freeman (1930), studying the concentration of diastase in non-stimulated mixed saliva in 193 subjects varying from 20 to over 60 years of age, found no significant change with age. The method he used is open to objection. His most interesting observation was that in 63 per cent of 27 subjects without teeth, the reaction of the oral secretions was either neutral or alkaline. This indicates that in edentulous subjects the mouth tends to be more frequently neutral or alkaline than acid in reaction.

Such a salivary deficiency in the aged is known to occur clinically, and might be anticipated on the basis of the atrophy of the salivary glands which is alleged to be found in old people. No data are available which indicate the age of onset of the morphological and physiological

TABLE 11

A comparison of salivary secretion in young and old adults

Number of subjects	Age	Ptyalin		Stimulated secretion	
		Basal secretion	Stimulated secretion	Specific gravity, average	Volume
	years	*units per cc.*	*units per cc.*		*cc.*
12	21–31	2.4–22.2	2–14.3	1.004	13.6–15.0
	Av. 25	Av. 10.15	Av. 8.2		Av. 14.2
27	69–100	0.19–0.48	0.18–0.42	1.009	1.5–15
	Av. 81	Av. 0.30	Av. 0.28		Av. 5.8

Compiled from data provided by Meyer, Golden, Steiner and Necheles, 1937.

decline of the salivary glands. Studies on lower animals, where the question might be more readily answered have not been made.

In view of the evidence persons above 70 years of age have a relative deficiency of starch digestion in the mouth and stomach. Normally at least 60 per cent of the starch of a meal, containing five ounces of bread or potatoes, is digested in the mouth and stomach (Bergeim, 1926; Ivy, Schmidt and Beazell, 1936). For example, two ounces of well-baked white bread would be digested easily and completely in the mouth and stomach of the young adult, whereas only 5 per cent of it would be digested by most persons over the age of 70. Of course, the pancreatic amylase, unless deficient in amount, is sufficient to digest all the cooked starch usually ingested. But, nothing is known concerning the secretion of pancreatic amylase in the aged, or the amount of starch that may be ingested by old persons without starch appearing in the feces.

2. ESOPHAGUS

No evidence worthy of mention regarding the effect of ageing on the esophagus is available. Schatzki (1932) who studied 30 old persons ranging from 65 to 83 years of age, believes that the esophago-diaphragmatic hiatus becomes with ageing a point of lowered resistance, which predisposes to the development of diverticula and herniae. The concept is interesting but not established as a fact by the evidence available.

3. STOMACH

1. *Growth and senescence of the stomach as indicated by the postmortem weight of the organ.*

The data (Scammon, 1919 and 1923; Boyd, 1861), show that the weight of the stomach increases up to the age of 20, after which it remains stationary and does not show a definite decrease in weight until after the age of 80. The biological significance of this observation is to be doubted, because the only reliable data would be obtained from cases of death due to accident. Chronic undernutrition increases rather than decreases the weight of the stomach (Miller, 1927). Further, all post-mortem weights of the stomach should be checked histologically, since the edema of gastritis would increase the weight of the stomach and mask an actual decrease in tissue. The factor of edema would best be determined by ascertaining wet and dry weights. Goodpasture (1918) found multiple polyps in the mucosa of the pyloric antrum in 7 of 50 old dogs; evidences of atrophic changes were not noted. Unchallengeable evidence pertaining to the effect of ageing per se on the morphology of the stomach does not exist.

2. *Gastric secretion.*

Considerable evidence is available concerning the relation of the acidity of the gastric contents after test-meals to age, especially in those decades above the second. Little evidence is available regarding the volume output and the peptic activity of gastric juice in the various age groups. The reasons for this are: (a) methods, which yield a fairly accurate value for the volume output of gastric juice, have been available only for a relatively short period; and (b) it has been generally assumed that whenever free acid is present, pepsin is also present; this is an assumption that is generally, but not always, true.

It is established that at birth the gastric mucosa of most mammals is differentiated sufficiently to secrete acid gastric juice. Concentration of acid and pepsin is lower than found later (Carlson, 1923). In fact, the stomach of the premature infant secretes acid juice (Pollitzer, 1921; Moritz and Schmitt, 1933), and the gastric glands of fetal cats and dogs shortly before term respond to histamine (gastrin) (Sutherland, 1921). The mechanisms for the gastric and intestinal phases of gastric secretion are ready to function at birth, and the mechanisms for the cephalic phase (appetite secretion) become functional during the first year (Taylor, 1917b; Dordi, 1931).

It is well established that the acidity of the gastric contents of new born infants and sucklings is low. The incidence of absolute achlorhydria as determined by the response to histamine has not been studied. Izumita (1930a) using a test-meal, which does not constitute a reliable test for absolute anacidity, found three instances of achlorhydria among 52 infants varying in age up to 72 hours. Five instances of achlorhydria were found among 36 sucklings up to 12 months of age.

A study of 330 children, ranging from 5 to 17 years, by Wright (1924) and Klumph and Neale (1930), who used a test-meal, yielded three probable but not proven cases of anacidity. The average acidity was lower than that of the adult. In the subjects used by Klumph and Neale, the average free acidity did not begin to approach the adult range until after 4 years of age.

Actual data (Neale, 1930; Dietrick and Shelby, 1931; Siemsen, 1932) on the results of histamine tests are available on only 63 children ranging from 0.5 to 14 years of age. No instances of achlorhydria are reported. It would be important to have data on a larger series of children to settle the question whether congenital or hereditary absolute achlorhydria ever occurs. *It is certain that most of the cases of anacidity or achlorhydria that occur in later life do not date from birth.* However, it is apparent from the histamine and test-meal data that a wide range of variability in response occurs in early life. The high and low secretory responses that occur in adults also occur in children. A high or low response is apparently a quality inherent in an individual at an early age.

The mean free acidity resulting from an Ewald meal has been determined from data in the literature by Vanzant and her collaborators (1932, 1933), for 162 boys and 203 girls ranging in age from 1 to 20 years. On referring to figure 29, it will be observed that the mean free acidity rises to a plateau about the age of 10 where it remains until the onset of puberty. From 3 years of age, the mean free acidity of the males is somewhat higher than that of the females. During puberty in males the mean free acidity rises rapidly to a plateau about the age of 18 or 19. In females a rise occurs with the onset of puberty but a plateau is not reached until about 25 years of age. The plateau of acidity is considerably lower in the female than in the male. After the age of 40 the mean acidity of the males gradually declines until it reaches the mean acidity of the females which has not changed since the age of 25 or 30 years. (Analogous data are presented by Sagal, Marks and Kantor, 1933.)

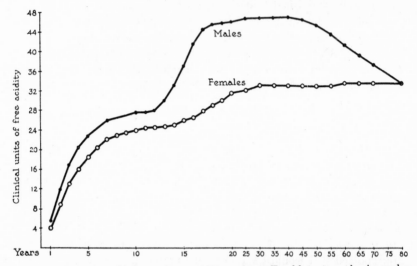

Fig. 29. Showing the mean free acidity values, Ewald test-meals, in males and females. The portion of the curve from 1 to 20 years of age includes tests on 203 girls and 162 boys; from 20 to 79 years of age includes tests on 3,381 subjects. The curves are made from data supplied by Vanzant, Alvarez, Berkson and Eusterman (1933).

Similar data of significance, obtained by means of the histamine test, are not available for the age group under 20 years. However, Polland (1933) provides valuable data for the various decades from 20 to 70 years. The essential features of his data are illustrated in figures 30, 31 and 32. When the mean acidity alone is considered (fig. 30), the instances of achlorhydria being excluded, it is evident that the mean acidity falls with age in males but not females. This result is analogous to that obtained with an Ewald meal (fig. 29). However, the histamine test permits a fairly reliable estimate of the volume of juice secreted.

On referring to figure 31, graph "A", it is clear that females secrete less juice at all decades above 20 years than males, and that the volume

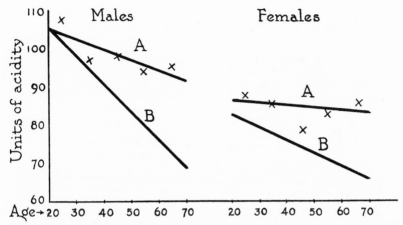

FIG. 30. Histamine test. Standards of normal of maximum acidity observed, showing the relation of total acidity to age in 384 males and 270 females. "A," excluding cases of anacidity; "B," including cases of anacidity. "A" includes 326 males and 224 females with free acidity after histamine (Polland, 1933).

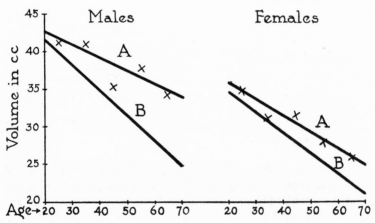

FIG. 31. Histamine test. Standards of normal of maximum quantity of juice secreted during any 10-minute period after histamine, showing relation of volume to age. "A," excluding cases of anacidity and "B" including cases of anacidity (Polland, 1933).

of juice decreases significantly as age advances. Knowing both the volume and acidity of the juice secreted, it is possible to estimate roughly the total amount of acid secreted at each decade. When this is done, an important observation is made, namely, that with advancing age a similar percentage decrease in acid production occurs in both sexes (fig. 32). If both volume and acidity are not considered, it would appear that total acid production decreased with age only in male subjects, which is indicated by the observations by Vanzant and her collaborators (fig. 29).

It has been definitely demonstrated that *the incidence of achlorhydria increases with advancing age.* This is well illustrated by the data

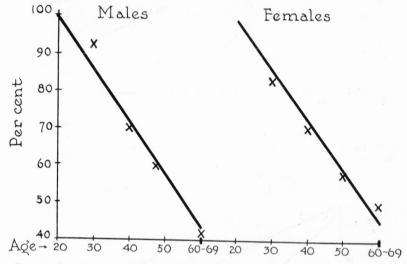

Fig. 32. Showing percentage decrease in total output of acid (volume times acidity) with age in normal persons. Note that when the volume of secretion is considered, the total acid secreted decreases with age similarly in both sexes. When acidity alone is considered, a decrease appears to occur only in the male, as indicated in figures 29 and 30 (Polland, 1933).

(table 12) obtained by Ewald test-meals and compiled by Bloomfield and Polland (1933). It is confirmed by the histamine data obtained by Polland (table 13) on 644 "normal" subjects. As might be expected the percentage of achlorhydria is less with histamine than with the Ewald test-meal.

A sex difference in the occurrence of achlorhydria has been observed by a number of investigators. Vanzant's data revealed achlorhydria to be present in 17.4 per cent of females and 12.9 per cent of males; Polland's (table 13) in 14.2 per cent of females and 10.8 per cent of males. Although the total incidence of achlorhydria is greater in females than males, the increase in achlorhydria with age is greater in males. The low mean acidity of females is apparently related to a higher general incidence of achlorhydria; and when the mean acidity of the males begins to decline after the age of forty, a rapid increase in achlorhydria in males occurs. These observations suggest that

TABLE 12

Percentage incidence of achlorhydria in various decades of life. Ewald test-meal (Bloomfield and Polland, 1933)

Age	Number of subjects	Number of cases of anacidity	Per cent with anacidity
years			
20–24	866	46	5.3
30–39	1,354	137	9.5
40–49	1,299	224	16.7
50–59	1,043	250	24.0
60+	642	227	35.4
	5,204	884	16.9

TABLE 13

Relation of achlorhydria to age and sex in 644 "normal" people. Histamine tests (Polland, 1933)

Age	Males			Females			Both sexes, per cent incidence
	Number of cases	Total anacidity	Per cent	Number of cases	Total anacidity	Per cent	
years							
20–29	70	2	2.9	43	2	4.7	3.5
30–39	86	3	3.5	67	5	7.5	5.2
40–49	107	12	10.0	68	13	19.1	14.2
50–59	65	9	13.9	50	9	18.0	15.6
60–69	35	11	31.7	32	7	21.9	26.8
70+	14	4	28.6	7	2	28.6	28.5
	377	41	10.8	267	38	14.2	12.2

achlorhydria is simply an exaggeration of the wide variations in the gastric secretory response of different individuals to a test-meal or histamine. That is, *achlorhydria apparently results from a "physiological" involution and becomes manifest first in those persons who are endowed constitutionally with a less responsive and a more vulnerable gastric secretory mechanism.*

The foregoing view is justified by the data obtained from the use of the histamine test. However, the data obtained by the Ewald test-meal may be interpreted differently. For example, the decline in mean acidity in males after 40 (fig. 29) is probably not due to a progressive senile atrophy of the gastric mucosa, because a similar decline does not occur in females. Also, the increase in the incidence of achlorhydria with age cannot be attributed to senile atrophy because the distribution curve does not show a parallel shift to lower values in men and women. For these reasons Vanzant and her collaborators (1932) believe that the process which gives rise to achlorhydria is different from the one which is concerned in the decline of acidity in males after 40 years. They believe the process which gives rise to achlorhydria is inherited.

Thus, one who believes that the test-meal method is the most physiological test has reason to hold a view, in regard to the way age influences gastric secretion, different from one who believes that the histamine method yields the best criteria of acid production. Neither method is accurate, because the response of the same individual to a test-meal or histamine varies considerably from day to day. Regardless of that fact, the number of subjects studied renders the trends observed highly probable. Since the author in his experience has found the histamine test to yield more constant data in man and dogs, and to be the most certain test of the capacity of the gastric glands to secrete acid, and to yield more accurate values of the volume of juice secreted, he is inclined to accept the interpretation of Bloomfield and Polland, which recognizes the probable existence of a constitutional factor.

When the apparent effect of puberty, particularly in males (fig. 29), and the decline in acidity that occurs after forty years are considered, an endocrine factor immediately comes to mind. It is known that relatively large doses of Theelin and Antuitrin S have no effect on gastric secretion in the male or female dog (Atkinson and Ivy, 1938); but the effect of testosterone and castration is not known.

The evolution of the secretory mechanisms and the morphological growth of the stomach are factors which undoubtedly account for some of the increase in the mean acidity from birth to maturity (Scammon, 1919). The mean free acidity increases about eight times, whereas the surface area of the gastric mucosa increases about seventeen times, the glandular bodies about twelve times (Scammon, 1919; Toldt, 1880; Vanzant, Alvarez and Berkson, 1936–37).

As has been indicated previously, the relative and absolute achlorhydria associated with advancing age has been attributed to senile atrophy of the gastric mucosa. Much of the data supporting such a claim has come from a study of the stomach of patients dying from all sorts of diseases. Lubarsch and Borchardt (1929), who view the matter critically, tacitly accept the claim. That such an atrophy actually occurs has not been proved; as a hypothesis it is reasonable.

In fact, no unanimity of opinion exists in regard to the relation of gastritis to the etiology of achlorhydria. Faber (1927, 1935) believes that achlorhydria is most commonly due to a chronic gastritis resulting from infectious diseases or the ingestion of irritating substances. It is well known from experimental and clinical observations that strong irritants and most infectious diseases produce a temporary achlorhydria. Continued or repeated insults, as with alcohol for example (Thomsen, 1925), may produce atrophic gastritis with achlorhydria. Martius, Hurst and others (Oliver and Wilkinson, 1933), present evidence on the constitutional origin of achlorhydria and cite its tendency to occur in many members of the family. In some instances the probabilities of multiple incidence in the same family, on the basis of the incidence of achlorhydria in the general "healthy" population, are not adequately considered. Much of the evidence, however, is adequate to show that certain families manifest an inborn defective gastric secretory mechanism. The view of Einhorn (1892) that achlorhydria is or may be neurogenic in origin also has its adherents among clinicians (Cheney, 1926; Schmidt, 1911; Oliver and Wilkinson, 1933). In this connection, it is of interest that Schnedorf and Ivy (1937) studied eight monkeys which manifested achlorhydria to histamine for a period of from two to eight months. They found that after one or two doses of mecholyl, a parasympathetic stimulating drug, the stomach of the monkeys became responsive to histamine.

Because of the numerous uncontrollable factors which may operate in man and contribute to the development of achlorhydria and chronic and atrophic gastritis, it would appear that the effect of age on the morphology and secretory activity of the gastric glands will have to be decided by carefully performed experiments on laboratory animals.

3. *The consequences of achlorhydria.*

It is well known that many persons may have achlorhydria for years and remain in good health. The effect of the condition on the life span is unknown. On the basis of experimental studies on animals, persons with achlorhydria should be more exposed to gastrointestinal infections because of the loss of the relative "sterilizing" action of gastric acid (Arnold, 1933); they should be more prone to develop a hypochromic microcytic anemia because of the rôle that gastric acid plays in the absorption of iron (Ivy, Richter, Meyer, and Greengard, 1934; Ivy, Morgan, and Farrell, 1931); and, they, especially growing children, should manifest defective calcification of the bones (Bussabarger, Freeman, and Ivy, 1938). Subacute combined degeneration of the spinal cord and pernicious anemia do not occur in animals rendered achlorhydric or achylic by total gastrectomy (Ivy, Richter, Meyer and Greengard, 1934). In man it is known that achlorhydria (*a*) occurs almost constantly in pernicious anemia and subacute combined degeneration of the spinal cord, (*b*) is frequently associated with hypochromic microcytic anemia, and (*c*) is sometimes associated with diarrhea and vague digestive complaints. The treatment of achlorhydria and its association with various diseases, such as allergic disease, certain dermatoses, glossitis, and rheumatoid arthritis has been reviewed by Oliver and Wilkinson (1933).

Atrophic changes of the mucosa of the tongue are apparently more frequent in elderly persons with achlorhydria than in those with normal acid values (Davies and James, 1930–31). This is more related to dietary deficiency than to achlorhydria (Hutter and Middleton, 1933). The relation of senile osteoporosis to anacidity is uncertain.

4. *Pernicious anemia.*

It appears to be well established that the etiology of pernicious anemia is at least in part due to a functional disturbance of the gastrointestinal tract. The stomach and probably the intestine secretes an "intrinsic factor" of the nature of an enzyme. The "intrinsic factor" acts on an "extrinsic factor" in the food so as to elaborate an "essential substance" for the normal maturation of red blood cells or for the prevention of pernicious anemia. This being the case, the process of ageing, or factors contributing to an atrophy of the gastrointestinal tract, may tend to decrease the elaboration of the intrinsic factor; and hence, an increase in the incidence of pernicious anemia would occur with ageing. Since in most cases of pernicious anemia it is known that the intrinsic factor is absent or markedly reduced in amount and that the administration of the "essential substance" (liver; the essential substance is stored in the liver) will control pernicious anemia, the bone marrow is not primarily at fault.

Achlorhydria is of great diagnostic importance in pernicious anemia

(Castle and Minot, 1936; Cornell, 1927; Davidson and Gulland, 1930). In some instances it is known that achlorhydria may be present for many years before definite anemia results.   There is no case on record in which achlorhydria appeared after the anemia, and in rare instances only has the achlorhydria disappeared after the relief of the anemia by liver therapy.   Further, numerous definite instances of familial pernicious anemia have been reported, but familial achlorhydria may apparently occur without pernicious anemia resulting in the family (Wilkinson and Brockbank, 1931).

Such considerations suggest that the age incidence of pernicious anemia might bear some relation to that of achlorhydria.   The results

TABLE 14

Pernicious anemia mortality

Age	Part A. Average annual death rates per 100,000—Dublin and Lotka Metropolitan Insured Group				Part B. Mortality Statistics Bureau of the Census, U. S. A.		
	Males		Females		Years	Deaths	
	1921*–1935	1931–1935	1921*–1935	1931–1935		Males	Females
1–74	2.4*	1.9†	3.3*	2.1†	1932	1,559	1,709
					1931	1,535	1,584
25–34	0.5	0.4	1.2	0.6	1930	1,564	1,706
35–44	1.9	1.0	3.3	1.6	1929	1,420	1,651
45–54	4.6	3.0	7.2	3.9	1928	1,440	1,682
55–64	12.0	9.5	15.4	9.3	1927	1,811	2,222
65–74	20.2	18.2	24.4	19.6		9,329	10,554
						47%	53%

* Thirty-seven per cent higher in females than males.
† Ten per cent higher in females than males.

of a study of 1071 cases by Cabot (1927), show that the disease is between six and seven times more common after the 35th year than before, and is rare under the age of 20 years.   This is confirmed by data provided by Davidson and Gulland (1930).   Although their data give an idea of the "clinical age incidence" of the disease, they do not provide information regarding the true age incidence.   They fail to consider the relation of the age of their patients with pernicious anemia to the number of persons surviving at the various ages.   That the "true incidence" of pernicious anemia increases with age is better indicated by mortality statistics (table 14, part A).   It can hardly be doubted that the incidence of this disease like that of achlorhydria increases with age.

Does a sex difference exist in the incidence of pernicious anemia as it does in achlorhydria? The clinical reports vary widely in regard to the sex incidence of pernicious anemia. In practically every report the male and female population of the clinic from which the report comes is not considered. So, in some instances the males with pernicious anemia markedly outnumber the females; for example, Cabot (1927), found that the disease was almost twice as common in males. In the anemia clinic of the Cook County Hospital, Chicago, from June, 1931 to December 1937, 490 patients with the disease were diagnosed and responded to liver therapy (Richter, 1938). Of these, 255 were males and 235 females. However, when the sex ratio is corrected for the male and female population of the medical service of the Hospital during the period, 0.415 per cent of males and 0.684 per cent of females had the disease. The mortality statistics from the Bureau of Census of the U. S. A. for the period 1927 to 1932, a period when the criteria for the diagnosis of the disease were quite well-known, show a ratio of 47 males to 53 females (table 14, part B). The mortality from pernicious anemia in the group insured by the Metropolitan Life Insurance Company for the period of 1931 to 1935, the most comparable period for which data were available, was 10 per cent higher in females (Dublin and Lotka, 1937). Data collected by Cornell (1927) from various countries other than the U. S. A. prior to the introduction of liver therapy showed a mortality from the disease of 47.5 per cent in males and 52.5 per cent in females, which difference is analogous to that shown by the Bureau of Census statistics. But, with the data available from the various sources, it is not possible by a legitimate statistical inquiry to determine whether the increased incidence of achlorhydria in females correlates well with the increased incidence of pernicious anemia in females.

Thus, it appears that a decline or disappearance of the "intrinsic factor" may occur with advancing age; but whether the decline is due to ageing *per se*, or is related directly to achlorhydria or to gastritis and their causes is uncertain.

5. *Gastric and duodenal ulcer, or "peptic ulcer."*

As indicated before, the mean acidity of the gastric contents and the incidence of gastritis are related to age and sex. Many believe that gastritis is a factor in the etiology of gastric ulcer, and that gastric acidity is a factor in the etiology of duodenal ulcer and contributes to the chronicity of both types of ulcer. It is widely maintained that "peptic ulcer" is due to some sort of dysfunction rather than to an infectious process. These considerations lead one to inquire whether "peptic ulcer" may be related to the ageing process.

Gastric and duodenal ulcer are diseases generally characterized by remissions and recurrences (Eusterman and Balfour, 1936). These diseases have frequently existed in the patient for from ten to twenty years before death results from hemorrhage or perforation with peritonitis, or before the patient seeks relief from surgery (table 15). Also, the ulcer may heal and not recur (Portis and Jaffe, 1938). It is well known that the incidence of and mortality from gastric and duodenal ulcer vary widely in different populations. These considerations, even though the onset of symptoms of and the death rate from "peptic ulcer" is related to age, indicate that ageing per se is not etiologically involved; in fact, much evidence indicates that these diseases are related more to the mode of living and eating.

Nevertheless, the death rate from gastric ulcer (table 16) becomes progressively higher with advancing age up to 75 years in both males and females (Dublin and Lotka, 1937). The death rate from duodenal ulcer also increases slightly with advancing age. These observations would at first glance indicate that age is a factor in the incidence of "peptic ulcer." However, it is commonly recognized and agreed, as shown by the data in table 15 that the onset of "peptic ulcer" rarely occurs after the age of 60, or during the more tranquil conditions of old age. This fact associated with the fact that "peptic ulcer" is a disease of relatively long duration explains the observation that the death rate gradually increases as age advances up to 75 years. Further, clinical observation indicates that the perforation of an ulcer and hemorrhage, the most frequent causes of death from "peptic ulcer," are more serious in old than in young persons (Allen, 1933; Bohmansson, 1934; Chiesman, 1932; Christiansen, 1935). This is ascribed to the general lowered resistance of the aged and to the greater tendency in the aged to extensive hemorrhage due to the sclerosis of their blood vessels (Allen, 1933). Sclerosed blood vessels would also increase the tendency to perforation by becoming thrombosed and relatively devascularizing the area. Also, gastric ulcer causes death more frequently than duodenal ulcer, although duodenal ulcer occurs clinically more frequently than gastric; this is chiefly because the perforation and hemorrhage in gastric ulcer are more serious than perforation and hemorrhage from duodenal ulcer, and because a duodenal ulcer is more likely to cause symptoms than a gastric ulcer (Portis and Jaffe, 1938). This is supported by the observation that as age advances the death rate from gastric ulcer increases more than the death rate from duodenal ulcer (table 17).

TABLE 15

Age of onset of symptoms and age of operation of patients who had duodenal ulcer and gastric ulcer

(Eusterman and Balfour)

Age	Duodenal ulcer—onset of symptoms						Gastric ulcer—onset of symptoms					
	All patients			Operated on			All patients			Operated on		
	Male	Female	Total	Male	Female	Total	Male	Female	Total	Male	Female	Total
years												
6–10	6	0	6									
11–20	72	21	93	2	2	4	4	1	5			
21–30	181	49	230	62	17	79	39	9	48	9	3	12
31–40	171*	45*	216*	195	45	240	74	11	85	43	2	45
41–50	76	26	102	160*	49*	209*	62*	14*	76*	92*	22*	114*
51–60	40	6	46	99	15	124	32	12	44	49	17	66
61–70	5	3	8	27	12	39	12	3	15	26	6	32
71–80				6	0	6				4	0	4
Total.....	551	150	701	551	150	701	223	50	273	223	50	273
Average age.....	32.7	32.9	32.8	42.7	43.5	42.8	40.7	43.1	41.2	47.8	49.8	48.2

* Decade into which fall the average ages.

TABLE 16

Averages of annual death rates per 100,000 in whites
(Dublin and Lotka)

Age	Duodenal ulcer				Gastric ulcer			
	Males		Females		Males		Females	
	1931–1935	1921–1935	1931–1935	1921–1935	1931–1935	1911–1935	1931–1935	1911–1935
years								
20–24	0.8	0.7	0.2	0.2	1.0	1.7	0.6	1.1
25–34	2.8	2.4	0.2	0.4	4.1	4.4	0.9	1.7
35–44	5.5	5.1	0.9	0.9	11.8	10.7	1.7	3.0
45–54	8.5	7.0	1.2	1.3	21.4	16.8	3.7	4.7
55–64	10.9	7.9	1.9	1.8	25.4	18.8	5.3	7.1
65–74	9.9	7.6	2.1	1.6	26.0	20.8	8.0	12.4

The recent report of Portis and Jaffe (1938) on the incidence of gastric and duodenal ulcer as observed at necropsy is illuminating in regard to the preceding discussion. Their necropsy data indicate that the peak of the incidence of peptic ulcer coincides with those decades of life in which arteriosclerotic changes occur. When peptic ulcer was not the cause of death but was found incidentally during the necropsy, it was most often associated with cardiovascular disease. Thus, clinical, necropsy and mortality-rate statistics apparently tell different stories or parts of a complete story. The clinical statistics give the

TABLE 17

Incidence and percentage of active ulcers of the stomach and the duodenum in 9,171 consecutive autopsies from January 1, 1929 to December 31, 1936 in whites according to sex

(Portis and Jaffe, 1938)

Age group	Stomach						Duodenum					
	Males			Females			Males			Females		
	Essential lesion	Incidental lesion	Percentage	Essential lesion	Incidental lesion	Percentage	Essential lesion	Incidental lesion	Percentage	Essential lesion	Incidental lesion	Percentage
years												
0–5	0	0	0	0	0	0	0	1	0.2	0	0	0
6–10	2	0	2.1	0	0	0	0	0	0	0	1	1.7
11–20	0	1	0.4	0	0	0	2	2	1.8	0	0	0
21–30	2	1	1.7	1	0	0.6	1	2	1.7	1	0	0.6
31–40	3	4	2.2	2	1	1.1	10	3	4.2	2	0	0.7
41–50	5	15	3.0	0	1	0.3	10	0	2.8	0	1	0.3
51–60	17	21	5.1	0	4	1.4	8	6	1.8	1	0	0.3
61–70	11	13	4.0	1	9	4.6	8	14	3.7	0	6	2.7
Over 70	1	12	3.7	1	5	3.5	4	7	3.1	0	3	1.7
Total.....	41	67	2.9	5	20	1.3	43	35	2.3	4	11	0.7

The expression "essential lesion" means that the ulcer was dominant in the diagnosis.

The expression "incidental lesion" means that the ulcer was active but incidental to another cause of death.

period at which the patient complains to the physician. The necropsy statistics give the age incidence of the presence of ulcer as a cause of death, as an incidental observation in which the ulcer is either concomitant with or in part due to an associated fatal disease, and as a healed lesion. The mortality statistics give the age incidence of ulcer as a cause of death.

The greater tendency of males to both gastric and duodenal ulcer has been ascribed to the greater mean acidity of the gastric contents of the male during the years that the onset of ulcer is most frequent, and to the greater stress of living to which males are subjected in modern life. The death rate from gastric ulcer from 1931 to 1935 is almost five times greater in white males than females, and is about twice as great in colored men as colored women. The same is true of duodenal ulcer. If gastric acidity is a factor contributing to the chronicity of "peptic ulcer," and the experimental evidence so indicates, then relatively few patients after the age of fifty should complain of a "peptic ulcer" of recent onset; this is supported by clinical observation (table 15). Of course, the mode of living is also concerned. In the special case of gastric ulcer, gastritis, because its incidence increases with age and because it is thought to delay or to prevent healing, would tend to increase chronicity and to favor perforation and hemorrhage. This gastritis factor, in addition to the factors given in the preceding paragraph, would be in part concerned in the cause of the higher death rate from gastric ulcer as age advances.

6. *Relation of gastric ulcer to gastric carcinoma.*

The question of the relation of gastric ulcer to the etiology of gastric carcinoma, which is well known to increase with age (Dublin and Lotka, 1937), has been debated extensively in the literature (Hurst and Stewart, 1929; Newcomb, 1932). The question is important because cancer of the stomach is an important cause of death in males and females (Dublin and Lotka, 1937), particularly in the males, who have gastric ulcer more frequently than females. Fifty-one per cent of observers present evidence which indicates that not more than 10 per cent of gastric carcinomata arise in ulcers; 74 per cent of observers consider that less than 20 per cent of gastric cancers arise in ulcers (Newcomb, 1932). Those who believe that the cause of cancer is related to chronic irritation point out the increased incidence of gastritis with age. Goodpasture (1918) records the presence of polyps, an overgrowth of mucosa, in the gastric mucosa of old dogs. In view of the importance of gastric cancer as a cause of death, the morphologic changes that occur in the gastric mucosa with age have certainly not received the attention they deserve.

7. *The relation of the occurrence of post-operative jejunal ulcer to age.*

That post-operative jejunal ulcer is less likely to occur when a gastro-jejunostomy is performed after the age of 50 is a clinical impression widely accepted. The impression is supported by some statistical evidence (Judd and Hoerner, 1935; Perman, 1935), and is usually ascribed to the decline in gastric acidity that occurs with age.

8. *Gastric motor activity. The position and peristaltic activity of the stomach.*

The position and shape of the stomach depends on the arrangement and development of the different muscular layers and their tone. Some believe that the relative amount of fat present in the abdomen, and the tone of the abdominal musculature are also concerned; such a view has been questioned, however (Hurst and Stewart, 1929; Moody, 1927; Moody Van Nuys and Chamberlain, 1923; Wright, 1924).

The shape of *the infant's stomach*, when filled, like that of the adult's is not fixed. It may manifest the form of a flask lying on its side, or it may be oval or globular (Scammon, 1923). It is more frequently located horizontally and obliquely than vertically. The more vertical position, or J-shape, characteristic of many children and most adults first appears about the age of 3 years.

Peristalses are difficult to observe in the infant's stomach, because the waves are not as deep as those which occur later. The peristaltic mechanism is present at or soon after birth because in the presence of hypertrophic pyloric stenosis, which may become manifest a few weeks after birth, visible peristalses are evident on inspection of the abdominal wall (Ivy, 1937). Active peristalses are evident at 3 months (De Buys and Henrique, 1918).

Wright (1924) has studied carefully the position and shape of the *stomach of healthy children* (243 subjects) ranging from 6 to 15 years. He found the shape and position to vary widely, but the variation became greater with the approach of puberty. The J-shaped stomach became the characteristic type at 12 years of age. The position of the stomach was the same in males and females up to the age of 11, after which the females manifested a tendency to have lower stomachs. Moody (1927) found the stomach to be higher in British boys 7 to 14 years of age than in men of medical school age. The foregoing observations and those of others show that "gastroptosis" and "gastric atony" are rare in children (Schiff, 1923), and that the shape and position of the stomach changes with age. The change to the characteristic adult type begins at the age of 3 and becomes definite after the age of 11, when the first evidence of a sex difference appears.

The position and shape of the stomach have been studied in 600 young adults of university age, equally distributed between the sexes, by Moody, Van Nuys, and Chamberlain (1923). The J-shaped stomach, reaching from 3 to 7 cm. below the interiliac line, was found in 80.6 per cent of the subjects. The average position of the greater curvature was 2.5 cm. and 4.5 cm. below the interiliac line in men and women respectively. In 25.6 per cent of the men and 13 per cent of the women the greater curvature was above the line. The hypertonic stomach (high, short and obliquely situated) was present in 17.1 per cent of men and 7.1 per cent of women; the hypotonic stomach (long markedly hooked) was present in 3.6 per cent of men and 15 per cent of women; the orthotonic stomach or the stomach of average length was present in the remainder. The hypersthenic person (broad and short thorax, wide intercostal angle, abdomen broad and large) tends to have a high-lying stomach and the asthenic person a low-lying stomach. For example, the fact that in 44 per cent of British and only 22.5 per cent of American young adults studied, the stomach was 2 inches below the interiliac line was found to be due to the difference in the body habitus; the British young adults had narrower chests and smaller intercostal angles (Moody, 1927). However, no constant relationship exists between the strength and build of a person and the shape and position of the stomach.

Data, similar to the foregoing, are not available for various decades after thirty. A start has been made by Moody (1927) who studied the radiographs of 100 British patients, 50 males and 50 females, with gastrointestinal complaints. The ages of the patients ranged from 40 to 81 years. It was found that low stomachs occur more frequently in healthy young British adults than in elderly British patients with gastrointestinal complaints.

An investigation of the change of the shape and position of the stomach in subjects above the age of 30 and devoid of gastrointestinal complaints should throw some light on the relation of age to the gastric motor mechanism. But, since the shape and position of the stomach is not always related to the rate of gastric evacuation, actual studies of the rate of evacuation at different ages are necessary to ascertain the effect of age on gastric motor functions.

9. *The motility of the empty stomach. Hunger motility.*

The studies of Carlson (1916) and his students have shown that the stomach of the human infant manifests greater hunger motility than the stomach of the adult. In the breast-fed infant, the first period of hunger motility starts 2.5 hours (average) after a meal; in the young adult from 4 to 6 hours after the meal. The periods of hunger motility occur more frequently in the infant, because the periods of quiescence of the empty stomach are shorter. In the infant the quiescent periods range from 10 to 60 minutes in length; in the adult from 1 to 3 hours. A study of the hunger motility of the human stomach by decades has not been made.

A study has been made of the hunger motility of the stomach of dogs at different ages (Carlson, 1916). The most constant difference occurs in the length of the periods of quiescence and activity. The periods of quiescence are shorter, and the periods of hunger activity are longer in young than in old dogs (table 18). Old dogs must also

TABLE 18

Gastric hunger contractions in dogs of different ages

(Carlson)

Dogs	Length of contraction period	Length of quiescent period
Old adult	30 minutes to 2 hours	1.16 to 3.66 hours
Adult	1.66 to 3.0 hours	1.16 to 2.0 hours
Young adult	2.75 to 3.75 hours	1 to 1.5 hours
Pup (age 5–6 months)	3 to 4 hours	5 to 10 minutes
Young pup (age 5–6 weeks)	4.5 to 5.66 hours	2.5 to 3.4 minutes
Prematurely born pups	Continuous	None

be fasted longer than young adult dogs before hunger contractions appear (Ivy, 1938).

The decrease in the hunger motility of the stomach with age may be due to two factors, namely, (a) the age of the musculature or the motor mechanism of the stomach, and (b) the decline in metabolism which may reduce the quantity of the blood-borne, chemical stimuli of the hunger mechanism. The latter is not primarily concerned because Patterson (1914, 1915) found that prolonged fasting, though it increased the hunger contractions some, did not lead to contractions which approached in vigor those of young dogs. Thus, it appears as if the irritability of the gastric motor mechanism concerned in hunger contractions decreases with age. To what extent the extrinsic nerves of the stomach may be concerned in the decrease in hunger motility with age has not been determined.

In acute gastritis the stomach is relatively atonic and hunger contractions do not occur (Carlson, 1916; Luckhardt and Hamburger, 1916). Hunger motility has not been studied in uncomplicated cases of chronic gastritis and achlorhydria. This is mentioned because the incidence of gastritis is alleged to increase with age (vide ut supra).

10. *The rate of gastric evacuation.*

It has been indicated above that the motility, and probably the tone, of the stomach is greater in the infant and child than in the adult. It is well established that increased motility and tone of the stomach and increased hunger, under normal conditions, cause the stomach to empty more rapidly. Thus, a relatively more rapid rate of gastric evacuation should be expected to occur in the infant and child than in the adult. But, since the quantity and quality of food also influence the rate of gastric evacuation, and since many different kinds of test meals have been employed, it is impossible to use much of the data reported in the literature. The X-ray method gives reliable results only when the same technique is employed; even then, a single examination is not very reliable. A single examination would be indicative if performed in a large number of subjects; but at present there are no data in the literature which establish the rate of gastric evacuation in the various decades of life. Certain comparisons, however, may be made.

It is generally agreed that the infant's stomach will evacuate 100 or 150 cc. of milk in from 1.5 to 3 hours, occasionally more rapidly (Ginsburg, Tumpowsky, and Carlson, 1915). In young adults 400 cc. of milk is evacuated in from two to three hours (Hawk, Rehfuss, and Bergeim, 1926). The same is true of the various types of barium meals used by roentgenologists, the maximum limit of normal in the adult being from five to six hours. Some roentgenologists have the impression that the stomach of persons, not complaining of specific dyspeptic symptoms, over the age of 65 empties more slowly than the stomach of the young adult, but definite proof is not available. It is generally thought that the J-shaped or long stomach empties more slowly than the steer-horn or short stomach; but there is no proof. Both types of stomach may be associated with dyspeptic symptoms, the short stomach when it is hypermotile and the long stomach when it is atonic and hypomotile. Of course, both types of stomach exist normally without producing symptoms, even when they empty at the same rate or at different rates.

Since gastric acidity declines and the incidence of achlorhydria increases after the age of 45 years, these factors may affect the rate of gastric evacuation. It is generally considered that in the presence of achlorhydria the stomach empties faster; but, this cannot be considered as established on the basis of the actual data presented in the literature. The data of Vanzant and her collaborators (1932, 1933) show that with advancing age less contents are aspirated after the Ewald meal. Dedichen (1924–25), who studied the stomach of 99 healthy old people from 67 to 92 years by the Ewald method and found the incidence of achlorhydria to be 66 per cent, states that the stomach of the aged empties more rapidly than that of the young adult. It is also claimed that the stomach of patients with pernicious anemia who have achlorhydria, empties faster than normal (Davidson and Gulland, 1930). However, Keefer and Bloomfield (1926) do not report a high incidence of rapid gastric evacuation in the achlorhydric patients they studied. Davies and James (1930–31) who present actual data obtained on 100 patients ranging from 65 to 90 years by the use of an Ewald-gruel meal, find that the stomach of elderly achlorhydric subjects empties faster than that of non-achlorhydric subjects. The clinical impressions of numerous other authors (Bloomfield and Polland, 1933; Poeschel, 1930), might be quoted, but the data available are inadequate to warrant compilation and definite conclusions. Even the extensive data of Vanzant (1932, 1933) referred to above, are not clearly interpretable because the reduction of the amount of gastric contents with advancing age may be due either to decreased secretion of acid or to more rapid emptying, or both.

It is of interest that 100 cc. of milk is evacuated from the infant's stomach at about the same rate that 400 cc. is evacuated from the adult's stomach. This may be related to two differences which exist between the stomach of the infant and that of the adult. The mean acidity of the adult's stomach is four times that of the infant (Vanzant, Alvarez and Berkson, 1936–37), and the "capacity" and weight of the adult's stomach at 20 years of age is approximately four times that of the infants at the age of 1 year (Scammon, 1919).

11. *Dyspepsia among men and women above 40.*

According to a recent report from the Mayo Clinic (Rivers, 1938), dyspepsia or "indigestion" is among the complaints of almost one-half of patients between thirty and sixty years of age. This evidence shows that complaints referable to the digestive system are the most common of all complaints, a fact that is generally accepted. This is because disorders of organs outside the digestive system cause functional disorders of the alimentary tract either by causing changes in the composition of the blood or by disturbing the activities of the tract reflexly through the nervous system.

In males aged forty and above who complain primarily of dyspepsia, peptic ulcer ranked first as the cause; in women gallbladder disease ranked first.   In 17 per cent of the males and 5.8 per cent of the females

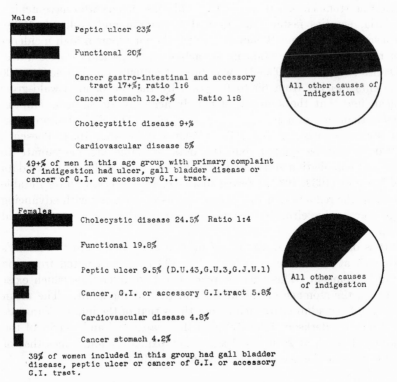

THE MOST FREQUENT CAUSES OF DYSPEPSIA AMONG MEN AND WOMEN AGED 40 AND OVER

Males

Peptic ulcer 23%

Functional 20%

Cancer gastro-intestinal and accessory tract 17+%; ratio 1:6

Cancer stomach 12.2+%   Ratio 1:8

Cholecystitic disease 9+%

Cardiovascular disease 5%

49+% of men in this age group with primary complaint of indigestion had ulcer, gall bladder disease or cancer of G.I. or accessory G.I. tract.

All other causes of Indigestion

Females

Cholecystic disease 24.5%   Ratio 1:4

Functional 19.8%

Peptic ulcer 9.5% (D.U.43,G.U.3,G.J.U.1)

Cancer, G.I. or accessory G.I.tract 5.8%

Cardiovascular disease 4.8%

Cancer stomach 4.2%

All other causes of indigestion

38% of women included in this group had gall bladder disease, peptic ulcer or cancer of G.I. or accessory G.I. tract.

Fig. 33. The most frequent causes of dyspepsia among men and women aged 40 and over (Rivers, 1938).

cancer of the organs of the digestive system, chiefly the stomach, was the cause of the dyspepsia.   In 49 per cent of the men and 38 per cent of the women in whom dyspepsia was the primary complaint, the dyspepsia was due to some disorder of the digestive organs that demanded careful diagnosis and early medical or surgical attention (fig. 33).

These observations show that the medical profession has the responsibility of educating laymen concerning the dangers of using therapeutic nostrums for dyspeptic symptoms and the responsibility of making an accurate diagnosis of the cause of dyspeptic symptoms particularly in persons above the age of 40 (Rivers, 1938).

4. PANCREAS

1. *Growth and senescence of the pancreas as indicated by the post-mortem weight of the organ.*

The growth of the pancreas of the rat has been carefully studied (Donaldson, 1924), but the effect of age has not been ascertained. Histologically the human pancreas at birth is relatively deficient, like the salivary glands, in parenchymatous tissue. Secretory granules are present after the sixth fetal month and evidences of secretion appear in the gland at this time (Scammon, 1923). Scammon (1923, 1926–27) finds the average weight of the pancreas of the newborn human to be 3.54 grams. The data (table 19) indicate that the weight of the pancreas decreases after the age of sixty. The effect of inanition, which probably existed in Boyd's (1861) subjects prior to death, on the acinar and islet cells of the pancreas is uncertain because of contradictory reports (Jackson, 1929). Wet weights, especially without histological study, yield unreliable data. As in the case of the gastric mucosa and salivary glands, statements are found to the effect that the pancreas in old persons is atrophic, but the evidence is not convincing. Goodpasture (1918) in his study of fifty old dogs found degenerative changes in the pancreas. Grossly its lobulations were more distinct and its consistency was firmer than in the young adult. Unchallengeable evidence of the effect of ageing per se on the morphology of the human pancreas does not exist.

2. *External secretion of the pancreas.*

The effect of the hormone, secretin, on the secretion of the pancreas of the newborn animal has not been adequately studied. Neither has the effect of ageing on the external secretion of the pancreas in animals been studied. If degeneration of the external secretory cells or the acinar cells of the pancreas occurs in the aged, less pancreatic secretion will be formed. This is based on the fact that the response of the pancreas to the hormone, secretin, is directly proportional to the amount of acinar tissue (Voegtlin, Greengard and Ivy, 1934). Further, functional regeneration of acinar tissue apparently does not occur in

TABLE 19

Pancreas

Age	Sex	Average weight	Number of cases	Body weight	Data from Vierordt
years		*grams*		*pounds*	*grams*
Newborn*		3.5	465		
Newborn		3.2	465		
Newborn {	M	3.1	39	5	2.85–4.0
	F	3.1	34	4.18	
6–12 months {	M	9.6	41	12.0	
	F	9.0	36	10.7	
1–2 {	M	12.4	30	14.3	
	F	13.8	32	13.0	
2–4 {	M	21.4	27	20.0	
	F	19.2	27	18.5	
4–7 {	M	22.6	26	25.5	
	F	22.6	19	24.5	
7–14 {	M	47.5	18	42.3	
	F	37.9	16	38.3	
14–20 {	M	62.0	17	68.0	78.0
	F	74.7	14	63.8	
20–30 {	M	99.9	100	92.5	56.0–88.0
	F	83.5	98	83.7	
30–40 {	M	98.1	164	100.0	89.7
	F	86.6	132	83.7	
40–50 {	M	104.0	207	105.0	90–105
	F	78.8	147	82.2	
50–60 {	M	99.7	158	104.6	97–99
	F	83.0	126	83.8	
60–70 {	M	91.7	161	104.5	
	F	79.5	186	84.8	
70–80 {	M	90.0	113	106.0	
	F	75.8	165	82.2	
80+ {	M	80.0	31	97.2	
	F	67.7	82	80.2	

* Computed by R. C. Scammon, 1926–1927. The remainder of the data from Boyd, 1861, but have been rearranged by the author.

the dog. (Functional regeneration does occur in the stomach and liver.) Whether the pancreas of man manifests functional regeneration is not known. The fact that the volume output of pancreatic juice and the total output of enzymes decrease after the destruction of pancreatic acinar tissue does not mean necessarily that a deficiency of pancreatic digestion in the intestine would occur. This would depend on the amount of acinar tissue destroyed. If all the acinar tissue is destroyed, it is known that appreciable steatorrhea (fat in the feces), creatorrhea (meat fibers) and sometimes amylorrhea (starch) occur. But, we do not know, even approximately, the amount of acinar tissue

TABLE 20

*Duodenal contents**

Age	Number of cases	Units of enzyme						pH
		Fasting			Test meal			
		Protein-olytic	Lipo-lytic	Amylo-lytic	Protein-olytic	Lipo-lytic	Amylo-lytic	
1–3 months	10	1.65	0.60	0.61	1.61	0.55	0.50	5.2
3–12 months	13	2.01	0.65	0.75	1.81	0.70	0.77	5.3
1–2 years	8	2.38	1.10	2.24	2.49	1.32	2.78	5.2
2–4 years	6	1.65	1.31	2.31	1.91	1.32	2.56	5.2
4–6 years	8	3.37	1.15	2.97	3.34	1.41	3.28	5.0
6–9 years	11	2.42	1.13	4.01	2.08	1.43	3.47	5.4
9–12 years	18	2.56	0.88	3.23	2.48	1.31	2.95	5.4
Adults†								
Average					2.8	1.6	2.2	

* Klumph and Neale, 1930.

† McClure, Wetmore and Reynolds, 1921; Jones, Castle, Mulholland and Bailey, 1921.

that must be destroyed to cause the first detectable evidences of incomplete pancreatic digestion (Ivy, 1936–37).

A deficiency of pancreatic secretion is known to occur in the child, adult and the aged. It causes marked inanition. It is only rarely diagnosed and at present its age incidence is unknown. As a rule only the severe cases are diagnosed. This is because considerable careful laboratory work is required to detect the mild or moderate cases. Since chronic pancreatitis is more frequently associated with biliary tract disease than with any other disease, and since biliary tract disease occurs most frequently (vide ut infra) after the age of forty, a deficiency of pancreatic secretion would be expected to occur more frequently after the age of forty. Helmer, Fouts, and Zerfas (1933) have found that patients with pernicious anemia, who show involvement of the central nervous system have decreased tryptic activity in the duodenal contents.

The best and most reliable data available regarding the relation of the concentration of the pancreatic enzymes in the duodenal secretions (obtained with a doudenal tube) to age are those shown in table 20. The starch digesting or amylolytic power is feeble under one year; beyond one year it is plentiful, exceeding the average for adults. The fat digesting or lipolytic power is feeble under one year after which it enters the range of adults; it does not reach the adult average until after the twelfth year. The proteolytic or protein digesting power is plentiful throughout infancy and childhood. The data referred to in the tables are superior to much other data reported in the literature, because good methods for the determination of enzyme concentration were used. None of the data, however, show the effect of old age per se on external pancreatic secretion.

Although the relation of the vitamin C content of the pancreas to external pancreatic secretion is not known, it is reported that as age advances the vitamin C content of the pancreatic tissue decreases (Yavorsky, Almaden, and King, 1934). To what extent this observation is related to a true age factor or to dietary intake or fibrosis is uncertain.

5. LIVER

1. *Growth and senescence of the liver as indicated by the postmortem weight of the organ.*

The growth of the liver of the rat has been studied carefully (Donaldson, 1923), but the effect of ageing has not been determined. The human liver grows quite steadily up to the age of 20 (Scammon, 1919, 1930). The average weight of the human liver at birth is 135 grams. Its weight is more than doubled the first year, and tripled in the third. By puberty the liver weighs about 10 times that of the natal weight. After the age of 20 the weight of the liver remains fairly constant in both males and females. At 25 years in the white male the median weight is 1820 grams. The weight decreases to a median of 1480 by 75 years. The liver of the white female ranges between a median weight of from 1460 to 1430 grams at from 20 to 60 years of age, after which it decreases 11 per cent to a median weight of 1180 grams at

75 years. These data were compiled by Edith Boyd (1933), and are the best available (fig. 34). They were obtained from cases of death from accident, and the factors of disease and inanition, which markedly affect the weight of the liver, were controlled.

Frischmann (1932), has reported the results of an histologic study of the effect of ageing on the connective tissue stroma of the liver in man. He concludes that the increase in connective tissue previously reported to occur in the liver of the aged is due to pathological processes and not to physiological senescence. He failed to find an increase in the connective tissue in Glisson's capsule and in the reticular lattice work of the liver in ten cases ranging in age from 60 to 86 years of age.

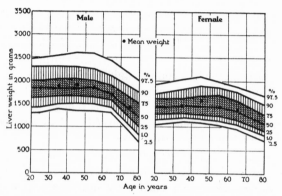

Fig. 34. Graphic standards of normal variability in weight of the liver of both the male and the female based on the data in figure 29. The percentage figures given at the side of each panel indicate the percentiles of weight. Fifty per cent of normal weights may be expected to fall in the heavily shaded zone, 80 per cent in the totally shaded zone and 95 per cent in the total zone limited by the 97.5 and the 2.5 percentile lines. For practical purposes, the last two percentile lines may be considered the usual upper and lower limits of normal variability in the weight of the liver (Edith Boyd, 1933).

2. Changes in functional activity and resistance to hepatotoxins with age.

Since the factor of safety of the liver is large, the decrease in the weight of the liver with age should not cause any evidences of hepatic insufficiency (Mann and Magath, 1922). In an adult dog four-fifths of the liver may be removed without evidences of hepatic hypofunction as tested by the ordinary tests of liver function. Unless ageing per se effects the functional activity of the liver to a greater extent than its weight, evidences of hypofunctioning of the liver should not become manifest with ageing. Further, in the adult it is known that the regenerative capacity of the liver is remarkable. After the surgical removal of 70 per cent of the liver, the weight and volume of the liver returns to about 75 per cent of the original within a few weeks. After central necrosis of the liver induced by chloroform, complete recovery occurs in a few days (Whipple and Sperry, 1909). After the exposure of the liver to various hepatoxins, the liver shows marked recovery and the regenerated cells manifest an increased resistance to these poisons (MacNider, 1935). Regeneration of liver cells occurs only when the blood supply of the liver is normal and the bile ducts are not obstructed (Mann and Magath, 1922).

The relative ability of the liver to regenerate after the surgical removal of a portion in old animals has not been determined. The resistance of the senile liver of dogs to chloroform poisoning has been studied by MacNider (1935, 1936). In 22 dogs ranging in age from 8 to 15 years, which had been kept under laboratory conditions for long periods, the liver manifested histologically a diffuse atypical epithelium much like that found in the liver of a young adult following the repair which occurs after uranium nitrate or chloroform poisoning. The liver cells and cords are flattened and stain intensely as though the cytoplasm is condensed; the nuclei are relatively enlarged and hyperchromic. In addition incompletely undifferentiated cells form syncytical structures. Atypical epithelium has also been described in the liver of old dogs by Goodpasture (1918). He has described the changes in much detail; the changes are characterized chiefly by degeneration which is associated with simplification of structure and regressive alterations tending in areas to manifest cellular overgrowth. The most characteristic degenerative change found was the presence of crystals in the nuclei which are insoluble in acids and soluble in strong sodium hydroxide. Similar crystals were found in the liver of old dogs by Brandts (1909).

In 13 of the 18 old animals subjected to experimentation by MacNider (1936), the liver reacted normally to the phenoltetrachlorphthalein clearance test. The liver of every animal manifested greater tolerance to chloroform than the liver of young adult dogs. Thus, dogs in ageing may naturally acquire an atypical hepatic epithelium similar to that which occurs as a repair process following liver injury induced experimentally with an hepatoxic agent.

There is no reliable evidence showing that the functional activity of the liver when examined by the ordinary tests of liver function decreases with age in man.   Serious studies of the bile volume output and the composition of the bile in the aged have not been made.   Warthin (1929) states that hyperbilirubinemia occurs in the aged, but the statement is not supported by evidence.   The results of such studies would have to be interpreted in the light of studies on the histology of the liver to render them truly significant in so far as ageing per se is concerned.   For example, cirrhosis of the liver interferes with hepatic function and this disease markedly increases in incidence with advancing years (Dublin and Lotka, 1937).

Like the pancreas, the vitamin C content of the liver apparently decreases with age (Yaborsky, Almaden and King, 1934).   The decrease appears to be significant after the age of 45; but, the relation of this decrease to dietary intake of the vitamin is uncertain.   Some very meager and poorly controlled observations indicate that the vitamin A content of the liver increases shortly after birth in the canine and human infant (Busson and Simonnet, 1933).

The effect of ageing on the glycogen content of the liver has been studied in the rat (Deuel, Butts, Hallman, Murray, and Blunden, 1933). The content of liver glycogen increases after birth up to 40 days of age when it exceeds 8 per cent.   It then decreases slowly to 4 per cent at the age of 75 days.   In rats from 19 to 24 months old the liver glycogen is approximately 4 per cent.   A sex difference does not exist in rats from 26 to 29 days old or from 17 to 24 months old.   In between the liver of the female contains less glycogen, the minimum value being found at 3 months of age.

6. GALLBLADDER

1. *Growth.*

The gallbladder of the newborn infant is relatively small.   During the first two years of life its capacity increases so that by the end of the second year "the capacity of the gallbladder to liver weight" yields the same general ratio as in the adult (Scammon, 1923).   After the second year, the gallbladder and liver tend to grow at the same rate. According to Gundobin (1912), the contents of the gallbladder (at autopsy) in infants from 1 to 3 months of age averages 3.2 cc. and from 1 to 3 years of age, 8.5 cc. of bile.   The functional capacities of the gallbladder at different ages are best determined by the method of cholecystography.   The data obtained by this method in so far as the method has been utilized will be given later.

2. *Functional activities.*

The activities of the gallbladder concerning which most is known, are concentration of the hepatic bile and evacuation (Ivy, 1934). The normal gallbladder concentrates the hepatic bile which enters it from 4 to 10 times; under conditions of stasis, 20 times. The gallbladder evacuates most of its contents after a meal containing fat, protein, and acids such as are found in gastric juice, vinegar and fruits. No facts are available regarding the capacity of the gallbladder to concentrate at different ages, although considerable is known regarding the effects of disease on its capacity to concentrate. More is known concerning the relation of age and sex to the rate of evacuation of the gallbladder.

The best data on the relation of age and sex to the rate of evacuation of the gallbladder have been provided by Boyden and Granthan (1936). Although the number of subjects employed in the three major age groups was small, the data were studied statistically for the significance of the differences noted. Eighty-four subjects were used, ranging from 6 to 78 years of age; 16 boys and 12 girls, average age 9; 12 young men, average age 23, and 12 young women, average age 24; 14 elderly men, average age 67, and 10 elderly women, average age 65. In childhood the rate of evacuation was found to be faster than in early maturity, the difference being due to a faster rate in boys than in girls. After puberty the male gallbladder emptied slower than that of the female. The gallbladder of elderly women emptied faster than that of elderly men. Thus, it appears that the gallbladder of the female empties at a rather constant rate from childhood to old age, and at the onset of puberty some influence operates in the male to slow down the rate so that from puberty on, the gallbladder of the male empties more slowly than that of the female (figs. 35 and 36).

Since gallbladder disease increases definitely with age and in chronic colecystitis the gallbladder cannot be visualized, Boyden's group of elderly persons represents those subjects whose gallbladder had escaped pathological alteration. This fact obviously increases the value of the data in so far as the effect of ageing per se on the gallbladder is concerned, and indicates that the power of evacuation does not lessen with age per se.

In regard to the size of the gallbladder, the data of Boyden and Granthan (1936) show that it is not significantly related to the rate of evacuation. This is important because the mean cholecystographic volume of the elderly women was 29.0 cc., of the elderly men 33.4 cc.,

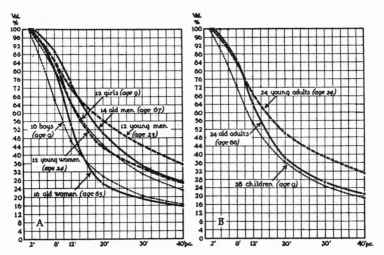

FIG. 35 Assembly drawings illustrating the mean rate of evacuation of the gallbladder. (*A*) 6 groups divided according to age and sex; (*B*) 3 groups divided according to age alone (Boyden and Grantham, 1936).

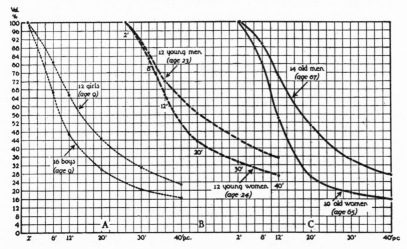

FIG. 36. The three age groups arranged for comparison of six differences (Boyden and Grantham, 1936).

of the young women 24 cc., of the young men 30.8 cc., of the girls 13.5 cc., and of the boys 13.9 cc. The average for boys and girls (average age 9) is 13.7 cc., for young men and women (average age 24), 27.4 cc. and for elderly women and men (average age 66), 31.5 cc.[1] Regardless of the differences in size, the mean differences between the rate of emptying of the gallbladder in childhood and old persons are not significant, and the gallbladder of the young adult empties slower than that of both of the other groups (figs. 34 and 35).

So, it would appear as if the gallbladder of the old person returns to that of the child in regard to rate of emptying. It would be necessary to have data on a larger number of children and old people before such an observation could be considered to be a fact. Yet, it is clear that if the gallbladder of old persons escapes disease, it will evacuate well. It may be that the gallbladder which empties well throughout life is the one more likely to escape disease.

If it be true that the gallbladder of old persons evacuates as rapidly as that of a child, and more rapidly than that of a young adult, it follows that the gallbladder of the old persons should either manifest hypertrophy of the musculature, or the resistance offered to the flow of bile from the common duct into the duodenum should be less than in the young adult. (Of course, the gallbladder of the young adult may be more subject to reflex or hormonal inhibitory effects.) No evidence is available concerning the latter possibility, and the evidence concerning the former is contradictory. Lütkens (1926) could not substantiate Charcot's belief that the musculature of the gallbladder is atrophied in the old person. In fact, he gained the impression that the gallbladder of old persons manifested some hypertrophy of the entire wall with some sagging. He thought the sagging might be due to weakening of elastic fibers. In some instances sclerosis of the blood vessels and atrophy of the mucosa of the gallbladder may be found in old persons, the effect of which on gallbladder function was not determined. In fifty old stray dogs, Goodpasture (1918) found the mucosa of the gallbladder to be thickened and to manifest a polypoid overgrowth with dilated glandular crypts filled with a substance staining like mucus. The rate of emptying and the concentrating ability of the gallbladder of old dogs has not been studied.

It would appear from the evidence now available as if the greater susceptibility of the female gallbladder to disease (vide ut infra) is due to metabolic disturbances, which alter the composition of the bile, or to infection, or to stasis resulting from disturbance of the sphincter of

[1] In a personal communication, Boyden gives an average volume of 30.3 cc. for the gallbladder of 32 young men, average age 25.7 years, and of 30.6 cc. for 36 older men, average age, 60.1 years.

Oddi mechanism, rather than to motor insufficiency of the gallbladder. This is because the gallbladder of the non-pregnant adult female tends to empty faster than that of the adult male. Considerable evidence

TABLE 21

Biliary calculi

Averages of animal death rates per 100,000 (Dublin and Lotka)			Data from 2,621 consecutive autopsies, Cook County Hospital, Chicago, 208 cases of gall-stones, 1929-1932 (Jaffe†)		
Age periods	Males, 1911-1935	Females, 1911-1935	Age periods	Males	Females
Whites					
years			*years*	*per cent*	*per cent*
1-74*	1.4	4.9	Average in-	6.76	17.57
45-74*	5.8	19.3	cidence		
20-24	0.1	0.5	21-30	0	5
25-34	0.4	2.3	31-40	1.45	11.51
35-44	1.4	5.9	41-50	4.24	21.90
45-54	3.5	13.3	51-60	6.75	17.07
55-64	6.5	22.4	61-70	11.20	29.03
65-74	10.6	30.0	Above 70	13.90	24.44
Colored					
1-74*	0.7	1.9	Average in-	1.04	10.23
45-74*	2.6	6.8	cidence		
20-24	0.3	0.5	21-30	0	3.28
25-34	0.5	1.4	31-40	0.73	7.50
35-44	0.8	2.8	41-50	0	12.24
45-54	1.8	5.1	51-60	1.86	16.27
55-64	3.0	7.2	61-70	4.34	25.0
65-74	3.9	10.6	Above 70	6.66	20.0

* Standardized for age—Dublin and Lotka, 1937.

† Jaffe, 1933. The deaths in this series were, of course, not necessarily due to gall stones. The number of cases of gallbladder disease in relation to the number examined in each age and sex group are considered by the author. Among the colored persons the pigment variety of stone predominated; among the white the mixed variety predominated.

exists (Ivy, 1934) showing that the gallbladder of pregnant women empties more slowly than normally and tends to be distended (Potter, 1936). Gerdes and Boyden (1936) have shown quite definitely that during pregnancy the gallbladder does not empty as rapidly or as completely as before or as in nulligravidae. The cause or causes of gallbladder retention in pregnancy is not known, but Westphal (1923) has performed certain experiments, the results of which indicate that a hypertonus of the sphincter of Oddi exists during pregnancy. This is a field of investigation that deserves more attention than it has received, because of the high incidence of cholecystopathy, including cancer of the organ, in women who have borne children.

3. *Gall stones.*

Although it is well known that gall stones may occur in children, all observers agree that less than one per cent of the cases of cholelithiasis occur in persons under 20 years of age. The incidence of gall stones increases with each decade above 20, and becomes marked above the age of 40. This is illustrated by the data in table 21; the data are based on mortality and autopsy statistics which yield the most reliable data. The clinical data manifest the same increase of the incidence of gall stones, if the data are properly treated, which is so infrequently done in clinical reports. There is a marked variation in the statistics from different countries and races (Jaffe, 1933), but the increase with age holds true. The increased incidence of gall stones in the female is true of most occidental peoples, but in Japan, for example, where the pigment type of stone predominates, a sex difference does not seem to exist (Jaffe, 1933). A racial difference is manifest between the white and colored people living in Chicago. The observation that cholelithiasis is more common in whites than in negroes is truer of the males than the females (table 21), and it does not seem reasonable to ascribe the differences to diet, occupation and incidence of infection. It would appear that the most favored theories of diet and infection do not hold, and that some functional disturbance is concerned, for example, endocrine and reflex nervous influences, which appear to predispose to biliary stasis in pregnancy (vide ut supra).

The clinical evidence (Crump, 1931; Deaver and Bortz, 1927; Graham, 1928; Mentzer, 1926), indicates that all types of cholecystopathy increase with advancing age. The exact incidence with each decade is uncertain.

7. SMALL INTESTINE

1. *Growth and senescence.*

The growth of the small intestine has been studied in the rat (Donaldson, 1923); the effect of senescence has not been studied. The growth of the small intestine of the human fetus has been studied by Scammon and Kittelson (1926–27). At birth the small intestine of the human infant measures about 340 cm. in length; its length is doubled by the age of puberty, and in the adult (14 cases only) its average length is about 760 cm. The data given by Vierordt (1906) indicate that the weight of the human intestine increases up to the age of 42, after which it decreases. The data are so meager that it cannot be concluded that the weight of the intestine in the aged is less than that of the mature adult. The same is true of the effect of age on the length of the small intestine. It is generally stated and believed, however, that the intestine of old persons manifests atrophy of the mucosa and musculature. Inanition in rats results in an increase in the weight of the intestine due to edema and an atrophy of the cells of the mucosa (Miller, 1927); the same is true of human infants (Jackson, 1929). It would appear, then, that reliable data regarding the effect of ageing on the weight and histology of the intestine could be obtained only from persons dying from some sudden cause of death.

2. *Functional activities.*

Few data are available on the rate of passage of inert materials through the small intestine in the young and mature adult; none are available for infants and children, and none for the aged. The secretion of succus entericus and the rate of absorption of food from the small intestine in old animals have not been studied. Takashina (1932) presents some evidence indicating that adrenaline is absorbed more rapidly from the intestine of the infant and child than of the adult, but the significance of his observations is questionable.

Except for early childhood (1 to 4 years), deaths from intestinal obstruction is chiefly a condition of advanced age (above 50 or 55 years). This fact does not necessarily indicate the existence of some weakness of the intestine in elderly persons. This is true for two reasons. (a) The incidence of hernia markedly increases above the age of 55, and, although hernia is more likely to become strangulated during the period of active adult life, it is the most common cause of intestinal obstruction. (b) Abdominal adhesions are the second most frequent cause of intestinal obstruction. Abdominal adhesions occur most frequently as an early or a late result of operations on the appendix and pelvic organs. Abdominal and pelvic operations have increased in recent years. Operations on the appendix are frequent at all decades and operation on the pelvic organs are most frequently performed on mature or elderly adults. These facts explain the increase in deaths from intestinal obstruction observed during recent years. Neoplasms of the colon rank third as a cause of intestinal obstruction and, of course, occur more frequently with advancing years (Dublin and Lotka, 1937; McIver, 1932; Wangensteen, 1937).

8. APPENDIX

1. *Growth and senescence.*

Although the growth of the appendix in the human fetus has been studied, relatively little is known concerning the effect of age on the organ, when the frequency of its disease is considered. In infancy and childhood it contains relatively a large amount of lymphoid tissue, which resembles that of the tonsil. Although considerable lymphoid tissue is present in the appendix at birth, the amount increases during the first year which is true of the other portions of the intestinal tract. The amount of elastic tissue in the appendix and intestine increases greatly during the first year (Scammon, 1923).

The appendix in the newborn infant is usually connected to the cecum by an enlarged base, the conus appendicis, i.e., in the infant the cecum frequently tapers into the appendix without there being a clear line of demarcation. The appendix measures from 2 to 6 mm. in diameter, and from 2 to 8 cm. in length at birth. It usually increases rapidly in length during the first year, reaching usually a length of from 8 to 10 cm. and becomes a more discrete organ. After the first year its growth is very slow and irregular (Scammon, 1923). Its content of lymphoid tissue is said to diminish with age as is generally true of lymphoid tissue throughout the body and in the alimentary tract. The appendix possesses a lumen extending to its tip in all infants and children. According to Ribbert (1893), the lumen shows a tendency to undergo obliteration as age advances. This obliteration starts at the tip and gradually extends toward the cecal end or base of the appendix. In 25 per cent of 400 cases the lumen was more or less obliterated; in adults over 50, it was obliterated in one-half of the cases. This is said to occur in the absence of the evidences of existing or previous inflammation, and to be a true process of involution associated with ageing. However, this is uncertain.

2. *Appendicitis.*

The great immunity of the nursing infant to appendicitis has been attributed to diet and also to the anatomy of the appendix; the cecal end of the appendix is more patent in the infant. In the infant, the wall of the appendix is relatively thin due to the slight development of the mucosa and lymphoid tissue (Royster, 1927; Schmidt, 1911; Schlossmann, 1922). The alleged relative infrequency of appendicitis in the latter years of life has been attributed to obliteration of the lumen and a diminution of lymphoid tissue. However, in recent years the mortality rate from appendicitis in the aged has increased, so that the mortality rate is apparently quite uniform from the decades above the third (Dublin and Lotka, 1937). The disease in the aged is regarded as peculiar or atypical in type and as having a higher mortality. This is attributed by Maes (1925 (a) to the atrophy of the protective lymphoid tissue, the atrophy of which predisposes to rapid gangrene and to a more rapid spread of the infection to veins and surrounding tissue, and (b) to the "naturally lowered resistance of elderly patients."

The clinical experience that the incidence of appendicitis is higher in males (about 25 per cent) than females, is confirmed by the mortality rates (Dublin and Lotka, 1937).

9. COLON

1. *Growth and senescence.*

The growth of the large intestine in the human fetus and in infants has been studied rather thoroughly (Scammon and Kittelson, 1926–1927; Scammon, 1923). At birth the large intestine weighs approximately 16 grams and is 65 cm. in length. At 3 years it weighs approximately 150 grams and is 90 cm. in length. In the adult it weighs about 450 grams and is 160 cm. in length. In the adult, however, it varies greatly in regard to position and length. The length of the pelvic or sigmoid portion of the colon is relatively greater in the fetus and infant than in the adult. This is also true of the rectum. The sacculations and the three longitudinal bands (tenia) of muscle, so evident in the adult colon, are not very evident in the newborn, and develop during the first six months. The sacculated cecum typical of the adult does not appear until the third or fourth year. Although it is frequently stated that the colon atrophies and its musculature becomes thin and atonic with age, real evidence supporting the view is wanting (Vierordt, 1906).

2. *The activities of the colon.*

The activities of the colon are absorption, secretion and motility. The colon by absorbing water and inorganic salts concentrates the material entering from the ileum. Relatively little food material, other than water and salts, is absorbed from the colon of the dog and man, although some glucose and other soluble substances may be absorbed to a variable and a rather insignificant extent. Drugs are sometimes administered per rectum. The colon secretes mucus which serves to protect the mucosa and to lubricate the feces. At times the secretion of mucus may become very marked, a condition called mucous colitis. The motor activity of the colon serves to increase the condensation of the fecal mass, to move the feces downward and to effect defecation.

There is no evidence indicating that the absorptive and secreting capacity of the colon is decreased in old persons. It is claimed by some that one of the causes of constipation in the aged is a decreased secretion of mucus. This claim is not supported by actual evidence. The claim that the colonic musculature becomes atonic with advancing years has not been established by actual studies on the time of passage of marked contents through the colon or by barium enemata.

3. *The effect of ageing on the musculature of the colon. Diverticulosis.*

Perhaps the best evidence regarding the thinning of the colonic musculature of man with advancing age is afforded by the increased incidence of diverticulosis of the colon with age. That the incidence of this condition increases with age is agreed to by all authors; further, this condition is said to be the most common pathological lesion of the colon seen by the surgeon and roentgenologist. When the diverticula become infected (diverticulitis), the condition is quite serious; when not infected, they may contain fecoliths. Diverticulosis is rare below the age of 35. The majority of cases are seen clinically by the physician in the sixth and seventh decades. But in the clinical reports which are reviewed up to 1935 by Lunding (1935), the incidence in relation to the number of patients in each decade examined by the physician is not considered. Fifield (1927), who examined the colon in 10,167 consecutive autopsies, found that most of the cases occur between the age of 60 to 90; unfortunately he does not give the percentages in regard to age and sex in relation to the number of cases of each sex and decade examined. Kocour (1937), who studied the incidence of the condition in 7,000 consecutive autopsies, gives the percentage of diverticula in relation to the number of autopsies performed in each age decade. His data (table 22) show that the condition increases markedly after the age of 40, and becomes relatively stationary in the seventh and eighth decades. Telling and Gruner (1916–1917) arrive at a similar conclusion when the clinical incidence observed by them is corrected to show the proportion of diverticulosis to the population surviving at the various ages. Their estimates indicate a decreased incidence above the age of 75, which may be due to the mortality incident to infection of the diverticula. It is of interest that Kocour found the incidence of lesions of the gallbladder in persons above 40 years of age to be doubled in those having diverticula.

TABLE 22

Age incidence of diverticulosis of the colon

From a study of 7,000 consecutive autopsies (Kocour)

Age	Autopsis		White male	White female	Colored male	Colored female	Total
years							
21–30	566	Number	0	2	0	2	4
		Per cent*	0	1.9	0	1.19	0.7
31–40	895	Number	0	2	1	0	3
		Per cent	0	1.0	0.45	0	0.34
41–50	1,178	Number	4	3	5	3	15
		Per cent	0.8	1.5	1.9	1.6	1.27
51–60	1,024	Number	10	5	5	3	23
		Per cent	1.9	2.8	2.5	3.0	2.24
61–70	711	Number	28	9	4	5	46
		Per cent	6.4	6.9	4.4	9.3	6.47
70 up	437	Number	18	16	1	1	36
		Per cent	7.1	15.2	2.0	3.0	8.2

* The figures give the percentage of diverticula in relation to the number of necropsies performed in each class. Number of cases above 20 years of age examined total 4,811. The remainder under the age of 21 amounted to 2,189 and in this group no cases of diverticulosis were found.

The most widely held theory of the cause of diverticulosis is that the diverticula are due to pressure from gas in the colon associated with weakness of the elastic or muscular tissue. This is supported by the report of Hausemann (1896) that diverticula may be produced experimentally by distending at autopsy the senile, but not young colon, with water under pressure, and by the observation that in a number of cases the diverticula are very numerous above a stricture of the colon.

Constipation or colon stasis is considered to be a factor by some.   In this regard constipation is generally considered to be more frequent in women than in men, but a summary of the clinical cases of diverticulosis reported in the literature shows a frequency of 64.9 per cent in the male.   Since many of the cases of diverticulosis are symptomless, it would appear that data from consecutive necropsies in which special attention is given to the condition would be more reliable.   The data provided by Kocour (1937) which is the largest series of necropsies performed in which data on the true percentage incidence is given, show that diverticulosis was about 33 per cent more frequent in the female.   Although diverticula may be found throughout the colon, excluding the rectum where they rarely occur perhaps because the musculature of the rectum is more plentiful and uniformly distributed than in the colon, they are usually more frequent in the sigmoid than in the remainder of the colon.   It is of interest in this connection that Kantor (1931, 1932) who has studied his cases of constipation in relation to the form, position and abnormalities of the colon, has found that the cause of most of the varieties of constipation lies in the distal colon. For example, redundancy of the sigmoid was one and one-half times more frequent in patients complaining of constipation than the general incidence of redundancy.   Many physicians (Case, Soper, Hurst, Boas), who have given the subject special study, emphasize the importance of distal-colon stasis or malfunction as a cause of ordinary habitual constipation.   Of course, some believe that pressure in the colon causes diverticulosis only in those persons who have inherited, or have constitutionally, a colon with areas anatomically deficient in elastic and muscular tissue.   No attempt has been made to produce diverticulosis experimentally in such animals as the pig and monkey, which have a colon like that of man.

4. Gastro-intestinal passage time.

The average gastro-intestinal passage time in breast-fed "normal" infants is about 15 hours; it varies from 4 to 28 hours.   The time is usually longer in bottle-fed infants because cow's milk tends to constipate (Ivy, 1937).   The gastro-intestinal passage time varies widely in adults complaining of no symptoms.   The time of appearance of an orally ingested test material in the feces varies in most adult subjects from 20 to 72 hours; the time of final appearance varies from 2 to 7 days (Alvarez, 1928; Burnett, 1923; Hellebrandt and Miles, 1934). Similar data for elderly persons are not available.

The frequency of defecation in breast-fed infants during the first four months usually varies from two to four times daily; after this period the infant may be trained to defecate once daily. In a study of 527 males and 598 females ranging from 19 to 30 years of age, average 22, 96 per cent of the males and 92 per cent of the females defecated one or more times daily, the remainder from one to three times per week (Walsh, Ivy, Laing and Sippy, 1938). According to Humphry's study (Humphry, 1889), the bowels acted daily without assistance in 69 per cent of 824 persons between 80 and 100 years of age.

5. Constipation or colon stasis.

It is impossible for several reasons to evaluate the extensive clinical literature on the subject of constipation, particularly in regard to its age incidence.

The term constipation has many connotations. It may be a real or an imaginary complaint of a patient; or it may be a symptom arising from a faulty diet, an atonic or hypomotile colon, nervous factors, a cathartic or enema habit, real pathology, etc. Further, many habitually and truly constipated patients give a history of the complaint as present since infancy or childhood. Also, by simply correcting the diet or by improving gastro-intestinal hygiene, by removing cathartics and enemas, etc., frequently constipation, as a complaint, is relieved.

The only way that the true age incidence of that type of constipation which results from decreased motor activity of the colon might be determined would be to determine the gastro-intestinal or colonic passage time after placing the subjects on an adequate diet associated with proper hygiene. Then, some such plan of investigation as outlined recently by Kegerreis (1937) should be employed. The same plan would serve to determine the mean gastro-intestinal-passage time of persons not complaining of constipation or gastro-intestinal disturbances.

6. Constipation as a complaint.

According to Grulee (1923), constipation is one of the most common gastro-intestinal disorders in infancy. It may be present in the youngest infant and exist throughout infancy and childhood. Griffith and Mitchell (1934) state that age has little influence on the frequency of constipation in infancy and childhood. But data, worthy of consideration are not provided by the literature regarding the actual frequency of constipation as a complaint in infancy and childhood.

In a study of 1082 persons, 582 females and 500 males, between the age of 19 and 30 years, average age 22, Walsh and his collaborators (1938), found that 24.3 of males and 38.1 per cent of females complained of constipation. The subjects surveyed were college and medical students and nurses; only about 2 per cent had consulted a physician directly because of the complaint, and none of the males and only 1.5 per cent of the females resorted to aperients oftener than once per week. Of course, all persons who complain of constipation do not show an "abnormal delay" or slow passage time (72 hours is considered a normal average) of barium through the alimentary tract; about one-fifth do not (Kantor, 1931). On the other hand, Spriggs (1930–1931) found "abnormal delay" in the bowel in 1,000 patients out of 2086 complaining of colonic disorders. Of the 1,000 only 764 complained of constipation. Of these 670 took aperients and 431 took them every day.

In 3,000 ambulatory adult patients living in New York and complaining of gastro-intestinal symptoms, constipation was complained of in 46.5 per cent (Kantor, 1931). More recently Kantor (1938) has found that 54.2 per cent of 4,700 patients with dyspeptic symptoms complained of constipation; of course, in some of those with dyspeptic symptoms, the symptoms were probably caused by a cathartic habit. Of those complaining of constipation, 93.5 per cent had had the complaint longer than one and one-half years. Kantor has remarked, a remark that is not uncommonly made, that "in the majority of cases constipation is a life-long condition beginning during the youth or childhood of an individual." "Recent constipation" is at least five times as common in cancerous (alimentary tract cancers) as in non-cancerous patients. However, the age incidence by decades of constipation as a complaint in Kantor's large series is not provided; in fact, the author has not been able to locate such data except that given above for the third decade. Humphry (1889) states that very few (31 per cent) of the 824 persons above the age of 80, whose accounts he studied, complained of constipation or took aperients. The foregoing reports vary somewhat from the report of Stroup (1909) who found that 23 per cent of 134 men and 39 per cent of 96 women over the age of 60 suffered from constipation of more or less recent onset. The average of onset was 73 years in the males and 66 years in the females. Such variations in observations simply indicate that a careful study of many cases will be required before it can be concluded that ageing predisposes to the development of true constipation.

It is believed that rectal constipation or impaction of feces in the rectum occurs not uncommonly in the aged (Rolleston, 1932). No data are available, however, to show that this condition is more frequent in the aged than in the mature adult. Miles (1932) regards the development of the "pecten band," which limits the distention of the anal canal (Miles, 1919) to be a pathological development of advancing years.

7. Colonic malfunction.

In the clinical literature dealing with the colon, the statement is rather frequently made that colonic malfunction (constipation, non-ulcerative colitis, mucous colitis, or the so-called irritable or unstable colon) occurs most frequently from 20 to 50 years of age, generally in the fourth decade (Eggleston, 1934). The average age of Spriggs' (1930–1931) 242 cases of colonic malfunction was 44 for males and 42 for females. Eighty-three per cent of 200 cases of irritable colon observed by Jordan (1929, 1932) occurred between the age of 20 and 60 years, and 68 per cent between the age of 20 and 50, the largest number occurring during the fourth decade. The fact that the old and young are so immune is attributed to the relative tranquil conditions of living to which they are exposed. Ulcerative colitis has an age incidence not unlike that of functional disturbances of the colon. Brust and Bargen (1935), who report on a study of 1291 cases of ulcerative colitis, found that only 1.9 per cent of their patients were more than 60 years of age, and in these elderly patients the disease was relatively mild and limited to the distal colon.

10. RECTUM

1. Hemorrhoids.

Although hemorrhoids are associated with very definite local organic changes, some (Lockhart-Mummery, 1934) believe that the frequent occurrence of the condition in man in contrast to lower animals is the result of the erect posture. In view of the general changes in the tissues associated with ageing, one might expect hemorrhoids to increase with age. Further, the opinion is widely held that hemorrhoids frequently result from constipation.

In regard to the general incidence of hemorrhoids, Kantor (1931) made a study of 1,892 patients, the results of which give some indication of the occurrence of the condition as observed in gastro-intestinal medical practice, and not that of a proctologist. In this group 9 per cent manifested active hemorrhoids and an additional 17 per cent "healed hemorrhoids" on physical examination. His study showed further that hemorrhoids were as frequent in patients complaining (29 per cent) of colitis, a condition associated with diarrhea, as of constipation (26 per cent), and that the condition was more frequent (38 per cent) in the presence of the cathartic habit than in any other group. Although with such evidence it is not possible to separate cause and effect, such evidence supports the opinion that the most important predisposing cause of hemorrhoids is the abuse of the rectum and anal canal with purgatives, or abnormal and frequent defecation, i.e., a functional disturbance.

Hemorrhoids are seldom seen in infants and children. The condition rarely occurs before the third and fourth year of age, and is usually associated with constipation in children (Goodman, 1923). The condition was found to be present in 10.3 per cent of 283 males and 6.8 per cent of 305 females between the ages of 19 and 30. At the Mayo Clinic 3.4 per cent of all patients that enter have hemorrhoids; whereas 48.8 per cent of those who present complaints referable to the bowel have hemorrhoids (Buie, 1938b). In 23,443 patients with hemorrhoids the condition was clinically found most frequently in the fifth decade. Unfortunately, however, the true age distribution was not estimated (Buie, 1938a).

It would appear that ageing may be a factor in increasing the incidence of hemorrhoids, but in view of the several other factors which predispose or contribute to their cause, it will be difficult to ascertain the truth regarding the effect of ageing *per se* on the condition.

11. SUMMARY

On considering the digestive system, three questions of prime importance to the ageing person arise. These questions are: What is the likelihood of death from disease of the digestive system? What is the likelihood of one of the digestive organs wearing out prematurely? And, what may the ageing person do to prevent or delay the onset of disease and wearing-out processes of the digestive organs? The first two questions have been answered on the basis of the evidence available. The third question will be briefly considered; it can be answered only by very general and appropriately qualified statements.

No scientific data are available which show that those diseases and atrophic changes of the digestive organs associated particularly with ageing can be prevented or postponed by any general method or procedure. The trite recommendation to eat and live wisely and not to over-indulge in food, drink, irritating condiments, to seek a periodic health examination and to advise with the physician at the onset of digestive symptoms is undoubtedly rational. Chronic irritation should predispose to premature atrophy of any mucosa and may explain the greater incidence of buccal and gastric cancer in the male and of cancer of the gallbladder in the female. Early diagnosis and operation for cancer of the operable digestive organs is obviously important. Although the cause of cirrhosis of the liver is unknown, it would appear that various toxic substances exaggerate the process and that the symptoms of the disease and possibly its progress respond to dietary management. Pernicious anemia and its complications are subject to control in the majority of coöperative patients. The same is true, but to a less degree, of gastric and duodenal ulcer. Intestinal obstruction, appendicitis and hernia are frequently amenable to early surgical intervention. Diarrhea and enteritis are avoidable by observing careful dietary precautions and are amenable to early medical care.

In the aged the quantity of saliva secreted and the amount of starch digesting enzyme it contains is less than that of younger persons. This shows that the salivary glands tend to involute with age. Evidence obtained from old dogs indicates that this functional change is due to atrophic changes in the cells of the glands. To what extent the dimunition of salivary secretion in the aged interferes with starch digestion is uncertain.

Unchallengeable evidence pertaining to the effect of ageing on the morphology of the gastric mucosa does not exist. However, after the age of 20 the production of hydrochloric acid by the stomach of both sexes decreases. The percentage of persons whose stomachs secrete no hydrochloric acid, a condition known as achlorhydria, markedly increases after 40 years. Above the age of 60 about 35 per cent of people have a stomach which does not secrete acid when they eat a meal; and 28 per cent have a stomach which does not secrete in response to the drug histamine, a powerful excitant of gastric secretion. This decline in the capacity of the stomach to secrete acid is apparently the result of a physiological involution and becomes manifest first in those persons who are endowed with a less responsive and a more vulnerable gastric secretory mechanism. To what extent the eating and drinking habits and the previous health of the individual contribute to the development of achlorhydria is unknown. Irritating foods and infections may produce chronic gastritis which may in turn cause achlorhydria; or, achlorhydria secondary to a constitutional factor may predispose to gastritis. Achlorhydria is compatible with good health, but it may predispose to several serious conditions, such as anemia, pernicious anemia, inadequate calcification of bone, and enteritis and diarrhea. In pernicious anemia, a disease that afflicts elderly people chiefly, achlorhydria is nearly always found. This disease is at least in part due to the failure of the stomach and intestine to secrete an essential enzyme. Whether the failure of the stomach and intestine to secrete the enzyme adequately is due to ageing or an atrophy secondary to gastritis is uncertain.

Although the death rate from gastric and duodenal ulcer increases with age, much evidence indicates that these diseases are related more to the mode of living and eating, and are commonly acquired some ten or twenty years before they cause death. The onset of ulcer of the stomach or duodenum rarely occurs after the age of 60, or during the more tranquil conditions of old age. But, when an elderly person starts to bleed from an ulcer, the hemorrhage is likely to be more serious because of sclerosis or hardening of the blood vessels. The greater incidence of these diseases in the male is generally ascribed to his higher mean gastric acidity and the greater stresses of life to which he is exposed. Whether gastric ulcer is a common cause of gastric cancer is still debatable. This is important because in persons above 45 years, cancer of the stomach causes death six or seven times more frequently than gastric ulcer. Seventy per cent of observers consider that less than 20 per cent of gastric cancers arise from ulcers.

Although considerable factual data are available regarding the shape, position and the rate of evacuation of the stomach in the infant, child and adult, none are available for the aged. In regard to the hunger motility of the stomach, the evidence shows that the irritability of the gastric motor mechanism decreases with age. The truth of this statement depends chiefly on observations made on the dog, since the hunger motility of elderly persons has not been studied. Also, since the incidence of gastritis is alleged to increase with age and gastritis diminishes hunger motility, hunger motility should be less in the aged than in the mature adult.

As is true for the stomach, the secretion of the pancreas is relatively poor in the infant and increases during childhood. But, whether the secretion of the pancreas declines, as the weight of the organ apparently does after the age of 60, is unknown. On the basis of the decline of salivary and gastric secretion, one would predict that pancreatic secretion also declines with age. To what extent the associated decline of gastric and pancreatic secretion, the most important digestive juices, accounts for the senile inanition that is sometimes observed in the aged has not been studied. This would be revealed by appropriate metabolic studies. The factor of the effect of age on absorption from the intestine would also be involved, but, nothing is known regarding the effect of ageing on the absorptive processes of the small intestine.

It is clear that the liver manifests morphologically a period of growth, maturity and involution. Data are not available, however, to warrant a similar statement in regard to the secretion of bile. It would appear that the increase in connective tissue reported to be present in the liver of the aged is due to pathological processes rather than to physiological senescence. The capacity of the liver to regenerate in the aged has not been determined, and there is no evidence indicating that the functional activity is decreased by ageing *per se* sufficiently to cause death. Ageing probably decreases the factor of safety of the liver so that it may be more vulnerable to diseases of the liver which produce death more frequently in elderly than in young persons. It is clear, however, that dogs in ageing may naturally acquire an atypical hepatic epithelium like that which occurs as a repair process following liver injury produced experimentally with certain hepatic poisons. Whether this change is due to minor insults of the liver received as a result of the exigencies of life or is a direct result of ageing, cannot be stated. There is reason for believing that the liver, if protected from pathological processes, may serve the body much longer than the usual span of life.

Available data show that the gallbladder of elderly persons, if it escapes disease, evacuates well. After puberty the gallbladder of females, except during pregnancy, empties faster than that of males. It would appear that the factor of pregnancy, which tends for some unknown reason, to cause stasis in the gallbladder, is chiefly responsible for the higher mortality of females from diseases of the gallbladder.

There is no good evidence indicating that the small intestine atrophies morphologically or functionally with age. The fact that after early childhood intestinal obstruction causes more deaths above the sixth decade than in previous ones does not necessarily mean weakness of the intestines. It must be remembered that herniae, abdominal adhesions, and neoplasms, the more common causes of intestinal obstruction in the aged, increase with age.

The mortality rate from appendicitis is relatively high in the aged.

This is attributed to the atrophy of lymphoid tissue and the lowered resistance of elderly persons.

There is no evidence indicating that the capacity of the colon for absorption and for the secretion of mucus is decreased in elderly persons. Neither does evidence exist showing that the rate of passage of contents through the gastrointestinal tract or colon is changed by ageing. The best evidence indicating that a weakening of the muscular and elastic tissue of the colon occurs with age, is the increased incidence of diverticulosis in elderly persons. Diverticulosis has a general incidence of about 7 per cent in persons over 60, and is about 33 per cent more frequent in females than in males. The condition becomes serious when the diverticula become inflamed and infected, or diverticulitis occurs.

There is no reason to believe that constipation is more common in the aged. The concensus of opinion is that constipation is generally a life long or a long standing condition or complaint. If of recent onset in the aged, it may indicate the presence of a neoplasm of the colon. It is striking that 31 per cent of a group of 1082 college students complained of constipation and that only thirty-one per cent of 824 persons above the age of 80 complained of constipation. It must be remembered that constipation as a complaint may be present in a patient when true constipation is not.

Ageing may be a factor in the etiology of hemorrhoids, but in view of the several factors which contribute to their cause, the data available does not permit a conclusion.

On reviewing the evidence of ageing in the digestive system, one gains the impression that the organs of the system manifest the elements of growth, maturity, and senescence. The evidence supporting such an impression is very incomplete. In most instances the evidence requisite for establishing the impression may be obtained readily by carefully planned though time consuming studies.

Death in the aged is apparently only rarely due to a wearing out of the organs of the digestive system. Most elderly persons die with a digestive system, when not directly affected by cancer, a toxic or an infectious process, that is capable of functioning beyond the ordinary life span. Atrophic changes as a consequence of ageing or of injury by external agents may cause death or serve as a contributory cause. Whether these changes contribute to neoplastic growth, which is so common in the digestive system, is, of course, uncertain. Even though the consequence of ageing per se in the digestive system are not serious, it is striking that during life, symptoms referable to the gastrointestinal tract occur more frequently than those referable to any other system in the body (fig. 33). This is because the alimentary tract is so readily influenced reflexly by mental states and by disease elsewhere in the body, and because many of the symptoms of disturbance of the tract are functional in nature and tend to respond readily to diet and rest. This is probably why Josh Billings wrote: "I have finally kum tu the konklusion that a good reliable sett of bowels is worth more tu a man than enny quantity of brains."

REFERENCES

ALLEN, A. W. 1933. Bleeding duodenal ulcer. New England J. of Med., **208**, 237–241.

ALVAREZ, W. C. 1928. The mechanics of the digestive tract. New York: Paul B. Hoeber Inc., 447 pp.

ARNOLD, L. 1933. Bacterial flora within stomach and small intestine; effect of experimental alterations of acid-base balance and of age. Am. J. M. Sc., **186**, 471–480.

ATKINSON, A. J., AND IVY, A. C. 1938. Further attempts to produce achlorhydria. Am. J. Digest, Dis. & Nutrition (in press).

BERGEIM, O. 1926. Intestinal chemistry. Arch. Int. Med., **37**, 110–117.

BLOOMFIELD, A. L., AND POLLAND, W. S. 1933. Gastric anacidity: its relation to disease. New York: Macmillan, 188 pp.

BOHMANSSON, G. 1934. On the diagnosis and treatment of severe hemorrhages from peptic ulcer. Acta chir. Scandinav., **74**, 476–477.

BOYD, R. 1861. Tables and weights of the human body and internal organs in the sane and insane of both sexes at various ages, arranged from 2614 post-mortem examinations. Phil. Trans. Roy. Soc., **151**, 241–262.

BOYD, E. 1933. Normal variability in weight of the adult human liver and spleen. Arch. Path., **16**, 350–372.

BOYDEN, E. A., AND GRANTHAM, S. A., JR. 1936. Evacuation of the gallbladder in old age. Surg. Gynec. & Obst., **62**, 34–42.

BRANDTS, C. E. 1909. Über Einschlüsse im Kern der Leberzelle und ihre Beziehungen zur Pigmentbildung beim Hund, beim Menschen. Ziegler's Beitr. z. pathol. Anat., **45**, 457–475.

BRUST, J. C. M., AND BARGEN, J. A. 1935. Chronic ulcerative colitis among elderly persons. Minnesota Med., **18**, 583–585.

BUIE, L. A. 1938 a. Personal communication.

———— 1938 b. Practical Proctology. Philadelphia; W. B. Saunders Co 512 pp.

BURNETT, F. L. 1923. The intestinal rate and the form of the feces. Am. J. Rontgenol., **10**, 599–604.

BUSSABARGER, R. A., FREEMAN, SMITH, AND IVY, A. C. 1938. The experimental production of homogeneous osteoporosis by gastrectomy. Am. J. Physiol., **121**, 137–149.

BUSSON, A., AND SIMONNET, H. 1932. Variation de la reserve en Vitamie A der Foie Suivant l'age chez le chien. Compt. rend. Soc. de biol., **109**, 1253–1254.

CABOT, R. C. 1927. Pernicious anemia. In Osler's Modern Medicine. Re-edited by Thomas McCrae, Vol. V, Chapt. 2, Philadelphia: Lea and Febiger.

CARLSON, A. J. 1916. The control of hunger in health and disease, Chicago, University of Chicago Press, 316 pp.

———— 1923. Secretion of gastric juice in health and disease. Physiol. Rev., 3, 1–40.

CASTLE, W. B., AND MINOT, G. R. 1936. Pathology, Physiology and Clinical Descriptions of the Anemias. New York: Oxford University Press, 205 pp.

CHENEY, W. F. 1926. Significance of achlorhydria. J. A. M. A., 87, 22–25.

CHIESMAN, W. E. 1932. Mortality of severe hemorrhage from peptic ulcers. Lancet, 2, 722–723.

CHRISTIANSEN, T. 1935. On massive hemorrhage in peptic ulcer. Acta med. Scandinav., 84, 374–385.

COCCHI, C. 1924. Richerche sull'amilasi nella saliva del bambino battante nei primi mesi di vita. Riv. di clin, pediat., 22, 449–457.

CORNELL, B. S. 1927. Pernicious Anemia. Durham: Duke University Press, 297 pp.

CRUMP, C. 1931. The incidence of gallstones and gallbladder disease. Surg., Gynec. & Obst., 53, 447–455.

DAVIDSON, L. S. P., AND GULLAND, G. L. 1930. Pernicious Anemia. London: H. Kimpton, 305 pp.

DAVIES, D. T., AND JAMES, T. G. I. 1930–31. An investigation into the gastric secretion of 100 normal persons over the age of sixty. Quart. J. Med., 23, 1–14. (Also Lancet, 1930, 2, 899–901.)

DEAVER, J., AND BORTZ, E. L. 1927. Gallbladder disease, a review of 903 cases (operated). J. A. M. A., 88, 619–623.

DE BUYS, L. R., AND HENRIQUE, A. 1918. Effect of body posture on the position and emptying time of the stomach. Am. J. Dis. Child., 15, 190–195.

DEDICHEN, L. 1924–25. Anacidity in old persons. Acta med. Scandinav., 61, supp. no. 7, 345–350.

DEUEL, H. J., JR., BUTTS, J. S., HALLMAN, L. F., MURRAY, S., AND BLUNDEN, H. 1933. The effect of age on the sex difference in the content of liver glycogen. J. Biol. Chem., 119, 617–620.

DIETRICH, H., AND SHELBY, D. C. 1931. Gastric analysis in childhood. Am. J. Dis. Child., 41, 1086–1099.

DONALDSON, H. H. 1924. The Rat. Philadelphia: Wistar Institute Press, 2nd ed., 469 pp.

DORDI, A. M. 1931. Richerche sperimentalli sull'azione del riflesso psichico visivo e del succhiamento sulla secrezione gastrica del lattante. Riv. di clin. pediat., 29, 791–802.

DUBLIN, L. I., AND LOTKA, A. J. 1937. Twenty-five years of health progress. New York: Metropolitan Life Insurance Co., 611, pp.

EGGLESTON, E. L. 1934. Functional disorders of the colon. J. Michigan M. Soc. 33, 378–382.

EINHORN, M. 1892. On achylia gastrica. Med. Rec., 41, 650–654.

EUSTERMAN, G. B., AND BALFOUR, D. C. 1935. The stomach and duodenum. Philadelphia: W. B. Saunders Co., 958 pp.

EWING, James 1931. Neoplastic diseases. 3rd Ed., Philadelphia, W. B. Saunders Co., p. 1127.

FABER, K. 1927. Chronic gastritis; its relation to achylia and ulcer. Lancet, 2, 901–907.

———— 1935. Gastritis and its consequences. Copenhagen: Gyldendolske Boghandel Nordick Foslog, 119 pp.

FIFIELD, L. R. 1927. Diverticulitis. Lancet, 1, 277–281.

FREEMAN, E. B. 1930. A study of the hydrogen ion concentration and diastase content of mouth secretion. Trans. Am. Gastroenterol. Asso., 151–156.

FRISCHMANN, F. 1932. Das Verhalten des Bindegewebsergüstes der Leber des Menschen beim Wachstum und Altern. Zeitschr. f. mickr. anat. Forsch., 31, 635–648.

GERDES, M. M., AND BOYDEN, E. A. 1936. Retardation of the gallbladder in pregnancy. Proc. Soc. Exper. Biol. Med., 35, 393–394.

GINSBURG, J., TUMPOWSKY, I., AND CARLSON, A. J. 1915. The onset of hunger in infants after feeding. J. A. M. A., 64, 1922-25.

GOODMAN, A. L. 1923. In Abt's Pediatrics, Vol. III, Chapt. 50, Philadelphia: W. B. Saunders Co.

GOODPASTURE, E. W. 1918. An anatomical study of senescence in dogs, with especial reference to the relation of cellular changes of age to tumors. J. Med. Research, 38, 127–190.

GRAHAM, E. A. 1928. Diseases of the gallbladder and bile ducts. Philadelphia: Lea and Febiger, 477 pp.

GRIFFITH, J. P. C., AND MITCHELL, A. G. 1934. Diseases of infants and children. Philadelphia: W. B. Saunders Co., 1155 pp.

GRULEE, C. G. 1923. In Abt's Pediatrics, Vol. III, Chapt. 46, Philadelphia: W. B. Saunders Co.

GUNDOBIN, A. P. 1912. Die Besonderheiten des Kinderalters, Berlin: Allgemeine Medizinische Verlagsanstalt, 592 pp.

HAMPERL, H. 1931. Beiträge zur normalen und pathologischen Histologie Menschlicher. Ztschr. f. mikro.-anat. Forsch., 27, 1–55.

———— 1933. Über besondere Zellen in alternden Mundspeicheldrüsen (Onkocyten) und ihre Beziehungen zu den Adenolymphonen und Adenomen. Bemerkungen zu der Arbeit von G. Steinhardt. Virchow's Arch., 291, 704–705.

———— 1937. Über das Vorkommen von Onkocyten in Verschiedenen Organen und ihren Geschwülsten. Virchow's Arch., 298, 327–375.

HAUSEMANN, D. 1896. Über die Entstehung falscher Darmdivertikel. Virchow's Arch., 144, 400–406.

HAWK, P. B., REHFUSS, M. E., AND BERGEIM, O. 1926. Response of normal human stomach to various standard foods and a summary. Am. J. Med. Sci., 171, 359–369.

HELLEBRANDT, FRANCES A., AND MILES, M. M. 1934. The influence of exercise on the rate of passage of inert material through the digestive tract. Research Quart., 5, 73–79.

HELMER, O. M., FOUTS, P. J., AND ZERFAS, W. G. 1933. Pancreatic enzymes in pernicious anemia. J. Clin. Invest., 12, 519–532.

HUMPHRY, G. M. 1989. Old age: the results of information received respecting nearly nine hundred persons who had attained the age of eighty years, including seventy-four centenarians. Cambridge: Macmillan, 218 pp.

HURST, A. J., AND STEWART, M. J. 1929. Gastric and duodenal ulcer. New York: Oxford University press, 544 pp.

HUTTER, A. M., AND MIDDLETON, W. S. 1933. Vitamin B deficiency and atrophic tongue J. A. M. A., 101, 1305–1308.

IVY, A. C. 1934. The physiology of the gallbladder. Physiol. Rev., 14, 1–102.

————— 1936–37. Certain aspects of the applied physiology of external pancreatic secretion. Am. J. Digest. Dis. & Nutrition, 3, 677–682.

————— 1937. Physiology of the gastro-intestinal tract of infants and children. in Brennemann's Practice of Pediatrics, Vol. 1, Chapt. 20.

————— 1938. Unpublished observations.

IVY, A. C., MORGAN, J. B., AND FARRELL, J. I. 1931. Effects of total gastrectomy; experimental achylia gastrica in dogs with occurrence of spontaneous anemia and anemia of pregnancy. Surg., Gynec. & Obst., 53, 611–620.

IVY, A. C., RICHTER, O., MEYER, A. F., AND GREENGARD, H. 1934. The relation of gastrectomy to anemia. Am. J. Digest. Dis. & Nutrition, 1, 116–119 and 560–561.

IVY, A. C., SCHMIDT, C. R., AND BEAZELL, J. M. 1936. The gastric digestion of starches. J. Nutrition, 12, 59–83.

IZUMITA, T. 1930a. Über die Azidität des Magensaftes bei gesunden Neugeborenen und Säuglingen. Jahrb. f. Kinderh., 129, 319–334.

————— 1930 b. Über die Form des Magens des japanischen Säuglings, insbesondere die Formveränderung bei dem Entleerungsvorgang. Jahrb. f. Kinderh., 129, 153–170.

JACKSON, C. M. 1929. The effects of inanition and malnutrition on growth and structure. Arch. Path., 7, 1042–1078; 8, 81–122 and 273–315.

JAFFE, R. H. 1933. Cholelithiasis. A statistical study with special reference to its frequency in the colored race. J. Lab. & Clin. Med., 18, 1220–1226.

JONES, C. M., CASTLE, W. B., MULHOLLAND, H. B., AND BAILEY, F. 1925. Pancreatic and hepatic activities of duodenal contents of normal man. Arch. Int. Med., 35, 315–336.

JORDAN, S. M. 1932. The irritable colon and neurosis. J. A. M. A., 99, 2234–2237.

JUDD, E. STARR, AND HOERNER, M. T. 1935. Jejunal Ulcer., Ann. Surg., 102, 1003–1018.

KANTOR, J. L. 1931a. The practical significance of digestive tract anomalies. J. Michigan M Soc., 30, 820–828.

————— 1931b. Hemorrhoids—medical aspect. Am. J. Surg., 14, 620–623.

————— 1931 c. Anomalies of duodenum and colon. J. A. M. A., 97, 1785–1790.

————— 1932. Roentgen diagnosis of diseases and abnormalities of the colon. Radiology, 19, 269–281.

————— 1938. Personal communication.

KEEFER, C. S., AND BLOOMFIELD, A. L. 1926. The significance of anacidity. Bull. Johns Hopkins Hosp., 39, 304–329.

KEGERREIS, R. 1937. A method of determining and recording human intestinal motility. Am. J. Digest. Dis. & Nutrition, **4**, 432–438.

KLUMPF, T. G., AND NEALE, A. V. 1930. The gastric and duodenal contents of normal infants and children. Am. J. Dis. Child., **40**, 1215–1229.

KOCOUR, E. J. 1937. Diverticulosis of the colon. Am. J. Surg., **37**, 433–436.

LOCKHART-MUMMERY, J. P. 1934. Diseases of the Rectum and Colon, 2nd ed. Baltimore: W. Wood & Co., 605 pp.

LUBARSCH, O., AND BORCHARDT, F. 1929. In Henke-Lubarsch, Handbuch der speciellen pathologischen Anatomie and Histologie, Berlin, IV, part 3.

LUCKHARDT, A. B., AND HAMBURGER, W. W. 1916. Contributions to the movements of the empty stomach. A note on the movements of the empty stomach in certain pathologic states. J. A. M. A., **66**, 1831–1833.

LUTKENS, ULRICH. 1926. Aufbau und Funktion der extra-hepatischen Gallenwege mit besonderer Bezugnahme auf die primären Gallenwegsstauungen und die Gallensteinkrankheiten. Leipzig: Vogel, 205 pp.

LUNDING, K. 1935. The symptomatology of diverticulum formation of the colon. Acta med. Skandinav., **72**, 1–286.

MACNIDER, WM. DE B. 1935. The resistance of fixed tissue cells to the toxic action of certain chemical substances. Science, **81**, 601–605.

——— 1936. The resistance to chloroform of a naturally acquired atypical type of liver epithelium occuring in senile animals. J. Pharmacol. & Exper. Therap., **56**, 383–387.

McCLURE, C. W., WETMORE, A. S., AND REYNOLDS, L. 1921 a. Physical characters and enzymatic activities of duodenal contents. J. A. M. A., **77**, 1468–1471.

——— 1921 b. New methods for estimating enzymatic activities of duodenal contents of normal man. Arch. Int. Med., **27**, 706–715.

McIVER, M. A. 1932. Acute intestinal obstruction. Arch. Surg., **25**, 1098–1134.

MAES, U. 1925. Appendicitis in aged. New Orleans M. &. S. J., **78**, 117–122.

MANN, F. C., AND MAGATH, T. B. 1922. The production of chronic liver insufficiency. Am. J. Physiol., **59**, 485–486.

MAYER, W. B. 1929. A comparison of the amylase concentration in the saliva of infants and adults. Bull. Johns Hopkins Hosp., **44**, 246–247.

MENTZER, S. H. 1926. Clinical and pathological study of cholecystitis and cholelithiasis. Surg., Gynec. & Obst., **42**, 782–793.

MEYER, J., GOLDEN, J. S., STEINER, N., AND NECHELES, H. 1937. The content of human saliva in old age Am. J. Physiol., **119**, 600–602.

MILES, W. E. 1919 Observations upon internal piles. Surg., Gynec. & Obst., **19**, 497–506.

——— 1932. Rolleston, Medical Aspects of Old Age, 2nd ed., London: Macmillan, 205 pp.

MILLER, S. P. 1927. Effects of inanition on the stomach and intestines of albino rats underfed from birth for various periods. Arch. Path., **3**, 26–41.

MOODY, R. O. 1927. The position of the abdominal viscera in healthy young British and American adults. J. Anat., **61**, 223–231.

MOODY, R. O., VAN NUYS, R. G., AND CHAMBERLAIN, W. E. 1923. Position of the stomach, liver and colon. J. A. M. A., **81**, 1924–1931.

MORITZ, D., AND SCHMITT, A. 1933. Magenfunktionsprüfungen bei Frühgeborenen. Arch. f. Kinderh., **99**, 23–27.

NEALE, A. V. 1930. Gastric secretion in infants and children. Arch. Dis. Child., **5**, 137–145.

NEWCOMB, W. D. 1932. The relationship between peptic ulceration and gastric carcinoma. Brit. J. Surg., **20**, 279–308.

NICORY, C. 1922. Salivary secretion in infants. Biochem. J., **16**, 387–389.

OLIVER, T. H., AND WILKINSON, J. F. 1933. Achlorhydria, a critical review. Quart. J. Med., **26**, 431–462.

PATTERSON, T. L. 1914. The variations in the hunger contractions of the empty stomach with age. Am. J. Physiol., **33**, 423–429.

———— 1915. The cause of the variations in the gastric hunger contractions with age. *Ibid.*, **37**, 316–329.

PERMAN, E. 1935. Surgical treatment of gastric and duodenal ulcer. Acta chir. Scandinav., **77**, supp. 38, 1–333.

POESCHEL, R. 1930. Magenfunktion bei alten Leuten. Ztschr. f. klin. Med. **113**, 379–386.

POLLITZER, R. 1921. Gastric secretion in newborn. Pediatrica, **29**, 253–259.

POLLAND, W. S. 1933. Histamine test meals, an anlysis of 988 consecutive tests. Arch. Int. Med., **51**, 903–919.

PORTIS, S. A., AND JAFFE, R. H. 1938. A study of peptic ulcer based on necropsy records. J. A. M. A., **110**, 6–9.

POTTER, M. G. 1936. Observations of gallbladder and bile during pregnancy at term. J. A. M. A., **106**, 1070–1074.

RIBBERT. 1893. Beiträge zur normalen und pathologischen Anatomie des Wurmfortsatzes. Virchow's Arch., **132**, 66–90.

RICHTER, OSCAR 1938. Personal communication. Data to be published.

RIVERS, A. B. 1928. The dangers of treating "indigestion" by advertised nostrums. Proc. Mayo Clinic, **13**, 87–88.

ROLLESTON, H. 1932. Medical Aspects of Old Age. 2nd ed., London: Macmillan, 205 pp.

ROYSTER, H. A. 1927. Appendicitis. New York: Appleton, 370 pp.

SAGAL, Z., MARKS, J. A., AND KANTOR, J. L. 1933. The clinical significance of gastric anacidity. A study of 6679 cases with digestive symptoms. Ann. Int. Med., **7**, 76–88.

SCAMMON, R. E. 1919. Some graphs and tables illustrating the growth of the human stomach. Am. J. Dis. Child., **17**, 295–296.

———— 1923. A survey of the anatomy of the infant and child. In Abt's Pediatrics. Vol. 1, Chapt. 3.

———— 1926–27. The prenatal growth of the human pancreas. Proc. Soc. Exper. Biol. & Med., **24**, 391–392.

———— 1930. In the Measurement of Man. Minneapolis: University of Minnesota Press, 215 pp.

SCAMMON, R. E., AND KITTELSON, J. A. 1926–27. The growth of the gastrointestinal tract of the human fetus. Proc. Soc. Exper. Biol. & Med., **24**, 303.

SCHATZKI, R. 1932. Die Beweglichkeit von Ösophagus und Magen innerhalb des Zwerchschlitzes beim alten Menschen. Fortsch. a. d. geb. d. Röntgenstrahlen., **45**, 177–187.

SCHLOSSMANN, E. 1922. Age incidence of appendicitis. Arch. f. Kinderh., 71, 208-214.

SCHMIDT, A. 1911. Leitsätze über die Diagnose, Pathogenese und Aetiologie des Chronischen Darmkatarrhs. Med. Klin. Berlin, 7, 50-51.

SCHNEDORF, J. G., AND IVY, A. C. 1937. The incidence and permanence of unexplained gastric anacidity in the Rhesus monkey after histamine and mecholyl, with hematologic studies. Am. J. Digest. Dis. & Nutrition, 4, 429-432.

SCHIFF, E. 1923. Asthenic children. Monatschr f. Kinderh., 26, 1-16.

SIEMSEN, W. J. 1932. Histamine test of gastric secretion with particular reference to its practicability in childhood. Am. J. Dis. Child., 44, 1013-1025.

SMITH, R. R. 1912. A study of children with reference to enteroptosis. J. A. M. A., 58, 385-392.

SPRIGGS, E. I. 1930-31. Functional disorders of the colon. Quart. J. Med., 24, 533-565.

STEINHARDT, G. 1933. Über besondere Zellen in den alternden Mundspeicheldrüsen (Onkocyten) und ihre Beziehungen zu den Adenolymphomen und Adenomen. Virchow's Arch., 289, 624-635.

SORRMONT, D. L. 1928. The salivary glands. Cowdry's Special Cytology, Vol. 1, Chapt. 5 New York: Paul B. Hoeber.

STROUP, A. 1893. Recherches sur la constipation chez le vieillard. These de Nancy, (loc. cit. Hurst, A. F. Constipation and Allied Intestinal Disorders, London, 1909, 344 pp.)

SUTHERLAND, G. F. 1921. The response of the stomach glands to gastrin before and shortly after birth. Am. J. Physiol., 55, 258-276 and 398-403.

TAKASHINA, O. 1932. Studien über die entrale Adrenalinesorption mit besonderer Berucksichtigung des Alters. Jap. J. Med. Sci., IV. Pharm., 6, 35-113.

TAYLOR, R. 1917 a. Hunger in the infant. Am. J. Dis. Child., 14, 258-266.

———— 1917 b. Hunger secretion. Am. J. Dis. Child., 14, 233-257.

TELLING, W. H. M., AND GRUNER, O. C. 1916-17. Acquired diverticula, diverticulitis and peridiverticulitis of the large intestine. Brit. J. Surg., 4, 468-530.

THOMSEN, E. 1925. Neurogenous and cellular achylia. Acta med. Scandinav., 61, 377-432 and 522-569.

TOLDT, C. 1880. Die Entwicklung und Ausbildung der Drüsen des Magens. Sitzungsb. d. bk. Skad. I. Wissenschi. Mo. Naturwlk., 82, 57-128.

VANZANT, FRANCES R., ALVEREZ, W. C., EUSTERMAN, G. B., DUNN, H. L., AND BERKSON, J. 1932. The normal range of gastric acidity from youth to old age. Arch. Int. Med., 49, 345-359.

VANZANT, FRANCES, R., ALVAREZ, W. C., BERKSON, J., AND EUSTERMAN, G. B. 1933. Changes in gastric acidity in peptic ulcer, cholecystitis and other diseases. Arch. Int. Med., 52, 616-631.

VANZANT, FRANCES R., ALVAREZ, W. C., AND BERKSON, J. 1936-37. The relation in man between the gastric acidity and height and weight. Am. J. Digest. Dis. & Nutrition, 3, 83-86.

VIERORDT, H. 1906. Daten und Tabellen für Mediziner. 3rd ed., Jena, G. Fischer, 616 pp.

VOEGTLIN, W. U., GREENGARD, H., AND IVY, A. C. 1934. The response of the canine and human pancreas to secretin. Am. J. Physiol., 110, 198–224.

WALSH, E. L., IVY, A. C., LAING, G. H., AND SIPPY, H. L. 1938. On the behavior of the average human colon: age group 19 to 30 years. In Press.

WANGENSTEEN, O. H. 1937. Bowel Obstruction. Springfield, Ill.: Thomas, 360 pp.

WARTHIN. A. S. 1929. Old age; the major involution; the physiology and pathology of aging process. New York: Paul B. Hoeber Inc., 199 pp.

WESTPHAL, K. 1923. Muskelfunktion, Nervensystem und Pathologie der Gallenwege. Zeitsch. f. klin. Med., 96, 22–150.

WHIPPLE, G. H., AND SPERRY, J. A. 1909. Chloroform poisoning. Liver necrosis and repair. Bull. Johns Hopkins Hospital, 30, 278–289.

WILKINSON, J. F., AND BROCKBANK, W. 1931. The importance of familial achlorhydria in the etiology of pernicious anemia. Quart. J. Med., 24, 219–238.

WRIGHT, C. B. 1924. Gastric secretion, gastrointestinal moiltity and position of the stomach. Arch. Int. Med., 33, 435–448.

YAVORSKY, M., ALMADEN, P., AND KING, C. G. 1934. The vitamin C content of human tissues. J. Biol. chem., 106, 525–529.

Chapter 10

URINARY SYSTEM

JEAN R. OLIVER

Brooklyn

As a biological problem ageing of the kidney derives interest more from its theoretical implications than from the practical aspect of ill effects produced by the senescent processes. The relative small place that disturbances of renal eliminatory function occupy in the picture of old age is however not due to any lack of senile change in the kidney but rather to the fact that, like most glandular organs, it contains so large a reserve of functioning tissue as to be rarely exhausted to the point of appreciable dysfunction.

1. GENERAL EVIDENCE OF RENAL SENESCENCE

That the kidney does grow old and lose its youthful adaptability to demands upon its powers of structural and functional growth is evident from the experiments of MacKay, MacKay and Addis (1924). In this investigation there was not observed with old rats the same response of compensatory renal hypertrophy following the removal of one kidney as was found with young animals. During the first month of life for example, there was a 52.6 per cent increase in the weight of the remaining kidney over half the weight of the kidneys of a control group, whereas at one year the final replacement was only 32.3 per cent.

When an exact determination of the physical basis of this senescence is attempted a problem of difficult solution arises, for in the kidney, as in all tissues and systems of higher mammals, there occurs the complication of incident "pathological" disease that must be separated from the "normal" processes of ageing. The varied alterations in the human kidney that follow vascular change, the so-called benign and malignant nephroscleroses of the clinician, are examples of such difficulties. In these questions the final decision as to what are to be considered phenomona of normal senescence will depend on the interpretation of the nature of the primary arteriosclerosis, an interpretation subject to wide variation, since it is often conditioned by the metaphysical aspects of the problem. For example, the implication of certain authorities that arteriosclerosis should be considered a "disease,"

257

since the acceptance of its involutional nature leaves no hope for prophylaxis and treatment.

The guiding thread that runs through all modern studies of senescence is the concept that its phenomona mark the orderly downward slope of a curve that ascended to maturity. It is indeed possible to construct graphs representing the waxing and final wane of the renal tissue with the passage of years that have the general configuration of such a curve. Figure 1 shows the weight of the kidney of man (Roessle and Roulet, 1932) and the number of glomeruli in the rat's kidney (Arataki, 1926) from birth to senility. We are to be concerned therefore in this discussion, not with the fortuitous accidents of accumulated years, but only with changes "normal" to the life history of the individual and which fit with no disturbing effect into such an ideal curve.

If the problem of senescence is examined from this standpoint, the kidney proves to be a peculiarly fortunate example for study. For the "kidney" is not a specific and definitive organ but a genus of organs whose basic structures and functions are similar but whose individual forms vary widely with enviromental conditions. Not only is this true in the phylogenetic series of the lower organisms but also ontogenetically in man. A large comparative material is therefore available for study. Only certain illustrative examples can be considered.

2. PHYLOGENETIC AND ONTOGENETIC EVIDENCE

A most striking case of involution in the kidney resulting from ageing is the transformation that occurs in the mesonephros of the daddy sculpin (Grafflin, 1933). In the young fish the kidney is both structurally and functionally a "glomerular" organ but as it grows older alterations in both glomeruli and tubules change it to an aglomerular type. The glomeruli undergo various forms of degeneration some becoming avascular and shrunken, others cystic or transformed into a necrotic mass of débris. Tubular disruption also is frequent, a constriction developing either at the origin of the tubule from the glomerulus or at some distance from this point. In this manner the glomerulus is separated from the tubule whose remaining portion persists as a functioning aglomerular nephron that is analogous to those units normally found throughout life in other fish.

Ageing in this instance has transformed the kidney so that the old individual possesses an organ that is structurally and functionally different from that with which it began life. In other fish analogous though less complete degenerations are noted in the glomeruli with increased age (Grafflin, 1937). It is interesting to note in passing that the investigator of these lower forms was also confronted with the

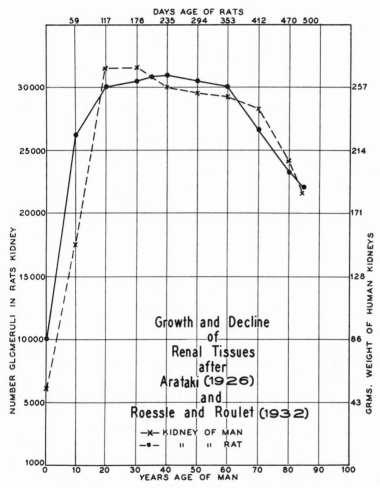

FIG. 37. The growth and decline of the renal tissues after Arataki (1926) and Roessle and Roulet (1932).

problem of separating pathological lesions from physiological involutions, for the kidneys of fish are commonly infected with parasites.

In mammals involutional change may be studied not in one kidney but in three, for the mammal has outlived two of his kidneys by the time of his birth. Our knowledge of the ageing and ultimate disappearance of the mesonephros is more complete than the life history of the poorly developed pronephros. The work of Altschule (1930) is of particular interest for his description of the dedifferentiation of the nephron of the ageing mesonephros will be referred to later in discussing the senile involution of the nephron of the metanephros of the adult mammal. The number of capillaries in the glomerular tuft becomes smaller but simultaneously the cells of the secretory tubule begin to decrease in size so that the tubule becomes thinner, shorter and loses some of its convolutions. Disruption of the tubule is next observed, occurring either at the junction with the glomerulus or at some lower point in the nephron. The epithelium of these disrupted tubules may retain its normal appearance so that it is impossible in the histological section to distinguish between aglomerular tubules or vesicles and the intact nephrons. The ultimate result is the complete disorganization of the mesonephros and the incorporation of its remnants in other organs.

In the studies of Grafflin and Altschule the cause of the degeneration and disappearance of structures is left unexplained. The involution of the organ is so completely accepted as an integral part of its life history that the mechanism of its destruction by implication at least is included in the processes of its growth and development. As a consequence of their living properties and characteristics the cells grow and differentiate and then in due course decrease and atrophy. To one whose interest has been turned toward the pathological aspects of vital phenomona, it would seem that, since these involutionary changes are distinctly degenerative, some disturbing mechanism must lie at the base of their inception and so be susceptible of examination. This idea receives support in the recent work of Gersh (1937) who has correlated the structural and the functional involutional changes that occur in the mesonephros of embryo mammals. In this study it was found that the processes of elimination are continuous in the mesonephros and metanephros so that renal function is not interrupted by the involution of the mesonephros. The cause of the functional and structural degeneration of this organ is moreover directly examined, for in the words of Gersh, "the gradual loss of function (. . . and the structural change . . .) may be correlated with the disappearance or transference to other growing zones (sex organs, adrenals, diaphragm) of the arterial supply of the mesonephros. The shunting off of the arterial supply and the consequent reduction of the glomerular blood pressure is probably the primary cause of nephron dysfunction and degeneration."

By this concept the reciprocal degeneration and development of mesonephros and metanephros is made dependent on the relative change in the arterial supply of the waxing and waning organs, an observation first made by Hill (1905). The theoretical importance of this hypothesis will become apparent when the involution of the final kidney of man has been considered.

3. RENAL SENESCENCE IN MAN—INVOLUTION OR SCLEROSIS?

So far it is evident that ageing of the kidney in lower forms and in the embryonic mammal is in the strict sense of the word an involution in which pathological disease plays no part. When ageing of the kidney of man is considered, the problem becomes more complex. Two questions must be answered; first, is there a primary abiotrophic involution characterized by a simple regression in size and differentiation of cells and nephrons; and secondly, are the alterations in the aged kidney that result from vascular change part of the normal life history of the organ or are they to be considered an aspect of vascular disease.

The second of these questions has been answered definitely by Jores (1903) who has shown that the structure of the arteries varies with the passage of years from birth to senility. The sclerotic artery of the aged is as normal to that period of life as the thin and flexible vessel is to childhood, and the age of the individual can be roughly estimated by the histological appearance of his arterial walls. Any effect in the renal parenchyma secondary to such arterial alteration is therefore not pathological but as true a condition of senescence as the simpler and more direct involutionary degenerations that are so clearly manifested in lower forms and in the embryonic life of mammals.

Admitting the validity of the vascular (arteriosclerotic) component in the genesis of the senile kidney, the question remains if the simpler abiotrophic involutional changes also occur and if they can be recognized and distinguished from the effects of vascular disturbance. A priori, this would seem doubtful for the involutional processes of atrophy, disruption and degeneration are just those that also result from vascular sclerosis.

In their study of the senile rats' kidney Moore and Hellman (1930) have confirmed the earlier observation of investigators who found a decrease in the number of glomeruli. This reduction was apparently due to a process of gradual atrophy and complete disappearance of the structures which left no trace of their former state, so that the possible effects of vascular sclerosis are precluded. A similar mechanism may also exist in the atrophy observed in the old dog's kidney, for here arteriosclerosis is uncommon. However, since the dog is peculiarly

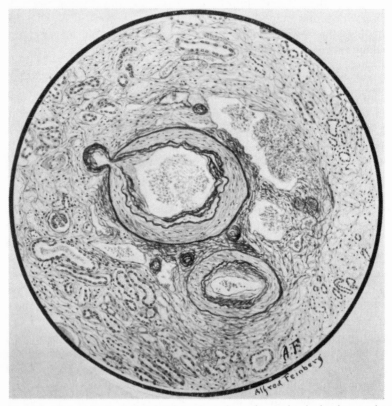

FIG. 38. Hyperplastic intimal thickening of renal arteries in benign nephrosclerosis (after Addis and Oliver, 1931). Magnification 50 ×.

susceptible to a true chronic interstitial nephritis the question is less clear than in the rat.

When past judgements concerning the problem in the human kidney are reviewed wide difference of opinion is found.

Fahr (1925) dismisses the "senile kidney" of man in a paragraph as a "benign nephrosclerosis" due to vascular change. Kaufman (1911), on the other hand, devotes considerable space to the description of a

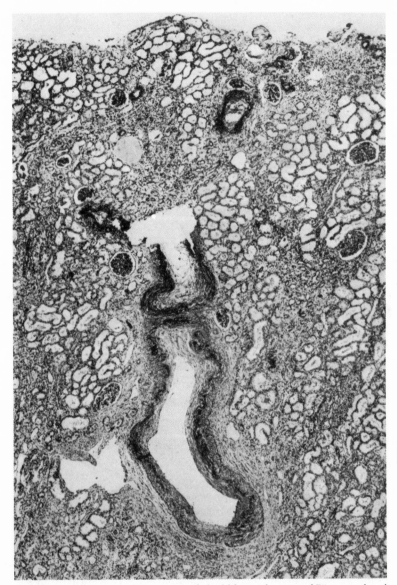

FIG. 39. General view of the cortex of the kidney of a man of 75 years showing the changes of a benign nephrosclerosis. The artery is greatly thickened and throughout the parenchyma areas of collapsed and atrophied tubules enclosed within fibrous scar alternate irregularly with regions of tubular persistence and hypertrophy. The glomeruli are reduced in number though some have maintained their normal size and structure. Magnification 25 ×.

senile kidney in which a peculiar primary atrophy of the tubules is
followed by a disappearance of glomeruli.   The description is general
and no specific evidence is offered in support of such an hypothesis,
though reference is made to the work of Furno (1909).   This investigator found in 70 old individuals 10 instances of what he terms "a

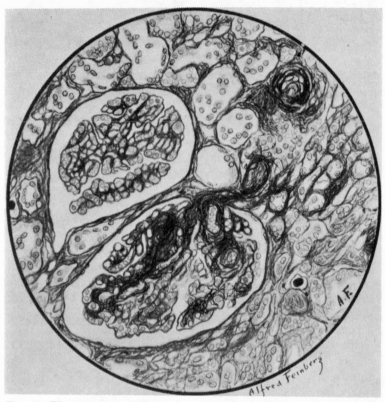

FIG. 40. The extension of fibrosis from the thickened efferent arteriole (shown
in two sections) into the glomerular tuft.   Tubular collapse and atrophy are
also present (after Addis and Oliver, 1931).   Magnification 200 ×.

typical senile kidney."   The descriptions are also given in a general
way that allows no detailed critical examination.   It is stated that some
organs weighed as little as 80 grams, while others were only slightly
reduced in weight; that the tubules were diminished in size by an apparent reduction in their epithelial cells; that the stroma was arranged
in orderly fashion.   The arteries of some showed slight arteriosclerosis

but in others arteriosclerosis was altogether absent. No indication is given of the correlation of these alterations. The remaining kidneys of the series showed various forms of vascular sclerosis. Furno's conclusion is that, though the arteriosclerotic kidney is the one most frequently observed in old people, it is not constant. The less common form of pure renal atrophy, which is never found except in old people, is therefore the typical senile kidney.

Between the extreme positions of Fahr and Furno stands Councilman (1919). Though "three-fourths, certainly" of the kidneys examined by him showed arteriosclerosis, he nevertheless states that he hesitates to assign to this cause the alterations observed in the parenchyma. No changes not easily explicable by such a conclusion are described however, nor are other more likely causes for the alterations offered.

These studies leave great uncertainty in the mind of the reader largely on account of the general manner in which the data are presented. For his personal satisfaction therefore the writer has examined histologically the kidneys from a general autopsy series of the last unselected 75 individuals over 70 years of age in whom no complicating renal disease was present. Every one of these kidneys showed an arteriosclerosis sufficient in his estimation to account for all the atrophic and degenerative changes that were present in the parenchyma. Apart from any possible variation in personal interpretation of the histological appearance, the vascular lesion was certainly of such degree as to make impossible the picking out among the varied pattern of arteriosclerotic scarring, atrophies and degenerations that might be due to some other cause.

Since, therefore as Fahr has stated, it is impossible to separate benign nephrosclerosis of vascular origin from any simple senile atrophy of the kidney a consideration of the arteriosclerotic kidney will describe in realistic terms at least the typical kidney that is found in aged man.

4. STRUCTURAL CHANGES OF SENILE NEPHROSCLEROSIS

1. Regressive processes.

The large and middle sized arteries are frequently affected though the changes may extend into the arterioles. Any sharp separation between the two forms of distribution as distinct morphological entities seems unwarranted, because gradual transitions are noted between the two extremes and the functional disturbances, at first inconsequential, also rise gradually to the level of clinical appreciation with the increasing involvement of the arterioles.

The alterations in the renal arteries are part of processes occurring generally throughout the arterial system with the advance of years. As Jores has shown there is a continuous modification of the structure of the vessel wall which may be regarded as a normal adaptive process. One of the most striking anatomical expressions of this evolution is the duplication of elastic fibrils and the development of a "hyperplastic" intimal thickening (fig. 38). The change in the terminal arterioles is of simpler nature, consisting of a thickening and hyalinization of the vessel wall. Accompanying the sclerosis in both large and small vessels there may occur a deposition of lipoidal material. Oppenheimer (1918) has studied these changes in detail and found that they begin in infancy and can be observed in ever increasing degree with advancing years.

The parenchymal modifications that follow the vascular change are the result of disturbances in the nutrition of the tissues and may be considered examples of ischemic atrophy. The distribution of these effects throughout the organ are determined by the distribution of the vascular change, so that a kidney not greatly reduced in size with a relatively smooth surface and scattered retracted scars is found when the larger and middle arteries are irregularly affected, while a general reduction of the size of the organ and a more diffuse granular scarring follows the involvement of smaller vessels and arterioles. The details of this distribution of the various changes in the different branches of the renal artery and their relation to the parenchymal modifications are fully described by Zacharjewskaja (1936).

The parenchymal change may be followed in both histological section (fig. 39) and by microdissection of macerated tissue (Loomis, 1936). The glomerulus is affected either by collapse of its capillaries when

Fig. 41. The parenchymal changes in nephrosclerosis (Arch. Path., 1936). Magnification 15 ×.
1. Atrophy of glomeruli and proximal convoluted tubules. Note the lack in correlation of glomerular and tubular size.
2. A complete atrophied nephron with almost a total lack of differentiation in the various segments of the tubule.
3. Fragments and cysts arising from the disruption of tubules.
4. A complete nephron with a portion of its collecting tubule. The glomerulus is large, the proximal convolution hypertrophic and hyperplastic. The loop of Henle is normal and the distal convolution is somewhat dilated. There is considerable scattered fat change in proximal convolution.
5. An hypertrophied and hyperplastic proximal convolution arising from an atrophied glomerulus.
6. Hypertrophied and hyperplastic proximal convolution. The corresponding ascending limb and distal convolution do not show this progressive change.
7. Irregular atrophy and dilatation of proximal convolutions.

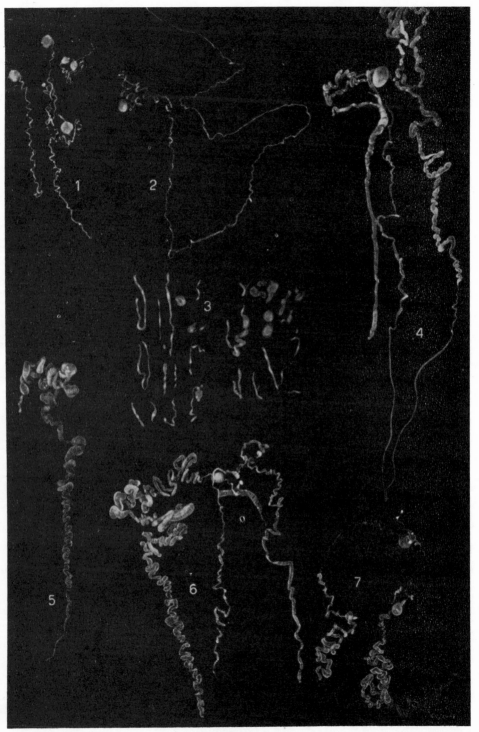

FIG. 41
267

the afferent arteriole is obliterated or hyalinization may extend into the tuft from the arteriole (fig. 40). By either process the tuft is transformed into a fibrous nodule and in the end may disappear (fig. 39). Quantitative examinations of the senile kidney of man have shown that in the seventh decade the number of glomeruli equals only two-thirds to one-half the early adult count (Moore, 1931). Atrophy of the tubules also occurs, recent past theory assuming that this is due to glomerular destruction. A criticism of this hypothesis has been given in another place (Oliver and Luey, 1935) where it was shown that when examined in the continuity of dissected material there is little correlation between the size of glomerulus and tubule (fig. 41, *1*) and that the tubule of the nephron does not constantly degenerate after glomerular destruction. The writer therefore sees no reason to suppose that atrophy of the tubule is not the result of the same factor that causes atrophy of the glomerulus, namely the ischemia due to vascular obliteration. The epithelial cells of the tubule decrease in size (fig. 40), it narrows to a shortened tenuous thread and the coils of the proximal convolution lose their complexity (fig. 41, *1*, *2*). So great may the reduction in its diameter be that thirty nephrons have been found in microdissected material to occupy the space formerly filled by three (Loomis, 1936). The ultimate fate of the shrunken nephrons is similar to that of the functioning elements of the kidney (mesonephros) of lower forms and the embryo. Tubular disruption occurs and the scars are filled with detached vesicles and cysts which lie among dense connective tissue (fig. 41, *3*).

Besides retrogressive alterations in the shape and contours of the nephrons degenerations are noted in the constituent cells of the tubules. These take the form of the milder expressions of cellular regression such as cloudy swelling and fatty metamorphosis. The proximal convolution is particularly prone to such damage so that either its entire extent or irregularly isolated coils of its loops appear a glistening refractile white in the isolated specimen (fig. 41, *4*).

The atrophy and disruption of the parenchyma, occurring in scattered areas among better nourished and preserved tissue, is the essential mechanism in the formation of the arteriosclerotic scar. As a consequent result of the reduction in the bulk of the nephrons the fibrils of the interstitial connective tissue framework are approximated and condensed. There is little evidence of an inflammatory component, such as round cell infiltration, in early arteriosclerotic scars. As they increase in extent and age such a reaction does occur along with an irregular proliferation of fibrils, though throughout their course the chief histological distinction between the changes that characterize the simple senile arteriosclerotic kidney and pathological malignant nephrosclerosis of vascular disease is the relative absence in the former of inflammation and its destructive effects on the parenchyma of the organ.

2. *Adaptive changes.*

So far the changes described in both vessels and parenchyma have been retrogressive and their presumable effect is to decrease the function of the organ. It is less well recognized that in both elements of the kidney and not in parenchyma alone progressive changes occur and since the direction of their functional effect is converse to the destructive lesion and the degree of their development is proportional to the sum of the retrogressive changes it seems reasonable to suppose them adaptive in nature and compensatory to the destruction of functioning tissue.

In the parenchymal nephrons hypertrophy of the tubules that lie outside the sclerosed vascular beds is observed (fig. 39). Its extent and distribution can only be properly appreciated by microdissection of the complete nephron from glomerulus to collecting tubule (fig. 41, 4). Under these conditions of examination it is interesting to note that the change is limited almost entirely to the proximal convoluted tubule, other portions of the nephron remaining esssentially unaltered. Hyperplastic lengthening of this segment may also increase its volume (fig. 41, 5, 6) so that in the end one proximal convolution may equal in amount of functioning tissue that of 12 or more normal units. There is no constant relation noted between the size of the glomerulus and its proximal convolution in either tubular hypertrophy or hyperplasia; the corpuscle may be normal in size, enlarged, atrophied or destroyed (fig. 41, 4, 5).

Progressive change in the arteries takes the form of a growth and new development of vascular channels (fig. 42). It is the generally accepted theory that in the normal kidney all the blood passes through the glomerular capillary bed before reaching the intertubular network for no significant number of direct branches from the renal artery to the tubular capillaries exist. It should be noted in passing that there has not been at all times agreement among anatomists in regard to this concept of indirect tubular blood supply and that some have claimed that direct branches do occur. The problematical existence of arteriae rectae verae is a well known example of such uncertainty and to this question we shall return after a description of the vascular apparatus of the arteriosclerotic kidney has been given.

In a kidney that shows a well developed sclerosis of its arteries there are found a great number of direct arterial branches to the intertubular network (Loomis, 1936). The new paths consist of the following sorts. (1) Ludwig's vessel, a small branch of the afferent arteriole that leads to the intertubular network (fig. 42, *1, 2*); (2) lateral branches from the interlobular artery (fig. 42, *3, 4*); (3) arterial branches from the arcuate arteries and deeper interlobular vessels that, passing to the medulla, form arteriae rectae verae (fig. 42, *5, 6*); (4) anastomoses between the afferent and efferent arterioles (fig. 42, *7*). Associated with these changes in the arterial tree is a growth of new capillaries that surround tubules and glomeruli in an adventitious network and so vascular connections are formed between structures not originally united.

To return to the problem as to whether the "normal" vascular bed of the kidney includes direct branches, the solution of a long continued

---

Fig. 42. The vascular changes in nephrosclerosis (Arch. Path., 1936). Magnification 15 ✕.

1. Fragment of interlobular artery from outer cortex showing Ludwig's vessel and its termination in the intertubular network.

2. Ludwig's vessel ending in a capillary brush.

3. Direct branches of interlobular artery breaking into capillaries. Nodular fatty change has occurred in the new formed vessels.

4. Sclerotic arcuate and interlobular arteries with irregular fatty deposits. The terminal branches of the interlobular artery show many kinds of change: tortuosity, changes in diameter, spiral turns, deposits of fat in rhythmic pattern or in irregular masses, diminution of terminal branches to tenuous threads and obliteration of the lumen with opaque fat. Vessels are present which end directly in capillary branches without intervening glomerular tufts. Most of the glomeruli are contracted, some to minute structures, and show extreme fatty change.

5. Fragment of an interlobular artery dividing to form an afferent arteriole with an arteria recta with long capillary divisions.

6. Arcuate artery from which arise afferent arterioles and arteriae rectae verae. The latter have undergone fatty degeneration.

7. Capillary branches from the cortex arising from end branches of the interlobular artery and from efferent arterioles. One clearly shows the union of the afferent and efferent arteriole in a continuous vessel with the glomerulus attached to its side.

8. Interlobular artery ending in capillaries. Severe fatty change in beadlike formation thickens the arterioles and extends to the capillaries. One of these vessels shows a sharp bend and thickening and the other a tuft, which are all that remain of the glomeruli. One glomerulus gives rise to an efferent arteriole in the normal fashion.

9. Capillaries arising from vessels with no sign of formerly existing glomeruli. Other abnormalities are beading with fat and the apparent obstruction of the lumen of the main vessel.

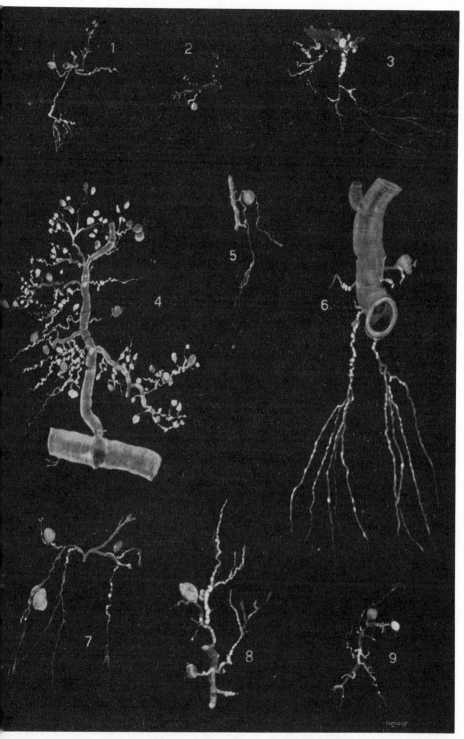

FIG. 42

controversy is found in the realization that the normal life history of the arteries includes the development of sclerotic changes. As previously mentioned Oppenheimer (1918) has shown that they begin early in life and that they are found constantly in latter years. The conclusion is obvious, therefore, that the adaptive and probably compensatory development of new vessels must also be considered a part of the life history of the renal arteries and characteristic of the structure of the senile kidney. Vasa rectae verae, therefore, are not "normally" found in significant numbers in the kidney of the young adult, though in the kidney of 70 years they are "normal" constituents of the arterial tree. It is of interest that all the new formed arteries eventually may undergo the same sclerotic changes that were in the first instance the cause of their development (fig. 42, *3, 4, 8*).

5. FUNCTIONAL DISTURBANCES OF SENILE NEPHROSCLEROSIS

Structurally the kidney of the aged is an organ whose original parenchyma and vascular supply is reduced, but which presents a varying, usually proportional, degree of compensatory change in both of its constituent elements. In theory a functional balance might be expected. A complication, however, is found in the fact that though the parenchymal changes of atrophy and of hypertrophy may be considered quantitative in their functional effect, with the development of new vessels there has occurred a qualitative change in the sense that a different sort of blood supply has developed. The blood that formerly passed first through the glomerular capillaries, and which there underwent certain modifications, is now being directed in ever increasing amount directly to the tubules. What change in renal function results from these altered conditions we can not even surmise.

The complexity of the changed structure of the kidney would be enough to make hazardous any attempt at a detailed interpretation of the functional disturbances noted in renal function of the aged, but they are only a part of the complications that make our understanding of the situation difficult. For the change in the renal arteries in Gull and Sutton's (1872) classic phrase is only part of a general "arterio-capillary fibrosis" of the vessels of the body and this disturbance of vascular balance reacts upon the function of the kidney. It is with a very considerable hesitation, therefore, that an attempt is made to discuss the function of the senile kidney in the brief confines of the present chapter.

Due to its great reserve of tissue, the eliminatory capacity may be normal or any part of normal depending on the balance of parenchymal scarring and compensatory change that have occurred within the organ. In the majority of aged people depreciation of kidney function is not a major difficulty for other systems, such as heart or brain, similarly involved by vascular change fail more rapidly and more disastrously. It is perhaps true that those urinary disturbances that do occur are more the result of circulatory abnormality than of the change that senescence has produced in the kidney. Albuminuria and cylinduria may be so slight as to be within the normal limits of earlier years. The concentrating power of the kidney is not greatly affected. No disturbance may be noted in the elimination of water, though the aged often complain of the inconveniences of a nycturia. In part this may be more apparent than real, a result of lighter sleep or of irritations of the bladder. When actual, it is, according to Volhard (1931), a polyuria compensatory to a lessened day output that in turn is the result of incipient cardiac failure and circulatory embarrassment. The ability to eliminate nitrogen may be decreased, as evidenced by a lowered urea clearance, but an abnormal rise of blood urea does not commonly result.[1]

If this is the picture of the function of the average and therefore "normal" senile kidney, it seems paradoxical to the writer, a pathologist, that a little more of the same change in kidney and heart and the gradually resulting disturbances of renal function that ensue should be placed in the category of the "abnormal" or pathological and therefore not be considered a part of senescence. Every gradation may be seen from what has been described above as "normal" to those cases where in the very aged altered structure and disturbed function may lead to nitrogen retention and other evidences of renal impairment. These cases, as Vohard has shown, cannot be considered examples of the so-called malignant hypertension and nephrosclerosis. And if, as many pathologists believe, the changes in the kidney of malignant nephrosclerosis are not so much qualitatively different as due to differences of tempo and distribution of the vascular lesion, then where is the line to be drawn between the "normal" and "pathological"?

Such questions are perplexing enough when only the eliminating function of the kidney, concerning whose mechanisms we are relatively well informed, are considered. But there are other activities of this organ whose importance recent investigation is confirming.

[1] Since this writing the study of Lewis and Alving (1938) has appeared. The reader is referred to their findings for a detailed confirmation of the description given above.

6. GENERAL EFFECTS OF RENAL-VASCULAR SENESCENCE

It has been stated that the disturbance in renal function is more the result of circulatory dysfunction than of renal structural change. The common cardiovascular disturbance of old age is the result of or associated with or expressed by a hypertension, and the speculations that originated in Bright's first suggestion that renal abnormalities were concerned have received their final objective and experimental confirmation in the demonstration of Goldblatt (1937) that restriction of blood flow through the renal arteries results in a continued elevation of general blood pressure. Is then hypertension, so frequent to some degree in old age as to be in a sense physiological, the result of arterial change in the kidney?

Moritz and Oldt (1937) studying arteriolar sclerosis in a series of hypertensive and non-hypertensive individuals have found that though the arterioles of the body generally are affected in increasing degree with age, the changes in the arteries of the kidney alone are constantly associated with hypertension. Of 100 non-hypertensives, one-third of which were over 61 years of age, none showed a severe alteration in the arterioles of the kidney and in 16 the changes were only mild. In 100 hypertensive individuals on the other hand 97 per cent showed renal arteriolar involvement, in 47 per cent the change being severe. In the words of these investigators it would seem that "the effect of the renal arteriolar sclerosis in human hypertension appears to be the functional analogue of the renal arterial clamp in experimental hypertension. In both instances hypertension appears to be produced by reduction in renal blood flow which does not necessarily lead to a sufficient degree of ischemia to impair renal function measurably."

There is with increasing age a slow elevation of blood pressure that commonly is considered a "normal" process (Saller, 1928). Again comes the question, at what point is this to be considered "pathological" or "malignant"? Moritz and Oldt see no need for qualitative distinctions in the problem, but state, "The factor which determines that some cases of essential hypertension will run a more rapid course with early death from renal insufficiency does not appear to be the degree of the hypertension but rather the rate of renal destruction incident to the progressive character of the renal vascular disease."

The result of recent investigations is therefore to place senescence of the kidney in a distinctive position among the ageing processes, for apparently by reactions originating in this organ may be determined the nature of the old age that an individual is to have and even the manner in which that last period is to close. If a theoretical description may be permitted, and no other is possible at the present, the train of sequences might be described as follows.

As a part of the senescent process there develops a generalized sclerosis of the smaller arteries. Other factors fortuitous or "pathological" may influence the course of the vascular alteration, but with this we are not at present concerned. The vascular change within the various tissues and organs may be severe, but there is no evidence that compels the conclusion that these lesions produce an elevation of blood pressure. If the arterial change within the kidney is sufficient to produce renal ischemia however, hypertension follows. Depending on the degree of renal arterial involvement the hypertension may be "benign" and senility ends with mild circulatory difficulties and a benificent broncho-pneumonia; more grave, and cardiac failure or cerebral accident, depending on the condition of the local vessels, terminates in more dramatic fashion life's last episode.

By such a concept it is not so much vascular senescence, common to all organs and tissues, that determines the ultimate outcome, but a disturbance within the kidney and peculiar to its functions that is the final and actuating mechanism of senile circulatory failure and accident.

A man's arteries may then be old, but only if his kidneys are spared does his senescence approach the biological ideal of a gradual and peaceful decline.

7. SUMMARY

In lower vertebrate forms and in the embryonic mammal degenerative changes are observed with ageing of the kidney. Senescence in these instances has been looked upon as a primary parenchymal involution due to a decrease in the vital energy of the cells.

If such a primary senescent involution occurs in the kidney of man, it is obscured and its effects over-shadowed by secondary tissue changes that develop as a result of the normal ageing of the renal arteries. Ageing of the human kidney becomes therefore a special case of ageing of the vascular system.

A possible solution of this antithesis may ultimately be found in a further extension of those investigations which have shown that the supposed "primary" structural involutional changes in the ageing kidney of the embryo mammal are correlated with the retrogression of blood vessels and the transference of the blood supply to other growth zones. Vascular alteration would thus become the determining factor of the senescent change in the kidney of both man and the lower forms.

The disturbance of renal function in aged man is determined less by the degree of change in the functioning parenchyma of the kidney than by circulatory failure, an accompaniment of similar senescent changes in the cardio-vascular system. In only the unusual instance is the factor of renal failure important, and such an eventuality is not a part of "normal" old age.

A disturbance within the ageing kidney that may determine the entire course of a senescence is that which follows renal ischemia and results in hypertension. Its importance may be judged by the fact that over half of the aged die by its effects.

REFERENCES

ALTSCHULE, M. D. 1930. The changes in the mesonephric tubules of human embryos ten to twelve weeks old. Anat. Rec., **46**, 81–91.

ARATAKI, M. 1926. On the postnatal growth of the kidney, with special reference to the number and size of the glomeruli (Albino rat). Am. J. Anat., **36**, 399–436.

COUNCILMAN, W. T. 1919. The conditions presented in the heart and kidneys of old people. Contrib. to Med. and Biol. Research. Dedicated to Sir Wm. Osler, **2**, 918–928.

FAHR, Th. 1925. Pathologische Anatomie des Morbus Brightii. Henke and Lubarsch, Handbuch der speziellen Pathologischen Anatomie und Histologie. Berlin: J. Springer, **6**, (1), 374–

FURNO, A. 1909. Ricerche Anatomo-Patologiche intorno al Rene Atrofico Senile, Lo Sperimentale, **63**, 99–129.

GERSH, I. 1937. The correlation of structure and function in the developing mesonephros and metanephros. Pub. Carnegie Inst. Wash., Contrib. to Embry., **153**, 33–58.

GOLDBLATT, H. 1937. Studies in experimental hypertension III. The production of persistent hypertension in monkeys (Macaque) by renal ischemia. J. Exper. Med., **65**, 671–675.

GRAFFLIN, A. L. 1933. Glomerular degeneration in the kidney of the Daddy Sculpin (Myoxocephalus Scorpius). Anat. Rec., **57**, 59–79.

——— 1937. Cyst formation in the glomerular tufts of certain fish kidneys. Biol. Bull., **72**, 247–257.

GULL, W. W., AND SUTTON, H. G. 1872. On the pathology of the morbid state commonly called chronic Bright's Disease with contracted kidney ("arterio-capillary fibrosis"). Med. Chir. Tr., London: **55**, 273–329.

HILL, E. G. 1905. On the first appearance of the renal artery and the relative development of the kidneys and Wolffian bodies in pig embryos. Johns Hopkins Hosp. Bull., **16**, 60–64.

JORES, L. 1903. Wesen und Entwickelung der Arteriosklerose. Wiesbaden: J. F. Bergmann, 172 pp.

KAUFMANN, E. 1911. Lehrbuch der speziellen Pathologischen Anatomie fur Studierende und Ärzte. Berlin: G. Reimer, 6 Aufl., **2**, 815–818.

LEWIS, W. H., JR., AND ALVING, A. S. 1938. Changes with age in the renal function in adult men. I. Clearance of urea. II. Amount of urea nitrogen in the blood. III. Concentrating ability of the kidneys. Am. J. Physiol., 123, 500–515.

LOOMIS, D. 1936. Plastic studies in abnormal renal architecture. IV. Vascular and parenchymal changes in arteriosclerotic Bright's Disease. Arch. Path., 22, 435–463.

MACKAY, L. L., MACKAY, E. M., AND ADDIS, T. 1924. The effect of various factors on the degree of compensatory hypertrophy of the kidney after unilateral nephrectomy. J. Clin. Invest., 1, 576.

MOORE, R. A. 1931. The total number of glomeruli in the normal human kidney. Anat. Rec., 48, 153–168.

MOORE, R. A., AND HELLMAN, L. M. 1930. The effect of unilateral nephrectomy on the senile atrophy of the kidney of the white rat. J. Exper. Med., 51, 51–57.

MORITZ, A. R., AND OLDT, M. R. 1937. Arteriolar sclerosis in hypertensive and non-hypertensive individuals. Am. J. Path., 13, 679–728.

OLIVER, J., AND LUEY, A. S. 1935. Plastic studies in abnormal renal architecture. III. The aglomerular nephrons of terminal hemorrhagic Bright's disease. Arch. Path., 19, 1–23.

OPPENHEIMER, F. 1918. Über den Histologischen Bau der Arterien in der Wachsenden und alternden Niere. Frankfurt. Ztschr. f. Path., 21, 57–84.

ROESSLE, R., AND ROULET, F. 1932. Mass und Zahl in der Pathologie. Berlin and Wien: J. Springer, 144 pp.

SALLER, K. 1928. Über die Altersveraenderungen des Blutdruckes. Ztschr. f. d. ges. exper. Med., 58, 683–709.

VOLHARD, F. 1931. Die doppelseitigen hamatogenen Nierenerkrankungen. Bergman and Staehelin, Handbuch der innere Medizin, Berlin, J. Springer, 2nd. Aufl., Bd. Vi, Th. II, 1665.

ZACHARJEWSKAJA, M. 1936. Über die Pathologischen Veränderungen im Arteriensystem der Niere, deren gegenseitige Beziehungen und Bedeutung für die Entstehung der Nierenschrumpfung. Beitr. z. path. Anat. u. z. allg. Path., 98, 1–23.

CHAPTER 11

SKELETON, LOCOMOTOR SYSTEM AND TEETH

T. WINGATE TODD

Western Reserve University

To the popular mind the ageing of Man is expressed in skin and hair and nails and teeth, in bones and muscles, in the body that has to perform the command of the will. But whereas ageing in skin and teeth, in hair and nails may take place without necessarily affecting the body as a whole, ageing in muscles and bones bites into Man's pride and gives him a sense of the passage of time which he fain would conceal even from himself. Conscious of waning strength and endurance, he seeks for substitutes, accepting with difficulty the limitations imposed by Time and inferring therefrom a suggestion of infirmity.

Age changes and age infirmities are so interwoven that it is not easy to segregate the former from the latter. This is largely due to the fact that we notice only phenomena of short duration. Infirmities of adult life progress more rapidly than ageing does. They seem to us therefore to be the expression and not the interruption of ageing. This is a false deduction. There are diseases characteristic of advanced age as there are of mature life and of childhood (Kotsovsky, 1935). We do not confuse the diseases of childhood with the progress of maturity in the child because both phenomena are of short duration and define themselves clearly against the background of the years.

Biological time is not synonymous with sidereal time which is divided by years or months or days. Biological time is measured by changes in the organism itself. Five years cover the span of life of a rat, thirty years the life span of most mammals but in thirty years a Man's body has barely passed its acme in muscular strength and agility. Time passes speedily for the rat when viewed from the standpoint of a man. Time passes swiftly for the child when considered from the standpoint of his parents. Since the rate of biological change is great in childhood much is accomplished in a few years for ageing is rapid. Sidereal time therefore seems long to the child. In the final period of maturity ageing is very slow and sidereal time appears to take wings to itself. Only if infirmity intervenes does the victim of disease find sidereal time again drag itself wearily with heavy feet towards the inevitable end.

Measured in units of physiological time, infancy is very long and old age very short but, as Carrel (1935, p. 169) points out, when infancy and old age are expressed in solar years, infancy appears to be very short and old age very long.

Time genes and rate genes have been claimed to account in part for the phenomena of ageing along with other controlling factors (Goldschmidt, 1927; Ford and Huxley, 1929) but these are less tangible than the actual expression of ageing shown in histological studies.

The impact of environment brings injuries in its train, injuries which are met by tne process of repair in the organism. Ageing implies therefore an unending alternation of injury and repair. In the very process of repair the tissues change but so long as repair is efficient adaptation increases, immunities are developed and the relation of environment to the organism is constructive in its influence. The tissues of the body are replete with mechanisms for the renewal of youth. Some tissues, epithelia particularly, show rejuvenation or physiological regeneration by mitosis. Others, like skeletal muscle, connective tissue and glia cells, respond by amitotic division. In smooth muscle there is neither mitosis nor amitosis yet smooth muscle has the power of repair (Wetzel, 1932). But with the progress of age physiochemical changes occur. Collagenous fibers increase in number, water content is reduced, the pH changes. Obscure biochemical alterations diminish both speed and effectiveness of repair. A wound of forty square centimeters heals in forty days in a patient of twenty years but requires seventy-six days in a patient forty years of age. In a man of sixty years a wound takes five times as many days to heal as it does in a child of ten years (Lecomte du Noüy, 1937, pp. 88, 155). Carrel and Ebeling (1921) have shown a similar effect of age on the growth of connective tissue. This tissue, cultivated *in vitro*, in plasma of a chicken six weeks of age, was not inhibited in growth in any way. But, by the addition of serum from a nine year old rooster, growth was greatly retarded. Whereas the culture lives forty-six days or more in the plasma of a six week old chicken it lives but four to six days in that of the nine year old rooster. Further, it was found that when the culture medium contained 70 per cent serum from the old rooster, the tissue fragment practically always contracted and showed very little activity. The cells contained more fat granules than they showed in lower concentrations of rooster serum. Evidently the serum of an old animal induces certain changes in tissue not detectable by mere measurement of proliferation rate.

Age is expressed then not merely in histological changes but chiefly through biochemical modifications. The immunity of any tissue stands in direct relation to its physiological equilibrium (Kotsovsky, 1935). Biochemical modifications are shown by the decline in immunity of tissues against injurious agents from within and from without. Disease further increases the disturbance of physiological equilibrium. Thus it is that the phenomena of ageing are also those of infirmity but infirmity accentuates them and robs them of that orderly control of differentiation which modulates the effectiveness of the organism in its environment, modulation being the essential principle of the ageing process.

It will be the aim of this chapter to illustrate this differentiation between true features of ageing and the characteristics of infirmity so far as they relate to the skeleton, the locomotor system and the teeth.

In connective tissue itself nothing is known of changes undergone in specific relation to adult life. It would seem indeed that throughout the life span, connective tissue is capable of going through the successive phases of its own ageing pattern. Sylvia Bensley (1934) has described these successive phases very clearly in her experimental studies on the pancreas of the guinea pig. Ligation of the pancreatic duct in this animal results, after fourteen to nineteen days, in a pancreatic fibrosis. At first the pancreas becomes oedematous, the stroma and its elements being spread apart by this oedema. After ten to fourteen days the pancreas becomes more gelatinous; there is a proliferation of fibroblasts and the ground substance, which hitherto would not stain metachromically with toluidine blue, now takes the stain, and is seen to fill the tissue spaces between the cells and fibers. New reticular or arygrophile fibers are specially abundant at this stage. By the end of nineteen days the pancreas has lost its viscid consistency; it is much firmer and more fibrous. Sections stained with toluidine blue show ground substance in which clear newly formed tissue spaces begin to appear. Within the ground substance the reticular fibers group themselves and some are continuous with collagenous fibers. In late stages the tissue spaces and collagenous fibers are conspicuous, the ground substance appearing to be reduced or modified but still evident in the neighborhood of the collagenous fibers.

Cyclic changes in the stroma of the human uterine mucosa are identical with those described above in illustration of the ever renewable life history of connective tissue wherever it is found.

Connective tissue has an importance in the nutrition of other tissues about and between which it lies. The amount of intramuscular connective tissue for example is claimed by Schiefferdecker (1911) and Kohashi (1937a) as giving a rough guide to the nutritive supply of the muscle which is of great significance in its early development. No change is to be noted in the reticular sheath of muscular fibers as age advances (Buccianti and Luria, 1934). The rôle of connective tissue in defense mechanisms and in hydration of the body (see Maximow, 1927) indicates the necessity for preservation in this tissue of youthfulness of response despite advancing years. Such age changes indeed as are known to take place in connective tissue in relation to the life span are to be found in early life, not in later age. They are illustrated by the observations of Frischmann (1932). The first latticework of connective tissue in human liver is seen at the end of the eighth week of fetal life. By steady increase in the number of bundles a well marked network is reached at birth. By the age of six weeks the fibrils attain their definitive form and the collagenous connective tissue of Glisson's capsule has then completed its development; no further changes are evident in Glisson's capsule or in the intralobular reticular bundles even in advanced age. Changes in liver stroma claimed as senile are therefore pathological in nature and not related to physiological age. Not only connective tissue itself but other related tissues discussed in this chapter such as bursae, tendons, ligaments, synovial membrane and smooth muscle give no characteristic or clearly defined evidence of age changes.

When, at the end of this chapter, the reader shall ask himself what precisely are the characteristic age changes of those tissues comprising the soma itself, the skeleton, the locomotor system and the teeth, he will be impressed by their scantiness both in number and degree unless he is misled into confusing age, which by its very existence bespeaks enhanced resistance, with infirmity which may supervene at any stage of life. Dehydration of tissue with reduction in intracellular fluid and increase in intercellular fluid and, in addition, a certain faltering in the orderliness of tissue pattern summarize the most significant features and at the same time indicate the course of transformation from the orderly and reversible phenomena of health into the disorderly and irreversible which are the stigmata of disease. But if blood and the body fluids are regarded as a tissue of the soma, as they may reasonably be considered, then there are other obscure biochemical changes evident in increasing age by the effect which they produce, as recorded in a previous paragraph, on the cultivation of tissues *in vitro* and on the healing of wounds.

1. GROWTH IN THE ADULT BODY

Before discussing age changes in skeletal and other supportive tissues it is well to turn for a moment to the subject of possible bodily growth in adult life.

Growth of body, as commonly understood, is dominated by growth in the skeleton but of course there may be growth in parts composed entirely of soft tissues. We must deal with both phases of the subject.

Our information on growth in adult life is culled mainly from the writings of Pfitzner (1899) on the dead, Jarcho (1935) and Hrdlička (1925, 1935, 1936) on the living. Pfitzner and Hrdlička give no measures of variability and their claims therefore cannot be statistically analysed. Jarcho, whose observations are limited to the male sex, gives the standard errors of his mean values and we may therefore subject these to critical analysis. His nineteen measures, excluding indices, give 130 means for comparison with the means of his age groups of twenty to twenty-five years. The higher age groups comprise respectively ages twenty-six to thirty-nine years, and forty years and over. Of these means our statistician Miss K. Simmons points out that 92, or 67 per cent, show consistence in progressive increases with age whereas 38, or 33 per cent, do not. Miss Simmons calculated forty critical ratios on length of head, breadth of head, malar breadth, morphological facial length and stature. Of these 27, or 67 per cent are insignificant and 13, or 33 per cent, are significant. All differences between the age groups in stature and breadth of head are insignificant. In three of the four racial stocks the increases with age of head length and morphological facial length are significant but they are not the same three stocks. In two stocks increase in malar breadth is significant. There is here therefore no evidence that stature increases with years after early adult age is attained. Malar breadth and facial height involve measurements of soft tissues which are always subject to correction whether measured on the living or the dead. Head length, which is practically a measurement of bone, stands in another category and this increase remains to be explained. According to Graves (1925a, b), when we take samples of humanity differing in age by twenty years or more, we are not measuring comparable groups because many of those having a less longevity value have died leaving only, in the main, those of greater constitutional fitness between whom and the less fit there may be expected to be found differences in bodily measurements. According to Graves (1936) also this difference in measurement applies to soft parts such as nose as well as to bony dimensions.

That there are changes in soft parts, as Hrdlička claims, there seems no doubt. It is debatable however if these changes should be classified under the heading of genuine growth. The changes in nose, mouth, ears involve actual addition of substance but are in principle modifications in type and arrangement of tissue elements comparable to those also found in skin, subcutaneous tissue and joint structure.

Apart from those in the face the most notable changes in tissue structure of bodily parts occur in hands and feet. On these Hrdlička has touched. In some, as yet, unpublished investigations McGaw and I found actual changes in comparative length of great and second toes during adult life. This work is too long and involved for a report here but its underlying principle is a change in the tissues about the metatarso-phalangeal joint of the great toe. Its clearest illustration is to be found in the composite statues offering themselves for study in the Louvre and the Boston Museum of Fine Arts. Restorers have not always been careful to mount the head (and torso) of the statue upon lower extremities of comparable age. The distinction stands out distressingly when the observer's eye glances from face to foot.

2. SKELETON

Any study of the skeleton must contemplate three aspects, namely, bones as supporting structures and agents in locomotion; bones as a source of mineral, particularly a source of calcium for utilization in blood coagulability, muscle tone, kidney function and activity of the central nervous system; and bones in their rôle of blood forming organs through the agency of the red marrow.

The last mentioned may be dismissed in this chapter with a single paragraph as marrow is discussed elsewhere. The marrow forming organ is found in the metaphysis of the bone, that part of the shaft next the growing end which may or may not be covered by an epiphysis. Soon after increment ceases at the growing end the epiphysis, if there be one, unites with the shaft in primates but not necessarily in lower mammals (Todd, Rodents). At about the time of cessation of growth or union of epiphysis in Man, the metaphysis usually loses its capacity to form red blood corpuscles. There is therefore automatic retirement of the different metaphysial stations of the long bones in succession during adolescence, but patches linger on into adult life in the upper end of humerus and femur. Remaining also in adult age are the stations in ossa innominata, bodies of the vertebrae, ribs and sternum, but as life progresses the vertebrae gradually lose this function and, in advanced age, there may be no red marrow except in the bodies of lower lumbar vertebrae and sacrum (Piney, 1922).

3. NEW BONE FORMATION DURING ADULT LIFE

Changes in superficial texture of bones resulting from subperiosteal activity illustrate quite well the orderly control of differentiation characteristic of young adult life and the gradually increasing defectiveness of control already evident in mature life but so obvious in advanced age as to simulate the bizarre, unregulated overgrowths of pathological nature. These changes in texture are expressed in principle in skeletons of Man and all mammals. They are most readily seen in the skull. Inasmuch as any collection of human skeletons includes perforce a large number showing the evidence of malnutrition produced not only by dietary deficiency but also by chronic disorders, it is quite impossible, without expert knowledge and long experience, to differentiate them from low grade pathological processes. Nature has however provided us with a clearly defined example of age changes depicted on a scale large enough to be differentiated without difficulty by the naked eye and therefore useful as an introduction to the subject. The shield on which these changes are portrayed is the curiously expanded zygomatic arch and adjacent parts of the skull of Caelogenys paca, the Spotted Cavy, an animal allied to the guinea pig, living near the banks of the Rio Grande do Sul.

The greater part of the zygomatic shield of Caelogenys is formed from the maxilla. The posterior root only is formed by the squamous temporal. Between these two is interposed another bony element, the malar bone (Owen, 1866, pp. 371–372). Suture lines between maxilla, malar and temporal root are clearly evident. In an animal which still has its milk dentition the texture of the malar is finely granular. It lacks the shining smoothness of the squamous temporal and parietal bones, but is practically identical with the texture of frontal and nasal bones. It contrasts with the texture of the maxillary expansion which is lava-like in its granulation, pierced by innumerable fine vascular foramina, marked in its lower portion by a lattice-like tracery and scored beneath the orbital margin by a series of delicate parallel ridges. The facial surface of the lacrimal bone exhibits a pattern composed of high ridges like stalagmites. The postorbital process of the frontal bone displays a similar though less advanced pattern of ridging (B 760, fig. 43).

At the stage of eruption of the single premolar, after the three permanent molars have erupted but while occipitosphenoid suture is still patent, remarkable changes have taken place. The lacrimal tracery has no longer the well ordered pattern of the younger animal. A well ordered pattern is now characteristic of the tracery in the postorbital process of the frontal while the entire surface of the frontal bone and that area of the parietal not covered by temporal muscle are taking on a pattern which has reached the flat topped phase of the tracery seen on the postorbital process of the younger animal. On the maxillary shield the suborbital parallel ridges have disappeared and the lattice-like tracery of the lower portion has developed into an orderly system of ridges which has extended over almost the entire lateral surface of the malar and crept upwards on the maxilla itself

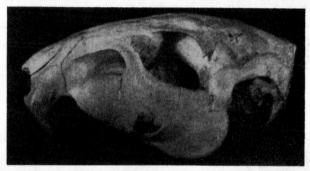

Fig. 43. Left side of skull, Spotted Cavy. B 760 W. R. U. Milk dentition. Lava-like texture of maxilla with innumerable vascular foramina, delicate parallel ridges beneath orbital margin and lattice-like tracery of lower part. Finely granular texture of malar. Pattern of raised "stalagmitic" ridges on lacrimal. Similar but less developed pattern on postorbital process.

toward the orbital margin. Despite all these fantastic embellishments of the outer surface of the skull suture lines stand out clearly without the least interruption or encroachment by the new bone formation (B. 761, fig. 44).

A fully adult specimen shows the tracery on the postorbital process of the frontal dwindling in its turn. But by this stage the lattice formations on maxillary shield and malar are exuberant. They cover the lateral surface of both bones completely and appear on the adjacent surface of the temporal root. The pattern on the two frontal bones resembles an arbor vitae with extensions not only to parietals as before but also to nasal bones. The later formed ridges are lower and flatter than those earlier formed which are seen to greater advantage in the

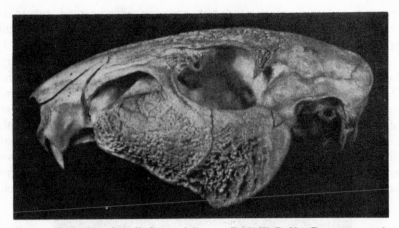

FIG. 44. Left side of skull, Spotted Cavy. B 761 W. R. U. Permanent molars erupted. Occipitosphenoid suture patent. Well-ordered pattern lost in lacrimal but fully developed in postorbital process. Frontal and part of parietal decorated by flat topped tracery like that of postorbital process in figure 43. On maxillary shield the suborbital parallel ridges have disappeared and lattice-like tracery of lower portion is now a well ordered system of ridges extending to almost the entire lateral surface of malar as well as maxilla.

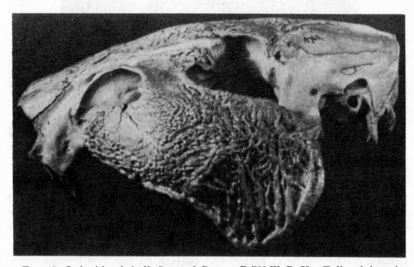

FIG. 45. Left side of skull, Spotted Cavy. B 762 W. R. U. Fully adult male. Dwindling tracery on postorbital process. Exuberant lattice-like tracery on maxilla and malar extending to squamous root of zygoma. Pattern on frontal resembles arbor vitae with extensions to parietal and nasal, later formed ridges being lower and flatter than those earlier formed.

younger skulls. It is worthy of notice that the regressing, earlier formed ridge patterns, as they dwindle, take on the structural characters of the later formed patterns (B 762, fig. 45).

The important principle illustrated by these three skulls of the Spotted Cavy is the age relationship of differentiation. During the growing period when the modelling process of the skeleton is in its prime the pattern is clear cut and orderly in its design. During mature age orderly differentiation is progressively diminished and the clear cut character of its features is lost.

As a skeleton progresses from mature to advanced age further textural changes are observable, always in the direction of diminution in orderly and clear cut differentiation. These, like the earlier age changes, are registered on human bones, but for their clarification we must seek an example of new bone formation occurring in later life as a regular

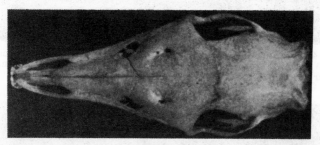

Fig. 46. Frontlet of young Okapi before formation of horn bosses. B 1659 W. R. U. Numerous fine vascular channels radiating from emissary foramina.

process of ageing and not pathological in nature. This is fortunately provided by the skull of the Giraffe, an animal which adds as many as seven horn excrescences to its equipment as it grows older. This peculiarity in the Giraffe contrasts outstandingly with the regular orderly pattern of horn development seen in its close relative, the Okapi. We may therefore carry this study of textural change from young adult life to advanced age by observation of the frontlet in these two animals. The frontlet of an Okapi before differentiation of the horn bosses (B 1659, fig. 46) shows veins communicating with diploe of the frontal bones. These veins lie in numerous fine channels which radiate from emissary foramina.

Horn cores underlying the permanent velvet are ossified but not yet united with the calvarium in the frontlet of a young Giraffe (B 474, fig. 47). Enlarged venous tracks are obvious on the frontal bones around the emissary foramina and the cores themselves show an orderly design in their vascular pitting.

An adult male Okapi differs from the Giraffe in that its horns possess petrous tips projecting through the permanent velvet. In B 894 (fig. 48) growth of horn cores has ceased and therefore vascularity is

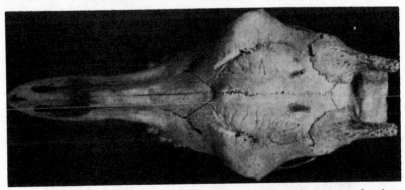

FIG. 47. Frontlet of young Giraffe before union of horn bosses to calvarium. B 474 W. R. U. Enlarged venous tracks round emissary foramina and orderly vascular pattern of horn cores.

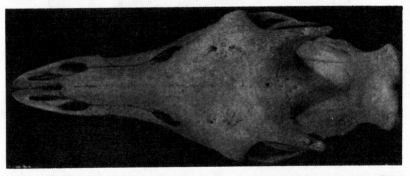

FIG. 48. Frontlet of adult male Okapi after cessation of horn growth. B 894 W. R. U. Vascular pattern reduced but still symmetrical and well ordered.

greatly reduced but there is still a symmetrical and well ordered pattern of grooves or tracks on base and surface of core for the vessels supplying the velvet. While the original horn cores of the Giraffe do grow in adult life, new horn cores appear, one in the center of the forehead over the metopic suture, several over the internasal suture, one from each postorbital process, one from each side of the lambda, smaller ones

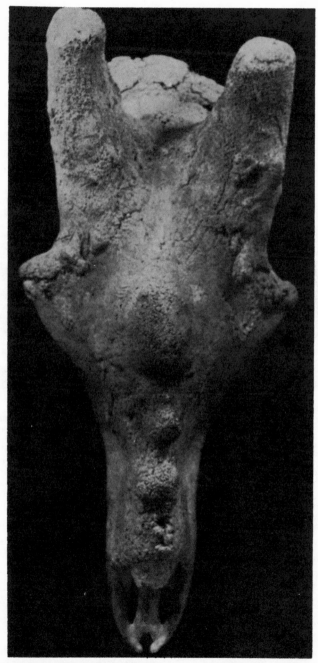

FIG. 49. Frontlet of old male Giraffe. B 1658 W. R. U. Commencing disorderliness of vascular pattern about horn cores and of ossification in subsidiary bony masses.

from the zygoma and base of the great horn above the ear so that the old Giraffe possesses several well marked and many rudimentary horns.

A glance at the frontlet of an old Giraffe, B 1658 (fig. 49), shows commencing disorderliness in vascular pattern and still more disorderliness in the ossification about the cores and the subsidiary bony masses and also in the very large venous tracks leading to the emissary foramina. It is indeed impossible to distinguish these bony and venous patterns from those of pathological origin. Nevertheless these are true features of the ageing process and in no way related to disease.

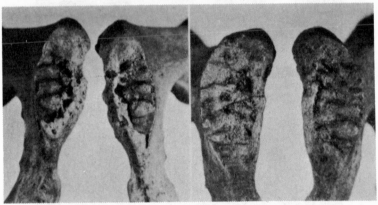

FIG. 50   FIG. 51

FIG. 50. Symphysial face, pubic bones. No. 744 W. R. U. Negro, male, aged 22 years. The billowed pattern of adolescence is now being covered by a finer textured epiphysial bone over upper and lower ends and ventral margin. These ossifications may occur separately as upper and lower nodules and ventral rampart. At this stage of maturity there is no sign of dorsal margin or transformation in surface texture.

FIG. 51. Symphysial face, pubic bones. No. 860 W. R. U. Negro, male, aged 23 years. Nodules and rampart are present but less clearly distinct than in figure 50. Dorsal margin and commencing textural transformation in surface are apparent.

With the knowledge of these examples from comparative anatomy corresponding changes in the human skeleton become intelligible. They are most clearly discernible in the symphysial face of the pubic bone. In post-adolescent and early adult life the subepiphysial symphysial face presents a transversely billowed surface with an increasing sharp dorsal margin and a bevelled ventral area. Overlying this subepiphysial face is a cartilaginous epiphysis, the ventral part of which alone ossifies. The close textured epiphysial ossification is apparent early in the third decade (fig. 50). It forms upper and lower extremities and a ventral rampart for the symphysial face with which it may or may not fuse at this time. Under the ventral rampart rarefaction appears in the billowed subepiphysial bone so that the epiphysial rampart may actually form bridges of bone.

Most frequently however the bony epiphysis, as it ossifies, fuses immediately with the underlying bone so that the billowed surface becomes glazed by close textured new bone (fig. 51). Distinction between epiphysial and underlying bone is often difficult (fig. 52).

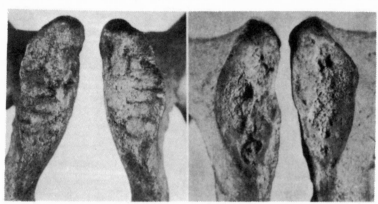

FIG. 52   · FIG. 53

FIG. 52. Symphysial face, pubic bones. No. 525 W. R. U. Negro, male, aged 22 years. All parts seen in figures 50, 51 are present in this example but are retrogressive in type. The cause of variants in ruggedness of expression in different bones is not yet known.

FIG. 53. Symphysial face, pubic bones. No. 791 W. R. U. Negro, male, aged 28 years. Upper and lower nodules and ventral rampart are now losing themselves in the general textural transformation.

In the latter part of the third decade the billowed texture is lost and a typical ovoid symphysial face results, formed dorsally by the pubic bone itself but ventrally, and at upper and lower extremities, by ossified fused epiphysial bone (fig. 53). Early in the fifth decade the symphysial face presents an oval surface of which the texture is relatively smooth, delimited by clearly outlined dorsal and ventral margins meeting at raised upper and lower extremities (fig. 54). Toward the end of the fifth decade a narrow beaded rim develops on the margins as in other articular surfaces of the skeleton (fig. 55).

During the sixth decade erosion of surface and breakdown of ventral margin begin to modify the configuration of the symphysial face (fig. 56). In the seventh decade this modification has progressed to the complete transformation of the surface into the irregularly eroded texture of advanced age (fig. 57). This terminal disorderly configuration is a true feature of the ageing process. It corresponds to the disorderliness described under ossification of the horns of the old Giraffe. Although the morphological features are indistinguishable from those of pathological origin it is not due to disease. It illustrates a blend of ageing and infirmity where orderly control of differentiation

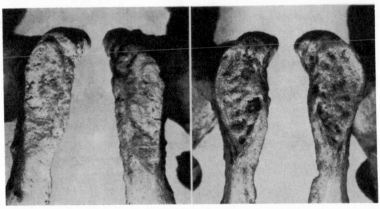

FIG. 54   FIG. 55

FIG. 54. Symphysial face, pubic bones. No. 314 W. R. U. White, male, aged 42 years. Relatively smooth and generally inactive surface with complete oval outline, clearly defined extremities, no "rim" or beading of borders and no lipping of margin.
FIG. 55. Symphysial face, pubic bones. No. 202 W. R. U. White, male, aged 52 years. A distinct narrow beading or "rim" round borders.

is lost although the bizarre and often grotesque overgrowth of frankly pathological origin is lacking (Todd, 1920, 1921).

4. SKULL

Cranial suture closure is a subject which illustrates very well the progressive emancipation from orderly sequence in differentiation characteristic of mature and advanced age. Bolk (1915, 1919) has shown that if premature obliteration of sutures occurs it takes place for the most part, if not entirely, before the age of seven years. Just why this "premature" obliteration should occur in a creature derived from anthropoid stock we shall not discuss at the moment. We simply

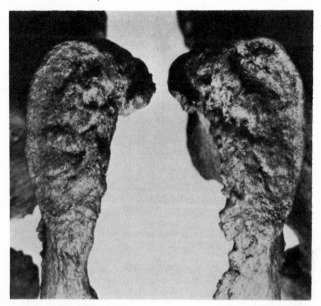

FIG. 56. Symphysial face, 1.5 pubic bones.   No. 253 W. R. U.   White, male, aged 58 years.   Marked erosion of surface and breakdown of ventral margin.

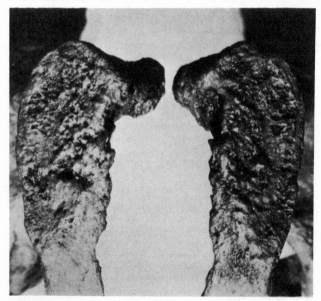

FIG. 57. Symphysial face, 1.5 pubic bones.   No. 359 W. R. U.   White, male, aged 63 years.   Complete transformation of surface into the irregularly eroded texture of advanced age.

set these aberrant skulls on one side and turn our attention to those more representative of human differentiation.

Closure of cranial sutures in Man is characteristic of mature age and always commences in and is more extensive on the endocranial surface. The period of most rapid progress in suture closure lies between twenty-six and thirty years, immediately after the termination of epiphysial union at the sternal end of the clavicle. From thirty to forty years progress is very slow and after forty years there is practical inactivity punctuated by bursts of renewed progress at approximately sixty-three and eighty years. Thus sagittal, coronal, lambdoid and sphenofrontal sutures begin to close on the endocranial surface at or before the age of twenty-six years. Union proceeds vigorously till thirty years of age by which time sphenotemporal, masto-occipital and sphenoparietal sutures have all begun to close. From then on progress in closure becomes progressively slower but does not cease for squamous and parietomastoid sutures begin to unite in the later thirties. Completion should occur in the sagittal suture by thirty years but the squamous may still be patent at more than sixty.

That there is some general or constitutional influence which modifies progress in suture closure, commencing approximately at thirty years, is evident since all sutural elements, whatever their degree of union, show arrested activity at this age. It is as if Nature grew tired of carrying on her morphological work to its completion and left the structure imperfect in appearance though not in function. Failure of union is much more frequent in sutural than in epiphysial closure and is characterized by a heaping up of bone tissue along the edges of the unclosed part. The edges therefore look "clawed" and inturned like the margins of trachomatous eyelids.

While bone along a suture edge is still in a state of active change it possesses a granular texture difficult to describe but easy to recognize. After activity has ceased the granularity gives place to a waxy smoothness of texture. Heaped up edges on an unclosed suture are characteristic evidence of quiescence which absolutely differentiates the suture from one still in a state of active closure. I have therefore called this condition lapsed union. It is very frequent in the sutures on the endocranial aspect of human skulls and is almost constant on the ectocranial surface where however it does not present the characteristic heaped up feature (Todd and Lyon, 1924, 1925).

Closure of sutures between the bones of the face commences in general later than but pursues its course parallel with suture closure in the cranium. No adequate description has so far been given of the age relationship of facial suture closure in Man though Schweikher (1930) has made a detailed record of the sequence of union between the several facial bones of the Hyaena as a type of mammal and Krogman (1930) has described the same process in anthropoids and Old World apes.

Age changes are also evident in the texture and markings of the cranium both without and within.

The texture of the young adult cranium is ivorine on both outer and inner surfaces but gradually, between thirty and fifty years, a change takes place. The surface assumes a matte appearance like that of an English biscuit. It is not coarse enough to deserve the term granular, though granularity may occur after middle life, and is often present in advanced age as evidence of nutritional deficiency. The muscular ridging on the exterior of the cranium, absent in the young, shows itself in temporal and occipital areas from twenty-five years. It does not become better marked during mature life nor does it diminish in advanced age. Similar muscular ridging appears and pursues an identical course on zygoma and masseteric area of mandible. Pitting of the parietal bones is not an age character but is evidence of a nutritional defect in childhood. From this the bones, once scarred, never recover so that the percentage showing pitting remains approximately constant in samples no matter what their age. The imprint of the sagittal venous sinus does not become more marked during mature or even advanced age nor does that of the left lateral venous sinus though there is some evidence, perhaps equivocal, of deepening in the imprint of the right lateral venous sinus after fifty years is reached. Contrary to general belief we have found no significant change occurring solely as a result of advanced age in depth or extent of Pacchionian depressions. The grooves for the meningeal veins (Wood Jones, 1912) do however show a deepening and sharpening of their margins as age increases. All these records are taken from data now being prepared for publication (Todd, Simmons and Nickerson).

Symmetrical atrophy of the parietal bones has been claimed as an age characteristic since Maier first adequately described it (Maier, 1854). It is however by no means frequent. Humphry (1858, pp. 242–243) found only one example in Cambridge, four in Paris and one in Berlin and hazarded, from the exact symmetry, similarity of deficiency in the several skulls and from the absence of any trace of disease, that the condition is congenital. Among more than 3000 contemporary skulls of White and Negro origin added to the Hamann

Museum since 1912 we have never seen it but it does occur once only as a well marked feature among the skulls collected for the Museum from the unclaimed dead of Cleveland since the year 1892. This skull is figured by Keen (1908, vol. 3, p. 43). Symmetrical thinning of the parietal bones was very common in Egypt between the fourth and nineteenth dynasties, occurring among the upper classes in people accustomed to wear wigs of enormous proportions and great weight (Elliot Smith, 1907). It is produced by a thinning successively of the outer table, diploe and inner table and never occurs under about thirty years of age. Meyer (1917), writing ten years after Elliot Smith, has doubts on the uniformity of causation but there was no history for any skull in Meyer's series to give indication of a probable cause. The skull (0.22 W.R.U.) in the Hamann Museum illustrates the fact that in symmetrical thinning of the parietal bones we may have to deal with diverse causes. Thinning in this skull started on the endocranial surface which shows sheaves of vascular channels radiating from the sides of the sagittal elevation along which the sagittal venous sinus coursed. Some of these are associated with Pacchionian depressions. The diploe has collapsed but the outer table is not directly affected. Meyer's contention is therefore borne out but this is a totally different type of thinning from that described by Elliot Smith. It is however equally pathological in origin and in no way a feature of age.

Wetzel (1932) speaks of an atrophy of diploe in old age. Schüller (1935) however describes this change as a transformation of the diploe into bone from fifty years onward. He also claims as age characters both symmetrical thinning of the parietals and general thickening of the vault. I have however just alluded to the cause of symmetrical thinning and in our very large collection of skulls of known age I have shown that there is no characteristic change in the thickness of the vault with advancing years (Todd, 1924). If there is a real and constant change in cranial thickness characteristic of age it is not conclusive enough to permit measurements.

The diploe of the cranium, which first makes its appearance in childhood at about the sixth year, continues to develop until young adult life and is evident in the roentgenogram as a fine mottling. Harris (1933) has pointed out that the diploe first becomes channelled by venous sinuses at about thirty-five years, possibly to provide a backwater connected with the cerebral circulation as these diploic sinuses form a communication between the venous sinuses of the dura and the veins of the scalp. Harris further points out that after the onset of the menopause in women and during the later fifties in men the diploic sinuses again disappear with the increase of bony deposit in the diploe. This of necessity means a reduction and final elimination of the safety factor provided for middle life by the presence of the diploic sinuses. The fine mottling on the roentgenogram now gives place to a more irregular open tracery or complete loss of mottling.

Halisteresis has frequently been described, both in cranium and face, as characteristic of old age. It is by no means invariable and is definitely an expression of the failure of adequate nutrition which so often supervenes as a mark of infirmity in the supportive tissues of advanced years. Pearce (1936) has described the diminution in oxygen consumption of excised organs in mice of a year or more in age when contrasted with the tissue respiration of growing animals of the same racial strain. No such experiments are extant to demonstrate a like distinction in bone or connective tissue. But Wolbach's researches on the influence of Vitamin C in the formation of collagen and reticulum (Wolbach, 1933, 1936; Wolbach and Howe, 1926; Menkin, Wolbach and Menkin, 1934) together with the investigations by Lanman and Ingalls (1937) on the resistance of healing wounds to the strain of rupture make very impressive the indispensibility of Vitamin C for the effective function of connective tissue. Good bone texture of proper strength is likewise the result of appropriate nutrition in adequate amount and suitable form. The infirmities of old age, implying malnutrition in diverse forms, are certainly associated with halisteresis. Further an osteoporosis indistinguishable from the halisteresis of advanced years is frequently present in persons of mature and even of youthful age when suffering from chronic impaired constitutional health. Many fractures of the skull are due less to the force of the injury than to the weakness or brittleness of the osteoporotic bone.

Age changes in the skull are, therefore, to be found in suture closure of cranium and face, in texture, in markings on outer and inner surface of brain case, and in the patterns of special embellishments such as the zygomatic shield of the Spotted Cavy and the horn cores of the Giraffidae. A description of these special characteristics in mammals is included to illustrate the fact that the texture of features newly formed in mature life is modified according to the age at which they appear. The permanent horns of Antelopes, Cattle, Sheep and Goats, the deciduous horns of the Pronghorn antelope, and the antlers of the Deer give more generally recognized though hardly better known illustrations of the same fact. Muscular ridges culminating in the great sagittal and lambdoid flanges of mammals, particularly the Gorilla, are features developing during the period of growth and early adult life. Like the corresponding muscular ridges on temporal and occipital bones of Man they show no evident textural changes and undergo no atrophy with the onset of old age.

No obvious age changes are to be found in the markings of venous sinuses or in Pacchionian depressions although deepening of channels and sharpening of margins do occur in the grooves for meningeal veins with advancing years. Changes due to age alone in thickness of cranium and in diploe are not sufficient to emerge on statistical analysis. The cause of obliteration of sutures in childhood must be sought in phylogeny and is not an age character. Granularity of surface of cranium, thickening or thinning of vault, multiple vascular pitting of parietal bones and gross changes in texture, often quite striking in the adult, are all features the cause for which must be sought in chronic nutritional defect or other constitutional infirmity. Halisteresis of cranial and facial bones, like halisteresis in the skeleton under which heading the process will be discussed, does set in after fifty years. This however is indistinguishable from the osteoporosis consequent upon constitutional defect and may indeed be a sign of supervening infirmity.

5. APPENDICULAR AND AXIAL SKELETON

Age changes in the skeleton can clearly be seen in the thin translucent scapula. These changes resolve themselves into three types, namely, modifications of vascularity, of surface texture, and of cancellous structure. For information on vascularity and surface texture we are indebted to Graves (1922).

The features of deep vascularity in the bone substance are best shown in photographs made by transmitted light which demonstrates also the atrophic spots in surface texture. Surface vascularity is easily seen by simple observation but the vascular tracks are small and the history of their modification is identical with that of deep vascularity.

Figure 58 shows the vascular pattern in adolescence. It is rich over entire noncancellous areas both above and below the spinous process. In the early twenties (fig. 59) it is equally rich but its pattern is more distinct. Leashes of vessels sweep over the axillary and vertebral borders and swirl inwards and downwards from the region of the spinous process. In the infra-spinous area leashes also enter through the glenoid base swirling upwards and downwards respectively to mingle with the leashes sweeping over the axillary and vertebral borders.

The lines of attachment of intramuscular tendinous bands are evident as narrow dark zones originating in the vertebral border and extending towards the glenoid base. By about the age of fifty years (fig. 60) the vascular pattern is no longer clearly marked. The lines of ten-

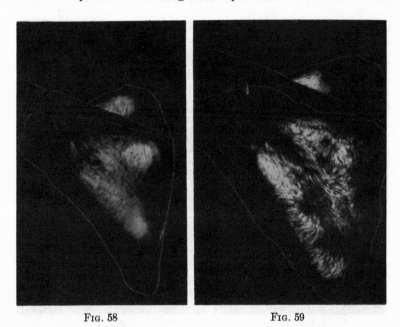

FIG. 58   FIG. 59

FIG. 58. Transilluminated scapulae. No. 633 W. R. U. Negro, female, aged 13 years. Note richness of deep vascularity as described in figure 59.
Fig. 59. Transilluminated scapulae. No. 423 W. R. U. White, male, aged 24 years. Leashes of vessels sweep over axillary and vertebral borders and swirl upwards and downwards from region of spinous process.

dinous insertion are more numerous and between them are clearer, irregular areas of bone atrophy. In old age (fig. 61) deep vascularity is indistinguishable by transmitted light and the thickened ridges of tendinous attachment appear as dense black zones extended into a bizarre pattern of local thickenings between which are the clear atrophic spots.

The surface texture of the bone changes with advancing age in a manner similar to that of the skull. In the thin scapular blade these changes are complicated by the appearance of areas or spots of atrophy, seldom seen before forty-five years but occurring with increasing frequency after fifty years. The bone, held up to the light, seems patchy, spotted or "moth eaten." Those areas in which the atrophy is more advanced are depressed below the level of the adjacent surface and plainly delimited by a sharp margin. By transmitted light the spots are pearly, granular and amorphous in appearance. They may

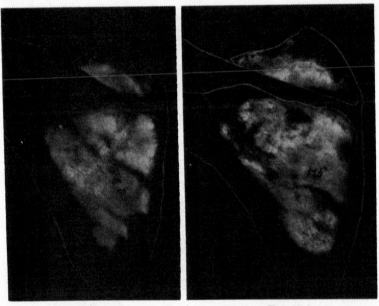

FIG. 60   FIG. 61

FIG. 60. Transilluminated scapulae. No. 285 W. R. U. White, male, aged 45 years. Vascular pattern no longer clearly marked. Continuity marred by development of "muscular" ridges radiating from vertebral border.

FIG. 61. Transilluminated scapulae. No. 115 W. R. U. White, male, aged 88 years. Vascularity indistinguishable. Both supra- and infra-spinous areas irregularly thickened with intervening atrophic areas. "Muscular" ridges extended and erratic.

be thin like parchment or their centers may be perforated. Thus they resemble the special symmetrical atrophic areas on the parietal bones.

Accompanying the bone atrophy are other features, namely, blistering, buckling or pleating of surface and distorsion of substance. A coarse wrinkle or pleat may be seen even in the thirties. It usually appears on the dorsal surface of the blade below the spine and parallel in a general way to the cristae of tendinous attachment. Buckling is more frequent in thin blades and increases in frequency with age. Blisters are local areas of paper-thin compacta raised above the surrounding surface. They cover venous enlargements and are seen only in advanced age. Distorsion implies deformity or warping of the entire thickness of the blade. It can be seen equally well in macerated and in fresh dissected scapulae of advanced age but never occurs in scapulae possessing a thick blade.

All the foregoing characteristics of age can be seen in roentgenograms of the scapula but they are less clearly evident than in transilluminated bones.

A roentgenogram of the scapula is particularly instructive for the study of cancellous tissue. This is illustrated by figures 62–65.

In adolescence (fig. 62) there are no cristae of tendinous attachment. Thickening has not yet taken place on the axillary border. Cancellous tissue is close textured with fine trabeculae along borders and attachment of spinous process. Lacunae of more open trabecular architecture occur between axillary border and spinous process. Trabecular lines paralleling glenoid surface have appeared in glenoid base but those radiating from glenoid surface have not yet arranged themselves into a formal pattern.

During early adult life (fig. 63) cristae for tendinous attachment are commencing to develop and the axillary border is thickening. Cancellous tissue is close textured; its trabeculae and lacunar formation are unchanged from those of adolescence. The trabeculae parallel to glenoid surface in the glenoid base are also unchanged; the radial trabeculae have now arranged themselves into a formal pattern. The glenoid rim, which is not evident until about thirty-five years, is absent.

During mature life, except for a possible further development of cristae, there are no significant changes in substance.

With the onset of old age (fig. 64) cristae for tendinous attachment are numerous and well developed. Cancellous tissue becomes more open and its lacunar formation becomes more extensive. Irregular areas of atrophy with surface pleating are evident. The articular margin of the glenoid surface no longer shows a beaded rim but has a sharp lipped margin. There is reduction in thickness and number of parallel and radiating trabeculae beneath the glenoid surface.

In senility all the features of old age are accentuated but if halisteresis or demineralization becomes severe (fig. 65), as it often does in advanced age, all the features already catalogued as characteristic of old age and senility become exaggerated except the cristae which cannot become sharper or more pronounced for lack of mineral.

These observations are, to a certain extent, heterodox. It must be remembered, however, that intensive study of age features in the

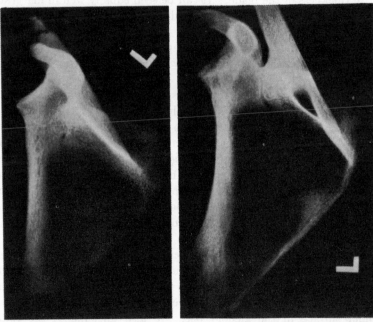

Fig. 62   Fig. 63

Fig. 62. Roentgenogram of left scapula. No. 633 W. R. U. Negro, female, aged 13 years. The rich vascular pattern is evident. There are no cristae of tendinous attachment. The axillary border is not thickened. Cancellous tissue is close and fine textured along borders and attachment of spinous process. It shows some lacunae between axillary border and spinous process. Radiating lines in glenoid base have not yet a formal pattern. Lines paralleling the glenoid surface are present. Glenoid rim is not yet formed.

Fig. 63. Roentgenogram of left scapula. No. 680 W. R. U. White, male, aged 23 years. Vascular pattern is less rich but more formal in design. Cristae of tendinous attachment are commencing. Axillary border is thickened. Cancellous tissue is close and fine textured along borders. Lacunar formation remains as in figure 62. Radiating lines are arranged in formal pattern in glenoid bone. Lines paralleling glenoid surface are the same as in figure 62. Glenoid rim is not yet formed.

skeleton was impossible until the utilization of the roentgenogram as a routine technical method for study and the establishment of the collection of skeletons of known age in the Hamann Museum. Cristae are not evidence of muscularity but merely of maturity. Whatever

the influences which determine the formal pattern of bone architecture
(Anseroff, 1934; Murray, 1936), the pattern itself is an age character
developing in childhood and youth, maintained during mature life and
lost as age advances or infirmity intervenes. The characteristics of

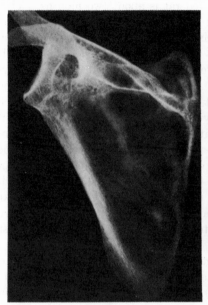 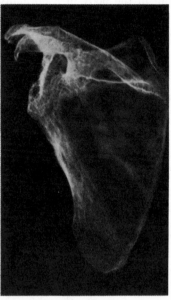

FIG. 64   FIG. 65

FIG. 64. Roentgenogram of left scapula. No. 3132 W. R. U. White, female,
aged 61 years. Entire bone is demineralized. Vascular pattern is no longer
distinguishable. Cristae are numerous but demineralized. Axillary border is
greatly demineralized. Cancellous tissue is open textured. Lacunar formation
has extended into base of glenoid. Radiating lines in base of glenoid are still
evident though reduced in number and limited in area. Lines paralleling glenoid
surface have disappeared. Glenoid rim shows sharp margin. Irregular areas of
atrophy are present above and below the spinous process. One very definite
area of radial buckling is evident below the spine.

FIG. 65. Roentgenogram of left scapula. No. 3053 W. R. U. White, female,
aged 70 years, constitutional deficiency. Entire bone greatly demineralized.
No vascular pattern. Cristae present. Axillary and vertebral borders and
acromion buckled and distorted. Cancellous tissue open; its trabeculae fragmented. Lacunar formation permeates all cancellous tissue. Glenoid surface
completely demineralized and disorganized. Radiating and parallel lines of
glenoid base lost. Distortion evident in acromion, coracoid and vertebral border.

articular areas will be discussed under the heading of joints (pp. 320–
322).

Details of interrelationship between the biochemical factors and the
histological elements in bone substance are still obscure. That bone

is in a state of constant change, however, is illustrated by the investigations of Chiewitz and Hevesy (1935) who, using as an indicator the radio-active isotope of phosphorus $_{15}P^{32}$ which has a half life of seventeen days, found that the average time spent by a phosphorus atom in the body of a normally fed rat is about two months. Their rats, killed about a month after the intake of phosphorus, contained only about half the active phosphorus found in those killed at the end of a week. About 30 per cent of the phosphorus deposited in the skeleton of an adult rat seems to be lost by the end of twenty days. Calculations of the phosphorus content of the different organs per gram of dried tissue showed that spleen and kidneys contain about 18 per cent per gram, brain nearly 15 per cent and liver 14 per cent. Muscles and fat contain 7 per cent but bone a little less than 3 per cent, despite the fact that the largest part of the phosphorus ingested goes into the skeleton. No conspicuous differences are found in the phosphorus content of different parts of the skeleton. On this analysis the bones are continuously taking up atoms of phosphorus which are wholly or in part lost again and are replaced by others, the phosphorus temporarily stored in the skeleton being utilized in the metabolism of organs.

The active biochemical changes constantly evident in the skeleton at all ages are reflected in the equally changing structure detectable both by roentgenography and by histological examination. Haversian systems, formerly thought to be characteristic of compact bone, were shown in 1913 to be present also in spongiosa or cancellous tissue (Todd, 1913), an observation later confirmed by Arey (1919). But haversian systems whether in compacta or spongiosa are not permanent: they undergo resorption and replacement with or without the accompaniment of osteoclasts (Todd, 1913). During pregnancy and the first six months after parturition, during infancy and adolescence, subsequent to fracture or bone disease, and in injuries of the soft tissues such as complete severance of median nerve or the tendons at the wrist, we have observed changes in mineralization of spongiosa to occur so rapidly that within six weeks the difference may be clearly evident in the roentgenogram. Analyses of the second phalanx of the little finger from hands of which roentgenograms have previously been made, show that a difference in structure discernible to the naked eye on the roentgenogram corresponds to a difference of 25 per cent in the amount of mineral per unit volume of bone (Todd and Hagemeyer). Lachmann and Whelan (1936) have stated that a difference of 7 per cent can be detected by roentgenography on dead bones experimentally subjected to the local action of acid. This is not strictly comparable to the process of demineralization or halisteresis during life, a subject on which I have made a preliminary presentation (Todd, 1937).

The degree of fluctuation in mineralization occurring in the ordinary vicissitudes of life is illustrated by selected roentgenograms of the left wrist (figs. 66–68). These show, respectively, the amount of mineral in the bones of the mother of one of our children the day before delivery, three months after delivery (the baby being breast fed for two months), and six months after delivery. In a well mineralized bone the interstices between the trabeculae of the spongiosa are filled with a gray sheen of labile mineral which to some extent obscures the tracery of the trabeculae. Owing to the demands of mineral for lactation, this gray sheen is less evident three months after delivery but is restored in another three months. Changes in the trabeculae themselves are limited to modifications of thickness and occasional fragmentation. Figures 69–73 typify the changes in bone texture characteristic of healthy life from adolescence onward and the demineralization incurred in constitutional deficiency. They demonstrate the hand textures of adolescence in a healthy girl of 13 years, in a girl of the same developmental age having a constitutional deficiency, in a healthy woman of 27 years, in advanced age and in the constitutional deficiency which usually accompanies senility.

In a healthy girl (fig. 69), a gray sheen largely obscures the trabeculae, the tracery of which is well on the way to adult pattern. Compacta is dense though still thin in radius, ulna and metacarpals and incomplete in phalanges as one expects of a child. Spongiosa of shafts of radius and ulna, of carpals and of metacarpal heads and bases already shows the closely arranged, fine trabeculae and interstitial gray sheen of labile mineral in normal adult life; but in phalanges, epiphyses and distal parts of metacarpal shafts it has not yet attained the adult pattern. Ossification is nearing completion in the sesamoids of thumb and index finger but has not yet started in the sesamoid of the little finger. The dense outlines of the bilateral bosses on metacarpal heads have not yet spread to the shafts. Radiating trabeculae are arranging themselves beneath articular surfaces but the surface outlines themselves are not yet dense nor are they accompanied by subjacent parallel trabeculae.

In the girl nineteen years of age but of retarded adolescent development and of constitutional deficiency (fig. 70), the trabecular pattern

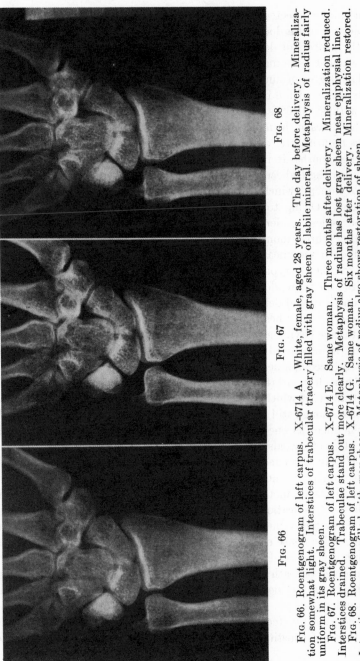

Fig. 66   Fig. 67   Fig. 68

Fig. 66. Roentgenogram of left carpus. X-6714 A. White, female, aged 28 years. The day before delivery. Mineralization somewhat light. Interstices of trabecular tracery filled with gray sheen of labile mineral. Metaphysis of radius fairly uniform in its gray sheen.

Fig. 67. Roentgenogram of left carpus. X-6714 E. Same woman. Three months after delivery. Mineralization reduced. Interstices drained. Trabeculae stand out more clearly. Metaphysis of radius has lost gray sheen near epiphysial line.

Fig. 68. Roentgenogram of left carpus. X-6714 G. Same woman. Six months after delivery. Mineralization restored. Interstices once more filled with gray sheen. Metaphysis of radius also shows restoration of sheen.

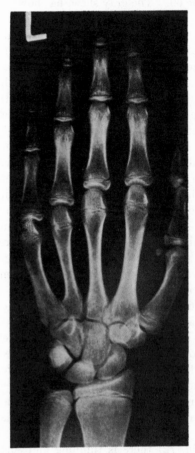 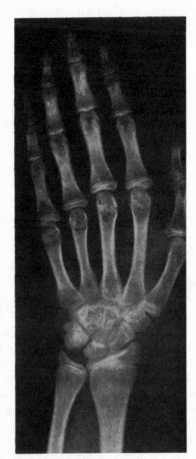

Fig. 69   Fig. 70

Fig. 69. Roentgenogram of left hand in early adolescence. White, female, aged 13 years. SS 171 H. Trabecular tracery of adult pattern in metaphyses of radius and ulna, in carpals and in metacarpal bases. Gray sheen of labile mineral fills interstices of trabeculae in carpus and metaphyses of radius and ulna. Compacta dense, thin, except in phalanges where it is still being formed. Articular surfaces not dense and subarticular radiating and parallel trabeculae incomplete.

Fig. 70. Roentgenogram of left hand in early adolescence. Retarded development; imperfect mineralization. White, female, aged 19 years. SS 3327 A. Trabecular tracery of adult pattern as in figure 29 but with thicker striae displaying "knots" or nodes of dense mineral scattered throughout the tracery. Sheen of labile mineral greatly diminished in all bones. Compacta thin, rather light, almost nonexistent in second and terminal phalanges. Articular surfaces not dense, subarticular trabeculae incomplete.

is almost identical with that in figure 69. The gray sheen has however largely disappeared from the interstices. The compacta of radius, ulna and metacarpals is lightly mineralized and thin. It is very light and retarded in development in phalanges. Spongiosa of radius, ulna, carpals and metacarpals shows a more open tracery of thicker trabeculae, fragmented indeed in places such as lower radius, its epiphysis and the carpals. In the tracery are irregularly scattered "knots" or little nodes of denser tissue. These are characteristic of bones in which restoration of adequate mineralization is still possible. One might define the condition as reversible halisteresis. We have not found these knots in the halisteresis of advanced age. A somewhat similar course of remineralization has been described by McLean and Bloom (1936) in experimental studies on the effect of parathormone in young growing rats. Trabeculae and knots are the more obvious because of the lack of interstitial labile mineral. Sesamoids, despite an outline characteristic for the age, show halisteresis. The outlines of bilateral bosses on metacarpal heads are also poorly mineralized. The radiating and parallel trabeculae under articular surfaces show a development characteristic of the stage in physical maturation.

The hand of the adult woman (fig. 71) shows the closely arranged fine trabeculae and interstitial gray sheen characteristic of health. Compacta is dense, thicker than in adolescence and is now well developed in all phalanges. The sesamoid for little finger is fully ossified. The bilateral bosses on metacarpal heads have dense outlines extended on to the shafts. All articular surfaces are densely outlined and present a full complement of subjacent radiating and parallel trabeculae. The dense outlines of articular surfaces on carpals are somewhat obscured by the interstitial sheen.

In the hand of advanced age (fig. 72) there is thinning and some demineralization of compacta in all bones but the articular surfaces maintain their shell of dense tissue. Halisteresis is evident in all sesamoids. No reduction of density has occurred in the outlines of the bilateral metacarpal bosses. The subarticular parallel trabeculae have almost disappeared but the radiating trabeculae, though thin, maintain their formal pattern. Trabeculae of spongiosa are thin but not fragmented: they are not thick as in the demineralization of adolescence.

The skeleton of advanced age complicated by constitutional deficiency (fig. 73) presents a very different picture. Clinically it would be described as polyarticular atrophic osteo-arthritis. Compacta is paperthin or entirely absent. The dense compact tissue of the articular surfaces is reduced to a mere shell or has completely collapsed with consequent telescoping of bones and formation of exuberant articular flanges. Trabeculae in the spongiosa are very thin, are fragmentary,

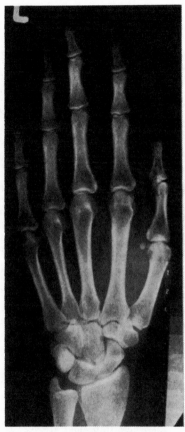 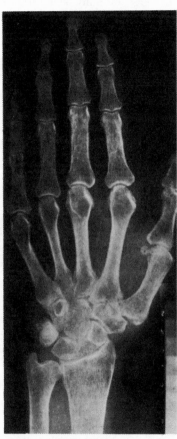

FIG. 71   FIG. 72

FIG. 71. Roentgenogram of left hand in mature life. White, female, aged 27 years. X-7929 A. Same fine closely arranged trabeculae and interstitial sheen shown in figure 69. Compacta thicker, dense and now is present in phalanges. Each articular surface consists of a shell of dense bone with full complement of subarticular radiating and parallel trabeculae.

FIG. 72. Roentgenogram of left hand in healthy advanced age. White, female, aged 78 years. X-9409 A. Thinning and some demineralization of compacta in all bones but articular surfaces maintain their shell of compact tissue though subarticular parallel trabeculae have almost disappeared and radiating trabeculae have lost their formal pattern. Trabeculae of spongiosa thin but not fragmented as in figure 73 except in lateral part of metaphysis of radius.

have completely lost their formal pattern and show no "knots." The gray interstitial sheen is almost entirely lacking.

Roentgenographic analysis of skeletal texture requires an adequate knowledge of bony structure in health and age but the reading of roentgenograms is greatly facilitated if proper precautions have been taken to insure uniformity of technique in processing (Todd, 1937).

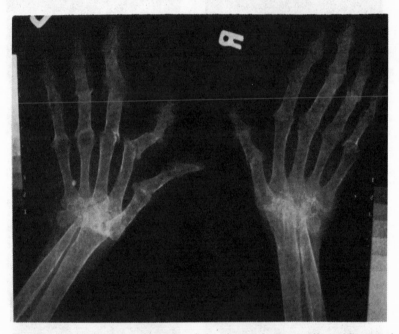

FIG. 73. Roentgenogram of both hands in advanced age complicated by constitutional deficiency. No. 3053 W. R. U. White, female, aged 70 years. X-8970. Compacta paper-thin or lacking. Articular shells of dense compact tissue have almost all collapsed with consequent telescoping of bones and exuberant articular flanges. Spongiosa of metacarpals and triquetrum, which have withstood deformation, is almost devoid of trabeculae. Elsewhere trabeculae are very thin, are fragmentary, have lost their formal pattern and show no "knots." The gray interstitial sheen is almost entirely lacking.

The gray interstitial sheen of labile mineral has not previously been emphasized by other writers but Bauer, Aub and Albright (1929) noted a diminution of trabeculae in kittens shortly after birth. They concluded from this that calcium is stored in the trabeculae against demands of postnatal growth. Burns and Henderson (1936) found this true also of cortical bone. Bone growth, they say, is largely determined by local factors, and not wholly by systemic blood supply. During growth bone is in dynamic equilibrium with its tissue fluids. This theme of bone change can be applied equally well to the phenomena of ageing. McCay, Crowell and Maynard (1935), describing the effect of retarded growth on the length of the life span, observed that the aged bones of their retarded rats were all demineralized despite the adequate ration for nutrition which they were careful to supply.

That there is a change in the collagenous matrix (Wetzel, 1932) of demineralized bone is evident from the brittleness of these bones. Intracapsular fracture of the neck of the femur is a good example: it usually occurs in the aged but may be seen also in children. Fracture of the bones in fragilitas ossium is another example. Probably the claim that 50 per cent of all fractures of the clavicle occur in children under five years, and the ease with which fracture of the skull occurs in some adults, are to be attributed to this brittleness. So many instances of greenstick and crushing fracture have occurred in the inadequately mineralized bones of allergic patients in my own experience that I believe this type of fracture should be considered a definite hazard of allergic children. Halisteresis however does not imply nonunion after fracture. The bony callus for repair of fractures is obtained though indirectly, from the adjacent areas of the shaft even though that shaft be relatively demineralized.

A study of ununited fractures shows that no rarefaction occurs in the neighboring areas of the shaft subsequent to the injury. This failure of adjacent bone to give up its mineral to the callus is not confined to the skeleton of advanced age. Nonunion is likewise to be found in fractures during infancy and even in "intra-uterine" fractures. Inasmuch as repair of demineralized bones readily takes place, there can be no impediment in these bones to cellular proliferation or to the normal biochemical processes of bone formation.

One of the characteristic features of advancing age is the increase in number of collagenous fibers (Wetzel, 1932). But if, as a result of constitutional deficiency, this does not happen, the matrix of white fibrous tissue in bone will be imperfect, perhaps replaced by some liquid material (Wolbach, 1936). The process suggests a deficiency of Vitamin C and, though vitamin deficiency has not so far been shown to be characteristic of ageing, it is certainly present in many old people (Ralli, 1938). The fact that the rats utilized by McCay, Crowell and Maynard (1935) showed demineralization despite an adequate ration is not inconsistent with this view. We know very little of the changing needs of the ageing organism for the several nutritionals.

The capacity of the body for handling bone salts is fundamental in that type of arthritis which increases in frequency and extent as age advances. This has been fully discussed by Willis (1924) whose description is a clear and convincing presentation of our knowledge of the subject. In Willis' chart of the frequency of atrophic joint lesions studied in the macerated bones of the dead, slender, lightly mineralized skeletons run a close second to those of average mineral density. These slender skeletons however tend to disappear from Willis' chart a full fifteen years before the others, probably because they represent the plus-potentially sick patients of Graves (1925b). This possibility was not fully explored when Willis' article was written. Ely (1922) noted the occurrence of lightly mineralized slender skeletons in patients suffering from frankly infectious arthritis. Chronic infection, indeed, seems to enhance the demineralization. In Willis' survey skeletons of good mineralization show the hypertrophic type of arthritis but these skeletons are far fewer at all ages below fifty years in the dead than lightly mineralized skeletons. The appearance of hypertrophic changes in the roentgenogram of a joint may signify only that the fourth decade of life has been passed.

For these age changes in bone it is possible to postulate arteriosclerosis as a cause. And indeed we may assume changes in intima, in muscle bundles of media and general thickening of wall in blood vessels to be phenomena of advancing age (see Chapter 7 by Cohn). But fatty degeneration and calcification clearly are not age changes. Furthermore there is characteristically in age an increase in number of capillaries (Wetzel, 1932). Doubtless the erratic changes described for scapula as blistering, pleating, buckling, distortion are on the borderline of infirmity and are therefore exaggerated if not caused by the presence of arteriosclerosis. Doubtless much, if not all, of the demineralization typical of advanced years is occasioned by defective nutrition, and that present in earlier life is due to constitutional deficiency of one or another type. But in all these expressions of disorder or disease the quasi-pathological features are erratic in time, bizarre in appearance and irregular in distribution. They lack the orderliness of that advance of the inevitable which typifies all genuine age changes.

Demineralization, or halisteresis, of the skeleton with advancing years is found first in the bones of the extremities, foot earlier than hand. Then in succession the innominate bones, vertebral column, sternum and ribs are affected. By this time the process has spread also to lower and upper tibia and fibula and subsequently to lower femur.

So definite are the changes in mineralization of spongiosa during mature and advanced years that they can be recognized in the sound produced by ribs as they strike the table when dropped from a height of a few inches. By this simple procedure it is possible to estimate within a few years the physiological age of a skeleton. It must be recognized however that the halisteresis of advancing years is indistinguishable from that of infirmity and the physiological age thus estimated is in reality a measure of the mineralization of the bone. The phenomenon has long been recognized; in a Druidical ceremony the rib of a deceased man was dropped into a large copper bowl. The sound emitted however was interpreted not as identifying the deceased but the murderer by whose hand the deceased met his death.

In summary we may say that, whereas orderly differentiation of age features in the skeleton is so clear cut in childhood and adolescence (Stevenson, 1924) that it can be used to assess maturation (Todd, 1937), no such definite progression is seen in advanced age. This I have illustrated by evidence from the symphysis pubis, cranial sutures, cranial texture, scapular substance and roentgenographic details in hand skeleton. Assessment of maturation in adult, and particularly in advanced age, is therefore correspondingly difficult. Assessment of maturation even in the young has indeed often been impugned, but never successfully for it is based upon features invariable in their sequence though their relationship to sideral time is modified by factors of pathological origin (Todd, Wharton and Todd, 1938). These factors may be the direct result of disease or the indirect consequence of poverty, malnutrition and domestic distress (Todd, 1931). The sequence of maturation is not affected by nationality, race, stock or sex (Todd, 1933b).

Progress in maturation is equally evident in the substance as on the surface of bones. It is expressed in both morphological structure and biochemical composition. Changes in the former can be studied by means of the roentgenogram and the microscope. For the latter new methods, physiochemical in type, are rapidly enlarging our understanding. The relationship of the vascular changes and the modifications in requirement of the several nutritionals in advanced age to the features of bone change is quite imperfectly known but orderliness of progress, faltering as it undoubtedly appears as life advances, still holds as a fundamental principle of true age changes.

6. CARTILAGE

Cartilage is largely a tissue of the growth period, hence its age changes and likewise its pathology are best exemplified in early life. With these we have nothing to do in this volume though it should be noted that the record of its early infirmity may remain throughout life in malformations and deformations of bony structure. There do occur permanent relics of disturbance of cartilaginous structure dating from its ageing process in early childhood. Such conditions are Schlätter's disease of the tibial spine; Köhler's disease of the navicular of the foot; subdivision of the navicular (scaphoid) of the hand; emarginate patella, split patella and accessory patellar ossicles; separate neural arch of the fifth lumbar vertebra. In the last mentioned there is a tendency to slipping forward of the fifth lumbar vertebra with its superimposed vertebral column upon the upper surface of the sacrum, a condition known as spondylolisthesis.

We do however see changes with age in cartilage during mature and advanced years and are mainly indebted for information on this subject to the researches of Amprino and Bairati (1933a,b, 1934, 1935). Hyaline cartilage, as exemplified in the trachea and costal cartilages (Amprino and Bairati, 1933a), adds to its substance by the transformation of connective tissue fibrils from the perichondrium, a process which is at its height at about the twentieth year. Costal cartilage reaches maturity earlier than tracheal cartilage and therefore shows regressive features much earlier. Among these features is albuminoid transformation which develops between the tenth and the twenty-fourth year in both types of hyaline cartilage and remains constant thereafter throughout life. Fibrillar changes also are found in the costal cartilages. Calcification is said to take place at different ages and is always present by forty years. In our roentgenoscopic examinations we have found it widespread and far advanced in costal cartilages of medical students and cadavera by the twenty-second year. Our roentgenographic and anatomical observations strongly suggest that if calcification does occur it is just as likely to take place in early adult life as later. Actual bony transformation is said to occur in the tracheal cartilages in about 22 per cent of bodies over forty years of age.

Among the most striking of age changes is the appearance of secondary new formations of cartilage developed from perichondrium in the trachea of bodies over forty years of age and within the fibrillar areas of costal cartilages. Thus cartilage is one of those tissues which maintains till late in life a mechanism for the renewal of youth to which allusion was made in the introduction to this chapter. New formation progresses side by side with regressive changes but it must not be assumed that this power of renewal is at all vigorous (Wetzel, 1932).

Histological details of the fibrillar transformation of hyaline cartilage as seen in the costal cartilages of the rat have been well described by Dawson and Spark (1928). A change in density occurs in the matrix with unmasking of fibrillae particularly in the axial region. Small scattered globules of fat and glycogen appear in the cells whose protoplasm is reticulated and stains lightly. Surrounding this now differentiated axial core is an intermediate zone of which the cells show a dense and homogeneous cytoplasm, with a lightly staining nucleus, a few large fat globules and a peripheral row of granules in vacuoles. The subperichondrial zone exhibits smaller cells without granules or globules. Next there appear clefts in the intermediate zone produced by local resorption of matrix in the region of atypical cells. A definite architectural pattern is developed in the disposition of these areas of resorption and in the fibrillae which cross the clefts. Modifications of the fibrillar systems rapidly follow resulting in a secondary fibrillar pattern which spreads eventually to the subperichondrial zone but not so distinctly into the axial zone. Occasionally, and particularly in older animals, the subperichondrial zone shows resorption of matrix and the cartilage cells freed from their matrix lie along the fibrils like fibroblasts. Vascular invasions, irruptions of active fibroblasts and even scanty ossification occur. All these features are deeply instructive, not only from the point of view of age changes, but also from the analogy they show to the stages in bone formation in those areas of the skeleton where local organizers determine the development of that tissue.

Elastic cartilage was studied by Amprino and Bairati (1933b) in the ear and epiglottis. It undergoes the same changes as hyaline cartilage though not to the same extent. Elastic fibers increase in number throughout life and may even form sheets but as the number increases the elastic quality diminishes.

For examples of fibrous cartilage Amprino and Bairati (1934) chose the intervertebral disc between second and third lumbar vertebrae and also the cartilage of the symphysis pubis: of the two, the cartilage of the symphysis, in mature years, is nearer hyaline cartilage in its structural characters.

By the age of twenty years intervertebral cartilage has reached full maturity of structure. This is attained in the symphysial cartilage at thirty years. Thence to about sixty years is the period of mature life. Regressive changes are thereafter predominant. These changes are penetration by connective tissue and blood vessels, degeneration, calcification, necrosis, lacerations and haemorrhages. Already at about thirty years a fibrous change invades the hitherto hyaline cartilage of intervertebral and symphysial areas beginning at the periphery and reaching the central portion by about sixty years. Changes in the cartilage are closely related to synchronous changes in adjacent bony surfaces. The textural changes on the symphysial face of the pubic bone have already been described (see pp. 290–292) as a typical example. The transformation of hyaline into fibrous cartilage is thus one of the earliest signs of ageing in the body (Uebermuth, 1930). The degree of this change can be approximately estimated by plunging a knife blade into the disc close to the body of the vertebra where the fibrosis first appears and noting the resistance encountered. With the onset of calcification the difficulty of inserting the knife is greatly increased: a second attempt nearer the midvertical point of the disc may be necessary or the procedure may even have to be abandoned. Starting at about ten years in the intervertebral disc and about fifteen years in the symphysis, the number of cells enclosed within a single capsule increases but this change commences in the depths and reaches the periphery at about forty years. Fibrous cartilage undergoes less natural retrogressive change than either hyaline or elastic cartilage but its power of repair is likewise small. Perhaps the greatly altered function of the vertebral column in Man, when contrasted with other mammals, predisposes the intervertebral discs to a regressive modification of the normal ageing process. Being cartilaginous structures however they tend to show degenerative processes at a comparatively early age in lower mammals as well as in Man.

For an adequate description of the life history of that very complex structure, the intervertebral disc, the account by Beadle (1931) should be consulted. I have made no mention of chorda cells of the nucleus pulposus for these have already disappeared before the adult or second period is reached (Uebermuth, 1930). There is some doubt as to whether the cavity which appears both in discs and symphysis during childhood is a genuine joint cavity.

The nucleus pulposus is a glistening, white, translucent cushion of fluid consistency forming the central part of the intervertebral disc, exceedingly firm and elastic and probably under considerable internal pressure from its own turgor. Enclosing the nucleus pulposus and forming the peripheral portion of the disc is the annulus fibrosus studied as an example of fibrous cartilage by Amprino and Bairati (1934). So densely fibrous is the annulus that one may have difficulty in identifying the cellular elements in a section examined with the microscope. The turgor of the nucleus pulposus depends on the fluid content of the tissue which gradually diminishes with age and may be completely lost in tissue degeneration. Püschel (1930) gives the water content at birth as approximately 88 per cent for the nucleus and 78 per cent for the annulus. It diminishes rapidly during the first year and by the age of three years has attained a value of 76 to 78 per cent for the nucleus and 70 per cent for the annulus. Thereafter the annulus remains steady until old age when its water content sinks a little lower. The nucleus however steadily diminishes in its water content which gradually approaches that of the annulus so that, in a woman of seventy seven years, its water content was 67 per cent while the annulus had maintained a value of 69 per cent. Compared with those of age, individual differences in water content are small and probably constitutional in origin. In degenerated discs the water content depends on the type and degree of change. A swollen and moist appearance of the disc on section is the earliest sign of degeneration but such discs do not register any change in water content. The appearance must therefore be due to a modification in the constitution of the tissue. But the dry, crumbling and fissured disc, more advanced in degeneration, shows a water content deviating in less or more degree from the normal.

A special though aberrant age change in cartilage so far recognized only in my own publications and in those of Dawson (e.g. Todd and Lyon, 1924; Todd and D'Errico, 1928; Todd, 1933a,b; Todd, Wharton and Todd, 1938; Todd, Todd, and Todd (unpublished as yet); Dawson, 1929) is that characteristic of cartilage which has remained at a site in the skeleton beyond the age when it usually disappears through transformation into or replacement by bone. This cartilage I have described as in a "lapsed" state for the reason that I first noted its occurrence in diaphyso-epiphysial planes where union should have already been perfected between shaft and epiphysis. It also occurs however in sutures of the skull and in all persistent symphyses like that of the pubis. The hyaline cartilage of the plane becomes increasingly fibrous and sometimes cystic in places. A thin lamella of bone forms over both faces of the cartilage capping the adjacent bone ends with a wax-like texture and shutting off the cartilage from the cancellous tissue. Dawson has described the histological features very well (Dawson, 1929). The condition is caused by any nutritional or other deficiency which retards the rate of skeletal maturation. It is observable in rachitic bones of young rats maintained for more than three weeks on a rachitogenic diet (Venar and Todd, 1934) where it is still a partially reversible phenomenon. It is evident also in the more profound deficiency caused by experimental endocrine disturbance (Todd, Wharton and Todd, 1938) where the phenomenon is irreversible. Eventually osseous bridges may erratically unite the periphery of the adjacent bones but never the deeper parts as in regular epiphysial union.

In a sense this is cartilage undergoing regular age changes in an irregular manner. It corresponds to the erratic bone formation in the horns which develop on the skull of the ageing Giraffe described in an earlier section of this chapter. It is not frankly pathological but is a borderline phenomenon and is of course characteristically seen in the long and often permanently patent sutures of the human skull. In the equally permanent human symphysis pubis its characteristic of a structural pattern changing as age increases has already been fully described.

Before leaving this subject some mention should be made of the vascular channels and their rôle in cartilage. Hurrell (1934) has summarized the literature and added thereto his own investigations and critical analysis. In Man the channels make their appearance in the third fetal month and it is only at a later stage that they are occupied by blood vessels. They are therefore primarily nutritive in character although when ossification of cartilage sets in, it is along the blood vessels in the course of these channels that the bony tissue is laid down. Linberg (1925) has made a study of the life history of these channels which reach their full development in the rib cartilages by thirty years. They are present according to this author up to about sixty years when atrophy of the marrow elements is accompanied by the formation of smooth-walled spaces and then by the disorganization of the vascular channels. Henschen (1925) has confirmed Linberg's work by his roentgenograms of rib cartilages. The blood vessels apparently remain present in advanced age unless the cartilage becomes ossified. It is claimed that vascular channels are developed in permanent cartilages in order to permit the persistence unaltered of masses of any size inasmuch as the vascular channels appear to form in response to the demand of the deeper cells for nutrition.

In summary it is obvious that cartilage though pre-eminently a tissue of the growth period, showing great power of activity in the early years, nevertheless persists as a tissue of adult and of old age and in consequence illustrates very clearly the types of transformation which characterize successive phases in the life span.

The hyaline cartilage of the bones (including the cartilages of the sternum, the costal cartilages, epiphysial cartilage, cartilage of the diaphyso-epiphysial plane and articular cartilage) and the hyaline cartilage of the respiratory passages (including nose, trachea, bronchi and most of those of the larynx), so closely related in their histological appearance, add to their substance by the transformation of fibers from their investiture of connective tissue. Where this transformation does not mean the development of bone, as in costal cartilages and trachea it reaches its height at about the twentieth year precisely like its counterpart in the subperiosteal bony growth. Indeed both fibrillar changes and calcification are common in costal cartilages though less so in the larynx early in the third decade and actual bony transformation can be seen in both skeletal and respiratory hyaline cartilages long before the age of forty years though perhaps more commonly after that age.

If cartilage is to remain relatively immune to these age changes, as in the ear, the auditory tube, epiglottis, corniculate and cuneiform cartilages, the apical and vocal processes of the arytenoid cartilages, it takes the form of elastic cartilage which becomes more fibrous with age changing in the structure and elasticity of its special tissue but showing no tendency to calcify or ossify with increasing age.

On the other side stands fibrocartilage comprising every intra-articular disc and meniscus, the labra of the articular rims, the intervertebral discs and the symphysis pubis. Here fibrous modification has occurred early but maturity of structure is attained as in hyaline cartilage at about the twentieth year. Fibrous transformation of a more vigorous type now begins to appear and intensifies its activity as the years pass with this exception that invasion of the symphysis is delayed for another decade. Doubtless this peculiarity is associated with the special sexual character of the symphysis (Todd and Todd, 1938). It is at the symphysis indeed that one can study most readily the correlated and synchronous age changes taking place in the chief types of skeletal tissue, namely, cartilage and bone.

The precise meaning and wider significance of age changes in hydration shown in the nucleus pulposus of the intervertebral discs, a process the progress of which is quantitatively measurable, are nevertheless still obscure.

The curious phenomenon of cartilage which has been retained in the skeleton beyond the date of its regular disappearance is seen in human cranial sutures and symphysis pubis. This "lapsed" form of cartilage presents precisely the pattern of transformation which one would expect, namely, increasing fibrous change with ultimate regressive modifications.

7. JOINTS AND BURSAE

The changes in joints during advanced age are for the most part a recapitulation of the phenomena already presented in preceding parts of this paper under the headings of articular cartilage, bony articular margins and bone texture. Infirmities in joint formation, which occur early in development, leave their mark, like those in cartilage, throughout life. Of these the most obvious examples are fusions of carpals, tarsals, vertebrae and of the sacroiliac joints. All are errors of differentiation and, as such, are not within our scope. Fusions of vertebral joints from spondylitis and of sacro-iliac joints from a like transformation of the ligaments do occur with increasing frequency after middle life but these are expressions of frank pathology and are in no way examples of the ageing process. Changes in articular cartilages with loss of water and atrophy of joint margins (Wetzel, 1932) are however so constant in advancing age as to fall within the true ageing category.

Keefer, Parker, Myers, and Irwin (1934a) have shown that changes occur in increasing frequency with advancing age at the knee joint. These changes are identical in both sexes. They are commonest in areas subjected to movement, strain, weight bearing and injury. They bear no relation to symptoms, to arteriosclerosis or to other particular disease processes. In the one hundred knee joints studied by these four authors age changes occurred in the patella in 81 per cent, trochlear surface 65 per cent, lateral condyle of tibia 64 per cent, medial condyle of tibia 55 per cent, medial condyle of femur 43 per cent and lateral condyle of femur 36 per cent. The same authors state (Parker, etc., 1934b) that the synovial membrane was essentially normal except in joints which showed changes in the cartilage. In these the capsule was thickened: there were papillary projections of synovial membrane and occasionally small collections of lymphocytes around the blood vessels. Changes in the cartilage comprised fibrillation, degeneration, destruction and in some areas regeneration such as Amprino and Bairati (1934) have described. Subarticular bone was thickened. Marrow spaces were frequently filled with fibrous tissue. Cysts and areas of cartilage were present in the bony tissue. There were also exostoses and projections of cartilage over the margin of the joint surface and depressions of cartilage below the original level which was caused by flattening or erosion of the joint surface and which gave the appearance of bony outgrowth. All these changes, which are identical with those of degenerative or hypertrophic arthritis, were found to occur in increasing frequency with advancing age. The initial features of rim formation and lipping, to which reference has already been made above are to be found in the article by Graves (1922).

Age changes in the joints of the vertebral column, not including spondylitis which is a pathological process, have been noted and are described in greater detail by Willis (1924).

One may not leave the subject of joints without mentioning in passing the clearly pathological though often quite localized changes which have been studied assiduously by Meyer (1922, 1924, 1931). These range from local superficial furring through fissuring and erosion of cartilage to erosion and polishing of bone. That there is an age factor in their progress there is no doubt but as this plays a minor rôle in their history they are not within our immediate scope. Meyer (1924) mentions one reference in the literature to their occurrence in the horse but they are found in anthropoids and in lower mammals in the large collection of comparative mammalian anatomy of the Hamann Museum.

For age changes in bursae we have the single article by Graves (1922) which describes changes in the subacromial bursa so far as these involve the acromion itself.

From the age of thirty years onward a plaque may be found on the under surface of the acromion varying in form, size and thickness. It is situated within an area bounded by the outer margin of acromion and a mesially curved line beginning at the metacromion and ending just lateral to the clavicular facet. It may prolong the acromion tip 8 mm. or more and, when it is large, usually extends beyond the outer deltoid margin. Its long axis ranges from 5 to 35 mm. and its transverse axis 4 to 25 mm. When prolonged beyond the acromial tip it lies parallel to the general direction of the coracoacromial ligament. Its surface is relatively smooth and often concave. When it extends as a plaque its dorsal surface is convex and its tip often serrated or digitated so that its margin is palpable through the skin and deltoid origin. It is obviously formed by ossification of the bursal wall. Graves gives good figures of its appearance at thirty-five and fifty years but one must not assume that these are in any way typical of scapulae at these ages. It is not a constant feature of the ageing scapula. When it is present, however, it is invariably associated with other evidences of advancing years. It is never found in young or relatively young bones and has been noted by Graves in every considerable collection of scapulae of whatever human stock and also in the giant anthropoids, provided they are old animals. This plaque may, however, be absent or rudimentary even in senile bones.

No other comparable structure related to bursae in the human body has ever been seen in the catacombs of the Hamann Museum. The plaque is therefore to be regarded as a formation of pathological origin which, when it is present, shows progressive features with advancing age.

In general bursae, like synovial membranes and connective tissue, show no age changes in the absence of factors of pathological origin.

In summary age changes in joints are confined to those characteristic of the hyaline articular cartilage and the fibro-cartilaginous labrum of the articular margin. In particular it should be noted that as age progresses there develops under the marginal labrum a rim of bone which has been described earlier in this section and illustrated in figure 55 on the articular face of the symphysis pubis. In old age the same dehydration and atrophy of articular cartilage with fibrillation, degeneration and destruction is to be seen as in other cartilaginous areas. Synovial membrane, like connective tissue, undergoes no age changes.

Bursae, like synovial membrane, show no age changes but bone underlying a bursa develops, as the years pass, a plaque which is the counterpart of the rim formed beneath the articular labrum.

8. TENDONS AND LIGAMENTS

Attached to the skeleton are tendons and ligaments which show no age changes. Nor do origins and insertions of muscles betray any evidence of age changes (Wetzel, 1932) except that, with increase in years these muscular attachments become interspersed with bony tissue so that the sites are more plainly marked by ridges or even numerous small osteophytic outgrowths which have been interpreted as indicating muscular strength or even the male sex. They probably result from the stress and strain of use, a form of injury and repair cumulative during life. But the fact that they increase in obtrusive-. ness as age advances, long after muscular strength and staying power have passed their zenith, is sufficient evidence of the erroneous character of this interpretation. Muscular ridges on bone are accompaniments in both sexes of advancing years not of muscular power.

Meyer (1924, 1928) and Batson (1928) have drawn attention to fraying, fasciculation and shedding of tendons, a process which they attribute to attrition. That tendon is readily repaired after the clean cut injury of tenotomy, even though a considerable segment has been removed, has been shown by Stewart (1936). In experimental animals there is a marked improvement in gait four weeks after operation and the movement of the affected limb becomes much freer. Evidently after this lapse of time sufficient regeneration has occurred to permit resumption of muscular function. It is during the third week after operation that the tissue filling the gap begins to resemble tendon in its histological structure. Not until the lapse of four months however does the regenerated tissue closely approximate normal tendon in its structure.

Accidental injuries to tendons and ligaments however are not as a rule so simple. In sprains there is a tearing accompanied by local hemorrhage. A soft tissue roentgenogram made immediately after the injury shows a local density and swelling both of the tendon or ligament involved and the adjacent connective tissue. This is particularly well demonstrated in sprains of the wrist. The clear differentiation of lateral ligament of the wrist and the adjacent tendons of abductor (extensor ossis metacarpi) pollicis and extensor brevis pollicis, which are so plainly evident in the uninjured wrist, is completely lost. A roentgenogram made after the subsidence of swelling demonstrates fraying of the ligament. This can be identified equally well a year or more later. It is evidence of the imperfection of repair and is accompanied by a definite disability in weakness and limitation of movement. Doubtless dissection, were that possible, would show precisely the fraying and fasciculation which Meyer and Batson have described. Inasmuch as sprains occur at all ages the changes consequent on injuries of tendons or ligaments cannot be attributed solely to age.

In certain unpublished studies on Vitamin C deprivation in guinea pigs Dr. Milton B. Cohen and I have found such weakening of ligaments that it is difficult to skin the animal without tearing the ligaments of joints particularly those of the knee and cervical vertebral column. The head of the animal indeed is very apt to be torn from the vertebral column by that ordinary force necessary to draw the skin over the cranium. Nutritional deficiency is probably responsible, in addition to local injury, for the production of structural defect in tendons and ligaments.

Ossification of the anterior common ligament of the vertebral column seen in the hypertrophic bone change known as spondylitis presents no features which could reasonably be interpreted as age changes.

It is accumulation of injuries with increase in years, followed by imperfect repair which results in the number of these lesions found in the bodies of the aged.

In summary then tendons and ligaments, like synovial membrane and connective tissue, show no clearly defined age changes. That changes of a destructive or degenerative type occur and are more frequent as age advances there is no question. These are the result however of imperfect repair after injury or consequences of constitutional defect perhaps of nutritional origin rather than of age itself.

9. MUSCLE

Although in this chapter we are concerned only with the skeletal muscles or "red flesh" of the body there are certain of these, the levator of the upper eyelid for example, which contain smooth muscle fibers in addition to the bundles of striated fibers which make up almost the total bulk of the muscle. We are not concerned with the Purkinje system or the true cardiac fibers of the heart or the specialized fibers of the tongue.

Smooth muscle need not detain us for Häggqvist (1931) reports that he can find no observations on age changes in this tissue. He himself investigated without positive result the musculature of the human caecum from autopsies of persons ranging in age from eight to seventy-four years. This negative result is to be expected since smooth muscle according to Wetzel (1932), despite the absence of mitosis and of amitosis, can regenerate itself. I have been unable to find in Wetzel's writings any details in substantiation of this claim but it is certain that smooth muscle, like cartilage and to a greater degree than that tissue, preserves its youthful character even in advanced age.

Perfectly coördinated functional activity of striated muscle is evident in the new born marsupial embryo which, by the directed activity of its own forelimbs and hands, climbs into the maternal pouch. The process has been actually observed in the Kangaroo (Goerling, see

Hartman 1920), the young of which are born after forty days of gestation (Jennison, 1927a,b) and in the opossum after twelve and a half days of gestation (Hartman 1920, McCrady 1938). For observations on the activity of fetal musculature we are indebted mainly to the writings of Coghill; Angulo y Gonzales, Hooker on the rat; Windle and Carmichael on the cat; Barcroft, Barron and Windle on the sheep and Hooker on Man.

The fibers of striated muscle reflect in their thickness and contour on cross section the functional activity of the muscle. In the newborn infant therefore the bundles of greatest development are those of the eye and of respiration while the arm muscle bundles are larger than those of the leg. In the newborn also the connective tissue of the muscle is of fine structure or only moderately developed and elastic fibers are absent (Kohashi, 1937c). The greater the intramuscular and intermuscular connective tissue the richer is the capillary network. Schiefferdecker (1911) therefore concluded that the amount of connective tissue gives a rough guide to the nutritive supply of the muscle which is of great significance in its early development. This conclusion was confirmed by Kohashi (1937a). Each muscle, as Schiefferdecker (1927) insists, has its own specific structural pattern, its own specific function and its own specific development. The nucleus is the controlling center for the fiber which originates through nuclear activity. In disease the nuclear substance shows changes first in bulk and then in arrangement. In atrophy there are changes in dimension. In the adult the number of nuclei is small compared with the number of fibers, much smaller than in childhood. There is therefore a reduction in amount of nuclear substance compared with fiber substance throughout the period of childhood. Exercise also has a profound effect so that, to avoid false deductions, one must know in general the functional activity of a muscle in order to interpret one's observations on its nuclear and fiber pattern.

In the adult, muscular bundles are polyhedral in cross section whereas at birth they are rounded (Kohashi, 1937c). The thickest muscle bundles in adult life are found in the gastrocnemius and longissimus dorsi and the thinnest bundles in the eye muscles and psoas major. Muscles which are in continual action like the diaphragm possess thin bundles and much intramuscular connective tissue. Flexors of both arm and leg have thicker muscular bundles than extensors. In general the thicker the bundle and the richer its connective tissue the greater the strength but it should be noted that a multipennate muscle like the deltoid, the strength of which lies in its short and multiple fibers, has rather thin bundles. A detailed description of the characteristic size of bundles in the skeletal muscles is given by Kohashi (1937a) while those of the face have been studied by Kato (1937) whose findings fall into line with those of his fellow worker Kohashi.

A very elaborate study of the age changes in striated muscle was recently made by Buccianti and Luria (1934) who describe, in addition to modification in size of fiber, a change in direction of myofibrils. These are originally parallel in their disposition. Then successively there appear oblique, spiral and even annular dispositions of myofibrils followed later by complete regression. No change occurs however in the reticular sheath of the fiber.

Buccianti and Luria (1934) also describe as age changes an increase in collagenous fibers and in pigmentation as well as an increase of elastic fibers about the bundles of myofibrils.

Elastic fibers are shown by Kohashi (1937b) to be most abundant in the diaphragm, the muscles of the abdominal wall and particularly in the longissimus dorsi, but the greatest development of elastic fibers is to be found in the muscles of the eyeball where the bundles are not only numerous but form an anastomotic network around the muscular bundles. The masseter also shows this typical anastomotic network of elastic fibers (Kohashi, 1937b).

A previous study of muscle bundle thickness in Man in comparison with the recorded measurements on various vertebrates was made by Halban (1894) who points out that the muscle bundles in adult women are on the average about three quarters of the cross section area typical of corresponding bundles in men. The effect of health and exercise is strikingly shown in thickness of bundle in the strong and active compared with that in the weak and ill. Papanicolaou and Falk (1938) have reported that general muscular hypertrophy can be induced experimentally by injections of testeosterone propionate into the castrated male or spayed female guinea pig. Progesterone or estrogen will not produce this effect though a gonadotropic hormone (follutein) will, provided the animal is not spayed. Hence the activating substance is the androgenic hormone of the interstitial tissue of testicle or ovary. Our own, as yet, unpublished studies on athletes and non-athletes in the high schools of Cleveland do show a greater density of muscular shadows on the roentgenogram of the hand in the athletes where the actual difference in thickness of muscle is insufficient to account for the increased density. Our roentgenographic studies of the contracted biceps show that whereas the industrial worker possesses a biceps both larger and of denser shadow than the white-collar worker there is increasing bulk of muscle and greater density of shadow progressively in both sexes at least to the age of approximately fifty years. The muscle in persons over sixty years is reduced in bulk and in density of shadow.

Inasmuch as striped muscle has the power of regeneration through amitosis one would not expect to find obvious structural changes as age advances though fatty infiltration and brown atrophy do occur. There is no atrophy in the muscular attachments of the old (Wetzel, 1932).

Age changes in striped muscle are to be sought by measures of function rather than of structure. Ufland (1933) has gathered together the information on the subject and has added thereto many observations of his own. According to his investigations on flexors and extensors of forearm, on hand muscles, on the muscles of the back and of respiration, all groups reach their maximum strength between twenty and twenty-nine years, usually nearer the higher than the lower limit of this age period. With the thirtieth year all begin to decline but each group has its own particular course of diminishing power.

In flexion of forearm and in hand grip the maximum power attained is 20 per cent above that at sixteen to nineteen years. Flexion of the thumb rises only 10 per cent; flexion of wrist 4 per cent, extension of wrist 6 per cent and extensors of the back only 2 per cent.

Between thirty and thirty-nine years, muscles of the back, of respiration and flexors of the wrist sink back to their value at twenty years. This occurs in biceps and extensors of wrist between forty and forty-nine years and in hand grip and thumb flexion between fifty and fifty-nine years.

After the age of sixty years the dwindling of muscular power is greatest in biceps and in muscles of the back. The average biceps strength of a man at sixty-five years is 54.1 per cent, the back muscle strength 64.3 per cent of the average strength of a man at twenty-five years. The average biceps strength of a woman at twenty-five is 46.8 per cent, the back muscle strength 54.2 per cent of the strength of a man at twenty-five years. Hence the strength of a man of twenty-five years bears the same relation to the strength of a man of sixty-five as it does to that of a woman of twenty-five years in the same occupation.

The power of sustained effort appears to dwindle during later mature life in approximately the same manner as maximum power.

Schochrin (1935), in a later communication, emphasizes his finding that the relationship between muscular power as shown in movements of forearm and of hand diminishes in relatively equal degree in both sexes until the sixth decade.

Kubo (1938) has recently investigated strength, speed of action and dexterity in Japanese men and women of ages ranging from 70 to 100 years. He found achievements high even at 72 or 73 years. There was surprisingly little decline with age, most in strength, less in dexterity and least in speed. The decline was not regular with increasing age and people of 90 years often showed ratings close to the highest. If the postulate be accepted that age implies health and experience, not infirmity, these results would be expected.

The cause of diminution in power and in sustained effort was sought with no very conclusive results by Mori (1936) in biochemical changes. Andrus (1936) attempted to find a change in the blood vessels of muscle but, though he records fibrosis of the media with increasing frequency in the pectoralis major from the thirtieth year onwards, many persons of advanced age exhibit only minimal degrees of fibrosis. No intimal disease of small arteries or arterioles is recorded by Andrus at any age.

In contrast with these inconclusive findings the observations by Ellis (1919, 1920) on the age changes in the cerebellum are very suggestive. Ellis points out that the Purkinje cells tend to disintegrate and disappear starting at about forty years. While the cells of the dentate nucleus suffer less than the Purkinje cells in advancing age they are more apt to show the presence of pigmentation: the failure to eliminate this pigmentation may be interpreted as an indication of defective function. There is often also a loss or shrinkage of myelinated fibers in the ageing cerebellum of which the right hemisphere tends to shrink first (compare age change in right lateral venous sinus, see p. 295). From these facts it seems apparent that we may find the cause of dwindling muscular strength and skill in the governing mechanism rather than in the structure of the muscles themselves.

That the composition of skeletal muscle changes during life is apparent from the studies on the ox made by Moulton, Trowbridge and Haigh (1922). The water content of the tissue gives a value of 87.5 per cent midway through fetal life, 80.0 per cent at birth and 77.0 per cent at five and a half months. Thenceforward it is constant. Nitrogen content is 1.4 per cent at miduterine life, 2.9 per cent at birth and 3.5 per cent at eleven months of age. Ash in the fat-free muscle is 1.05 per cent at birth, 1.11 per cent at six months and thereafter decreases gradually till it reaches 1.06 per cent at four years. The reason for the maximum at six months is not apparent from these studies.

Similar studies have been made of the iliopsoas muscle in two groups of human tissues by Simms and Stolman (1937). The tissues were obtained from autopsies of persons dying from accident, the younger group of eleven having an *average* age of thirty-five years, the older group of six having an *average* age of seventy-five years. In the senescent group there was an increase in water, chloride, total base, sodium and calcium and a decrease in potassium, magnesium, phosphorus, nitrogen and ash. The chemical changes in muscle in old age therefore suggest a decrease of intracellular fluids containing potassium and protein and an increase in intercellular fluids which contain sodium and chloride. It is interesting to note that, with the exception of the calcium decrease, the changes found in young tissue of pathological origin were similar to those noted in the senescent group but of less degree.

In summary we learn that age changes have not been recorded in smooth muscle but that the progressive changes with age are well known in striated muscle which reflects its functional activity in the thickness and cross section contour of its fibers. In the newborn infant the bundles of greatest development are those of the eye and of respiration while arm muscle bundles are larger than those of the leg. The proportions of course change during childhood so that in the adult the thickest bundles are those of gastrocnemius and longissimus dorsi and the thinest are those of eye muscles and psoas major.

In the newborn connective tissue is but moderately developed in muscle and elastic fibers absent. Both types of fiber however increase in number with age. During age also there are changes in the disposition of the myofibrils. In old age fatty infiltration and brown atrophy occur.

Muscles tend to increase in bulk and in roentgenographic density up to the age of about fifty years but maximal strength and staying power occur at about the thirtieth year. From the observations recorded by Ellis on the cerebellum it seems that the cause of dwindling muscular strength may be found in the governing mechanism rather than in the structure of the muscles themselves.

Chemical age changes in muscle suggest a decrease in intracellular fluid and an increase in intercellular fluid.

10. TEETH

The literature on teeth contains little of significance on changes characterizing age. This may be due, as Hellman (1937) suggests, to interference which necessarily follows the filling of teeth and the manipulations involved in orthodontic management. If there is significance in this suggestion age changes must be sought in long series of the teeth of primitive or ancient peoples in whom no mechanical interference has been carried out. Series of this type are not yet available for study but the increasing care with which skeletal remains are preserved in archeological investigation may provide the necessary material. The long series of gorilla and chimpanzee skulls housed in the Hamann Museum likewise provides opportunity for investigation of age changes in the teeth of anthropoids. Roentgenograms are of value in the study of teeth but their value lies in the information they shed on the effect of external wear on the structure (Hellman, 1937).

That the chemical composition of teeth in their growing period differs from that after growth is completed is indicated by the observations made by Chiewitz and Hevesy (1935) on the proportion of phosphorus in teeth to that of the skeleton. These observations illustrate the relation between active metabolism and phosphorus content. Rat incisors, which possess permanent pulps and are therefore constantly growing, contain a relatively large amount of phosphorus, the ratio to the average content of the skeleton being 10:1 in adult rats and 6:1 in half grown animals. Molar teeth, on the contrary, which have no permanent pulps and do not show continuous growth, are less rich in phosphorus per gram than the skeleton, the ratio in an extreme case being 1:2. It is to be hoped that this line of exploration will prove fertile enough to permit similar studies more extensive in nature.

There is no reduction in tooth vitality with increasing age except that secondary to arteriosclerosis (Orban, 1937). The enamel is permeable especially in the surface layers since dyes composed of small particles such as methyl blue can diffuse across the dentine into the enamel along the prism sheaths. The fluid path is not a free one and the permeability is reduced as age increases (Fish, 1931). The experiments upon which this fact is established were conducted on the teeth of dogs, the enamel of which is much more permeable than that of Man. The color of teeth grows more yellow with age though much less than commonly supposed (Webster, 1918). This is due to thickening of secondary dentine. Cementum also grows thicker (Orban, 1937). So far as calcium content is concerned the dentine of the crown is richer than that of the root and the dentine zone next the pulp has least calcium content. In the ageing of teeth the calcium content of all parts is increased but those parts which originally possessed less calcium approximate in value to that of the crown (Gerlach, 1930). With the changing calcium content there goes also a rebuilding of the fibrillar texture (Brodersen, 1930).

As the enamel wears the tooth is extruded further from the alveolar process and with the retraction of gum characteristic of advancing age more of the tooth is laid bare (Orban, 1937). Therefore loss of teeth both in men and women is closely related to advancing age (Lux, Lux and Stade, 1933), the canines tending to remain in place longest (Nagamine, 1932). Dental caries on the other hand is most frequent in the middle and late years of adolescence (Moore, 1936).

In summary the age changes in teeth, if we except those implicit in the relation between active metabolism and phosphorus content, confine themselves to diminution of permeability of enamel, to the changes in color consequent on the thickening of secondary dentine, to increase in calcium content and to rebuilding of the fibrillar texture.

11. SUMMARY

The tissues of the soma, if blood and the body fluids be excepted, conprise the skeleton, the locomotor system and the teeth. Age changes in these tissues are chiefly those of dehydration with reduction of intracellular fluid and increase in intercellular fluid and in addition a certain faltering in the orderliness of tissue pattern. These changes also indicate the course of transformation from the orderly and reversible phenomena of health into the disorderly and irreversible which are the stigmata of disease.

For actual growth in the body after adult age has been reached insofar as that growth implies growth in the skeleton itself no reliable evidence has been adduced.

Age changes in the pattern of bony deposition in the skeleton are evident in texture and in disposition of osseous material. These changes are very clearly illustrated in specific skeletal features which characterize certain mammals but they are evident also in the symphysial face of the human pubic bone, a site where changes in texture and substance are continued until old age.

As the impetus of growth declines in the skeleton the orderliness of control of progressive age change diminishes. Consequently in sites like the sutures of the skull where union occurs relatively late compared with the age of epiphysial union, fusion is usually imperfect and a characteristic texture develops on adjacent bony surfaces testifying to the absolute cessation of the impetus to change. Accompanying this development are changes in texture and on inner surface of cranium which, though not reliable as indicators of a particular time relationship, are useful as determiners of a stage in the life cycle.

Halisteresis of cranial and facial bones sets in after fifty years as it does in the rest of the skeleton but this is indistinguishable from the osteoporosis consequent upon constitutional defect and may indeed be a sign of supervening infirmity.

Age changes in the appendicular and axial skeleton resolve themselves into modifications of vascularity, of surface texture and of cancellous structure. They can be studied in flat bones like the scapula by transmitted light and in all bones by roentgenographic examination. The rapid change undergone by bone in the regular daily metabolism is illustrated by the observation that 30 per cent of the phosphorus deposited in the skeleton of an adult rat is lost by the end of twenty days. It is not surprising therefore that expert roentgenographic appraisal can detect changes in mineral shadow within six to eight weeks. The halisteresis which supervenes in advanced age is a measure of the failure of mineral replacement.

Cartilage is pre-eminently a tissue of the growth period but nevertheless persists as a tissue of adult and advanced age and illustrates very clearly the types of transformation which characterize successive phases in the life span. Just as the bony face of the symphysis pubis illustrates successive stages in bony pattern so also the superjacent symphysial cartilage gives clear cut evidence of the increase of fibrillar and then of regressive change associated with modifications in hydration. Costal and intervertebral cartilages amplify and extend the possibility of observations on age changes characteristic of hyaline and fibrocartilage. Elastic cartilage however shows but scant age changes and these in low degree.

In joints the age changes are confined to those of the hyaline articular cartilage and the fibrocartilaginous labrum of the articular margin.

Synovial membrane like bursae shows no age changes.

The bone under the labrum like that under a bursa develops in the course of time a characteristic pattern and texture.

Tendons and ligaments, like synovial membrane and connective tissue, show no clearly defined age changes but do present, as age advances, the cumulative effects of imperfect repair and constitutional defect.

Smooth muscle is another tissue for which no age changes have been recorded.

Striped muscle reflects its functional activity in the thickness and sectional contour of its fibers. As age increases both its connective tissue and elastic fibers multiply.

The bulk and roentgenographic density of skeletal muscle increase in both sexes to about the fiftieth year though muscular strength and staying power reach their maximum at about the thirtieth year. Observations on the cerebellum suggest that the cause of waning muscular strength may be inherent in the governing mechanism rather than in muscular structure itself.

Chemical changes in muscle with age indicate a decrease of intracellular fluid and increase of intercellular fluid.

Age changes in teeth, apart from those implicit in the relation between active metabolism and phosphorus content, confine themselves to diminution of permeability of enamel, to the changes in color consequent on thickening of secondary dentine, to increase in calcium content and to rebuilding of the fibrillar texture.

All else is infirmity. The criteria of healthy ageing are of necessity different from those of youth for our elasticity and resilience are lessened by the honorable scars of resistance and repair.

REFERENCES

AMPRINO, R., AND BAIRATI, A. 1933a. Studi sulle trasformazioni delle cartilagini dell'uomo nell' accrescimento e nella senescenza. I. Cartilagini jaline. Ztschr. f. Zellforsch. u. mikr. Anat., 20, 143–205.

——— 1933 b. II. Cartilagini elastiche. Ibid., 20, 489–522.

——— 1934. III. Cartilagini fibrosi. Ibid., 21, 448–482.

——— 1935. Nachtrag zu der Arbeit "Studi sulle trasformazioni delle cartilagini dell'uomo nell' accrescimento e nella senescenza." Ibid., 22, 484.

ANDRUS, F. C. 1936. The relation of age and hypertension to the structure of the small arteries and arterioles in skeletal muscle. Am. J. Path., 12, 635–652.

ANSEROFF, N. I. 1934. Architektonik der langen Knochen in Verbindung mit Alter und Konstitution. Ztschr. f. Konstitutionslehre, 18, 40–51.

AREY, L. B. 1919. On the presence of Haversian systems in membrane bone. Anat. Rec., 17, 59–61.

BATSON, O. V. 1928. The functional attrition of tendons. Anat. Rec., (Abstr.), 38, 3–4.

BAUER, W., AUB, J. C., AND ALBRIGHT, F. 1929. Studies of calcium and phosphorus metabolism. V. A study of the bone trabeculae as a readily available reserve supply of calcium. J. Exper. Med., 49, 145–161.

BEADLE, O. A. 1931. The intervertebral discs. H. M. Stationery Off.: London, 79 pp.

BENSLEY, S. H. 1934. On the presence, properties and distribution of the intercellular ground substance of loose connective tissue. Anat. Rec., **60**, 93–109.

BOLK, L. 1915. On the premature obliteration of sutures in the human skull. Am. J. Anat., **17**, 495–523.

———— 1919. Über prämature Obliteration der Nähte am Menschenschädel. Ztschr. f. Morphol. u. Anthropol., **21**, 1–22.

BRODERSEN, M. 1930. Altersveränderungen am Zahnbein. I. Die Umschichtung der Zahnbeinlamellen und Umbauten am Tuberculum dentale. Morphol. Jahrb., **65**, 465–480.

BUCCIANTI, L., AND LURIA, S. 1934. Struttura dei muscoli voluntari dell'uomo nella senescenza. Arch. ital. di anat. e di embryol., **33**, 110–187.

BURNS, C. M., AND HENDERSON, H. 1936. Influence of age on mineral constituents of bones from kittens and pups. Biochem. J., **30**, 1207–1214.

CARREL, A. 1935. Man the unknown. Harper: New York, 346 pp.

CARREL, A., AND EBELING, A. H. 1921. Age and multiplication of fibroblasts. J. Exper. Med., **34**, 599–623.

CHIEWITZ, O., AND HEVESY, G. 1935. Radioactive indicators in the study of phosphorus metabolism in rats. Nature, London, **136**, 754–755.

DAWSON, A. B. 1929. A histological study of the persisting cartilage plates in retarded or lapsed union in the albino rat. Anat. Rec., **43**, 109–123.

DAWSON, A. B., AND SPARK, C. 1928. The fibrous transformation and architecture of the costal cartilage of the albino rat. Am. J. Anat., **42**, 109–137.

ELLIS, R. S. 1919. A preliminary quantitative study of the Purkinje cells in normal, subnormal, and senescent human cerebella, with some notes on functional localization. J. Comp. Neurol., **30**, 229–252.

———— 1920. Norms for some structural changes in the human cerebellum from birth to old age. J. Comp. Neurol., **32**, 1–33.

ELY, L. 1922. Chronic arthritis. M. Rec., **101**, 223–227.

FISH, E. W. 1931. Age changes in the permeability of dog's enamel. J. Physiol., **72**, 321–326.

FORD, E. B., AND HUXLEY, J. S. 1929. Genetic rate-factors in Gammarus. Arch. f. Entwcklngsmechn. d. Organ., **117**, 67–79.

FRISCHMANN, F. 1932. Das Verhalten des Bindegewebsgerüstes der Leber des Menschen beim Wachstum und Altern. Ztschr. mikr.-anat. Forsch., **31**, 635–648.

GERLACH, H. 1930. Altersveränderungen am Zahnbein. II. Die Kalziumverteilung im Zahnbein und ihre Verschiebung mit zunehmendem Alter. Morphol. Jahrb., **65**, 481–496.

GOLDSCHMIDT, R. 1927. Physiologische Theorie der Vererbung. Springer: Berlin, 247 pp.

GRAVES, W. W. 1922. Observations on age changes in the scapula. Am. J. Phys. Anthropol., **5**, 21–23.

———— 1925 a. The relations of shoulder blade types to problems of mental and physical adaptability. Oliver and Boyd: Edinburgh, 35 pp.

———— 1925 b. The plus-potentially sick of the race. Glasgow M. J., **104**, 315–322.

———— 1936. Personal communication.

HÄGGQVIST, G. 1931. Die Gewebe. Springer: Berlin, 247 pp. (In v. Möllendorff, W., Handb. d. mikr. Anat. d. Mensch., 2, 3.)

HALBAN, J. 1894. Die Dicke der quergestreiften Muskel-Fasern und ihre Bedeutung. Anat. Hft., 3, 269–307.

HARRIS, H. A. 1933. Bone growth in health and disease. Oxford Univ. Pr.: London, 248 pp. Supp. 186–188.

HARTMAN, C. G. 1920. Studies in the development of the opossum Didelphys virginiana L. V. The phenomena of parturition. Anat. Rec., 19, 251–261.

HELLMAN, M. 1937. Personal communication.

HENSCHEN, C. 1925. Die Gefässanatomie der Rippenknorpel. Schweiz. med. Wchnschr. 6, 491–492.

HRDLIČKA, A. 1925. The Old Americans. Williams & Wilkins: Baltimore, 438 pp.

—— 1935. The Pueblos, with comparative data on the bulk of the tribes of the Southwest and Northern Mexico. Am. J. Phys. Anthropol., 20, 235–460.

—— 1936. Growth during adult life. Proc. Am. Philos. Soc., 76, 847–897.

HUMPHRY, G. M. 1858. The human skeleton. Macmillan: Cambridge, 620 pp.

HURRELL, D. J. 1934. The vascularization of cartilage. J. Anat., 69, 47–61.

JARCHO, A. 1935. Die Altersveränderungen der Rassenmerkmale bei den Erwachsenen. Anthrop. Anz., 12, 173–179.

JENNISON, G. 1927 a. Natural History: Animals. A. & C. Black: London, 344 pp. (see p. 323).

—— 1927 b. Table of gestation periods and number of young: Appendix to Natural History: Animals, A. &. C. Black: London, 8 pp. (see p. 8).

JONES, F. W. 1912. On the grooves upon the ossa parietalia commonly said to be caused by the arteria meningea media. J. Anat., 46, 228–238.

KATO, T. 1937. Über die Struktur der Gesichtsmuskeln bei dem Neugeborenen und dem Erwachsenen. Fol. anat. japon., 15, 297–307.

KUBO, Y. 1938. Mental and physical changes in old age. J. Genchè Psychol., 53, 101–108.

KEEFER, C. S., PARKER, F. Myers, W. K., AND IRWIN, R. L. 1934 a. Relationship between anatomic changes in knee joint with advancing age and degenerative arthritis. Arch. Int. Med., 53, 325–344.

KEEN, W. W. 1908. Surgery, its principles and practice. Saunders: Philadelphia, 3, 1132 pp.

KOHASHI, Y. 1937 a. Histologische Untersuchungen der Verschiedenen Skelettmuskeln beim Menschen. I. Untersuchungen beim Erwachsenen. Fol. anat. japon., 15, 175–188.

—— 1937 b. II. Elastische Fasern in den Muskeln. Ibid., 15, 263–271.

—— 1937 c. Über histologische Untersuchungen der einzelnen Skelettmuskeln beim Neugeborenen. Ibid., 15, 411–417.

KOTSOVSKY, D. Z. 1935. Allgemeine Symptome des Alters. Biol. generalis, 11, 87–106.

KROGMAN, W. M. 1930. Ectocranial and endocranial suture closure in anthropoids and Old World apes. Am. J. Anat., 46, 315–353.

LACHMAN, E., AND WHELAN, M. 1936. Roentgen diagnosis of osteoporosis and its limitations. Radiology, 26, 165–177.

LANMAN, T. H., AND INGALLS, T. H. 1937. Vitamin C deficiency and wound healing. Ann. Surg., 105, 616–625.

LECOMTE DU NOÜY, P. 1937. Biological time. Macmillan: New York, 177 pp.

LINBERG, B. E. 1925. Zur Pathologie der posttyphösen Rippenchondritis, Virchows Arch. f. path. Anat., 258, 367–404.

LUX, F., LUX, W., AND STADE, A. 1933. Zahnverlust und Lebensalter. Monatschr. f. Zahnheilkunde, 51, 28–35.

McCRADY, E. 1938. The embryology of the opossum. Am. Anat. Mem., no. 16, Wistar Inst.: Philadelphia, 226 pp.

MAIER, —. 1854. Beiträge zur pathologischen Anatomie einer Form der Schädelatrophie. Arch. f. path. Anat. u. f. klin. Med., 7, 336–340.

MAXIMOW, A. 1927. Über die Funktionen des lockeren Bindegewebes. 288–289. (In v. Möllendorff, W., Handb. d. mikr. Anat. d. Mensch., 2, T. 1. Die Gewebe. Springer: Berlin, 703 pp.)

McCAY, C. M., CROWELL, M. F., AND MAYNARD, L. A. 1935. The effect of retarded growth upon the length of life span and upon the ultimate body size. J. Nutrition, 10, 63–79.

McLEAN, F. C., AND BLOOM, W. 1937. Mode of action of parathyroid extract on bone. (Proc. Nat. Acad. Sciences 1936) Science, 85, 24.

MENKIN, V., WOLBACH, S. B., AND MENKIN, M. F. 1934. Formation of intercellular substance by the administration of ascorbic acid (Vitamin C) in experimental scorbutus. Am. J. Path., 10, 569–575.

MEYER, A. W. 1917. Notes on senile atrophy of the calvarium. Anat. Rec., 12, 69–76. In Spolia anatomica, 43–91.

———— 1922. Further observations upon use-destruction in joints. J. Bone & Joint Surg., 4, 491–511.

———— 1924. Further evidences of attrition in the human body. Am. J. Anat., 34, 241–360.

———— 1928. Spontaneous dislocation and destruction of tendon of long head of biceps brachii. Arch. Surg., 17, 493–506.

———— 1931. The minuter anatomy of attrition lesions. J. Bone & Joint Surg., 13, 341–360.

MOORE, M. M. 1936. Age incidence of dental caries. Am. Dent., 3, 77–83.

MORI, Z. 1936. Age and muscular exercise. Jap. J. Sc., 3, Biophysics, 309–365.

MOULTON, C. R., TROWBRIDGE, P. F., AND HAIGH, L. D. 1922. The composition of ox muscle on the protoplasmic basis. Studies in Animal Nutrition. III. Changes in chemical composition on different planes of nutrition. Missouri Agric. Exp. St. Research. Bull., No. 55, 1–87. See p. 24.

MURRAY, P. D. F. 1936. Bones. University pr.: Cambridge, 203 pp.

NAGAMINE, Y. 1932. Statistische Betrachtung der Zähne im Greisenalter. Nihon Shika Gk. Z., Tokyo, 25, 225–231. See Abst. in Jap. J. Med. Sci., I. Anat., 1934, vol. 4, p. (58).

ORBAN, B. 1937. Personal communication.

OWEN, R. 1866. Anatomy of vertebrates. Longmans Green & Co.: London, 3 vols., vol. 2, 592 pp.

PAPANICOLAOU, G. N., AND FALK, E. A. 1938. General muscular hypertrophy induced by androgenic hormone, Science, 87, 238–9.

PARKER, F., KEEFER, C. S., MYERS, W. K., AND IRWIN, R. L. 1934 b. Histologic changes in the knee joint with advancing age; relation to degenerative arthritis. Arch. Path., 17, 516–532.

PEARCE, J. M. 1936. Age and tissue respiration. Am. J. Physiol., 114, 255–260.
PFITZNER, W. 1899. Social-anthropologische Studien. I. Der Einfluss des Lebensalters auf die anthropologischen Charaktere. Ztschr. f. Morphol. u. Anthropol., 1, 325–377.
PINEY, A. 1922. The anatomy of the bone marrow. Brit. M. J., 2, 792–795.
PÜSCHEL, J. 1930. Der Wassergehalt normaler und degenerierter Zwischen-wirbelscheiben. Beitr. z. path. Anat. u. z. allg. Path., 84, 123–130.
RALLI, E. P. 1938. Personal communication. Proceedings Sixth Annual Conf. Milbank Memorial Fund.
SCHIEFFERDECKER, P. 1911. Untersuchungen über den feineren Bau und die Kernverhaltnisse des Zwerchfelles in Beziehung zu seiner Funktion, sowie über das Bindegewebe der Muskeln. Arch. f. d. ges. Physiol., 139, 337–427.
——— 1927. Vergleichende Betrachtungen über 116 von mir untersuchte Muskeln. Ztschr. f. mikr.-anat. Forsch., 9, 499–539.
SCHOCHRIN, W. A. 1935. Über die Beständigkeit des Altersverhältnisses zwischen der Muskelkraft der Strecker and Beuger. Arbeitsphysiol., 8, 607–609.
SCHÜLLER, A. 1935. Alters-und Geschlechtsbestimmung auf Grund von Kopf-röntgenogrammen. Röntgenpraxis, 7, 518–520.
SCHWEIKHER, F. P. 1930. Ectocranial suture closure in the hyaenas. Am. J. Anat., 45, 443–460.
SIMMS, H. S., AND STOLMAN, A. 1937. Changes in human tissue electrolytes in senescence. Science, 86, 269–270.
SMITH, G. E. 1907. The causation of the symmetrical thinning of the parietal bones in ancient Egyptians. J. Anat., 41, 232–233.
STEVENSON, P. H. 1924. Age order of epiphyseal union in Man. Am. J. Phys. Anthropol., 5, 53–93.
STEWART, D. 1936. An experimental study of the return of function after tendon section. Brit. J. Surg., 24, 388–396.
TODD, T. W. 1913. A preliminary communication on the development and growth of bone and the relations thereto of the several histological elements concerned. J. Anat., 1913, 47, 177–188.
——— 1920. Age changes in the pubic bone. I. The male White pubis. Am. J. Phys. Anthropol., 3, 285–334.
——— 1921. Age changes in the pubic bone. II. Male Negro-White hybrid. III. White female. IV. Female Negro-White hybrid. Am. J. Phys. Anthropol., 4, 1–70.
——— 1924. Thickness of the male white cranium. Anat. Rec., 27, 245–256.
——— 1931. The registration of life's handicaps. Brush Foundation Publication: Cleveland, O., no. X, 10 pp.
——— 1933 a. Human bodies and human beings. Sigma Xi Quarterly, 21, 123–140.
——— 1933 b. Chapter on Growth and development of the skeleton in White House Conference on Child Health and Protection, Growth and Development of the Child, pt. II, Anatomy and Physiology. Century Co.: New York, 76–130.
——— 1937. The mineralization problem in orthodontia. Angle Orthodontist, 7, 158–165.

TODD, T. W., AND D'ERRICO, J. 1928. The clavicular epiphyses. Am. J. Anat., 41, 25–50.

TODD T. W., AND HAGEMEYER, D. 1938. Chemical determination and roentgenographic discrimination of mineral in the human skeleton (in preparation).

TODD, T. W., AND LYON, D. W. 1924. Cranial suture closure: its progress and age relationship. I. Endocranial closure, White males. Am. J. Phys. Anthropol., 7, 325–384.

———— 1925 a. II. Ectocranial closure: White males. Am. J. Phys. Anthropol., 8, 23–45.

———— 1925 b. III. Endocranial closure: Negro males. Am. J. Phys. Anthropol., 8, 47–71.

———— 1925 c. IV. Ectocranial closure: Negro males. Am. J. Phys. Anthropol., 8, 149–168.

TODD, T. W., AND McGAW, W. H. 1938. Changes in comparative length of toes during adult life (in preparation).

TODD, T. W., AND OTHERS. 1937. Atlas of skeletal maturation. Part I. The Hand. C. V. Mosby: St. Louis, 204 pp.

TODD, T. W., SIMMONS, K., AND NICKERSON, R. Age changes in the texture and markings of the skull (in preparation).

TODD, T. W., AND TODD, A. W. 1938. The epiphysial union pattern of the Ungulates with a note on Sirenia. Am. J. Anat., 63, 1–36.

TODD, T. W., TODD, A. W., AND TODD, D. P. Epiphysial union in mammals with special reference to Rodentia (in publication).

TODD, T. W., WHARTON, R. E., AND TODD, A. W. 1938. The effect of thyroid deficiency upon bodily growth and skeletal maturation in the sheep. Am. J. Anat., 63, 37–78.

UEBERMUTH, H. 1930. Die Bedeutung der Altersveränderungen der menschlichen Bandscheiben für die Pathologie der Wirbelsäule. Arch. klin. Chir., 156, 567–577.

UFLAND, J. M. 1933. Einfluss des Lebensalters, Geschlechts, der Konstitution und des Berufs auf die Kraft verschiedener Muskelgruppen. I. Mitteilungen über den Einfluss des Lebensalters auf die Muskelkraft. Arbeitsphysiol., 6, 653–663.

VENAR, Y., AND TODD, T. W. 1934. The efficacy of vitamin D administration in aqueous preparation. J. Nutrition, 8, 553–568.

WEBSTER, A. E. 1918. The effect of time and wear on the human teeth. J. Nat. Dent. A., 5, 1019–1025.

WETZEL, G. 1932. Altersanatomie. Verhandl. d. anat. Gesellsch., 41, 15–36.

WILLIS, T. A. 1924. The age factor in hypertrophic arthritis. J. Bone & Joint Surg., 6, 316–325.

WOLBACH, S. B. 1933. Controlled formation of collagen and reticulum. A study of the source of intercellular substance in recovery from experimental scorbutus. Am. J. Path., 9, 689–699.

———— 1936. Vitamin C and the formation of intercellular material. New England J. Med., 215, 1158–1159.

WOLBACH, S. B., AND HOWE, P. R. 1926. Intercellular substances in experimental scorbutus. Arch. Path. & Lab. Med., 1, 1–24.

Chapter 12

AGEING OF THE SKIN

FRED D. WEIDMAN

Philadelphia

If there is any part of the human body which literally thrusts the evidence of its advancing years upon whomsoever may look, it is the skin. A child knows the significance of wrinkles, gray hair and baldness. As Cowdry says, employers and prospective husbands and wives have learned to call upon the skin as the indicator in respect to youth, to which I would add the man of the street. In short, the skin advertises both its chronologic (in terms of life periods) and biologic ages definitely and obviously in the given individual, thus permitting reliable reconcilements and comparisons of changes of various kinds. There is thus already supplied a starting point which is based upon a solid foundation. The skin is one of very few organs which has already arrived in this respect.

Although few cutaneous diseases are death dealing (even cutaneous cancer accounts for only 2.7 deaths per thousand), the psychological effects of appearances on the skin may be greater in the aggregate than the fear of disease or death. This constitutes one of the complications and problems of the old age complex.

The skin is more than a mechanical barrier between the tissues beneath and the outside world. Alterations in it exercise a profound influence on the body as a whole and vice versa. Moreover, the skin can be studied more directly, completely, and with greater ease than any other system. Consequently the ageing processes are susceptible of detailed analysis. These circumstances are real assets when studying a process, like ageing, which is progressive, years long, and in which examinations should be made accurately.

The pluriorganic composition of the skin should be appreciated at the outset. With its functions protective, thermotaxic, secretory, sensory, etc., it is obvious that the skin must be of diversified structure. Organs like the kidney (Chapter 10) also exercise multiple functions, but only a few are divided as definitely, anatomically speaking, into highly specialized and independent systems. As exceptions, the pancreas, adrenal and pituitary might be cited, but even in them the differently functioning cells are not as sharply separated anatomically. Apparently the pancreas approaches closest in its pluriorganic composition.

These circumstances indicate the necessity, when the time arrives, of distributing studies of cutaneous ageing into several different fields if it is to be done logically and analytically, e.g. as to sweat secretion, sebaceous secretion, fat storage, lipoid partitions, etc. We recall the diversity of studies which have been conducted on the pancreas.

1. HEREDITY AND CONSTITUTION

The main lead is in connection with xeroderma pigmentosum. According to Lynch (1934), "The course of this disease is progressive, the exposed parts of the skin undergoing all of the progressive changes of senility." "Its hereditary tendency is well known; it is recessive, with no sex difference. Consanguinity of the parents has been recorded in from 17 to 59 per cent of the cases and was regarded by Toyama as the reason for the high incidence in Japan." In short, for the exposed parts of the body, heredity is the basis for cutaneous ageing through the medium of one of the inborn errors of metabolism (Garrod, 1923). With hematoporphoryn established as the light-sensitizing agent in xeroderma pigmentosum, curiosity is aroused as to the rôle of analogous substances in normal ageing of the skin at large. That other light-sensitizing substances exist (eosin, methylene blue and acridine) is well established, but these of course are only used in experiments and are not factors in normal ageing.

In connection with the apigmentation of hair in ageing, note should be at least made of the hereditary excess of homogentisic acid in the urine which accompanies albinism, with alkaptonuria. The disturbance is one of metabolism of tyrosin and phenylalanin (Garrod, 1923). In 20 per cent of cases collected, the parents were consanguinous.

There does not appear to be any cogent relationship between constitutional habitus and the ageing of skin. Perhaps the most that can be suggested is the tendency for sandy complexioned types to exhibit precociously some of the features of senile skin such as pigmentation (freckling) of the exposed parts of the body. It is realized that this differs from true ageing; nevertheless, it appears advisable to call attention to this particular constitutional type as a promising one for further studies.

2. SYMPTOM COMPLEX OF CUTANEOUS SENESCENCE

A definite symptom complex for cutaneous senescence has become well established. Layman, general practitioner and dermatologist all know that it exists, and have at their command the shorter or longer list of items comprising the complex. Naturally, the dermatologist knows it best, and has, true to form, composed the adequate nomenclature which is necessary to express the particular conditions existing. He has done well, too, in integrating the senile skin with certain pathological processes, such as cancer.

It is regrettable, though, that thus far cutaneous senescence is little more than a clinical entity, and at that, one of morphology. For whatever reason, the demand has not gained much headway for systematic studies of the physiology and chemistry of the skin. The available data are scattered through reports in which the ageing factor was more or less incidental. This will explain why, in the paragraphs to follow, a wealth of factual information is indicated in the literature concerning the morphology of cutaneous ageing, but a dearth of other data. However, the latter is still worth recording, if only for its suggestiveness.

3. RETROGRADE TISSUE CHANGES

Soon after the age of 40 signs of ageing begin to appear in the skin, together with certain others like loss of teeth and failing eyesight. The list (table 23) is long, and obviously every item will not qualify as a member of normal ageing. In fact, strictly applying the 51 per cent rule, in the present state of our knowledge but few would survive, since factual, statistical information is so sadly lacking. Furthermore, it would certainly vary depending on the age level which supplied the data. For example, in the fifth decade only atrophy might be disclosed; in the sixth, atrophy, baldness, calvities and sebaceous hyperplasia; in the seventh, telangiectasis and seborrheic keratosis might be added; and, in the eighth, elastosis. Thus, if the eighth decade were the one selected as the basis for statistics, a large number of signs might rightly qualify. The writer feels that in the skin, the ageing of which has been directly observed by generation upon generation of physicians, general impressions have greater weight in comparison with statistics than in other organs. The situation is different for arteries, kidney and gonads, in which, even if the number of cases observed is not dwarfed by comparison, the *course* of the changes can not be followed for they are not exposed to view as in the skin. Consequently all the items in the table justify mention in following paragraphs, even though statistics might, and probably would, exclude them under the 51 per cent rule.

Speaking of the skin as a whole (for the time being its fibro-elastic tissue, essentially), the processes which occur most regularly and frankly in ageing are the regressive ones common to so many other organs and tissues; namely, atrophy and degeneration. They may be regarded tentatively as processes purely of ageing, i.e., uncomplicated

TABLE 23

Reconciliation of processes and symptoms in ageing

Processes	Symptoms
A. Purity of ageing unquestionable	
Atrophy (hair papilla)	Baldness
Atrophy (hair papilla)	Graying of hair
Degeneration and loss of elastic tissue	Wrinkles
Atrophy (epiderm)	Thinning of skin with smoothness (scaliness corollary)
Atrophy (epiderm)	Dystrophy of toenails
Withdrawal of subcutaneous fat	Leanness and wrinkles
B. Purity questionable	
Secondary to degeneration of collagenous tissue (?)	Telangiectasia
Epidermal hyperplasia	Seborrheic keratosis
General endocrine interrelationship (?)	Hyperpigmentation
Sebaceous hyperplasia	Yellowness, large pores
Hyperplasia of fibrous tissue with degeneration	Cutaneous tags (acrochordon)
Epidermal hyperplasia	Senile keratosis
Epidermal hyperplasia	Cancer

by other agencies like arteriosclerosis which are seen in so many other organs. As to the atrophy, it is the essential atrophy of unexplainable decadence. Thus, the thin skin upon the trunk of the man of 85 still exercises protection as it did at 20. Certainly it is not the atrophy of disuse, since the call for protection remains. Hyponutrition cannot be demonstrated to account for atrophy and degeneration; there is no evidence that the blood volume of the skin becomes insufficient— even in arteriosclerosis. Indeed, considering the thinness of the tissue to be nourished and its low nutritional requirements (probably), the expansive vascular bed in the subcutaneous parts to be drawn upon, and the free anastomoses within the skin (arteries not terminal in type), there appears to be a reasonable explanation why arteriosclerosis does not induce atrophy of the skin. Moreover, the flushed face of the hypertensive arteriosclerotic speaks for just the opposite. Long-continued pressure as a cause of atrophy cannot be invoked; it is doubtful that pressure operates on the senile skin more than on the juvenile. As to endocrine rôles, information in this direction should come from the endocrinologist; at this distance the relationships are so nebulous as to be of most limited value. In short, the atrophy is probably a pure, autochthonous atrophy.

As to the degenerations met with, a basophilic degeneration of both the collagenic bundles and elastic fibers is common—indeed almost invariable. Elastic tissue suffers far more regularly and severely, undergoing fragmentation and disappearance in addition. Changes begin at different ages, depending on the region, and are less intense in women than in men according to Ejiri (1936, 1937). The mechanism is probably the same as for atrophy. It appears safe to assume that enzymes are not abundant in the corium; at least this tissue does not autolyze after death to the extent that many others do (cf. leather).

The foregoing has to do with the skin as a whole and in which the tissues of the corium proper are particularly concerned. As to the epiderm, there is no doubt that it undergoes atrophy with age. Apparently this is also authochthonous atrophy, with the considerations similar to ones outlined above in some detail. The subepidermal connective tissues (papillae) concomitantly lose their special conformation and, flattening out, result in the smooth, shining cutaneous surface familiar in the aged. That is, the finer surface lines of the skin are lost, in contradistinction to the coarser folds and wrinkles which are developed *de novo* as the result of atrophy of the corium and subcutaneous fat.

The most spectacular prototype of precocious (presenile) ageing of the skin, morphologically at least, is encountered in the clinical entity, xeroderma pigmentosum. In it there is a congenital excess of porphyrins which leads to skin sensitiveness to actinic light (Lynch, 1934). Such a close counterpart of the senile skin is thereby developed that the suspicion at once arises whether the normal ageing of the skin also results from its exposure to light, albeit gradually over a longer period of years. Moreover we would like to know whether, if not porphyrin itself, some other form of light-sensitizing substance which develops incidentally to general ageing plays the contributory rôle. In passing, the writer thinks that the children he has seen with this disease exhibited as well something of the senile habitus constitutionally.

In any event, the skin in xeroderma pigmentosum becomes thin, dry, telangiectatic and hyperpigmented. Freckles, sometimes huge, form in addition to diffuse pigmentation. Cutaneous cancer almost invariably develops—in early childhood! Reflecting the unquestioned rôle of light, the face and hands are the parts most severely affected.

Information is not satisfactory in respect to the changes in the appendages of the skin. It is a handicap at once that the glands, both sebaceous and sudorific, normally vary in size within wide limits depending on the region of the body concerned (Way, 1931). The best information comes from regions where the appendages are highly developed, as on the scalp. It is evident that the hair undergoes atrophy. Microscopic studies show that, while the hair shaft can disappear completely, the sebaceous glands become only reduced in size. Yet, singularly, the hairs of the male beard increase in diameter throughout life (Trotter, 1922). The apocrine glands of the axilla and elsewhere are particularly inviting subjects for investigation because they are so large to begin with, their cells are more highly specialized than those of the exocrine sweat glands, and because there are suspicions of interrelationship with the endocrine-sympathetic duo.

Baldness. As an unquestionably senile phenomenon, that form which begins with thinning, and gradually proceeds to the more or less complete baldness is the only one which is unequivocal. It must not be confused with hereditary and other forms of baldness. Recalling that the hair shaft is an ametabolic,—dead, structure, just as is the bark of trees (Chapter 2), inquiries should be directed to the hair papilla when analyzing the processes concerned. The papilla, being homologous with the epiderm is essentially but a highly specialized and sharply localized focus of epidermal cells. It is necessary to envisage the atrophying processes as common to all epidermal cells and to remember the factor of specialization in order to understand that atrophy would make its more profound and earlier impress upon the hair than elsewhere. Indeed, it is doubtful that any structure in the body, except possibly the eye, signals the onset of senescence as obviously and as early as the hair.

Care should be exercised under all circumstances to distinguish senile baldness from the pathological ones occurring in syphilis and other diseases (e.g. the "gastric" hair of Wadsworth, 1915). There is a rich literature on the etiology of alopecia in general, in which the sympathetic, endocrines and nervous effects (shock in general) come under suspicion (Danforth, 1925). Males are far more extensively affected than females.

Canities. The graying of the hair, due to decrease of pigment, can doubtless be correlated with the same atrophying processes occurring in the hair papillae that account for baldness as just outlined. The order in which the apigmentation and atrophy of hair occurred, i.e., whether the graying or baldness came first, might, if analyzed in a large series of cases in respect to ageing in general, throw some light on the latter. Incidentally, melanin production and its dopa reaction are intimately related to adrenal function.

Wrinkles. There are probably two factors which explain the development of wrinkles. For one, the well-known withdrawal of fat from certain parts of the subcutaneous tissue concerns not only the levels below the corium, but also the extensions (columnae adiposae) which pass perpendicularly from it into the corium around the sweat glands.

The second factor is probably far more important, namely, loss of elasticity. If the skin on the back of the hand is pinched up into a thin fold and pulled strongly upward, it will return to its normal position less promptly in senile subjects than in young ones. It becomes permanently overstretched owing to movements of the body, and in the absence of elastic properties fails to return as it does in young subjects.

It is questionable whether yellow elastic tissue is really responsible for the elasticity of the skin. Some claim that it is the mesh-like arrangement of collagenous bundles, instead, that serves this function, in which case the guilt for wrinkles would lie more properly with the latter kind of tissue. Further, studies of the lines of cleavage in senility, as conducted by Batson (1928) employing awl punctures, would be in order. Do the lines deviate from the normal pattern?

Pityriasis. The scaliness is but scanty. It is diffuse and of a fine, almost powdery type. It can be observed to advantage on negro skin on account of the contrasting color. It is probably not due to increased keratinization since the epiderm is atrophic; more likely its presence is accentuated because retained in connection with the dryness of the skin.

Pseudohypertrophy of toenails. At first thought it might appear that the thick, deformed, opaque or black or sometimes horn-like toenails which frequently accompany senility are the results of hyperplasia. But the keratin is typically degenerative. For example, the old keratinous accumulations in long-standing ichthyosis and Darier's disease are black, but the recently developed lesions are not. Furthermore, the effects of pressure (atrophy) should become progressively exaggerated during ageing on a place like the toe.

Doubtless the abnormality is referable to impaired function of the epiderm consequent upon senility, thus involving an abnormality of keratinization, with decreased rate of production. It is likely that if adequate records were available of the growth rate of the nails of the aged (Heller, 1927), they would support the thesis that the increased thickness is due to retention rather than overproduction of keratin. This done, it would be simple to explain the deformity, opaqueness and changes in color on the basis of simple degeneration of keratin. As a matter of fact, statistics are available showing that the nails grow more slowly in the aged than in youth and much less rapidly on the toes than on the fingers and in winter than in summer. The differences in rate of growth are probably sufficient to explain the extreme changes met in old age.

4. PROGRESSIVE (PROLIFERATIVE) TISSUE CHANGES

All of these come under the heading of questionably senile processes (table 22), for other factors than those of ageing are involved. Such changes deserve mention, nevertheless, because they are met almost exclusively in senile skins.

The telangiectasis of Dubrueilh is the brilliant red, round, elevated focus that is familiar to every physician, located or confined to covered parts of the body like the chest. It appears for the most part after 40, often in goodly numbers. It has the architecture of a miniature cavernous hemangioma. Robertson (1934) has seen similar structures develop during episodes in cardiac decompensation and disappear with the episode. It is certain, though, that all do not originate in this way, since most of them develop far in advance, or in the absence of cardiac symptoms. They are generally regarded as nevi, but the basis for this idea appears to be only presumptive. Kyrle (1925) claims that senile degeneration of the connective tissue stroma is the deciding factor.

The seborrheic keratosis (verruca senilis) is the brown or black mole which commonly accompanies the telangiectases. Like the latter, it occurs on the chest, sometimes in large numbers, develops mostly after

40, and is regarded as nevic.[1] Histologically it approaches basal cell cancer, but is strictly limited within the epiderm. It is so commonplace and free from hazards to health that it has not received the

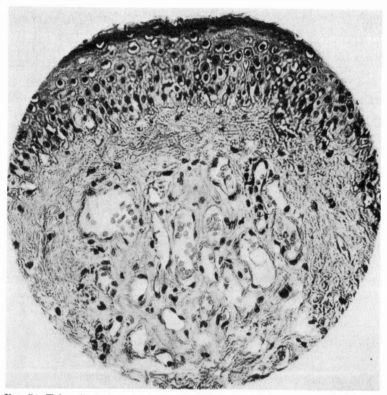

Fig. 74. Telangiectasis. A circumscribed focus of dilated capillaries located most superficially. There is not any evidence of degeneration in the stroma which could be claimed to predispose to their formation. Moreover, their endothelial cells are of normal appearance; the author regards the processes as purely hyperplastic,—at least in these materials. Aged 59.

attention it merits. What is it in the senile state that provokes its appearance? For the patient it is but a cosmetic defect. Being so palpable, it should constitute a valuable indicator or perhaps test object when studying senile influences of any sort,—whether humoral,

[1] It is worth while in this connection to reflect whether these structures are homologous with the embryonic or vegetative cells of invertebrates cited by Jennings, in Chapter 2.

nervous or endocrine. In spite of its name, it is essentially an epidermal hyperplasia; the keratosis is but secondary (commensurate with the cellular hyperplasia) and the sebaceous glands are not significantly changed.

Hyperpigmentation. It is difficult to specify or speak strongly on any of the phases of senile pigmentation. By and large, it would appear that the melanin of the epiderm in general is slightly increased, thus accounting for the somewhat ashy appearance of the skin of many old people. The accentuation of freckles is more unequivocal, even disregarding those on the face and hands where the continued rôle of light might be invoked etiologically. Old ones on the shoulders are in point.

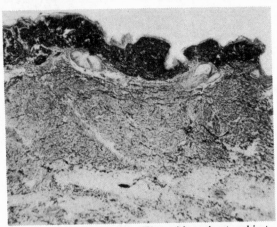

Fig. 75. Elastic tissue hyperplasia. The epiderm is atrophic to a degree, but immediately below it there is a broad band of elastic tissue. It stains black by Weigert's elastic tissue stain. Aged 73.

Sebaceous hyperplasia. Only anatomical considerations will be brought up at this time; the functional ones will appear later. After the age of 40, the sebaceous glands of the face commonly become enlarged, probably as the result of cellular hyperplasia. It is most unlikely that others elsewhere participate. This is reflected in a general yellower color, particularly of the nose, with accentuation of the outlets. As a result, larger "pores" appear. At times, in addition, special foci of yellowing can be made out on some subjects even by direct observation, and histologic examination confirms the presence of sebaceous hyperplasia to account for them.

Certain of the hyperplasias are so extreme and so definitely circumscribed that they have been (quite erroneously) regarded as adenomas or nevi. They occur more on the forehead than on the nose (Weidman, 1931). In any event, both as to the more diffuse and circumscribed, the frequent presence of Demodex folliculorum introduces a disturbing factor as to the sole etiological rôle of senescence (Gilman, 1937). By and large, then, the sebaceous hyperplasias are open to question as phenomena essentially of senescence, just as are senile keratosis and cancer. They occur in the senile skin beyond a doubt, but that they are fundamentally a part of ageing remains to be demonstrated.

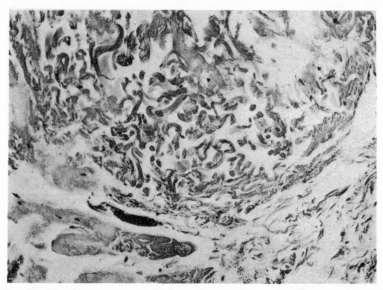

FIG. 76. Elastic tissue hyperplasia and degeneration. In this order of tissue change the collagenous bundles and elastic fibers mutually approach each other's morphology. The scarcity of nuclei is suggestive of the considerations mentioned in the text. Aged 73.

Senile elastosis. The elastic tissue of the skin all over the body undergoes some grade of degeneration in senescence. On exposed parts, especially the face and neck, it exhibits hyperplasia in addition (Ejiri, 1936, 1937). The amount of elastic tissue may be so great as to produce a strong orange yellow color of the skin surface and to form such thick wrinkles that the skin of the neck may be likened to that of a turtle. Analogous changes occur in the collagenic bundles, and inasmuch as both kinds of connective tissue undergo a basophilic degeneration and the approach to each other's morphology is mutual, it is difficult indeed to separate the two sharply for accurate analysis of the processes. However, the associated fatty changes which are grossly responsible for the yellow color are more definite in the elastic tissue (Weidman, 1931).

Recalling the scarcity of nuclei and the relative absence of capillaries in the corium, this accumulation of "hyperplastic" tissue does not appear to be consistent with the low metabolic state of cutaneous collagenous tissue. It is natural, therefore, to wonder whether there is a factor of infiltration concerned in this increase of elastic substance. Can it be that, as in amyloid infiltration, the disappearing elastic substance of lungs and arteries of senile subjects is deposited in the skin? Only the finest of chemical and histological research can answer this question.

Precocious senile elastosis. The senile elastosis which has been already discussed may also appear precociously—in young adults. The writer cannot speak positively, but thinks that the skin in these "patients" is also atrophic. Such cases are weak as bespeaking essential ageing because the elastosis occurs on the face and neck (although not necessarily in those exposed to vicissitudes of weather). The affection known as pseudoxanthoma elasticum also deserves analysis in respect to somatic ageing and is in point more certainly so because it is not the exposed parts that are outstandingly involved; covered parts of the body (axillae and abdomen) are affected, besides the neck. In addition, alterations which occur in the eye (angioid streaks of the retina) should be included in any thoughts about ageing.

In this connection, too (precocious ageing), consider records of molluscum fibrosum gravidarum under acrochordon, which naturally occurs mostly in adolescence.

Acrochordon. This is a small, soft, fleshy, skin-colored, wart-like affair which often dangles from the skin because its pedicle is so attenuated (Gr. *akron*, extremity, + *chordē*, cord). It may attain the size of a pea but is commonly only 1 to 2 mm. in diameter. It is particularly on the neck and upper part of the thorax and consists of degenerate fibrous tissue which is at times so soft as to suggest mucoid substance. There are intimations that similar structures (molluscum fibrosum gravidarum) are etiologically connected with processes occurring during pregnancy and after the menopause (Templeton, 1936). Knowledge on etiology is vague, but it is reasonable to assume that an initial hyperplasia of fibrous tissue occurs, succeeded by mucinoid degeneration. One of the gonadotropic hormones of the

anterior pituitary acts as an ectodermal stimulant in tissue cultures
of chick embryos (Danforth, 1925).

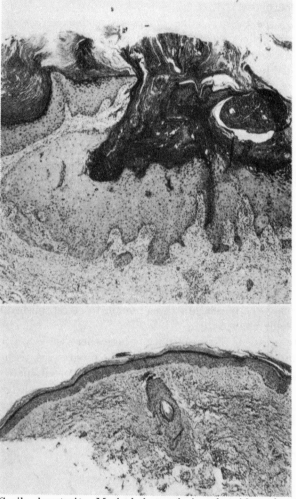

FIG. 77. Senile keratosis. Marked hyperplasia of epidermal cells, with
attendant hyperkeratosis. The illustration immediately below is of skin at the
farthermost edge of the same section and serves as a control when evaluating
the degree of hyperplasia. The two are magnified equally. Aged 55.

The senile keratosis. Since this occurs almost exclusively upon the
face and hands, together with other reasons, actinic light must play
some part in its production. Indeed, this is generally conceded. Since

the epidermal hyperplasia underlying the keratosis occurs only in senile skin the processes of senility would appear to at least predispose to the hyperplasia.

Review of progressive tissue changes in cutaneous ageing. It is in order now to collect the data which have been already recorded in this connection and to summarize them because, while retrogressive processes unquestionably dominate the scene in somatic ageing, there is still much uncertainty as to the genuineness of progressive ones. Doing this, it would appear that for the skin, not a single instance of progressive process can be summoned but which can be criticized when considered by itself. Hyperplasia of collagenous tissue does not occur except in acrochordon. As to an increase of elastic tissue, whereas it is frequently met on exposed parts of the body, it remains to be demonstrated that it is purely senile etiologically; however, studies of presenile elastosis and of pseudoxanthoma elasticum might shed other light in the case. The metabolism of keratin is fallaciously increased in senile keratosis; the excess is an accumulation secondary to epidermal hyperplasia. The same can be said of the pityriasis, and the thick, horn-like toenails can well be examples of retention only of keratin. If seborrheic keratosis be admitted to this category there is an unquestionable example of hyperplasia of epithelial cells, and the same may be said of sebaceous hyperplasia, but these remain to be established as autochthonous senile changes.

In spite of all of this negativity, where there is such a notable accumulation of instances of presumptively progressive tissue changes, it does not seem likely that every item will be eliminated on some count or other, when we acquire more complete knowledge of all of the intricacies of the processes involved. Indeed, there is very much of an outside chance that when each of the items is definitely classified either as true or pseudo ageing some of them will survive in the true ageing group.

5. PHYSIOLOGIC CHANGES

Rapport between the skin and the body at large. It is only necessary to mention the heat-regulating function of the skin as an example of the considerations that properly fall under this heading. Without it, the general body temperature would drop to levels incompatible with life. In addition to this function, it is possible that all of the other functions of the skin would, if sufficiently studied be found to bear upon internal processes in one or other respect. To be exhaustive, it is therefore quite in order to consider each function of the skin separately and catalogue its disturbances regarding ageing if only as a matter of record. At this time, though, it is impractical to do more than indicate the more unequivocally established effects of age upon cutaneous functions and submit other suggestive data.

Heat regulation. It is well known that senile subjects cannot tolerate cold as well as they did in youth. They suffer from chilliness. There is no readily available evidence that this can be accounted for on the basis of inadequate blood flow through the skin. As stated above, arteriosclerosis does not appear to seriously compromise the cutaneous circulation. Moreover, Ejiri (1937) stated that blood capillaries become dilated above the age 40–50. It is certain, however, that the insulation of the skin cannot be as efficient because it is atrophic and subcutaneous fat has been largely withdrawn. On the other hand, in view of the decreased sudorific function, it might be expected that elderly people would suffer more seriously from extremes of heat, and this does appear to be the case (see Chapter 23 by Cannon).

Sensation. Itchiness (pruritus) qualifies, beyond doubt, as a process in ageing. Indeed, it is the most common and conspicuous symptom of senile skins. The covered parts of the body suffer most, perhaps because sweat secretion is less abundant than on the hands and face. In any event, it is proper to assume that the abnormal dryness of the skin is largely etiologic. The well known "senile pruritus" of the dermatologist is treated by greasy or soapy applications, but the possibility that the secretions and products of the epiderm are abnormal and irritative must be kept in mind, particularly since the correction of the dryness does not always relieve the itching. The rôle of uric acid in pruritus was introduced by Schamberg and Brown (1923), who found the highest uric acid values between ages 40–80.

Sebaceous secretion. Immediately after puberty the faces of children become greasy. This is an important predisposing factor for acne vulgaris, with which even the layman is familiar. Moreover, infants often develop "milk crust"—really an accumulation of sebaceous secretion upon the scalp. Both of these "seborrheas" occur regularly enough to be regarded as physiologic and therefore qualify as items in ageing. Sebaceous activity is greatest in the latter months of pregnancy, at puberty and thence up to middle life (Way, 1931). The seborrheic dermatitis of adults occurs upon a seborrheic skin; while this is in the realm of pathology, it nevertheless connotes a skin that is greasy. Considered collectively, these data indicate some relation between certain definite age periods and sebaceous activity, of which the two first named are the more clear-cut in their age limitation. Hamilton (Chapter 17) postulates age 1-5 as one of sex activity, and there can be no question regarding sex in the puberty period. In short, sexual and sebaceous activities appear to be correlated.

Internal secretions. A number of claims have been made that the skin should be included as one of the active participants in the entire endocrinologic complex. In support of this thesis the rôle of the thyroid in inducing myxoedema, the low hair line in pituitary disease, the difference in the beards and in the distribution of pubic hair of males and females, suprarenal hirsuties, the rarity of baldness in eunuchs —to cite only a few of the items, are commonly quoted, but precise knowledge of the mechanisms involved is lacking. For example, for the hair Danforth (1925, p. 93) states that the endocrines condition in some way the intrinsic properties of hair papillae, but that we lack any useful knowledge of the way they act. Unfortunately the same has to be granted for the other structures of the skin which have been involved. It might be instructive to compare the well known postmortem growth of hair of the beard of juveniles and the aged of both sexes.

All of the evidence here advanced bears upon only one side of the supposed endocrine "interrelationship." That is, it is not a genuinely "inter" as far as the strictly endocrine phases are concerned. It is not reciprocal. In all of the citations, it is a non-cutaneous hormone that is the active partner, and it is upon a cutaneous structure which is not yet proven to be endocrinologic that the effects are exerted. In other words, while there is strong circumstantial evidence, there is not any convincing proof that there are epidermal or sebaceous or sudorific hormones that influence the thyroid, suprarenal, etc. Consequently we cannot claim that the skin, in any of its parts elaborates an internal secretion and thus participates in the endocrine balance. This, though, in no way detracts from the likelihood that cutaneous secretions include also endocrine ones. It is only the proof that is lacking.

However, these shortcomings of cutaneous endocrinology do not destroy its value in studies of ageing at large. It remains that some of the effects of general body endocrines become visible upon the skin and that the way is open to analyze them yet farther in respect to the way these endocrines behave at different age periods. It still stands as a field upon which general systemic endocrinologic changes may be signalled at different age periods.

Fat metabolism in subcutaneous fatty tissue. It is not sufficiently realized how this tissue has been neglected in medical research. Ordinarily, fat is fat and little more, whether the thinker is lay or medical. However, evidence has existed for a long time that fatty tissue is not quite homogeneous and passive; there is a difference between fat and fatty tissue. For example, for the female its distribution is different in childhood and maturity; it is responsible for what amounts to secondary sexual characteristics. The buccal pad of infants is comparatively temporary. Castration affects the development of the panniculus. It remains relatively constant upon the palms and soles and in the buccal pad of infants in spite of severe general emaciation. These should suffice to indicate that it is not entirely passive, but has individualities of more than one kind.

It is true that there is a wealth of data concerning fat metabolism in general, including the storage of fat in the main fat depots of the body; that is, the omentum and abdominal panniculus. For example, animals crammed with deer or other kinds of fat store the surplus as deer (or other) fat. However, the writer is unaware that analyses of the various lipid constituents of fat have been made for different parts of the same body, in which connection the skin of secondary sexual regions (hips and calves of the female) might be found to differ. This subject acquires fresh importance right now, with our increasing knowledge of vitamins, including the fat soluble ones like carotene. It is brought up on account of a possible bearing upon ageing, for the skin is an accessible fat depot very suitable for investigation.

Suggestive, too, are the cycles of fat storage that occur in man's lifetime because they correspond to some extent with his major endocrinologic cycles. The normal infant is fat, the child and adult leaner; in the fifty to sixth decade there is a tendency to fattening, while leanness supervenes in old age (see Chapter 17 by Hamilton). While on this subject, it would be interesting to learn whether, in the cases of impotence at age 37–40, any special changes, either anatomical or chemical (lipid partition of fats) take place consistently in the skin.

While pathological processes cannot be admitted to the subject of ageing proper, it is in order to cite one to indicate that the composition of subcutaneous fat can and does change. In sclerema neonatorum (Gray, 1926) confined to infants, the melting point of fat is raised so high that it is solid at body temperatures, resulting in hardness of the skin. Similar phenomena are not known for adults.

Water content of skin. Considering free and bound water together.

the skin is the dryest tissue of the body, except bone and fat,—72.74 per cent against an average of 78 per cent for other organs. Moreover, the figure is not so constant as it is for other organs. On the contrary, the absolute water is high, being only surpassed by muscle. If the entire body consists of 65 per cent water, the muscles account for 50 per cent of it and the skin 6–11 per cent. The skin of infants contains far more water than that of adults. For rats, 20 per cent is lost during the first 24 hours. Water appears to fluctuate in the skin in an almost unique way. It is intriguing that in spite of diarrhea, the skins of infants do not lose water.

These considerations are significant when we remember that one of the criteria of senility uniformly cited is water loss. For the skin atrophy and senility, the path is opened to speculation. Is the water shortage propter hoc or post hoc? Either way, in senility the water-storing function of the senile skin must be markedly reduced.

Sulphur metabolism and growth. As previously stated, nails grow more rapidly in the young than in the aged, and the fingernails faster than toenails. Since nails contain as much as 2.80 per cent of sulphur, in the form of the amino-acid cystine, it is possible that the general sulphur metabolism of the body might be implicated in cases of dystrophy of the nails. Hair, too, contains 3.83–8.23 per cent of sulphur (the latter figure is for red hair) with an average of 4.86 per cent (Brown and Klauder, 1933). Sulphur is particularly in point here in view of Hammett and Reimann's (1929) contentions that sulphydryl compounds, of which cystine is one, are important in the promotion of general growth.

Chlorides. The skin is an important depot normally, containing one third of those of the entire body. The quantity varies markedly in disease; during diuresis of rabbits, 42 per cent is extracted from the skin; on dry, rich diets in nephritis chloride increases. However, the chloride and water content do not run hand in hand. Values are not readily available in respect to ageing and the data submitted above are included here simply as suggestive leads in studies of ageing.

Arsenic. For the entire body, the skin is the chief site for arsenic deposition, keratin being the particular substance which holds it. It is in a fixed chemical combination which breaks up with difficulty. It increases with age; at age 23, 0.0095 mgm.; at 47, 0.01; and at 71, 0.017. That is, there is almost twice as much at 71 as at 23 (Rothman and Schaaf, 1929).

6. IMMUNOLOGIC CHANGES

There is a growing sense of the immunological importance of the skin. Tuft (1931), for example, comments on the "close relationship between the skin and processes of immunity in infectious and allergic diseases." In relation to ageing there is at least one clear-cut relationship in connection with ringworm of the scalp. This disease is excessively rare in adults. In children it spontaneously clears up as puberty is reached. It is not known whether tissue or humoral defenses are concerned or whether the composition of sebaceous fats changes at puberty in the direction of becoming fungicidal. These considerations do not hold for other forms of ringworm.

Both man and guinea pig are available as test objects for immunologic studies in ageing of the skin because they are susceptible to experimental favus induced by Achorion Quinckeanum—a mycosis which is readily amenable to treatment. Local resistance to reinfection develops which could be tested at different ages. Greenbaum (1924) used his own skin in his work.

The skin must mature to some extent before certain other immunologic functions become well developed. Thus, Pillsbury (1937) found increasing protection against bacteria as rabbits and dogs grew older. After injections of horse serum, Kahn reported (1937) that the skin of mature rabbits anchors diphtheria antitoxin more effectively than does that of immature ones—in the ratio of 1000 to 75 as measured by the specific antitoxin.

The self sterilizing property of the skin is said to be decreased where sebaceous secretion becomes deficient. On the face of it, this circumstance would seem to have a bearing on the problem of the dry skin of the aged. But clinical experiences do not indicate that the aged are more liable to cutaneous infection than others.

Effect of cutaneous ageing upon the general health of the individual. Except as a predisposing cause of cutaneous cancer, this appears to be nil—*at least in the present state of our knowledge.* The impairment of cutaneous processes which may influence general body functions is not severe enough to compromise them sufficiently to impair health. Thus, thin though the skin may be, it still suffices to protect against average environmental adversity; certainly it does not ulcerate. Heat regulation, too, still carries on. It is only speculation whether an additional load is thrown on the cutaneous vasomotor mechanism involving the overexercise of more than one part of the general nervous machinery of the individual.

The most likely, but at present undemonstrated rôle for the skin in regard to general health, lies in the possibilities of functions endocrinologic (sebaceous glands), metabolic (fat soluble and other vitamins), and immunologic.

7. SUMMARY

The skin is unique as a field for the direct observation of ageing processes and for furnishing tissue directly from itself for study, thus supplying the most unequivocal of signs of ageing, to say nothing of permitting a study of their development stage by stage. This gives a starting point that is definite, and removes many sources of error in the analysis of processes. A larger number of positive statements can therefore be made about ageing of the skin than about most other organs. The fact that few dermatoses are death dealing does not impair the usefulness of the skin in the investigation of ageing.

The following processes are concerned beyond question in cutaneous ageing: atrophy (graying of hair, baldness, thinning of skin with smoothness, and dystrophy of the toenails); degeneration of (particularly elastic) tissue (wrinkles); and withdrawal of some of the subcutaneous fat. As questionably senile changes—meaning that processes additional to senility may be concerned, a goodly number of progressive changes are listed—seborrheic keratosis, hyperpigmentation, sebaceous hyperplasia, and elastic and fibrous (but local) tissue hyperplasia (acrochordon). Telangiectasis also falls here, but may be due to degeneration of fibrous tissue. Precocious ageing of the skin is expressed in the form of elastic tissue hyperplasia and has a prototype in the disease xeroderma pigmentosum.

With retrograde processes dominating the picture during ageing of tissues at large, the senile skin contrasts with most other organs by presenting two unequivocally progressive lesions, namely acrochordon and seborrheic keratosis. In the absence of inflammatory features, endocrine factors should attract thought and investigation in connection with these, particularly since there are certain discrepancies between them and the nevi with which they are rather naively classified. At least an endocrine factor might contribute to their development. The same might be said of senile elastosis if it be true that the process concerned is really hyperplasia. Unfortunately, none of the progressive alterations are of the kind which would counterbalance the regressive changes met with in ageing.

Leads to the rôle of heredity in ageing of the skin, while tenuous, are attractive because a definite chemical, hematoporphyrin, is available as a base from which to start.

Physiologic changes are numerous. Chilliness and itching are familiar even to the laity. There are cycles of sebaceous activity at certain periods of life. Since endocrines are known to influence the distribution and quality of hair they may conceivably be the basis for senescence of hair. There is ample food for thought, too, in connection with the physiology of subcutaneous fatty tissue; in addition to special constituents of fatty tissue such as cholesterol which have been long known, the rôle of vitamins (particularly fat-soluble) attaches fresh interest and perhaps significance to this fat-storing tissue because so much knowledge has become recently available about them.

Certain chemicals (water, sulphur, chloride, and arsenic) are conspicuous in the skin and sufficiently involve factors of one or other sort (growth, drying) to merit attention in research on ageing. In short, it begins to appear that the skin is a storage place not only for fat but for a number of other substances. Lack of accommodation for them in the skin may possibly have a bearing upon general bodily welfare.

In any event, the observability of the skin, and its accessibility for study make it an ideal field for investigation of the processes of ageing, not only of itself but possibly also of important internal organs.

REFERENCES

BATSON, O. V. 1928. The anatomy of the corium. Science, **67**, 198–199.

BROWN, H., AND KLAUDER, J. V. 1933. Sulphur content of hair and of nails in abnormal states. Arch. Dermat. & Syph., **27**, 584–604.

DANFORTH, C. H. 1925. Hair. 152 pages. Chicago: American Medical Association, published serially in Arch. Dermat. & Syph., Apr.–Oct. 1925.

EJIRI, I. 1936. Histology of human skin: II. On differences in the elastic fibers of the skin according to sex and age. Jap. J. Dermat. & Urol., **40**, 216–217. Abst. in Arch. Dermat. & Syph., 1938, **37**, 664.

——— 1937. Histologic studies of human skin: III. Changes according to region and to age, of different elements of the skin, with particular consideration of changes of the elastic fibers with age. Jap. J. Dermat. & Urol., **41**, 8–12. Abst. in Arch. Dermat. & Syph., 1938, **37**, 666.

GARROD, A. E. 1923. Inborn Errors of Metabolism. London: Frowde and Hodder and Stoughton, Second edition, 216 pp.

GILMAN, R. L. 1937. Adenomatoid sebaceous tumors, with particular reference to adenomatoid hyperplasia. Arch. Dermat. & Syph., **35**, 633–642.

GRAY, A. M. H. 1926. Sclerema neonatorum. Arch. Dermat. & Syph., **14**, 635–654.

GREENBAUM, S. 1924. Immunity in ringworm infections (active acquired). Arch. Dermat. & Syph., **10**, 279–288.

HAMMETT, F. S., AND REIMANN, S. P. 1929. Cell proliferation response to sulfhydryl in mammals. J. Exper. Med., **50**, 445–448.

HELLER, J. 1927. The diseases of the nails. Berlin: Springer, Handb. d. Haut. u. Geschlkr. 13: Part 2, 34.

KAHN, R. L. 1938. The skin in immunity and allergy. To be published in J. Investig. Dermat.

KLAUDER, J. V., AND BROWN, H. 1936. Certain phases of sulfur metabolism of the skin. Arch. Dermat. & Syph., **34**, 568–581.

KYRLE, J. 1925. Histobiology of Human Skin and Its Diseases. Berlin: Springer, Vol. 1, 345 pp.

LYNCH, F. W. 1934. Xeroderma pigmentosum, a study in sensitivity to light. Arch. Dermat. & Syph., **29**, 858–873.

PILLSBURY, D. M., AND STERNBERG, T. H. 1937. Relation of diet to cutaneous infection. Arch. Dermat. & Syph., **35**, 893–906.

ROBERTSON, W. E. 1934. Physical diagnosis from the time of Roentgen. Ann. Med. Hist., **6**, 255–263.

ROTHMAN, ST., AND SCHAFF, FR., JADASSOHN, J. 1929. Handb. der Haut. u. Geschlechtskr. Berlin: Julius Springer, 1/2, 312–313.

SCHAMBERG, J. F., AND BROWN, H. 1923. A study of the blood uric acid in diseases of the skin with particular reference to eczema and pruritus. Arch. Dermat. & Syph., **8**, 801–817.

TEMPLETON, H. J. 1936. Cutaneous tags of the neck. Arch. Dermat. & Syph., **33**, 495–505.

TROTTER, M. 1922. A study of facial hair in the white and negro races. Washington University Studies, Scientific Series, **9**, 273–289.

TUFT, L. 1931. The skin as an immunological organ. J. Immunol., **21**, 85–100.

WADSWORTH, W. S. 1915. Post-mortem Examinations. Philadelphia: W. B. Saunders Co., 598 pp.

WAY, S. C. 1931. The sebaceous glands. Arch. Dermat. & Syph., **24**, 353–370.

WEIDMAN, F. D. 1931. The pathology of the yellowing dermatoses. Arch. Dermat. & Syph., **24**, 954–991.

CHAPTER 13

THE THYROID, PANCREATIC ISLETS, PARATHYROIDS, ADRENALS, THYMUS, AND PITUITARY

A. J. CARLSON

Chicago

As differentiation and specificity in the endocrine glands appear as marked in long life as in short life species, and since the "accidents of living," such as infections, dietary deficiencies or excesses and other forms of stress on the individual are on the whole probably not greater in the short life species, the primary "timer" of the life span is evidently hereditary factors not essentially conditioned on tissue differentiation. Accordingly, the hypothesis that the elements of senescence are inherent in the processes of differentiation does not seem fundamental. On this hypothesis the problem of ageing embraces the entire life span of the individual. Even if this hypothesis did express some truth, it is not very useful at the present stage of biology, in part because of the lack of adequate methods for testing it. We shall therefore focus our attention mainly on the late adult and the advanced age periods, since here we have both data and methods of testing their interpretation, albeit much of the data may be irrelevant or inconclusive, some of the methods need refinement, and most of the experimental material requires improved control.

1. NEED FOR CONTROLLED DATA

Well controlled data on age changes in the functions of the endocrines, apart from the gonads, is at present very meager. Most of the data relate to gross weight, and histologic structure of these glands relative to age. These structural findings cannot at present be given definite functional interpretations, partly because of the very large "factors of safety" in all of these glands. Great decrease in gross size, or great reduction in size or number of cells, may not therefore signify reduced output of hormones. Even the quantity of hormones per weight of glands, at different ages, cannot at present be related to hyper or hypo-activity, even were the methods of extraction reliably quantitative, because we do not know the precise relation between production, storage, and secretion. Before a significant chapter on ageing of the endocrines can be written, we must have data on the actual output of the hormones by age in controlled material. Observations on the concentration of the hormones in the blood, and in rare cases in the urine, in controlled material are urgently needed. We stress "controlled material" for the following reasons:

1. The structure, and probably the activity, of at least some of the endocrines is related to the diet, both as to quality and quantity. Controlled material would thus seem to call for an optimum diet throughout the period of observation. This is particularly the case with the vitamins, and with iodine, in case of the thyroid glands. The frequent, if not invariable impairment of the digestive processes with advanced age (see Ivy, Chapter 9) may, indeed, be a factor in slowing up hormone production through the dietary factor.

2. Some of the endocrines appear to be subject to histologic, if not functional, injuries by systemic or focal infections. When these cannot be avoided in controlled material, their number and relative severity should at least be part of the record when the data on change in endocrine function are to be related to age, directly or indirectly.

3. The factor of heredity might be ignored when observations are made on the hormone concentrations in the blood of the same individual, from youth to old age, or when the structural changes in these glands are followed in the same individual by the biopsy method. But heredity becomes important when random observations are on a mixed population, the observations, at that, being made on different individuals, for the different age groups. The fact that some individuals develop diabetes at the age of 10, others at the age of 50, while others may live to ninety or a hundred years without diabetes, may or may not be related to an hereditary resistance or endurance factor in the pancreas complex. Similarly, some do develop what appears to be spontaneous myxedema before 40, while others do not show it clearly even at 80. But we cannot assume at present that such hereditary "endurance factors" are not involved, even though they do not tell the whole story.

4. Since there is fairly good evidence that structural as well as functional changes in the endocrines are induced by impaired blood flow through these glands, "controlled material" implies not only parallel observations on the cardiovascular system, especially in individuals of advanced years, but renders observations on the endocrines on those individuals who reach very advanced age, with the minimum of vascular impairment, particularly important as the latter would serve as a check

on the endocrine age involution, if any, in the presence of inadequate blood flow.

5. In addition to diet, infections, heredity, and vascular adequacy, the attack on the rôle of the endocrine in the ageing process is further complicated by the growing evidence of some dependence, in the matter of structure and hormone output, of each endocrine on the hormone output of one or more of the other endocrine glands. In this respect the gonads seem to form a significant exception. While the very life of the gonads depend on hormones from the pituitary, the thyroids, and possibly the adrenal cortex, total loss of the gonad hormones, as by castration in early adult life, has so slight influence on the other endocrines in direction of impaired function, that no definite syndrome of hypofunction develops, there appears to be no premature ageing, physically or mentally, reliable established and there seems to be no shortening of the life span. But as to the complex interdependence of the other major endocrines (thyroid, anterior pituitary, adrenal cortex, the pancreas islets), there is now no doubt. And so our "controlled material" on the rôle of the endocrines in the ageing process involves simultaneous checking of the functions of at least five of the major endocrines at each age level.

The earlier theory that the gradual failure of the endocrines is the main factor in the ageing process (Horsley, 1884; Lorand, 1910; Gley, 1922; etc.) has not been substantiated by subsequent work, although it must be granted that this work is largely fragmentary and inconclusive. The clear case of the gonad atrophy with age, particularly the ovaries in the human species (see Chapter 14), has rendered this general theory plausible and attractive. But on closer analysis, the atrophy of no single endocrine or group of endocrines can by itself readily account for the ageing process. And in more recent years the glamour of the gonads has tended to ascribe ageing mainly to failure of these glands and has given rise to the spectacular pseudo-science of "rejuvenation" via the route of the gonad hormones or gonad implantation.

If the data so far adduced are even approximately reliable, and our reasoning so far sound, it should be apparent to the reader why past observations on the ageing of the endocrines, even by competent and industrious investigators, have so little scientific value for our present task. The past interest in the ageing process has centered largely on man, where we cannot, or specifically have not to date, controlled the factors of diet, heredity, infections, and vascular adequacy. And our information on the interdependence of the major endocrines is not only very recent, but is even now replete with gaps and guesses. The ageing processes in the endocrines alone make a full time or major biological problem, calling for large material resources and the long pull. Without both, the scientific perspicacity naturally turns to the things that can be done, with present facilities, even if these may seem less interesting and fundamental.

Obviously the central theme or problem is the hereditary "time clock" in the endocrine glands themselves. And this includes the endocrine interrelation factors. This is the direct endocrine timer of the adequate life span. But it is equally evident that diet, infections, and vascular inadequacy may so impair endocrine function as to render the hormone output inadequate for the optimum bodily needs. Thus, by indirection, the endocrine may also here act as one of the timers of the adequate life span. In fact, some of these relations seem to operate in the manner of the vicious circle. Thus, hypothyroidism and diabetes reduce the resistance to infection and repeated or prolonged infections appear to cause further weakening of the "factors of persistence." Hypoparathyroidism tends to unstabilize the nervous system, and this, in turn is probably not a good omen for digestion, metabolism, and the cardiovascular system. While we propose to analyze our present data from both points of view (the direct and the indirect endocrine timer of the adequate life span), the reader is urged to temper, and if possible, improve our conclusions by the contributions of the other authors of this book.

2. THYROID

No organ or tissue in the human or animal body seems to work up to par in the total absence of the thyroid hormone. This has been made out most clearly in the experimental animal, notably the rabbit, in which species accessory or aberrant thyroid tissue is rare, so that total thyroidectomy can be accomplished. Total absence of the thyroid hormone in man appears to be very exceptional, but varying degrees of hypothyroidism in man have been studied extensively, and in all essentials these data on man conform to the findings in the better controlled experimental animal. All organs do not seem to be impaired to an equal degree after total thyroidectomy. For example, the life of the gonads are more profoundly impaired than is the function of the pancreas islets. The central defect induced by total absence of the thyroid hormone appears to be the reduction in the rate of tissue oxidation. Impairment of growth, of repair, decreased resistance to infections, tendency to fatty degeneration in muscle and many other tissues may be sequelae of the impaired oxidation. The following, fairly well established data, are on the whole consistent with the theory, but are by themselves no proof, that the production of the thyroid hormone, after attaining its normal maximum at puberty, decreases with advancing age by the gradual running down of the hereditary time clock.

1. The slow, but gradual reduction in the basal metabolic rate in otherwise healthy man, after the age of 20 to 25, seems well established. There is no reason for thinking that other animals do not exhibit the same phenomenon, though actual data are not yet at hand. Is the lowering of the B.M.R. with age due directly to a parallel advancing hypothyroidism? If so, there should be other evidence of increasing myxedema with age besides the low B.M.R. Those who (like Lorand) argue that this is the case appear to us to give undue weight to superficial resemblances, such as occasional increased body weight, dryness of skin, and failure of hair growth on the scalp. In the total body oxidation as measured by the B.M.R. method, the skeletal muscles seem to contribute the major factor. Now, decreased skeletal muscle efficiency, muscle tone, etc., not to speak of fatty degeneration and other indices of muscle atrophy with advancing age, whatever be the cause or causes, appear to be on a firmer scientific basis, than is age involution of thyroid function. The primary thyroid responsibility for the age changes in the skeletal muscles is not established, and appears to us improbable, because were those the only causal relations, we ought to see a parallel impairment of brain function, as is the case in true cretinism and myxedema. On the contrary, intellectual processes may in man actually show an ascending curve, while physical capacity and endurance (mainly muscle efficiency) are descending.

2. There is a superficial resemblance between the impairments appearing in the skin and the hair with advancing age and those induced by varying degrees of hypothyroidism. But it is well known that loss of the hair color or even baldness of the scalp may occur in some people as early as the age of 25 to 30, with no other indices of hypothyroidism. It is further known that at the very time that the age involution of the human scalp hair is advancing, hair on other parts of the body (eyebrows, nares, ears, etc.) may exhibit increased growth. Moreover, the skin and hair defects due to true hypothyroidism can be largely checked by administration of the thyroid hormone. If the thyroid hormone has

the same efficacy in the case of loss of scalp hair or hair color with advancing age, the numerous and assiduous inventors of "hair restorers" have certainly overlooked a bet!

3. In the experimental animal at least marked hypothyroidism somehow produces a lowered resistance to infections, particularly infections of the respiratory tract, such as sinusitis, bronchitis and pneumonia. In man the incidence of infectious diseases in childhood, adult life, and advanced age is complicated by the immunities induced by several types of infections usually occurring in childhood. In infections where little or no immunity is induced, such as colds, pneumonia, and many of the streptococcal infections, the greater incidence of these with advancing old age is not yet clearly established. What appears to be indicated is a reduced capacity to combat these forms of infection in the old, and hence the greater prevalence of chronic arthritis or rheumatism, the higher mortality from pneumonia, etc., in the aged. This is consistent with the theory of primary hypothyroidism with advancing age, but since these facts can be otherwise interpreted, they constitute no proof of the theory.

4. In the experimental animal total absence of the thyroid hormone, or at least a very marked hypothyroidism induces weakness and atony of the skeletal muscles, accompanied by fatty degeneration in these muscles (as well as in the heart muscle). We are not acquainted with any data on biopsies on the skeletal muscles of human cretins and myxedematous adults, hence we cannot, at present view the skeletal muscle weakness atrophy, and signs of degeneration, or the myocardial degeneration in advanced age as causally related to a primary hypothyroidism. It seems to us the same caution is called for in relating other age involution or tissue atrophies, such as arterial sclerosis to thyroid function. A certain degree of chronic hyperthyroidism seems to induce myocardial degeneration and sclerosis, and is thought by some to be one factor in inducing or accelerating arterial sclerosis. The fact is that the primary relation of the thyroid hormone, hypo or hyper, to these usual tissue changes with advanced age is as yet an open question.

5. The literature contains considerable information on the usual gross and microscopic changes in the human thyroid gland from early intrauterine life to ripe old age. If we eliminate the instances of frank and possibly primary thyroid disease (hypo and hyperthyroidism, thyroid tumors) the gland appears to attain its maximum normal size (and possibly function) at the age period of 15 to 20. At this age

there appears to be considerable replacement of the epithelial cells, as indicated by the numerous cell divisions. The acini tend to be fairly round in outline, uniform in size, and lined with a single layer of cuboidal epithelium. According to Cooper (1925), based on human post mortem material, the thyroid of people from 60 to 80 years of age is reduced in size, the follicles and the cells are smaller, the vascular supply is reduced, there is much less mitosis seen in the epithelial cells, the colloid may be absent from many of the vesicles, and the colloid, when present, appears less dense. There is definite increase in the connective tissue (sclerosis). Less notable changes in the thyroid are described for the adult period of 40–50. McCarrison states that the human thyroid after the age of 40 shows less colloid, sclerosed blood vessels, and increased connective tissue. Dogliotti and Nizzi-Nuti (1935) report on the structure of the thyroid of 50 late adult and aged people, eliminating those of frank thyroid disease, and the thyroids of patients dying with severe infections. According to these authors, in the thyroid of the "pre senile" (50–65 years) the follicles are reduced in size and in colloid content, while during the "senile period" (over 65) the follicles are so reduced in size that the cavities are practically obliterated, with no colloid present, but there is some increase in the connective tissue. These authors interpret these age changes in the thyroid gland as indicating an increase in the output of the thyroid hormone with advancing age, the very opposite of the views of most authors on the thyroid-age problem.

There are some data indicating a reduced amount of iodine per weight of gland in aged human thyroids. This work requires repeating with our present superior chemical methods, and on controlled material, before it is worth while to even essay an interpretation. From the field of frank hyper- and hypothyroidism in man it appears that reduced iodine content per weight of gland may be present with lessened as well as with increased output of thyroid hormone. And the minimum iodine content of the gland commensurate with adequate thyroid hormone turnover for the age of the individual is not yet known.

Most anatomists, pathologists and, indeed, internists and physiologists are probably inclined to interpret the above gross and microscopic changes in the thyroid gland of late adult life and advanced old age in man as evidence of primary hypothyroidism. But we are impatient with mere interpretation where we may experiment and thus know. In view of the very large factors of safety in the normal thyroids, only controlled experiments can tell how far reduction in gross size of the gland, reduction in size and number of the epithelial cells, reduction in iodine and in colloid, reduction in vascularity, and increase in connective tissue can go before the output of the thyroid hormone falls below what may be determined as the normal or optimum rate.

6. Experimental as well as clinical evidence indicate that the thyroid hormone is one of the many factors concerned in the water balance in the tissues. At any rate in marked hypothyroidism there is a tendency to increase tissue water, while the initial reduction in body weight by hyperthyroidism is in part a matter of loss of tissue water through diuresis and sweating, followed by increased thirst, water ingestion, and a tendency to a continuous higher level of urine output. Now that tissue desiccation, rather than tissue hydration appears to be the rule in the ageing, the matter is referred to here, as one which by itself is not consistent with the view of significant hypofunction in the thyroid of advanced age.

7. While the possible rôle of the gonad hormones (especially the female) and the anterior pituitary so-called thyrotropic substance in the regulation of the normal rate of thyroid hormone secretion is by no means clearly established at least for the dog, yet we have these facts: in some species, at least, a temporary thyroid hyperplasia, and increased hormone output by something present in an extract of the anterior pituitary; the normally maximum thyroid size and possibly function in the adolescent years; the apparently more frequent occurrence of hyperthyroidism during the years of most active gonad function; the more frequent occurrence of hyperthyroidism in the human female than in the human male. The gonads atrophy with age. The ageing anterior pituitary exhibits some changes that may indicate but do not prove reduced hormone output. We advance no theory and offer no interpretation, as we do not know the facts. We merely refer to these indices as something to be considered in any well planned research project on thyroid and age.

8. Marine and Baumann (1922), and Scott (1922), report that in rabbits and cats adreno-cortical insufficiency raises the B.M.R. when the thyroid gland is intact, but not after thyroidectomy. This is being interpreted as an inhibitory action of the cortical hormone on the secretion of or on the systemic action of the thyroid hormone. The fact itself calls for re-investigation. The interpretation will probably not stand, for increased B.M.R. is not an element of Addison's disease in man, and Schachter has been unable to lower the B.M.R.

in normal dogs or in dogs rendered hyperthyroid by injecting large quantities of an active cortical extract (personal communication).

9. Some thyroid growth disturbances, and possibly disturbance of function may be prevented by iodine therapy and can therefore not be primarily hereditary. And yet both cretinism and myxedema do appear in populations where iodine ingestion seems to be at least minimal, and where iodine therapy is of little or no remedial value. In these cases defective hereditary thyroid potentials must at least be considered. Myxedema in man may come on in late adult life without previous history of earlier thyroid failure, even though frank myxedema appears not to increase with the advancing years beyond 40 or 50. It is, of course, entirely possible that these premature thyroid failures are not hereditary, but due to other types of injuries. If real thyroid heredity enters here, it is probably exceptional only in degree. That is to say, heredity may time the life span of all thyroid glands, but for the present, and excluding frank thyroid disease, the thyroid life span appears not to be the limiting link in the life, or rather the adequate life, of the aged. We say this despite the advocates of the use of thyroid substance as a helpful therapy for the years of decline, and even the reports of "curing senility" (!) by thyroid administration. When thyroid substance is found to have real value in the aged, its action is probably non-specific. The very aged may feel somewhat better temporarily after any stimulating therapy, such as a warm bath, massage, strychnine, ephedrine, caffeine, or even whiskey.

10. Many dietary factors, besides the quantity of iodine, appear to modify thyroid structure, if not function (McCarrison, 1917, 1920; Jackson, 1917, 1925; Marine, Baumann and Cipra, 1925; Herrington). These factors may play a rôle in the thyroid structure and function of the aged man and animal, where qualitative and quantitative food intake is in many cases likely to be less than the optimum. This will probably be a disturbing factor in the study of thyroid function in the very old individual, even in controlled populations, as appetite, hunger, digestive power, and metabolic efficiency may present barriers to conclusive experiments.

3. PANCREATIC ISLETS

1. Much water has gone over the dam on the pancreas-diabetes problem since the classical observations of von Mering and Minkowski on pancreatectomized dogs. The theory of pancreas hormone action

has mainly proved out, over the theory of a pancreas detoxication function, thanks largely to that other classical work of Banting, Best, Collip, and McLeod. But with growth of understanding has come increasing complexity: The islets and insulin are not the only factors. There is in all probability a second pancreas hormone, the lipocaic of Dragstedt, involved in the carbohydrate-fat interchange, at least in the liver. The work of Houssay and Biasotti (1931) showed a probable anterior pituitary factor, while the work of Soskin and others (1934) points to important relations of the liver and, in all probability, the blood capillary and muscle cell permeability. The possibility that the second pancreas hormone (lipocaic) is identical with the omnipresent cholin seems to be dispelled by Dragstedt's latest work, in which he has succeeded in so nearly completely removing the cholin from his extract that the trace of cholin left is too small to have any influence on the fatty livers of pancreatectomized dogs controlled by insulin (personal communication). But in experimental and in spontaneous human diabetes the pancreas islets and insulin still constitute the one indispensable link in the diabetic processes. All human diabetes appear to be influenced, in the direction of control, by insulin; and in the otherwise normal animal impairment or destruction of the pancreas appears to be the only sure way of reproducing true clinical diabetes. But we see no satisfactory explanation of the fact that the human diabetic needing even large quantities of insulin seems to get along without the lipocaic being supplied, and without developing a degree of fatty degeneration of the liver leading to death, while the pancreatectomized dog on adequate insulin control and without lipocoic dies within a few months with extremely fatty liver as a probable factor in the death. Of course, human diabetes is rarely absolute, some islet function usually remains. And there are indications that in the usually more severe form of juvenile diabetes fatty livers may develop, even under good insulin management. The lipocaic probably comes from the islets, as shown by the fact that on the nearly complete degeneration of the pancreas tissue producing the external secretion following ligation of the ducts, the islets remain relatively intact and neither diabetes nor fatty liver develop. If, as seems probable, the insulin and the lipocaic are produced by different islet cells, there may be a differential impairment of these two types of cells in human diabetes. Should this prove true, we may have to consider the pancreas factor (lipocaic) in other forms of fatty degeneration of the liver, not related to diabetes as we now think of this disease.

2. Before any generalizations are made anent the rôle of the pancreas islets in the ageing process, the following questions must be cleared up:

(a) While true spontaneous diabetes is not unknown in domestic animals, notably the dog, this disease appears to be distinctly more common in the human species. This may be a matter of lack of information in the case of the domestic animals. On the other hand, it may be due to a greater hereditary potential of the islet tissue in animals below man. There are some indications that the islets may be injured, temporarily or permanently by such factors as infections, extreme dietary disgression, marked hyperthyroidism, etc. But man is not the only species prone to overeating, and subject to all manner of infections, temporary and chronic.

(b) Again, in animals like the dog and the rabbit, there is normally so much excess islets present that from 9/10 to 15/16 of the islets may be removed before the sugar tolerance is so reduced that the Sandmeyer type of diabetes shows up. If a somewhat greater portion of the pancreas is left in the animal this remanent hypertrophies, in some cases to near the size of the original pancreas. We have no such accurate data on the factors of safety in the islets in the non-diabetic man, to be sure, but there is scarcely any exception to the rule that once a person, young or old, becomes a diabetic, he is a diabetic for life. The degree of diabetes may become more severe with time. Even under controlled conditions the diabetes rarely becomes less severe. That means, practically, the absence of regenerative capacity of the islet tissue (including the cells of the pancreatic ducts) in the human diabetic. Is this also true for the non-diabetic man? We are reluctant to accept, without better evidence, such a profound difference between man and the lower animals. There is, of course, a marked difference between surgical removal of part of the pancreas in the healthy animal, and the impairment of the pancreas islets by infections or overeating in man. The first procedure leaves the pancreas remnant normal, though possibly subject to overstrain; the latter may hit mature islet function and regenerative power with equal severity and permanency. To the extent that such injuries are favored by hereditary weakness in persistence, that weakness may be primarily in the capacity of regeneration.

(c) Statistics show unmistakably that obesity predisposes to diabetes in man (Joslyn, 1929). But which is the horse in this combination? The fact that overeating renders existing mild diabetes more severe, that partial starvation of a diabetic individual renders severe diabetes milder, that mass starvation reduces the incidence of new cases of diabetes in a population would seem to make the diet (overeating) the primary factor. Now, overeating to the point of marked adiposity is not unknown among animals (hogs, steers, some animals preparing for hibernation) without diabetes, or more specifically, without information that diabetes is the sequel. In the case of the domestic steer and hog, the answer may be that the time is too brief. The hibernating animal may give the islets a chance to recuperate in the subsequent months of starvation. But there are the permanently very obese marine mammals. Work could be done on the seal. The hog, as measured by alimentary glycosuria, indicates low sugar tolerance, but that does not necessarily mean reduced islet capacity and predisposition to diabetes. If it should turn out that the "prediabetic" glucose tolerance curve (John, 1934) really means eventual diabetes (barring death by accident), the glucose tolerance test might be a useful tool in securing data on the islet adequacy in animal populations.

The precise relation of direct and indirect nervous states to the islet-metabolism machinery is still an unknown. We have reports that "mental strain" may aggravate an existing diabetes, and call for larger doses of insulin, but even if so, such influences are probably both superficial (glycogenolysis) and temporary. We may assume that much of the acute but temporary fear of wild animals and primitive men has shifted to the prolonged anxieties of civilization. On a vascular basis the latter may do something to the pancreas islets, but hardly more so than to the liver and the gut.

3. Inadequate islet mechanisms, as indicated by lowered sugar tolerance, frank diabetes, and its control by insulin, may develop in man from earliest infancy on to the age of more than 90 years. The curve of incidence rises slowly, with the peak at the 40–50 age period. From the age of 60 on there is a very definite decline (Joslyn and Dublin, 1936; Dublin and Lotka, 1937). Since the onset of the defect may be gradual, and in its incipient stages may go unrecognized, the true curve of incidence (i.e., the beginning) fall probably further to the left (lower age periods) than present statistics indicate. The appearance of true diabetes in infants at the age of one or two years, and the absence of diabetes in men and women at the age of 80 would seem to indicate that hereditary persistence factors in the islet mechanisms are involved, irrespective of how much infections, dietary digression and other possible types of strain may be contributary. The latter may help to explain the increasing incidence of islet break-

down up to the age of 50, but neither heredity nor environment (internal and external) can account for the reduced incidence of diabetes in people past sixty. It can scarcely be gonad atrophy, since castration appears to have no such profound influence on the carbohydrate and fat metabolism. If, speaking in percentage of the age population, more people past sixty eat more sparingly, in relation to their physiological needs, than is the case in the population below sixty, we do not yet know it. We can conceive an hereditary persistence factor in the islets that would still be adequate even at the (alleged) age of Tom Parr. But even this assumption does not readily square with the reduced incidence of diabetes in old age. A "quantum theory" of inherited persistence might help, but such a concept does not fit the curve below sixty. Perhaps the present statistics are unreliable.

4. Atrophies, hydropic degeneration, sclerosis, etc., have been described in the pancreas (islets as well as the other tissue) of adult and old people, diabetic and non-diabetic (Opie, 1903; Allen, 1922). The earlier workers found more degenerative changes in the islets of the diabetics than in the non-diabetics of similar age groups. In man the pancreas as a whole seems to be labile or readily damaged, by dietary digression as well as by local and systemic infections. When the islet factor has been greatly reduced by surgery, high food intake seems to induce or aggravate atrophic or degenerative changes in the islet cells (Hedon, Allen, 1922). In regard to infections, it is assumed that these damage the prediabetic islets permanently, but the only thing we really know in the matter is this: infections, as well as many other things, increase temporarily but rarely permanently the insulin requirement of the diabetic man. This may or may not be solely a matter of depression of an already defective islet mechanism. It probably is not. At any rate it seems unlikely that infections by themselves should induce permanent islet damage in the prediabetic but not in the diabetic state. If it is infection, it must be infection plus. The earlier accounts of rather marked histopathology in the pancreas islets of human diabetics have been somewhat challenged by later observers, and it is fair to say that in some cases the islets, even of a patient dead in diabetic coma, may show less pathology than one would expect, on the basis of the large factors of safety in the islet mechanism of dogs and rabbits. But this is probably very superficial reasoning. For we do not know when and to what degree the anterior pituitary or the thyroid may render a moderate diabetes more severe, and we must know more about the state of the liver, and the degree of reduction in insulin output before

the islet cells show any histopathology. Even more to the point, we should know the amount of insulin in the blood of these people who are reported to die of diabetes, with so little evident pathology in the islet cells. Not that we would urge less work, or especially less quantitative work, on human diabetics and so-called prediabetics of all ages, but owing to the unsatisfactory control of human material even at best, a prime desideration now is a concerted attack on a controlled animal population through its entire life span, with the technique on tissues, body fluids, and hormone quantitation now available. Then, and not till then, will we be in position to say, for one species at least, whether or no the islet mechanism alters with age to such an extent that it becomes one of causative factors in the general ageing process. For the present the only thing we can say with certainty is that the depression of the islets mechanisms (causes unknown, but probably in part hereditary and dietary) leading to diabetes handicaps age and tends to shorten the life span of some people. For the optimum control of the diabetic state through diet, insulin, and possibly lipocaic, is not readily maintained throughout every day for months and years. Tolerance in the diabetic does fluctuate from causes so far unknown, and less than optimum control seem to reduce the resistance to infections.

Arterial sclerosis is a fairly constant phenomenon in ageing men, and in such other animals as have been adequately investigated to date (see Chapter 7). It may be noted in connection with islet function and diabetes that earlier or more extensive arterial sclerosis appears in many diabetic individuals of early adult age even when the diabetic condition appears adequately controlled by insulin and diet. The precise islet factor in this phenomenon is obscure. Since reduced islet function appears to predispose to infections, and infections stand at least accused in the etiology of arterial sclerosis, one of the causes may be disclosed up that alley.

4. PARATHYROIDS

1. According to Cooper (1925) the human parathyroids do not attain adult size and histologic structure until the period of puberty and adolescence. The importance of these developmental changes, as well as the reported appearance of relatively large cells with eosinophile granules in the parathyroids of young adults is difficult to evaluate, at present. The effects of parathyroidectomy do not seem to differ in youth from those in later years, except that they tend to set in earlier and be more rapidly fatal in very young animals. Only one hormone,

THE THYROID, PARATHYROIDS, AND PITUITARY

the chemical involved in calcium and phosphorus balance in the body, is even approximately known from these glands. The increase in connective tissue in the gland in early adult age and its fairly regular distribution around the epithelial cell groups tend to give the gland the appearance of embryonic thyroids. Colloid has been described both in and in between the gland cells, but whether this is a sign of secretion or of degeneration is not yet known. The difficulties in interpreting histologic findings in the light of function in these glands are illustrated by the fact that Houssay and others (1931) report impairment of the parathyroid after total hypophysectomy. Now it appears well established that no symptom of functional deficiency clearly related to the parathyroids follows ablation of the pituitary gland.

The earlier theory of identity in hormone function of the parathyroids and the thyroids had the support of apparent identity in embryonic origin. But nothing remains of that theory, except possibly the newer fact that massive doses of thyroid extract ameliorates the symptoms of parathyroidectomy in dogs. However, the mechanism of this action has not yet been satisfactorily worked out.

The potency of the theory of detoxication as a parathyroid function has been weakened by the discovery of the hormone mechanism. The greater susceptibility to systemic disturbances from gastro-intestinal disorder in the parathyroidectomized animal may be secondary to the upset in the blood-tissue calcium balance. According to Cooper (1925) the blood supply to the human parathyroids increases with age. This calls for verification.

Like most of the other endocrines the "factors" of safety in the parathyroids are very large, at least four to five times the minimum needs, and the parathyroids appear to have about the same growth and regenerative capacity as the thyroid tissue.

But several additional baffling facts remain to plague the workers in the parathyroid field: (a) the periodicity in the severity of some of the hypoparathyroid symptoms; (b) the gradual adjustment of the experimental animal (dog) to apparently total absence of parathyroid hormone and low (4–6 mgm. per 100 cc.) blood calcium, provided life is saved in the first 5–6 weeks after the total parathyroidectomy; (c) the lack of indication of a similar adjustment in man; (d) the temporary efficacy, but frequent failure after months, particularly in man, of calcium or parathyroid hormone therapy, especially the latter, in frank hypoparathyroidism.

2. The parathyroid hormone, together with vitamin D, appears to be involved in the absorption and elimination, as well as with the actual deposition or stability of the tissue calcium. The actual level of the calcium in the blood is in part a function of the concentration of the plasma proteins, the greater part of the blood calcium existing there as a calcium proteinate. Hypoparathyroidism lowers the blood calcium and increases its excretion, largely at the expense of the calcium in the bones. In hyperparathyroidism (which may occur spontaneously in man, in cases of hyperplasia of the glands) the blood calcium is elevated, also largely at the expense of the bone calcium. So we have, as is to be expected the opposite influence of the hypo and hyper states on blood calcium concentration, but the same effect (but not in degree), that is, depletion of the bone calcium. The level of dietary calcium seems not to play a major rôle in these complex parathyroid hormone relations, but it is, of course, important as a long run factor. Significant hypoparathyroidism seems always to lower the plasma calcium below the normal, and thanks to the good quantitative methods for estimating the calcium content of the blood now available, and the ease of securing, from man and animals, the quantity of blood needed for such determinations, we seem to have, provisionally at least, a good measure of parathyroid hypo-function in any species at any age. The situation is less satisfactory, as regards parathyroid hyperfunction, because information so far indicates that much calcium may be taken out of the bones, under excess parathyroid hormone influence, without raising the plasma calcium much above the high normal. We need not point out that present methods of parathyroid hormone isolation are too crude to yield anything of quantitative value either as to the blood or the parathyroids in youth and old age.

3. There are, at present, no clear indications either in the parathyroids themselves, or in the general course of the ageing processes, that hypo or hyperfunction of the parathyroids play any significant rôle in the impairments of the aged. Of course, we have no data on controlled material. But the blood calcium in man appears to remain within the normal limits up to 80 years and beyond. The calcium content of the bones of the aged may be "normal," increased or decreased, but there is no clear evidence that the failure or the excess of parathyroid hormone is involved in any deviations from the supposed "normal." There appears to be a definite decrease in the power of healing or repair of bones in old age, and the parathyroid hormone does seem to influence both osteoblasts and osteclasts, but changes in

the hereditary potentials of these cells must first be discounted before we can consider parathyroid hormone factors, as the land lies now. Various forms of nervous instabilities, such as paralysis agitans, are not infrequent sequelae of the ageing of man, and deficiency of parathyroid hormone produces instability in the nervous system. But hyper-excitable nervous states appear at any age, and despite much work to date clear involvement of the parathyroids seems limited to the tetany of hypoparathyroidism.

In the chronic hypoparathyroid animal (dog), certain dietary digressions, physiological and environmental strains seem to call for more parathyroid hormone, or at least, bring the state of hypoparathyroidism, or into clearer manifestations. But on the whole, these are strains of youth and younger adult life rather than those of old age. There are other indications (in the case of the rat) that diet and environment (temperature) both influence the severity of some symptoms of hypoparathyroidism.

Because of the importance of the parathyroids in the calcium metabolism, the query: What rôle (hyper or hypo) does parathyroid hormone play in the increased deposition of calcium in so many tissues, notably the blood vessels and the lens, with age, is to the point, and must be included in any real solution of the ageing problem.

5. ADRENALS

Armchair biologists have found little difficulty in pointing out the almost perfect parallel between the symptomatology of ageing (in absence of specific disease) and that of impaired adreno-cortical function, such as general asthenia, impairment of digestion, tendency to increased pigmentation of the skin, low basal metabolic rate, etc., and thus make out a plausible case for adreno-cortical failure as an important causative factor in the decline of the organism as a whole in what we consider advanced age for the species.

The usual hypertension in advanced age does not fit this picture, for one of the cardinal symptoms of significant impairment of hormone production by the cortex is profound and lasting hypotension. Turning to the adrenal medulla, and ignoring for the moment the above theory, excess adrenalin output was for a time seriously thought to be one of the significant factors in inducing or accelerating the usual arterial sclerosis found in the aged. Hence, the cortex contributes to the ageing process via hypofunction, the medulla via hyperfunction. Turning another intellectual summersault, we could drag the emergency theory of medullary function into the ageing nexus, for surely the aged individuals or at least those of very advanced age are progressively less able to meet all manner of physiological emergencies. They can't stand up in a fight even to a junior Dempsey or Louis, and in a marathon they will lose to a Nurmi, even when allowed a twelve mile handicap. Thus, the medulla could contribute to the general ageing process, but this time via hypofunction. What are the *facts*?

1. *The medulla and adrenalin.*

For some years the theory of an adrenalin factor in arterial sclerosis has seemed exceedingly anemic from lack of factual sustenance. Stopping nearly all secretion of adrenalin in patients and experimental animals by adrenal denervation or by bilateral section of the major and minor splanchnic nerves does not induce hypotension nor does it seem to significantly or lastingly reduce hypertension. There is no reliable evidence of a change in the rate of adrenalin output with age either in man or animals. The significance of assays for adrenalin content of the glands secured at post mortems, even when reliable methods are employed, is obscured by the fact that adrenalin rapidly disappears from the gland or is altered after death and that infections per se seem to deplete the adrenalin content of the medulla.

We would expect reduced content and output of adrenalin in advanced sclerosis of the gland, but even in this case, in animals, the content and output are found to be in the normal range if age alone is the variable and no infection or disease prevails (Rogoff and Marcus, 1938).

The supposed adrenalin factor in diabetes is still without adequate proof, and its alleged factor in hypertension, except when associated with tumor of the medulla, has been fairly well disproven (Dragstedt, Prohaska and Harms, 1936; Rogoff and Marcus, 1938). We are, therefore, forced to conclude that valid data as to the ageing process in the medulla, and hence the medullary factor in the general nexus of ageing are not yet even on the horizon.

It is conceivable that although the function of the adrenal medulla is not indispensable for life or health (Stewart and Rogoff, 1919), since it can be removed surgically or its epinephrine secretion suppressed, epinephrine may exercise a rôle which over long periods may be reflected in the processes concerned with the development and course of senescence.

Epinephrine may be in some way related to mineral metabolism. It has been found that injected epinephrine is capable of modifying the reactions produced by calcium salts. Furthermore, epinephrine may be concerned with the distribution of potassium in the body (Camp, 1937). Thus, there might be postulated a possible functional interrelationship between cortex and medulla, if these observations can be said to represent the activity of physiologic quantities of epinephrine.

Constant injection of epinephrine, in physiologic quantities, have been found to augment the blood sugar and lactic acid (Cori, Cori and Burchwald, 1930). While such quantities as may cause this effect are rapidly destroyed in the circulation, it is conceivable that a prolonged or chronic state of mild hypersecretion (i.e., in the upper physiologic range) of epinephrine, might by these effects have an influence on the ageing processes of tissues or organs.

There is evidence that the ordinary secretion of epinephrine may exert an influence on the heart, perhaps on the irritability of heart muscle (Stewart and Rogoff, 1919). Quantities of epinephrine corresponding to the amounts secreted physiologically, when introduced at a constant rate can cause hemodynamic effects (Dragstedt et al., 1928). Whatever the underlying factor may be which gives rise to the development of the so-called sympathicoblastoma or phaeochromacytoma, in these conditions it seems almost certain that paroxysmal hypertension is in some way associated with excess epinephrine production. But we must also consider the possibility of an increase of the adrenalin-like "sympathin" in this condition. In fact, the probable production of adrenalin-like chemicals in most, if not all peripheral sympathetic nerve endings, necessarily weakens and questions much of the older work and interpretations anent the rôle of the adrenal medulla in the cardio-vascular processes in health and disease.

2. *The cortex.*

The extraordinary metamorphosis (degeneration and regeneration) of the human adrenal cortex the first few months after birth (Lewis and Pappenheimer, 1918; Cooper, 1925) needs no restatement in this chapter. The physiological significance of this is at present unknown, especially since it appears to be absent in the new born of many of the lower mammals. These profound cortical changes apparently go on hand in hand with the secretion of the life sustaining hormone or hormones, because so far as is known the cortical hormone is as necessary for health and life in early infancy as in later years; the well known adrenal apoplexy in the new born is a fatal condition.

In the healthy experimental animal at least one entire adrenal can be removed without inducing any deficiency symptoms whatsoever. As little as approximately one-twentieth of one gland, or less, if supplied with adequate blood circulation, suffices to maintain life and normal health (Rogoff and Stewart, 1926, 1928). And in species like the rat, with fragments (sometimes microscopic) of cortical tissue along the abdominal aorta, or elsewhere, the two chief adrenals may be removed without bringing on any recognizable symptoms of Addison's disease. There appears to be no reasons for thinking that the healthy man is not equally well provided with cortical tissue way above his minimal needs. Indeed, accessory cortical tissue is not at all uncommonly found if careful search is made at human autopsies. If this is so, we need not wonder that the cortex may show extensive injury incident on vascular sclerosis, local hemorrhage, systemic and local infections, etc., without recognizable symptoms of cortical deficiency.

While the adrenal cortex is labile to the extent that systemic infections, vitamin deficient diets, removal of the anterior pituitary, etc., induce changes that may signify depressor injuries, the hereditary persistence and resistance of the cortex is apparently great, for frank Addison's disease is much less common than are for example, diabetes, and myxedema in man, and, so far as we know, spontaneous Addison's disease is unknown in the lower animals.

The isolation of the life sustaining cortical hormone has been in progress for years. A slight storage of the hormone in all glands so far tested is unquestionable. The hormone appears very unstable under ordinary conditions. The methods of isolation and assay available at present are not sufficiently quantitative to yield data of significance in the assay of the hormone content of the blood or of the cortex itself at different ages.

Owing to changes in the adrenal cortex induced by such conditions as systemic infections, prolonged asthenia, malnutrition, pituitary gland ablation, etc., the histopathology of the mine run of post mortem adrenal glands is difficult to interpret. But apparently normal (or even hyperplastic!) adrenal cortex has been described in persons past 90 years of age (Salimbeni and Gery, 1912).

The most significant fact suggesting an important rôle of the adrenals in geriatrics is the indispensability of the adrenal cortex for life and health, at all ages (Rogoff and Stewart, 1926, 1928) (dogs, cats, guinea pigs, rabbits, rats and a few monkeys). That the cortex is related to metabolic processes in the period of senescence, is indicated by changes in lipoid content, in the mitochrondria, siderophilia and other cytologic elements (Mulon, 1910, 1912; DaCosta, 1913), and by the greater deposit of pigment granules in the cortex ("Abnutzungsprodukten"— Landau). The juxtamedullary zone of the cortex has been claimed to be related to gonadal function and has been alleged to be endowed with androgenic qualities.

The adrenals have been supposed to influence, significantly, important oxidative processes in the body; e.g., an influence on the amount and behavior of glutathione in the blood and tissues (Zunz, 1932; Ferrari, 1935). The relation of the glands to vitamins is not well understood, but it may be significant that the cortex is rich in vitamin C.

Calcium metabolism has been shown to be related to adrenal function, probably through interrelation with the parathyroid (Rogoff and Stewart, 1928; Taylor and Caven, 1927; Pugsley and Collip, 1936; Schour and Rogoff, 1936); this may have a bearing on arterial changes, especially those involving calcification—more important in the smaller arteries and renal arterioles.

Chiefly, in relation to senescence, might be considered the as yet only vaguely known metabolic function of the adrenal cortex; acute, subacute and chronic insufficiency are characterized by changes in the composition of the blood and by pathologic manifestations in important organs (Rogoff and Stewart, 1926, 1928; Cleghorn and McVicar, 1936) viz., nervous system, circulatory apparatus, alimentary canal, pancreas, parathyroid and probably hypophysis and other endocrine organs. These indicate a profound "intoxication," which in milder form (i.e., probably resulting from chronic functional insufficiency) may represent retention of metabolities or toxic substances which might influence the processes of senescence. Toxic substances have been alleged to have been found in the blood of adrenalectomized animals (Abelous and Langlois, 1892; Loewi and Gettwert, 1914; Putschkow and Kubjakow, 1927; and others). Changes have been found in the blood leucocytes (Zwemer and Lyons, 1928; Fox and Whitehead, 1935).

Sodium chloride was found to be related to the activity of salivary amylase and also to that of the pancreatic and hepatic diastase (Glatzel); this may be related to the moderate disturbances in carbohydrate metabolism associated with adrenal insufficiency.

Changes in the mineral metabolism, viz. sodium chloride (Rogoff and Stewart, 1928; Loeb et al. 1933) potassium (Zwemer and Truszkowski, 1936) and in the nitrogenous metabolism (Rogoff and Stewart, 1928), as well as water balance, carbohydrate metabolism, etc., have a bearing on the question, although these are but little understood as yet. Probably the alleged influence of the adrenals in cholesterol metabolism (Troisier and Grigaut, 1912) has a greater influence on senescence than is recognized.

The subject can include even our vague knowledge of important *interrelationships* between the adrenals and other endocrine glands, especially in regard to growth and other metabolic functions in which the hypophysis, gonads, and thyroids participate (probably also the liver and pancreas, at least more indirectly). The singular combination of persistent hypertension and hypertrichiasis (virilism) that may appear in adult women, usually associated with an hyperplasia or tumor of the adrenal cortex, suggests that some cortical hormone, rather than the medullary, may operate on the vascular mechanism. Such a view is consistent with the profound and persistent hypotension following cortical ablation. Of course, one must recognize that an adenoma of the adrenal cortex may produce chemicals different from those secreted by the normal gland.

Perhaps the only condition primarily associated with abnormal premature age phenomena is "progeria." In this condition one complete autopsy on record records definite atrophic and sclerotic changes in the adrenals; however, since other endocrine organs, particularly the anterior hypophysis also showed abnormal changes, the disease cannot be said to be primarily the result of adrenal disease.

The characteristic complex of Addison's disease (disturbance of the K, Na balance, the water balance, and possibly the sugar metabolism, the hypotension, alimentary tract and general body asthenia), irrespective of the primary or secondary character of the several factors, is not clearly established even in very advanced age in man. The fact that high NaCl and a low K ingestion appears to control the major cortical deficiency symptoms in patients as well as in animals fairly well, at least for a time, might be made use of in the asthenias of the aged. Should the asthenia of the aged be amenable to this salt therapy (as a specific rather than a drug), we would have the first clear indication of a cortical involvement in the ageing process. But for the present we must say: *not proven.* And yet, we hasten to add: the adrenal cortex should nevertheless be included in any comprehensive experimental attack on the problem of ageing. The gonadotropic cortical factor should also be looked into as to its persistence and rôle, past the period of active gonad life, and its possible relation to the several growth anomalies at that period.

6. THYMUS

A hundred years of research on the thymus has built up a fairly complete story of its morphological changes with age, but it has given very little valid information in regard to the functional significance of these thymus changes for the organism as a whole especially in late adult life. Developing from essentially the same embryological anlage as the anterior pituitary, the thyroid, and the parathyroids, and being, up to puberty, made up in part of what seems to be glandular epithelium (Hassal corpuscles) the thymus is by most people suspected to have endocrine functions in the usual sense. But hormone production by the thymus is still an open question. Earlier extirpation experiments seemed to indicate some influence of the thymus on growth, particularly on bone and calcium metabolism. But the more recent work of Park and McClure (1919) appeared to dispose of that possibility, at least for the dog. Riddle reports interference with the production of the egg shell after thymectomy in birds. The onset of a more rapid involution at puberty, and the reported delay of this involution by prepubertal castration has suggested some mutual influence between the thymus gland and the gonads. In a recent preliminary communication Gershon-Cohen et al. (1938) report that X-ray destruction on the thymus in very young rats leads to nearly complete atrophy of the testes (and complete sterility) in the male, but is without influence on the ovaries of the female. Retarded growth of the body is given by these authors as one effect of X-raying the thymus.

Possibly the most significant reports in the thymus field in recent years are the several papers by Gudernatch (1937), by Asher (1930), and by Rowntree and their co-workers. These investigators fed or injected variously prepared extracts of the thymus to young rats, and to female rats throughout their reproductive cycle, and report some stimulation of the rate of growth of the young rats, and, in the work of Rowntree et al., in addition, precocious maturity, somatic and gonadal. The composition of these thymic extracts are not known, but they probably contain peptids, essential amino acids, and possibly glutathione (Gudernatch). The effects reported may therefore be due to an abundant supply of growth stimulating foods (Andersen) rather than to giving excess thymus hormones. This interpretation seems justified, at least until the reverse of these feeding and injection effects are definitely established by total removal of the thymus in young animals.

While a few of the peculiar Hassal corpuscles are reported to persist in the thymus into old age, the greater part of the fetal and prepuberty epithelium of the thymus is replaced by apparently ordinary lymphocytes, beginning with the age of puberty, and from that age on the ups and downs of the thymus appear to parallel that of other lymphoid tissue, as in infections, status lymphaticus, etc.

Thus it would seem, on the basis of fairly consistent cytological findings (Hammar, 1932, 1936), and in the absence of even definite indications of thymic hormone functions at least past the puberty age, that there is probably no thymus factor in ageing, using the term in our restricted sense. To be sure, complete thymic involution is probably not reached till some somatic ageing processes are under way, but to relate these as cause and effect would be idle speculation, at present. The conception of "sudden death," ("Mors thymica") rather than slow ageing, as related to a persistent, enlarged, or "overactive" thymus, is probably untenable.

From the above it seems clear that for the processes of senescence that make their clear appearance in man from the age of 40-50 on, the thymus gland is not even one of the minor prophets in Israel. But the ageing of the thymus itself is a problem of first importance and it may have hitherto unsuspected significance for the organism.

7. PITUITARY

1. A scientifically valid evaluation, and therefore useful rather than confusing, of the very extensive as well as conflicting literature, clinical and experimental, on the pituitary gland, and especially the anterior lobe, in line with the aims of this volume, seems today almost beyond human capacity. At least one anterior pituitary hormone forms an essential link in growth, and hence in repair, if not in the processes of immunity (which, surely, have growth aspects), presumably at all stages of the life span. The theory that such a hormone is an important regulator in the processes of senescence is almost too tempting to reject, even in the absence of valid evidence in its favor. This same lobe produces other hormones on which the activity, if not the very life of such organs as the ovaries, the testes, and the mammary gland depend. The latter organs wane with advancing years. Could we

settle relations in nature by logic alone, what is more logical than that this waning of the gonads and the mammary glands is caused by an antecedent hypofunction of the pituitary? Again, the anterior pituitary appears to have in some species, at least, a chemical driving machinery acting on the thyroid, and probably on the hormone production of the adrenal cortex, though in neither case is the pituitary machinery absolutely essential for all the functions of these organs. Slight but gradual failure of the thyroid and adrenal cortex activities in advanced years could very well induce some of the gradual decline in physiological processes known as "normal ageing." No doubt, that horse could pull this cart. But does it? And we have actual evidence that the different hormones of the anterior pituitary may not be secreted at parallel rates; that the production of some of them is, indeed, ruled by different chemical masters; that the output of one may go up while that of another goes down (as appears to be the case of the growth and the gonadotropic hormones in acromegaly). So we may, logically, call on the pituitary in middle life for excess production of the hormone driving, somehow, in the direction of diabetes. And, presto, we have the increasing incidence of diabetes up to the age period of 50 to 60 years. And, coming even closer to the actual phenomena of senescence, do we not have the apparent premature senility of Simmonds disease with its reported parallel, if not antecedent, atrophy of the anterior pituitary, not to mention the Cushing disease, or syndrome, (including persistent hypertension), with its reported indications of war inside the anterior pituitary hormone family? Considering the histochemical literature on the whole pituitary gland by itself, there is sufficient variety of findings to give comfort to almost any kind of hypothesis, and a mere physiologist is poorly qualified to winnow the chaff from the grains of wheat.

2. Were we permitted to rely on such accounts of the gross and microscopic structure of the presumably "normal" human pituitary from early intrauterine life to ripe old age as those given by Parsons (1936), and by Cooper (1925), this phase of the pituitary story would seem provisionally simple. According to these authors the eosinophile, the basophile, and the neutrophile cells make their appearance from the third month of fetal age on, apparently differentiated from the original non-granular cells. The latter persist, however, in slowly increasing numbers throughout life. The eosinophile cells increase in size during childhood. The basophile cells also increase in size, and in later adult years invade both the intermediate and the posterior

lobes in considerable numbers. The neutrophiles appear to be most numerous in the pituitary gland of old people. Parsons' paper is based on a cytological study of 107 human (male and female) pituitaries, ranging in age from childhood up to 78 years. The gross weight and size of the whole pituitary changes but little in either men or women, between the ages of 20 to 80. The average for both sexes is from 0.60 to 0.75 grams. In Parsons' series there is a slight decline in pituitary weight in women after 60, and a slight increase in pituitary weight of the men past 40. According to Simmonds (1914) data on a very large series (800) of human pituitaries well dispersed as to age, there is on the average a slight decrease in gross pituitary weight both in men and women after the 40th year of life. But considering the unknown relations between endocrine gland size and rate of hormone output, this is a very precarious foundation for a theory postulating anterior pituitary involution as a causative factor in normal ageing. This invasion of the posterior lobe by the basophile cells, and the usual increase in the pigmentation in this lobe appear to be the main histochemical feature of ageing in the posterior pituitary.

The invasion of the posterior lobe by the basophile cells has been considered by Cushing and others as a sign, if not a causal link, in ageing. In Parsons' cases this invasion roughly paralleled the age from 40 on, both in men and women, the invasion being somewhat less extensive in women past 40 who had hypertension. Some increase in the number of the neutrophile cells, and a slight increase in the connective tissue of the anterior pituitary are also described in older people.

Some vacuolization appears in the basophile and the eosinophiles in older people. According to Cooper, the unusually great vascularity of the anterior pituitary attained at puberty, is retained until the age of 50 or 60 years, when a slight but progressive diminution of the blood supply of this part of the gland appears to set in.

In the absence of frank pituitary gland disorders (tumors, cysts, etc.), and generalized and excessive vascular sclerosis involving also the pituitary, this gland appears, anatomically, and cytologically, remarkably stable, from the age of 20 on to 80. We should pause and ponder before ascribing either hypo or hyperfunction with ageing to this gland on these changes in structure, as we are able to interpret them at present. If, as appears to be the case, the anterior pituitary has differentiated from a common anlage (embryonic pharyngeal

epithelium) into a factory producing five or more distinct chemica-
substances, the relative anatomic stability of the gland is, indeedl
striking, in view of the indications that recent evolutionary achieve,
ments tend to be labile.

3. For the present we may consider at least five anterior pituitary
hormones as fairly well established, the growth promoting, the gonad
stimulating, the mammary gland stimulating, the thyroid stimulating,
and the substance acting with or via the pancreatic islets in carbohydrate metabolism. However, the evidence for the actual secretion
of some of these substances by the gland is both meager and indirect.
If there be only four types of cells in the anterior pituitary some of
these cells are evidently producing more than one hormone. There
appears to be a more or less independent rate of production of these
several hormones. At any rate cystic or other types of degeneration
of the anterior pituitary may affect the gonadotropic factor primarily,
leaving the growth factor, at least, unimpaired, in which case, we have
sexual infantilism but normal body growth. But gonad involution, or
more to the point, castration before or after puberty, appears not to retard the secretion of at least one of the gonadotropic factors (Prolan A).
Pregnancy, castration and total thyroidectomy induce some variable
(depending in part on species and sex) cytological changes in the
anterior lobe. The precise causes and functional consequences of
these are still largely conjectural. Since hypothyroidism and hypopituitarism each impair body growth and gonad activity, and since
one pituitary hormone stimulates the thyroid, another the gonads,
and, from the castration effects, the thyroid hormone appears to have
some (probably stimulating) effect on the pituitary, as well as on the
gonads, the possible primaries in this complex are several, and still
await solution.

In a certain sense, the involution of the human ovaries in late adult
life, the gradual reduction in secretion capacity of mammary glands,
the more gradual involution of the mammalian testes, are a part of the
picture of ageing. In the life of these several organs anterior pituitary
hormones form important, if not, indeed, essential links. If the age
involution of these organs is primarily a matter of specific hypopituitarism, we should be able to definitely prolong their life span by
pituitary hormone therapy. This is, at present, uncertain, but seems
a promising line of attack, given controlled materials. In the case of
the human female, whether the factor be primarily ovarian, or pituitary

(or what have you?), the fairly definite timing of the involution in normal women, and the more gradual gonad involution in the human male, points in the direction of sex-linked heredity in gonad ageing.

As to growth and repair, pituitary growth hormone, and ageing, except in such special cases as neoplasms, the male prostate (man), local hair follicles in hypertrichosis, and local foci of bone hyperplasia in some types of arthritis, growth and tissue repair slow down with age, though not in strict parallel. This slowing down tends to be marked in advanced old age. The pituitary gland may, indeed, produce more than one growth hormone. The pituitary action on the ovary and the thyroids may be, and is, by some, so interpreted. But as to the pituitary influence on the other organs of the body, present evidence indicates only one growth hormone. And there is no clear evidence that the reduction in the rate of production of this hormone is primary in the slowing up of growth and repair with age. Nor is there evidence, except for the special situation of acromegaly, of such excess production of this growth hormone as would account for the increased tendency to neoplastic growth in old people. Special carcinogenic chemicals are, so far, indicated from the gonads, not from the pituitary gland. This Gordian knot is not solved by postulating a primary hereditary factor in neoplastic growth, for heredity does not operate without chemical machinery.

Future work with more accurate quantitative methods of chemical and bio-essay studies of the blood, the urine, and the anterior pituitary in controlled populations may disclose variations with age in the hormone output, qualitative and quantitative, not evident from the literature of today. At present, the anterior pituitary seems a relatively stable organ. Such variations in pituitary functions as shown in acromegaly in early adult life, and in gigantism in youth, both very probably due to an excess production of the growth hormone; and sexual infantilism, and dwarfism of pituitary origin, due clearly to deficient production of the gonadotropic and the growth hormones respectively, are clearly exceptions and should be looked upon as disease. They are of significance for the problem of ageing only to the extent that they furnish clues to the machinery of hormone production and hormone action.

In 1926 Hirsch concluded that valid evidence for hypofunction of the anterior pituitary in old age had not yet been produced. This appears still to be a true verdict, with the addendum that valid evidence for hyperfunction of anterior pituitary in the aged is equally lacking.

4. The anterior pituitary was at one time, and is still by some investigators, held to be in some way concerned with the regulation of deposition of fat in the animal. The Fröhlich syndrome (partial hypopituitarism) in human youths is frequently associated with excess deposition of body fat. In the hands of many, especially the earlier workers in this field, attempts at total hypophysectomy in adult dogs, frequently produced very fat dogs, when they survived the operation. Excess or unusual obesity is not a necessary element in ageing. Very old cattle, horses, dogs, and men are more apt to be emaciated than excessively fat. But this is probably due more to defective teeth and other impairments of the digestive machinery, than to the age factor itself. In the human species, in the absence of serious disease, the tendency to excessive adiposity during the 4th and 5th decades is fairly common, but this is likely to be due to social and economic rather than to endocrine factors. At any rate, the following facts seem to dispose of any definite relations of hypopituitarism (anterior lobe) to fat metabolism or adiposity, except to the extent that a slightly lowered B.M.R. may be concerned in those processes: (a) experimental hypopituitary dwarfs have been produced (dog, rat) showing no unusual adiposity; (b) excess adiposity, bordering on the condition of adiposa dolorosa in man, has been produced (rat, dog) by destruction injuries to the base of the brain in the hypothalamic region, and without direct injury to the anterior pituitary. But it cannot be denied that such surgery is likely to sever the nerve tract connecting the hypothalamus with the posterior pituitary. The influence of this tract on the anterior pituitary is not yet clear (Ransom, 1937). (c) These types of adiposity in man and experimental animals are not definitely influenced by pituitary therapy (either or both lobes).

It may still turn out that some region of the hypothalamus enters the fat metabolism complex via the hormone route. But even should this be the case, the tendency to adiposity does not at present seem a significant element in the ageing problem.

5. None of the anterior pituitary hormones has as yet been completely isolated (except the prolactin), chemically identified, or synthesized. This unfortunate fact is partly responsible for some of the conflicting data in this field. More progress in this direction has been made with the anterior pituitary like substances in the urine. The assay of hormone concentrations in the urine appears much simpler than in the blood, or in the gland. Unfortunately only the gonadotropic pituitary hormones appear to spill over into the urine in sufficient

quantities for practical study, and there is even some uncertainty as to the pituitary origin of the urinary "pituitary like" substances. Discouraging as it appears now, we must nevertheless keep at the search for better hormone assay methods both for the blood and the gland. We think it is distinctly worth while even now to work with the best methods of extraction, and the most quantitative bio-assays, using different age pituitaries of controlled animals. There is, undoubtedly, more gold in that little pocket in the sphenoid bone.

6. The posterior pituitary presents neither the cytologic nor the hormonal complexity of its bed fellow. The only reason for considering it at all, in view of the aims of this book, is the possibility of this portion of the gland having something to do with, (a) the water balance in the tissues, (b) the regulation of blood pressure, (c) the regulation of pigmentation, all of which appear to be involved in the ageing nexus.

(a) *Water balance.* The earlier attempts at total hypophysectomy, if the animal survived, often lead to at least a temporary diabetes insipidus. The excessive diuresis of this condition appears to be primarily due to much water entering the blood from the tissues, causing a hydremia, or to altered renal physiology, rather than to primary water drinking caused by excess thirst. But more work is needed to establish or refute these points. We now know, for some species at least, that the posterior lobe may be excised up to the base of the brain, without inducing this polyuria, and that it is produced by destructive processes in the hypothalamus. The further important fact is this: a relatively crude extract (pituitrin) of the posterior lobe, or of the stalk, hypodermically administered, checks this diuresis temporarily. The rare cases of spontaneous diabetes insipidus in man, at times following basal skull fracture or other forms of basal brain injuries, is similarly controlled by pituitrin. But we have, to date, no conclusive evidence that the active anti-diuretic substance is ever secreted into the blood, the lymph, or into the cerebrospinal fluid. So it may be a drug rather than a hormone. While it appears to be true that measurable tissue dehydration parallels advancing age there is no evidence that this is causally related to posterior pituitary hypofunction, or that it can be checked by administration of pituitrin. Nor is increasing thirst (for water) a symptom of ageing.

(b) The same extract (pituitrin) induce relatively prolonged contraction of most, if not all the smooth muscle in the body. This, of course, raises the arterial blood pressure, by increasing the peripheral resistance to the flow of the blood. But again, no valid evidence is at hand to show that excess production of pituitrin by the posterior hypophysis is a factor in the arterial hypertension complex at any age. A new way of testing these possibilities seems to open, by the Goldblatt technique (chronic renal eschemia) of producing chronic arterial hypertension in dogs. Will posterior lobectomy relieve this condition? This does not seem probable, but if it does, we are on the way. According to Page (1938) the arterial hypertension of Goldblatt is not maintained after complete extirpation of the adrenal cortex. But, if confirmed, this fact cannot be, at present, ascribed directly to a cortical hormone factor in that form of hypertension, and the fact itself is questioned by recent experiments of Rogoff.

(c) The problem of cell pigmentation (surface, and body cells) in the ageing process, and the relation of the posterior pituitary as well as the pars intermedia thereto appears to be a matter of comparative physiology and pathology. We do not think it can be settled on mammals alone. In some of the lower species the posterior hypophysis (and the pars intermedia) seem to influence not only the chromatophores, but also general cell pigmentation. But the mosaic distribution of skin and hair pigmentation is such that no hormone circulating in the blood can be the only primary factor. The ageing white man usually loses the color of his hair (on the scalp only) before he loses the hair itself, while some of the body cells develop more pigment, and the skin becomes darker. If this is hormonal action, it becomes complicated, indeed. As regards the skin of the ageing white man, it seems more probable that the increased pigmentation with time is more a matter of chronic effects of the ultra violet light, than a plus or minus hormone action. Perhaps the work of Geiling on the whale pituitary, where two of the pituitary lobes are geographically separated, will bring some light into this perplexing situation.

8. SUMMARY

In the preceding paragraphs of this chapter we dealt with the problem of endocrine control (dietary, vascular, hormonal, metabolic, nervous) only incidentally. But this question seems so fundamental, especially in the rôle that decreased or increased hormone production may play in the ageing processes of the other physiologic machinery, that this brief space, given to recapitulation and attempts at greater clarification, may be useful.

1. In the matter of food factors, the fact that the thyroid glands depend on iodine, and the gonads on vitamin E seems well established,

and in the case of the iodine-thyroid relation, the mechanism appears as simple as that of iron to erythropoiesis. Several endocrines (thyroid, gonads, adrenals) exhibit cytological and probably functional, changes in general starvation (Jackson). High caloric diets seem to put a "strain," probably via increased hormone production, on the islets and the thyroids; especially by high carbohydrate intake in the former, and by high protein in the latter. The phenomena themselves need further study, especially in the comparative field, in search for the causal steps.

2. The dependence (within limits) of the rate of hormone output on the vascularity of the specific endocrines seems both reasonable and probable, but, so far, this dependence rests largely on assumptions, such as the usual increased vascularity in the hyperplastic endocrine gland; the periodic increase in the vascularity of the gonads, parallel with periods of increased hormone secretion; the dependence of urine output, muscle contraction, cardio efficiency, etc., on the blood flow through these respective organs, etc. But to what extent the ordinary vaso-motor mechanisms of the endocrines indirectly modify hormone production is still unknown. Nor do we know how great a reduction in local vascularity must be induced, before hormone output is decreased. In the case of the liver (in cirrhosis, fatty infiltration, etc.) we have an example of the danger of reasoning "on general principles," in the absence of actual tests. The attempts to control hyperthyroidism in man by partial ligation of the thyroid arteries have been less successful than one had a right to anticipate on theoretical grounds. So this virgin field invites invasion via the experimental route. Until experimental and observational data on this aspect of hormone output control are at hand, speculations anent the influence of endocrine sclerosis on the rate of endocrine function may be interesting, and even true, but they are not science.

3. The matter of mutual control among the endocrines presents fundamental but extremely complicated questions for solution. The influence of the thyroid hormone, and at least one anterior pituitary hormone on the gonads may be on metabolism and growth rather than on gonad hormone output, as seems to be the case with the anterior pituitary influence on the mammary gland. The influence of the gonad hormones on at least one of the anterior pituitary hormone factories appears to be inhibitory rather than stimulatory. The temporary influence of the anterior pituitary on the thyroid gland appears to be both on gland growth and hormone output. The apparent

influence of some anterior pituitary factor on the carbohydrate metabolism may be on organs other than the islets, for it operates in the absence of the pancreas. Evidently, we are here concerned either with a pancreas factor keeping some process in the anterior pituitary in check, or else with some type of balancing action by insulin and the pituitary factor in the liver, the muscles, and possibly other organs. The factual interpretation, as regards hormone production, of the several cytological changes induced in several endocrines by total ablation or total atrophy of any one of these glands constitutes a major research task of tomorrow.

4. The easy and plausible assumption that the rate of the hormone output in general is controlled by the involuntary nervous system via direct secretory nerves, and action on these nerves by such substances as adrenalin, sympathin, etc., has acted as a soporific rather than as a spur, in some quarters. Should this assumption turn out to be superficial and essentially incorrect, it will look worse than foolish. What appears to be true secretory nerve control, in the case of the endocrines, has been made out for the adrenal medulla-adrenalin alone. And in this case we have the additional and curious fact that when these secretory nerves are severed from the central nervous system the medulla no longer puts out adrenalin. So here we have not only secretory nerve control, but, apparently, exclusive nerve control. However, the medulla does not seem to atrophy after such denervation. It is precisely this nerve control of adrenalin secretion, and the stimulation by adrenalin (in a certain concentration) in sympathetic nerve endings in general that has made the assumption of sympathetic nerve control of all the endocrines so alluring to some colleagues.

The search for such secretory nerve mechanism has centered mainly on the thyroid gland. Here Cannon and his collaborators has reported data from many ingenious experiments, data consistent with but not proving secretory innervation of this gland. More recently Cannon et al (1929) have reported that total, or nearly total sympathectomy (in the cat), does not lower the B.M.R., showing that even if secretory nerves to the thyroid gland are present, the essential drive of even this gland is in this species directly chemical. And since total sympathectomy induces no sequelae referable to hypofunction of any of the other endocrines, the chemical control appears to hold for all of them, except the adrenal medulla, and possibly the anterior pituitary, as the nerve-path collecting the anterior pituitary and the hypothalamus remains intact in the Cannon experiment. But important as these findings are, they do not dispose of the question of endocrine secretory nerve control, for it is well known that the normal gastric glands, after section of both vagi nerves, secrete enough gastric juice to meet the digestive needs of the animal, and yet we know that the vagi carry secretory nerve fibers to the gastric glands. This question seems particularly pertinent for the endocrine phase of the ageing problem, since instability in the nervous machinery is part of the ageing process, and if we have nerve control of hormone output, disturbance of this control in the aged is, at least, a probability. And, finally, no one can critically examine the difficult literature on the endocrines in senescence without being disturbed by the indications of at least quantitative differences in the control mechanisms and, in the resistance, and in the persistence of the endocrines, not only in different species, but also with sex. Until these variations are cleared up as to cause (hereditary or environmental), we will continue to commit sins against science, especially in our generalizations in this field.

REFERENCES

ABELOUS, J. E., AND LANGLOIS, P. 1892. Note sur l'action toxique du sang de mammiferes apres la destruction des capsules surrenales. Compt. rend. Soc. Biol., 44, 165.

ALLEN, F. M. 1922. Microscopical studies of the pancreas in clinical diabetes. J. Metab. Res., 1, 193–219.

ASHER, L. 1930. Der Einfluss der Thymus auf das Wachstum und die Herstellung der Thymocresin. Endocrinologie, 7, 321–327.

CAMP, W. J. R. 1937. Influence of epinephrin on the distribution of potassium in the body. Proc. Inst. Med. 201.

CANNON, W. B., NEWTON, H. F., BRIGHT, E. M., MENKEN, V., AND MOORE, R. M. 1929. Some aspects of the physiology of animals surviving complete exclusion of sympathetic nerve impulses. Am. J. Physiol., 89, 84.

CLEGHORN, R. A., AND McVICAR, G. A. 1936. The chemistry of blood and urine in adrenal insufficiency. Canad. Chem. and Metal., 18.

COOPER, E. R. A. 1925. The Histology of the More Important Human Endocrine Organs at Various Ages. Oxford Press.

CORI, C. F., CORI, G. T., AND BURCHWALD, K. W. 1930. The mechanism of epinephrin action. VI. The changes in the blood sugar, lactic acid and blood pressure during continuous intravenous injection of epinephrin. Am. J. Physiol., 93, 273–283.

DACOSTA, A. C. 1913. Recherches sur l'histo-physiologie des glandes sur renales. Arch. de Biol., 28, 111–196.

DOGLIOTTI, G. C., AND NIZZI NUTTI, G. 1935. Thyroid and senescence. Endocrinology, 19, 289–292.

DRAGSTEDT, C. A., WIGHTMAN, A. H., AND HUFFMAN, J. W. 1928. The haemodynamic action of minimal effective doses of epinephrin in the unanesthetized dog. Am. J. Physiol., 84, 307–313.

DRAGSTEDT, L. R., VAN PROHASKA, J., AND HARMS, H. P. 1936. Observations on a substance in pancreas (a fat metabolizing hormone) which permits survival and prevents liver changes in depancreatized dogs. Am. J. Physiol., 117, 175–181.

———— 1937. Epinephrine hypertension: effect of continuous intravenous injection of epinephrine on blood pressure: experimental investigation. Ann. Surg., 106, 857–867.

DUBLIN, L. I., AND LOTKA, A. J. 1937. Twenty-five years of health progress, New York, 319.

FERRARI, R. 1935. Behavior of glutathione in blood after excision of the adrenals. Arch. di fisiol., 34, 364–373.

FOX, C. A., AND WHITEHEAD R. W. 1935. Effect of adrenal cortical extract on leucocytes in blood of normal adult rabbits. Proc. Soc. Exp. Biol. and Med., 32, 756–757.

GERSHON-COHEN, J. ET AL. 1938. Studies in the physiology of the thymus. Science, 87, 20.

GLEY, E. 1922. Senescence et Endocrinologie. Bull. de l'Acad. Med., 87, 285–291.

GUDERNATCH, F. 1937. The present status of the thymus problem. Med. Record, 146, 101–112.

HAMMAR, A. J. 1932. Ueber Wachstum und Ruckgang. Zeitschr. f. Miko.-Anat. Forsch., 29, 1–540.

———— 1936. Die Normalmorphologische Tymusforschung. Leipzig.

HIRSCH, S. 1926. Das Altern und Sterben des Menschen vom Standpunkt seimer normalen und pathologischen Leistung. Berlin: Handb. d. Norm. u. Path. Physiol., 17 (3), 752–797.

HORSLEY, V. 1884. On function of thyroid gland. Proc. Roy. Soc., 38, 5–7.

HOUSSAY, B., AND BIASOTTI, A. 1931. Hypophysis, carbohydrate metabolism, and diabetes. Endocrinology, 15, 511–523.

JACKSON, C. M. 1917. Effects of inanition and refeeding on the growth and structure of the hypophysis in the albino rat. Am. J. Anat., 21, 321–358.

———— 1925. The effects of inanition and malnutrition upon growth and structure. Philadelphia.

JOHN, H. J. 1934. Glucose tolerance studies in children and adolescents. Endocrinology, 18, 75–85.

JOSLYN, E. P. 1929. Diabetic Manual. Philadelphia.

JOSLYN, E. P., AND DUBLIN, D. I. 1936. Studies in diabetes mellitus; etiology. Am. Jour. Med. Sc., 191, 759–775.

LEWIS, R. W., AND PAPPENHEIMER, A. M. 1918. A study of the involutional changes which occur in the adrenal cortex during infancy. J. Med. Res., 34, 81–94.

LOEB, R. F., ATCHLEY, D. W., BENEDICT, E. M., AND LELAND, J. 1933. Electrolyte balance studies in adrenalectomized dogs with particular reference to excretion of sodium. J. Exp. Med., 57, 775–792.

LOEWI, O., AND GETTWERT, W. 1914. Ueber die Folgen der Nebennierenexstirpation. Arch. f. d. Ges. Physiol., 158, 29–40.

LORAND, A. 1910. Old age deferred. Philadelphia.

MARINE, D., AND BAUMANN, E. J. 1922. Effect of suprarenal insufficiency in thyroidectomized rabbits. Am. J. Physiol., 59, 353–368.

MARINE, D., BAUMANN, E. J., AND CIPRA, A. 1925. Studies on simple goitre produced by cabbage and other vegetables. Proc. Soc. Exp. Biol. and Med., **26**, 822-824.

McCARRISON, R. 1920. The effects of some food deficiencies and excesses on the thyroid gland. Ind. J. Med. Res., **7**, 633-647.

———— 1917. The thyroid gland. London.

MULON, P. 1910. Sur les mitochondries de la surrenale. Compt. rend. Soc. Biol., **68**, 772.

———— 1912. Mode de formation du pigment figure dans la corticale surrenale. *Ibid.*, **72**, 176-179.

OPIE, E. L. 1903. Disease of the pancreas, its cause and nature. Philadelphia.

PAGE, I. H. 1938. The effect of bilateral adrenalectomy on the arterial blood pressure of dogs with experimental arterial hypertension. Am. J. Physiol., **122**, 352-358.

PARKS, E. A., AND McCLURE, R. D. 1919. The results of thymus extirpation in the dog. Am. J. Dis. Child., **18**, 317-524.

PARSONS, R. J. 1936. Medical Papers, dedicated to H. A. Christian. Baltimore, 366.

PUGSLEY, L. I., AND COLLIP, J. B. 1936. The effect of parathyroid hormone upon the serum calcium and calcium excretion of normal and adrenalectomized rats. Biochem. J., **30**, 1274-1279.

PUTSCHKOW, N. W., AND KIBJAKOW, A. W. 1927. Toxic substances in the blood after adrenal extirpation. Arch. f. d. Ges. Physiol., **218**, 83-88.

RANSOM, L. W. 1937. Some functions of the hypothalamus, Harvey Lectures, Baltimore, **32**, 92-121.

ROGOFF, J. M., AND STEWART, G. N. 1926. Studies on adrenal insufficiency In dogs. I. Control animals not subjected to any treatment. Am. J. Physiol. **78**, 683-710.

———— 1928. Studies on adrenal insufficiency. VII. Further blood studies (cholesterol and calcium) in control and adrenalectomized dogs. Am. J. Physiol. **86**, 25-31.

ROGOFF, J. M., AND MARCUS, E. 1938. Supposed role of the adrenals in hypertension. J. A. M. A., 2127-2132.

SALIMBENI, A. T., AND GERY, L. 1912. Contribution á l'etude Anatomopathologique de la vieillesse. Ann. de L'Inst. Pasteur, **26**, 577-609.

SCHOCKAERT, J. A., AND FOSTER, G. L. 1932. Influence of anterior pituitary substances on the total iodine content of the thyroid gland. J. Biol. Chem., **95**, 89-94.

SCHOUR, I., AND ROGOFF, J. M. 1936. Changes in the rat incisor following bilateral adrenalectomy. Am. J. Physiol., **115**, 334-344.

SCOTT, W. J. M. 1922. Effect of suprarenal insufficiency in cats. J. Exp. Med., **36**, 199-217.

SIMMONDS, M. 1914. Ueber embolische Prozesse in der Hypophysis. Arch. f. Path. Anat., **217**, 226-239.

SOSKIN, S., ALLWEISS, M. D., AND COHN, D. J. 1934. Influence of the pancreas and the liver upon the dextrose tolerance curve. Am. J. Physiol., **109**, 155-165.

STEWART, G. N., AND ROGOFF, J. M. 1917. Quantitative experiments on the liberation of epinephrin from the adrenals after section of their nerves, with special reference to the question whether epinephrin is indispensable for the organism. J. Pharm. Exp. Therap., **10**, 1–48.

———— 1919. Further observations showing that epinephrin from the adrenals is not indispensable. Am. J. Physiol., **48**, 397–410.

TAYLOR, N. G., AND CAVEN, W. R. 1927. The serum calcium after adrenalectomy. Am. J. Physiol., **81**, 511–512.

TROISIER, J., AND GRIGAUT, A. 1912. Contribution á l'etude de l'origine Endocrine de la Cholesterine sanguine. Presse Med., 1081.

ZUNZ, E. 1932. Influence of cortical extract on reduced glutathione content of the blood. Compt. rend. Soc. Biol., **111**, 651, (also Rev. Soc. Argent. de Biol., 1934, **10**, 555).

ZWEMER, R. L., AND LYONS, C. 1928. Leucocyte changes after adrenal removal. Am. J. Path., **86**, 545–551.

ZWEMER, R. L., AND TRUSZKOWSKI, R. 1936. Potassium: Basal factor in syndrom of cortico-adrenal insufficiency. Science, **83**, 558.

Chapter 14

FEMALE REPRODUCTIVE SYSTEM

EDGAR ALLEN

New Haven

Ageing of the female reproductive system is of especial interest because (1) it occurs while other systems may still be in their prime, (2) one stage of ageing of this system is marked outwardly by menopause, a clearly terminal milestone in reproductive history, (3) there have been many instances of menopause in young women due to disease, operative removal of ovaries or reduced function by X-ray therapy, and these are similar in many respects to the natural menopause and (4) there is much experimental evidence bearing upon the endocrine control of menstruation and other reproductive functions which helps explain disturbances and cessation with advancing age.

The viewpoint of a man studying this problem is one thing—that of a woman herself approaching the climacteric may be quite different. The realization that old age is approaching in one's life, changes ageing from an abstraction applying to those of the previous generation to an urgent personal problem. A woman's viewpoint at this time is dependent on her past reproductive or sexual experience. To the "old fashioned mother" who has had many children, who does not use contraceptives, the menopause may be welcome as bringing relief from fear of another and probably more difficult pregnancy. For instance, a clinician of wide experience writes, "I have met many harassed mothers of the working class who positively welcome the arrival of the period of infertility." To the married woman of forty, enjoying moderate sex function with the use of contraceptives, approach of menopause brings the realization that this phase of life is closing; not suddenly, but still inevitably. Although sexual intercourse may occur after menopause, clearly established atrophic changes in the genital organs indicate that sexual function is waning. The viewpoint in this case may be "regretful, but resigned to the inevitable."

From one masculine viewpoint it would seem that most women might welcome cessation of the burden of menstruation, but this does not seem general. On the contrary, menstruation is to some synonymous with functional femininity, as virility often is with manhood.

1. MENOPAUSE AS A SIGN OF AGEING

The decrease in function of sex organs has frequently been associated with other signs of ageing in the body. They need not be related. There is little evidence to show that removal of the sex glands early in life reduces longevity. Frequently one finds animals whose external characteristics indicate senility and whose gonads still show signs of moderate function. But with advancing age difficulties appear in lactation and in carrying pregnancies to full term. Reduction in size of litters is common.

The menopause in primates is one of many signs of ageing of the female genital organs. In its strictest definition, it means the final cessation of menstruation. Before this occurs there is sometimes irregularity of menstrual rhythm, usually some decrease in sex function and frequently the appearance of other symptoms generally associated with menopause. While many women, probably a majority, pass through this time of life without major inconvenience; others, perhaps as many as fifteen per cent, experience accentuation of menopause symptoms which may incapacitate them for their usual round of daily activity. These symptoms may appear before the actual cessation of menses and may continue for several years afterward. The term "climacteric" is used to embrace all symptoms during this longer interval, including the menopause. Common usage justifies the interpretation of "menopause" defined broadly, as synonymous with "climacteric." (See Pratt and Thomas, 1937; Pratt, 1938; and Frank, Goldberger and Salmon, 1936.)

The most constant symptom is probably the occurrence of hot flushes, vaso-motor symptoms similar to blushing, which may prove very uncomfortable and embarrassing. Hot flushes may be followed by chills. The number may vary from a few a week to many each day. They may be more intense and more frequent at times coinciding with the former menstrual rhythm. Many other symptoms associated with the climacteric, such as irritability, emotional instability, headaches, digestive disturbances, languor, depression, numbness of extremities, and so on, have been listed. The frequency of various symptoms is summarized from a study of menopause in 1187 English women, both married and single, as reported in *Lancet* (1933, p. 106). The age at menopause varies a great deal. In the study just mentioned it ranged from 23 to 60 years, with 65 per cent falling between ages 45 and 55. One woman menstruated until her 73rd year, and a second until her 66th year. Menopause occurred before 40 years in 8 per cent.

An interesting record of what may be regarded as a normal menopause is reported by Engle (1938). A calendar of menstrual cycles was kept by an unmarried teacher from age 37 until age 48, when irregularities were first noted. These irregularities affected duration and amount of flow and length of total cycle. Hot flushes appeared at the age of 48 and continued for several years except at the time when menstruation occurred. To quote from her diary, "Hot flushes very regular. At times every 40 minutes, never lasting more than 3 minutes. At other times flushes seemed to come every 2 hours." At age 49 there was a period of 128 days without menstruation,—then a return of several cycles. This woman missed only 5 days from work during five years of "climacteric." Engle emphasizes the gradual nature of the change at the time of menopause.

There is some evidence to indicate that women who have had difficulties with menstruation during their active sexual life are more prone to serious symptoms at climacteric. There are exceptions, however, and it is difficult to generalize. It is popularly supposed that women who have not had children reach the menopause earlier than those who have had children. A few outstanding examples may give this impression where adequate data are not available for clear-cut conclusions. The study of English women already mentioned reports, "Childbearing in no way influenced the age at the menopause."

Not only may the number of children which a woman has had influence onset and seriousness of climacteric, but also whether or not she has nursed those children may have a bearing. Recent studies of the endocrine association of the reproductive organs with the pituitary and other glands of internal secretion provide a basis for the logic of this assciation.

During the years immediately following menopause there is a gradual but extensive atrophy of vagina, uterus, breasts and ovaries (Rossle, 1923). Atrophy of the ovaries is especially significant because of their endocrine dominance over other female genital tissues. Although sexual relations may be continued past this time, it is clear from the declining condition of the sexual organs that they are not in the proper condition to function at maximum. Extreme atrophy may develop in genital skin and continue as a chronic condition very difficult to treat satisfactorily. As signs of senility, various students of ageing have described sluggishness, uncertainty of movements, change in postural reflexes, a great reduction in activity, irregular respiration, and thinning of fur or hair.

There is much experimental evidence which can be brought to bear upon factors in ageing of the female reproductive system. There are many cases in the medical literature where it has been necessary to remove the ovaries, following disease or tumor growths, or where sterilization, either temporary or permanent, has been accomplished by X-rays.

2. CASTRATION OF WOMEN

Removal of the ovaries is followed by a premature menstrual·period, usually within a few days after the operation, and then a complete cessation of menstruation. This might be called an "operative menopause," and it is similar in many respects to the natural one. Hot flushes may appear within a month or six weeks after operation and other symptoms usually associated with natural menopause may occur with even more marked severity. Since these symptoms occur in young women, it is quite obvious that they are not dependent upon inadequacies of other systems, such as vascular or nervous, due to lowered functions because of ageing.

The uterus, mammary glands and vagina atrophy after ovariectomy in young women just as they do after natural menopause, but more rapidly. There is usually a decrease or loss of sex drive, although some cases are on record in which little change occurred in this particular for some time after operation.

It is now well established that removal of the ovaries affects the pituitary gland, for there is an increased excretion of its gonadotropic hormone (Albright, 1936). This has an important bearing, as will be shown later, on conclusions as to the primary cause of menopause.

It is now possible to treat women, from whom the ovaries have been removed, with ovarian hormones and thereby again induce menstruation. Werner and Collier (1933) first reported this in women. Many instances of successful replacement therapy with ovarian hormones, using return of menstruation as the criterion, are now on record in the medical literature. Two patients are reported after treatment with estrogenic material (Frank, Goldberger, Salmon and Felshin, 1937). They were given 1800 units daily for several months to alleviate menopause symptoms. "From four to six days after stopping medication, these women were surprised and alarmed by the appearance of profuse uterine bleeding, which did not recur." Sometime after menopause women experience a spontaneous sexual rejuvenation. This is frequently associated with growth of the lining of the uterus and sometimes with development of tumors. The condition is attributed to increased secretion of hormone by "reactivated" ovaries. Not only can menstruation be restored, but considerable alleviation of menopause symptoms can be obtained by endocrine therapy. To quote Dr. E. L. Severinghaus (J. A. M. A., **109**, p. 1878, 1937), "All these vasomotor and psychic symptoms may occur in patients before the menopause; but the significant thing is that after castration of a woman who has no other disturbances, these are the symptoms reported. They occur frequently in the spontaneous menopause. There is, conversely, the experience that all these symptoms can be abated and usually completely relieved by the use of an adequate dose of estrogenic chemicals."

Since many of the menopause symptoms are subjective, the question arises as to the extent psychological factors may enter into the results reported. The difficulty of adequate controls for clinical experiments is cited. To meet these valid objections, periods of treatment with ovarian hormone are alternated with periods of treatment with "dummy" doses,—similar material which does not contain the hormone (See Pratt and Thomas, 1937). This method seems to be the only adequate way to control clinical therapy. There can be little doubt that just the fact that the doctor is prescribing something for severe symptoms of climacteric may help some patients. When beneficial results are reported during injections of "dummy" doses, it must be admitted that the effects are psychic. On the other hand, when treatment with estrogenic hormones alleviates conditions, and then when hormones are supplanted by the "dummy" doses without the patient's knowledge and these fail to do so, evidence for the effect of the hormone is undoubtedly clear. Surely, resumption of menstruation in ovariectomized women after treatment with ovarian hormone is an objective criterion and extremely convincing.

Before further discussion of use of ovarian hormones in the restoration of menstruation and the alleviation of menopause symptoms, it may be well to consider briefly some of the basic experimental work on which this clinical treatment rests. Also, before considering why menstruation stops at menopause, some of the experimental evidence bearing on its cause should be reviewed.

The first step required studies of the changes in the genital organs due to removal of the ovaries. At one time removal of ovaries seemed to be almost as popular as appendectomy, so there are many descriptions of ovarian deficiency following ovariectomy in women. These studies have shown beyond a doubt that ovarian hormones are necessary to maintain the reproductive organs in good physiological condition. The tissues of vagina, uterus, and mammary glands are entirely dependent for retention of function upon these secretions. When this became fully realized, there were attempts to transplant small pieces of ovaries in other parts of the patient if it was necessary to remove her ovaries. When a piece of her own ovary can be transplanted in some other part of her body, it sometimes functions for at least a short period, in the production of the essential hormone. Transplants of tissue from animals to women, however, are usually resorbed quickly and are not effective. Another point of interest in this connection is that eggs in these ovarian transplants are very sensitive to even a temporary loss of blood supply. There are relatively very few eggs in the ovary of an adult woman anyway, and when this supply is further limited by transplantation involving delay of ingrowth of new blood vessels, the transplanted ova may be seriously injured. Other ovarian cells of the transplant may continue secretion of hormone.

3. ACTION OF OVARIAN HORMONES

The next advances involved isolation of the ovarian hormones. The first one, the follicular hormone, theelin, was obtained from the ovaries of pigs. It was recognized by its ability to reproduce the sexual (estrous) cycles in mice and rats after removal of their ovaries (Allen and Doisy, 1923). This hormone reaches a high concentration in the fluid which forms in the ovarian follicle as the egg ripens and it was therefore also called folliculin, or female sex hormone. It is really a growth hormone especially active upon the genital organs, for it causes increase in size, involving multiplication of cells in the vagina, uterus and mammary glands. As an example sections of vaginal epithelium of the monkey, normal and castrated before and after stimulation with estrogen are shown in figures 78–80. The atrophic vagina after menopause is similar to that of the castrate.

Using rats and mice to test and measure this hormone, it was extracted chemically from ovaries and crystallized (Doisy, Veler and Thayer, 1929). It has recently been synthesized in the chemical laboratory, but the hormone used clinically is still obtained from organic sources. It was found that injections of this hormone not only stimulate growth but also produce sex drive or mating reactions in castrated animals (estrus or heat). This led to the adoption of the names "estrin" or "estrogen" (estrus producing) for the follicular hormone.

Water balance and tissue fluids are recognized as extremely important in the study of causes of ageing. Estrogen plays a part in control of these factors in female genital tissues. The atrophic uterus after ovariectomy contains very little water. The cells are packed tightly together. Within a few hours after injection of follicular hormone there is an increase in blood supply and in the amount of tissue fluid. The connective tissues are flooded with fluids and become spongy and edematous. Cell division accompanies or follows soon after these changes. Somewhat similar effects are produced by estrogens in the "sexual skin" of monkeys and by male sex hormone in the cock's comb. For further details reference is made to Allen, Hisaw and Gardner (1939).

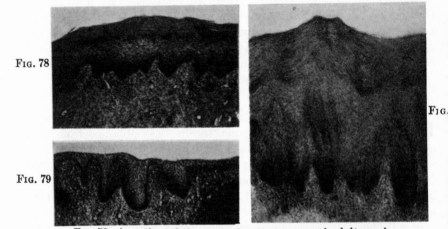

FIG. 78

FIG. 79

FIG.

FIG. 78. A section of the vaginal wall of a normal adult monkey
FIG. 79. A similar section several months after removal of ovaries
FIG. 80. A similar section after the castrated monkey has received 195 rat units of estrogen in 12 days.

Soon after injections of this stimulating hormone are stopped, degenerative changes begin in the genital organs. Therefore, in its simplest form, the sexual cycle in these rodents is really (1) a period of growth, which leads to (2) sex function, and is followed by (3) periods of retrogression or involution.

During these waves of growth in the genital organs there is marked increase in the blood supply and in the tissue fluids. Then a wave of cell multiplication runs through the genital tissues and this is followed by secretory activity in some (Allen, Smith and Gardner, 1937). The stimulation is not limited to the sex organs but reverberates throughout the body; for it is possible to induce periods of spontaneous activity,—

running in rotary cages in the case of the rat (Wang, 1923)—by injections of this ovarian hormone (Richter and Hartman, 1934). It is also interesting in this connection to note that the function of different organs requires varying amounts of this hormonal stimulation. For instance, maximal growth can be induced in the vagina with a certain amount (1 vaginal unit), but it may require considerably more to induce full growth and secretory activity of the uterus (5 to 20 or more units). It not only requires increased amounts of hormone, but longer intervals of time to produce full growth of the mammary glands. To be specific, it requires 8 months of estrogenic stimulation to grow the rudimentary mammary glands of a young *male* monkey to a size equivalent to those of an adult non-pregnant female (Gardner and van Wagenen, 1938). Thus there are quantitative stair-like thresholds of hormone for different reproductive activities.

The studies in the rodents are very interesting, but since rodents do not menstruate it was necessary to study the action of these hormones in primates. The monkey has a sexual cycle which is very similar to that of woman—menstruation of three to five days duration occurring on an average of every 28 days (Corner, 1923). In addition there is in monkeys a reddening and swelling of the "sexual skin" which also depends upon ovarian hormones and is a good outward sign of their high concentration.

Removal of the ovaries from monkeys is followed by degenerative changes in the vagina, uterus and mammary glands, as in women, and by disappearance of the reddening and swelling of the "sexual skin." If the ovaries are removed at about the mid-point between two menstrual periods, a menstrual period follows the operation in from 4 to 7 days and then menstrual function disappears.

Menstruation was first produced experimentally in monkeys after removal of ovaries by injections of ovarian follicular hormone from pigs' ovaries (Allen, 1927). Treatment for 10 days to 2 weeks stimulated growth in the uterus and other genital tissues and the return of color and swelling in the "sexual skin." After injections were stopped, an interval of 4 or 5 days ensued and then menstruation began. This experimental menstruation was similar to normal in both duration and amount of flow. It is possible just by lengthening the time of injections to lengthen the cycle. It is also possible to produce menstruation experimentally in very immature monkeys. From these experiments it is obvious that the injected hormone replaces ovarian endocrine function for a while and builds up growth in the uterus (and other genital organs), and that after hormone stimulation is stopped the tissue degenerates and menstrual bleeding begins. A detailed description of the changes in the walls of the uterus and their internal secretory control will be found in "Sex and Internal Secretions" (Allen, editor, 1939). This hormone treatment must be repeated before another experimental period can be induced.

Soon after the experimental production of menstruation in ovariectomized monkeys, the actual process of menstrual bleeding was visualized by microscopic observation in pieces of menstruating uterus transplanted into the eye. The principal points in Markee's description (1933) of this accomplishment are extremely interesting. The operation consists of transplanting small pieces of the lining of the monkey's uterus into the anterior chamber of her eye, where the blood vessels of the eye grow into the transplants and afford a new blood supply. Until just before menstruation is due, the transplanted tissue looks slightly pink becuse of the rich blood supply. A day or even less before menstruation appears, the circulation of the blood is impeded by general constriction of the superficial vessels. After this vasoconstriction and lack of blood supply has persisted for from 4 to 20 hours, a few vessels in different parts of the transplants open again. They have apparently been damaged during the previous few hours and blood escapes into the surrounding connective tissue where it forms small lakes directly under the surface. New hemorrhages add to these lakes and the blood then escapes into the anterior chamber of the eye (as it does into the cavity of the uterus). A few vessels spurt for a short period then close,—and others open, bleed and close. This type of individual action undoubtedly explains why the amount of blood usually lost during menstruation is limited. It also explains why students of the menstruating uterus have described great variations as to the amount of hemorrhage in different parts of the same uterus (Bartelmez, 1933).

We know that regular menstruation may not mean that eggs are being ovulated. Less than ten years ago our best text books taught otherwise and carried the statement that menstruation occurred because an egg was not fertilized and therefore did not need to implant in the wall of the uterus which had been especially transformed to receive it. In 1923, however, Corner demonstrated conclusively in monkeys that ovulation need not occur at all, and still normal menstrual cycles may continue. Therefore these two phenomena are not necessarily related. (See also Corner, 1932–33.)

When ovulation does occur, it usually falls at the midpoint between onset of two menstrual periods. Hartman (1932) has accumulated much evidence for the time of ovulation in monkeys and the greatest number of ovulations falls on the 13th or 14th days after onset of previous menses. Human eggs have been recovered from the uterine tubes at this time (Allen, Pratt, Newell and Bland (1930), and several days later in the cycle (Lewis, 1931; Pincus, 1937). Recently recording of ovulation in rabbits and women by sharp change in electrical potential has supplied a new method for study (Burr, Hill and Allen, 1935; Reboul, Friedgood and Davis, 1937; and Burr, Musselman, Barton and Kelly, 1937). This should make it possible to locate the exact moment of ovulation in women.

Beside actually describing the process of menstruation, Markee's observations have allowed him to settle another very important point: namely, that the menstruation which occurs after ovulation is similar in all essentials to the menstruation which occurs in the absence of ovulation. From the experimental evidence, then, menstruation is probably a bleeding during a degenerative phase of the cycle, and means that the ovarian hormone which has previously been causing growth of the uterus is no longer sufficient to sustain that organ in a growing condition.

Additional evidence was shortly forthcoming. It was shown that if the dosage of ovarian hormone injected was increased and maintained at a sufficiently high level, the uterus could be maintained in a growing condition for long periods without menstruating. For instance, Zuckerman (1936) reports daily injections of estrogenic ovarian hormone for a year in an adult ovariectomized monkey without the appearance of menstruation. The uterus was in an active growing condition at the end of this period.

Apparently as the follicles develop after the end of a previous menstrual period, enough hormone is produced to cause growth in the uterus. The added tissue grown requires more hormone and if the threshold is not raised sufficiently to continue growth, or if there is a decreased production of hormone, degenerative changes begin and in primates menstrual bleeding is one of the terminal phases of this degenerative process. Consequently, the menopause can be interpreted from these experiments as merely a failure in production of the ovarian follicular hormone to the point where enough growth is induced in the uterus so that, when periodic involution does begin, it will be followed by menstruation.

Many observations of the human ovary show that its function of producing follicles wanes markedly as the fortieth year approaches, or even before in some cases. In fact, one of the things which always surprises the medical student as he studies sections of the human ovary is the difficulty in finding normal follicles. Some students favor ageing of the ovary as the primary cause of involution of other genital organs such as the uterus. The deficiency may not be altogether in the ovary. It is now well known that organs which react to growth producing hormones frequently lose their reactivity. It becomes more difficult to awake growth in these organs after periods of stimulation. It is

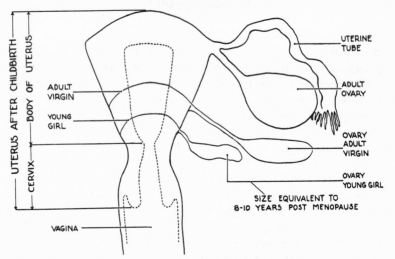

FIG. 81. Diagrammatic representation of the sizes of uterus and ovaries at several stages of life (see also table 24). The proportion of cervix to body of uterus changes also.

clear that there is a decrease in the amount of ovarian hormones with age, but there may also be a loss of reactivity of the uterus.

The lining of the uterus possesses remarkable ability to regenerate. Hartman (1937), in attempts to recover early embryos of monkeys at the times they were implanting in the uterus, has found it possible to open the uterus each month and to remove young embryos. On one of these occasions he completely removed the lining of the monkey's uterus, scraping it out very thoroughly to the muscle layers, and then sponging the cavity further with gauze. This was a normal monkey with functioning ovaries. He opened this same animal's uterus 16 days later to find the lining completely regenerated. This would be easily credible if it concerned the arm of a starfish. In an animal as high in the scale as the monkey, it is a truly remarkable instance of regenerative ability. The average size of the human uterus at different reproductive periods is shown diagramatically in figure 81. The size of the pregnant uterus, large enough to inclose a new born baby and placenta is indicated in table 24, in which other sizes and weights are listed for comparison. Decrease in size in old age reduces these organs to their size during childhood. Similar degenerative changes occur in the vagina and mammary glands.

4. OVARIAN FACTOR OF SAFETY AND ITS REDUCTION WITH AGEING

Another series of experiments bearing upon this point is of especial interest in this connection. This is the extremely large factor of safety which many organs have and which the endocrine glands share. For instance, it has long been known that if one ovary is removed from an animal like a rat or mouse which may produce seven to nine eggs at an estrous period, the remaining ovary will double its production to replace the function of the one removed. At least it does so in young animals. Wiesner (1932) has recently reported that after one ovary is removed from old animals, there is not an equal amount of compensation. This might be interpreted as demonstrating that the ovary has lost some of its productivity—that its factor of safety is reduced,—with ageing. It might be possible to show that similarly a loss of responsiveness appears in the uterus with advancing age. As yet, the writer knows of no experiments designed to test this point. There is so much interrelation in endocrine function that it is difficult to decide whether ageing factors are inherent in a particular gland or in others, whose secretions are required for support.

The above statements apply to the endocrine regulation of the non-pregnant cycle. If ovulation occurs the walls of the follicle from which the egg has been extruded undergo transformation into a corpus luteum. The cells involved change their type of secretion and produce a second ovarian hormone, progesterone. This hormone quickly begins to induce a change in the lining of the uterus which makes implantation of the embryo possible. W. Allen and Corner (1929) were first to succeed in endocrine replacement of this ovarian function during pregnancy. They removed the ovaries from rabbits after they had ovulated and then induced the animals by injections of progesterone to carry their litters to term and give normal birth. Another hormone from the corpus luteum serves a special function in animals like the guinea pig. This relaxes the pelvic ligaments, enlarging the birth canal and easing labor (Hisaw, 1927). It is named "relaxin." Therefore, a supplementary endocrine mechanism—superimposed upon that which is adequate for non-pregnant sexual cycles, and probably involving not only the corpus luteum but also the placenta—is required in some animals for the completion of normal pregnancy.

If the embryos are carried through a normal gestation period to birth, still another endocrine adjustment is required to start and sustain lactation. This involves not only the ovaries and the placenta but also the anterior pituitary gland. The last mentioned gland has recently

TABLE 24

Sizes and weights of the uterus at several stages of life

(from William's *Obstetrics*)

Stage of life	Length	Breadth	Depth	Weight
	cm.	cm.	cm.	grams
Infant.............................	2.5-3			
Adult virgin.......................	5.5-8	3.5-4	2-2.5	40-50
Adult, after childbirth.............	9-9.5	5.5-6	3-3.5	60-70
At end of pregnancy...............	32±	24±	22±	1,000

* At the end of pregnancy there may be an increase of more than 500 times in capacity of the uterus as compared with the non-pregnant adult.

There is also a change in proportion between cervix and body of the uterus: in the child the cervix may be twice as long as the body of the uterus, in the adult virgin, they are equal in length, and in the multiparous woman, the body of the uterus is 3 times as long as the cervix (fig. 81).

After menopause there is a progressive atrophy which reduces the uterus in extreme old age to a small fibrous stump.

been shown to secrete the lactation producing hormone, prolactin, which induces secretion of milk (Greuter and Stricker, 1929) after the mammary glands have grown under the influence of ovarian hormones (Turner, 1938). Prolactin also controls production of the crop milk of pigeons (Riddle, Bates and Dykshorn, 1932). It has been crystallized recently (White, Catchpole and Long, 1937).

To summarize this experimental work on the endocrine control of the female reproductive system we might say that the primary hormone of the ovary, estrogen, causes spurts of growth in the genital organs. These spurts of growth lead to transient sexual functions. After the functions have been sustained for adequate periods of time, there occurs either decrease in hormone, or the hormone present is not adequate to sustain the reaction, and periods of degeneration or involution occur in the sexual organs. In brief, (1) spurts of growth, leading to (2) transient functions, and then to (3) periods of involution. Several supplementary hormones, progesterone and prolactin and in some animals "relaxin," are necessary to complete the mechanism of pregnancy and lactation. The regular non-pregnant cycle, however, need involve only the action of the single hormone from the ovarian follicles, although progesterone is an added factor after ovulation. Since menstruation terminates the involutionary phase of the primate sexual cycle, its cessation at menopause is best explained by failure of this hormone (estrogen) to reach an adequate level for menstruation.

5. AGE INVOLUTION OF DIFFERENT PARTS OF THE SYSTEM

1. *During embryonic and fetal life.*

There are many other instances of involution of genital structures or of their failure to grow. These are by no means limited to old age. In fact, many occur in prenatal periods, even in very early stages of embryonic development. Outstanding examples should include death of the follicle cells which immediately surround the ovum, and degeneration of the polar bodies which are undoubtedly potential ova. These occur soon after ovulation.

The disappearance of the zona pellucida before implantation of the embryo in the wall of the uterus is another example. The zona pellucida is a clear gelatinous envelope around the ovum. The fertilized ovum as it passes down the tube does not increase in size but merely segments into smaller cells. When it reaches the uterus its stored food is exhausted and it must tap the maternal supply. To increase in size it must escape from this envelope, as an insect or crustacean moults from its shell. This escape is effected through a slight increase in acidity of the uterus, which dissolves the zona and permits rapid growth and implantation (Hall, 1936). This is of interest in connection with the discussion of acid-alkali balance in the chapter on homeostatic mechanisms by Cannon, although in the present instance it involves a secretion rather than the blood.

It is so obviously necessary for a structure to grow before it can undergo involution, that mention should be made of some of the instances of failure to grow. It is well known that the embryo starts with bi-sexual potentialities. In the female, rudiments of male organs are present but fail to grow, apparently from lack of genetic determination or endocrine stimulation. These things are appreciated when intersexes develop in embryos. They are brought even more clearly to mind by the experimental modification of sex, by injections of hormones into developing eggs or into pregnant mothers. It is possible not only to stimulate the rudimentary female organs in male embryos with the female sex hormone and to produce sex reversal (Willier, Gallagher and Koch, 1935), but also to prevent the growth of the female reproductive organs by injecting male sex hormone. Recently Hamilton and Wolfe (1938) have shown that injections of male hormone into pregnant rats will prevent proper formation of the embryonic vagina which fails to open, and also prevent the formation of the nipples of the mammary glands. Males of this species normally have no nipples. This is apparently a case of hormonal prevention of growth, or perhaps induction of premature involution in organs of the opposite sex.

Other examples of structures which complete their function before birth and undergo involution include the yolk sac with its rich plexus of blood vessels and also some of the chorionic villi, which at first completely cover the outside of the embryonic membranes. The normal chorions of different species show all stages of partial disappearance of these villi. For instance, the chorion of the horse has persistent villi all over its surface. In the cow and sheep the villi disappear from the surface except in spots or patches. In the monkey only two patches of villi persist to be included in primary and secondary placentas. In man there is usually persistence of only one disc-like patch which contributes to the single human placenta. The determining factors which decide whether or not villi shall persist or disappear in certain parts of the chorion, are partially conditioned by the relation of these parts to adjacent structures. For instance, in the sheep and cow, swellings appear on the inside of the uterus and the villi opposite to them develop well and persist while those in other regions retrogress and disappear. In the human embryo the source of blood supply to part of the adjacent chorion is undoubtedly a determining factor. The blood vessels in the villi which disappear undergo changes remarkably like old age changes in systemic blood vessels, but it cannot be concluded that sclerosis of the vessels of certain villi is the cause of their involution.

The placenta itself ages and begins degeneration before birth. This has been known for a long time. Loss of the elasticity of the vessels, patches of necrotic tissue, fibrosis, and other alterations similar to ageing changes, have been described in placentas from normal human pregnancies at term. This has led to the concept that the placenta, derived from both maternal and embryonic tissues, has a definite life span which is limited by the gestation period (See Warthin, 1929). There is some experimental evidence to support this explanation. For example, if the wall of the uterus is traumatized within 4 or 5 days after ovulation, a growth forms like the maternal part of the placenta (Loeb, 1907–8). A similar reaction involving epithelial tissues has recently been produced in the monkey's uterus by injecting ovarian follicular and luteal hormones and then traumatizing the uterus (Lendrum and Hisaw, 1936). These experimentally produced placentomatas have a definitely restricted span of life less than the length of pregnancy.

If embryos are killed by crushing and rupturing the membranes, the placentas may live on to full term (Newton, 1935). There is also experimental evidence that they may continue the production of an internal secretion. This concept of course involves a definite life span of the placenta as a factor in birth. Snyder and Wislocki (1931) were able to lengthen the period of pregnancy by inducing another ovulation and development of a second set of corpora lutea in the ovaries of the rabbit just before the birth of a litter was due. The extension of the gestation period could be carried on for several days. This idea of a definite life span of the placenta has been tested by attempted growth of placental tissues in tissue culture. The writer knows of no successful experiments of this kind.

2. Postnatal involutions.

There are several instances of involution of organs soon after birth which appear analogous in some aspects to the major involution of the female reproductive organs after menopause. There seems to be a spurt of growth of the uterus, vagina, and mammary glands of girl babies before birth. It is well known that at this time there is a high content of estrogenic hormone in the blood of the mother and that this passes through the placenta into the blood of the baby. Growth of both vagina and uterus has been produced in embryos by injecting hormones into the mother guinea pig during late pregnancy (Courrier,

1924). Within a few days after birth, girl babies may bleed slightly from the uterus. There may frequently be a slight watery secretion, "witch's milk," from the mammary glands of both girl and boy babies. There is much evidence to show that there is a drop in the level of estrogens before the onset of menstruation and before lactation in adults. Therefore, reduction of stimulating hormone due to severance of the baby's connections with the maternal blood supply seems to be a true explanation for these postnatal events.

The size of the uterus of the newborn decreases rapidly so that the uterus of the year old girl is considerably smaller than it was at the time of birth.

One of the most interesting examples of involution and atresia is to be found in the ovary. It occurs during embryonic life and is greatly accentuated before the attainment of puberty. Many more eggs than can be ovulated are formed and enormous numbers die and are resorbed in the ovary. Arai (1920) counted 35,000 eggs in the rat's ovary at birth; there had been a reduction to 10,000 or 11,000 at 22 days, the age of weaning, and a further reduction at the time of puberty to 5,000. Similar conditions have been described for the human ovary. Students of the ovary have often wondered just what factor it is that determines whether one egg shall live and grow to maturity while another dies. Undoubtedly hereditary factors are very important here as in all animal populations. Also availability of blood supply in the ovary must be a factor. There are no signs, however, that this elimination of follicles is due to age changes in the vessels of the ovary itself, such as might be interpreted as contributing factors in ageing of other organs during old age.

This elimination of ova is an instance of involution occurring throughout the life of the individual;—the involution being compensated for by formation of new eggs. The marked decrease in the number of eggs in the ovary of the ageing individual might then be explained by a decrease in replacement, rather than an increase in death rate. This recalls Minot's emphasis upon the fact that involution might go on more rapidly in the young individual or in the embryo than in the old person, but that it was compensated for by replacement of cells in the young individual, whereas the replacement factor declines as old age advances. As far as the uterus, vagina and mammary glands are concerned, the factor which promotes cell division in these tissues is available in the estrogenic hormone.

3. *At adolescence: pituitary secretions stimulate the ovaries.*

To appreciate properly the factors involved in ageing of the female reproductive system, one should have some conception of the factors involved in the attainment of puberty. There is now much experimental evidence on this point. As a girl approaches puberty the follicles in the ovary attain more advanced stages of growth. One of the most important discoveries of the last decade has been the demonstration that this can be hastened experimentally by increasing the amount of anterior pituitary secretion. This was done simultaneously by Smith and Engle (1927) and by Zondek and Aschheim (1927). The former, by implanting several pituitary glands into female rats at about 20 days of age, were able to produce ovulation of many follicles several weeks before the first ovulation would ordinarily have occurred. Since then many confirmations have been reported following injections of extracts of anterior pituitary glands. Apparently anterior pituitary secretions do not influence the early growth of ovarian follicles, but after these have attained medium size, the pituitary stimulates them to full pre-ovulation growth. This ovarian follicle stimulating effect of pituitary hormone is used to diagnose pregnancy, for there is an increase of this material in the urine very soon after conception.

Then it was discovered in some birds and mammals which breed seasonally that if the number of hours a day during which light were available to the animal were increased as winter set in, that ovaries and testes would begin to develop their sex cells and internal secretions (Rowan, 1925). This occurred at times when otherwise the sex glands were quiescent. It has since been shown that the added light affects the pituitary gland and induces it to secrete the hormone which stimulates the ovaries and testes. This is now a commonplace in poultry husbandry.

Not only does the anterior pituitary hormone affect the sex glands, but ovarian and testicular hormones in turn react upon the pituitary. Injection of the ovarian follicular hormone causes changes in the pituitary which can be seen microscopically. Therefore there is an intimate interrelation between these endocrine glands. Some students of adolescence have inquired if it might be possible that growth of the follicles at the time of puberty was the initiating factor influencing the pituitary which then began a reaction upon the ovary. At present, however, the evidence seems to point to increased pituitary function initiating a change in the ovaries. At least it can be truly said that it is possible to produce certain degrees of precocious maturity in the female sex organs experimentally;—to awaken by injections of pituitary hormones the immature ovaries, and then they awaken the immature vagina, uterus and mammary glands through secretion of ovarian hormones. It follows logically that a deficiency of this pituitary hormone might be a primary factor in decreased function of the ovaries such as occurs at menopause.

An example of involution of an organ associated with reproduction is found in the thymus gland which begins involution at the time of puberty. If maturity of the gonads is inhibited, involution of the thymus is delayed. For instance, if young male rats are injected with estrogenic hormone, the testes fail to grow and do not descend into the scrotum and the thymus remains large. When hormone injections are discontinued, the testes grow rapidly and descend into the scrotum and, coincident with this, the thymus undergoes involution. This has been done experimentally by Golding and Ramirez (1928). A similar inverse relation exists between ovaries and thymus.

Another interesting change depending upon hormones has recently come from the study of adolescence in children. Greulich (1937) has reported the development of certain skin glands, especially axillary and pubic, at the time of adolescence. The spurt of growth of certain hairs and other skin glands is well known to be associated with these endocrine changes. Measurements of ovarian hormone excreted in the urine of girls show an increase during adolescence (Dorfman, Greulich and Solomon, 1937). Conversely, decrease in hormone secreted at menopause would explain involution of these glands of the skin.

4. *Involutions during maturity.*

The instances of involution in genital organs during embryonic and pre-adolescent phases of life make it less difficult to understand the periodic involution which follows spurts of growth in adult female reproductive life. Failure of ovarian follicles to complete development and ovulate has already been cited. Continuation of this condition in adults explains some forms of sterility.

In case growth of follicles does bring one or a few of them to successful ovulation, the development, function, and involution of the corpus luteum in the ovary is worthy of note, for this structure undergoes involution after a brief period of function. As in the case of the placenta, the corpus luteum apparently has a definite life span which can be lengthened experimentally. It is possible to increase its length of function by supplying a hormone from the pituitary which apparently is necessary for continuing the life of these cells.

Some insight into the early life of the cells which make up the corpus luteum is essential. Before ovulation the follicle cells which surround the ovum multiply rapidly. They serve as "nurse" cells to the ovum, for all of the food which is stored in the egg must be passed through them. They are intermediaries,—bucket brigade performers,—between the blood stream and the egg. During the early growth of the follicle these cells are massed solidly around the ovum. In later development, fluid starts to form between them until the follicle becomes a blister distended with fluid. This fluid contains the ovarian follicular hormone in high concentration, which is good evidence that the second function of the follicle cells is to secrete this hormone and pass it out to the blood stream.

When the ovum is extruded from the follicle at ovulation its demand upon the follicle for food ceases. The cells in the walls of the ruptured follicle apparently continue to store food, because there is a marked accumulation in them of lipoid material. There is a rapid decrease and perhaps cessation of cell division and they begin a new phase of life as luteal cells;—the transition from follicle to corpus luteum is now well under way. As the cells change from follicular to luteal, their internal secretion changes, and the second ovarian hormone, progesterone, may be obtained by extracting them. In case the ovum is not fertilized and the animal fails to become pregnant, the life span of the corpora lutea is relatively short, but still in most animals it is several times the length of the non-pregnant cycle. In the human ovaries, scars of old corpora lutea may be found for 8 months or even longer after ovulation. Their secretory function rapidly declines and degeneration requires only a month or two at most. In case pregnancy occurs the life span of the corpus luteum is lengthened considerably, in the majority of animals it persists for the greater part of pregnancy. In women there are clear signs of degenerative processes in it before birth. It stops secreting estrogenic material before late pregnancy, for assays of corpora removed at the time of Caesarian section have given negative tests. Many of the changes described in corpora lutea toward the end of gestation are similar to old age changes described in other tissues.

Whether these cells have a definite life span beyond which they cannot continue is still a question. They persist longer in the guinea pig if the uterus is removed (Loeb, 1923). Attempts to prolong the life of luteal cells in tissue culture have not yet been successful. It seems probable that they lose their power to divide soon after ovulation.

In this connection the involution of the blood vessels in the degenerating corpora lutea deserves comment. Surely they do not involute because of ageing of the vessels themselves, for they are still young vessels; but rather through some loss of function of the cells which depend upon this vascular supply. One hesitates to ask if loss of the elasticity of the blood vessels of the corpora lutea is a factor in their involution.

The brief periods of involution which follow spurts of growth in short sexual cycles become long periods of extreme retrogression in animals where annual or seasonal breeding is the rule. Involution of the oviduct of the sparrow makes this organ almost threadlike during the winter. In some seasonally breeding mammals the ovaries and other genital organs undergo extreme involution out of mating season.

5. *Postpartum and postlactational involutions.*

The postpartum involution of the uterus is an amazing change. It involves predominantly vascular and muscular tissues. After the uterus is relieved of the baby and the afterbirth, continued contraction of the muscles reduces the size and helps control the hemorrhage caused by separation of the placenta. In the next few weeks the muscle fibers shrink and the uterus returns almost to its size before onset of pregnancy. The previously pregnant uterus can, however, usually be distinguished from the non-pregnant. The blood vessels decrease in size, but may remain quite tortuous following the first pregnancy.

Students of reproduction have sought earnestly for evidence of participation of the nervous system in sexual and generative functions. They have demonstrated that conception and pregnancy may occur after section of the spinal cord. Cutting the nerves to ovaries and uterus does not prevent the periodic recurrence of menstruation. We know that nervous system and genital system affect each other, that nervous tension may affect the menstrual rhythm, but nerve connections are not essential to many reproductive functions. Therefore it seems doubtful if ageing of the nervous tissues can be a very important factor contributing to ageing of the genital system.

Involution of the mammary glands after a baby is weaned is a remarkable change. It is almost as striking as the complete loss of foliage from trees in the fall. Secreting alveoli shrink to insignificance and almost completely disappear, and only the main branches of the duct system persist. This is so similar to the involution of the mammary glands in old age and following ovariectomy, that a clear parallel seems established. To fully appreciate these conditions, one should study whole mounts of the mammary glands of animals like the mouse or the monkey (See Gardner and van Wagenen, 1938). Here the glandular tissue can be spread flat, stained and cleared so that it can

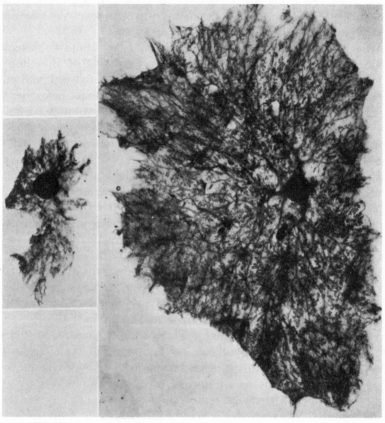

FIG. 82 FIG. 83

FIG. 82. Mammary gland from an adult monkey after removal of the ovaries. This is similar to the atrophic gland of old age.
FIG. 83. The other mammary gland from the same animal after 12 days of stimulation with estrogenic hormone from human placenta.

be examined just as one would examine ivy on the side of a building. If the ovaries are removed, secretory alveoli disappear leaving the branches of ducts as though the leaves had dropped from the twigs. There may be an actual regression of some of the smaller branches as shown in figure 82. This involution is similar to that of old age.

Injections of the primary ovarian hormone in such animals induce growth of the branching mammary ducts and the budding of new secretory alveoli. Figure 6 shows less than 2 weeks of growth in response to estrogenic hormone. The nipples also are stimulated to grow. The pituitary gland may be an essential intermediary between the ovaries and mammary glands in the growth reaction for Gomez and Turner (1938) have reported mammary growth following injections of pituitary extracts into castrated animals.

After the mammary glands have grown, the pituitary hormone, prolactin, starts their secretion of milk. Extension of the time of secretion by the mammary glands in the domesticated cow and goat is common knowledge. It is also known that this cannot be carried on indefinitely. The cow "goes dry" once a year and involution occurs in spite of all that can be done. It is apparently necessary for a spurt of growth to renovate the mammary apparatus before lactation will be resumed. Does this mean that these tissues too have a relatively short span of life and function,—a span extendable by increased function, but one which has definite limits notwithstanding?

A subject of frequent comment by students of reproduction is the apparent proportion between the length of sex cycles, gestation periods and life span. Where these are known, there frequently seems to be some correlation. In the mouse, the duration of the sex cycle is four to five days, the gestation period twenty days and the life span usually less than three years. In man, the sex cycle averages 28 days or a lunar month, the gestation period ten lunar months from onset of previous menses (nine and one-half, from conception), the life span three score and ten, plus or minus. There is much variation, of course, and in seasonally breeding animals the non-pregnant cycle frequently cannot be correlated with the other two periods. The whole question takes on added significance, however, when one emphasizes possible limited life spans of particular reproductive tissues.

6. *Evidence from malfunction and disease.*

Malfunction through disease, deficiencies of food, or excessive or deficient endocrine secretions contributes its part to the evidence for interpretation of ageing of the reproductive system. Clinicians speak of primary hypo-ovarian conditions in which the ovaries for some reason fail to produce adequate levels of hormone. Hereditary factors may be responsible in such conditions for certain endocrine states are genetically determined, as Stockard (1931) has shown by interbreeding dogs of contrasting types. If the ovaries are involved secondarily, the supporting secretions of the pituitary and thyroid are possible factors. Since hypo-pituitary effects upon the ovary can be produced experimentally by hypophysectomy, there has recently been much experimental study of this endocrine deficiency. Anterior pituitary secretion is necessary for late growth of the ovarian follicles, ovulation and formation of corpora lutea.

The anterior pituitary gland, like many other organs, has a wide factor of safety. This was realized in some of Rogers' experiments in rats (1937). He attempted to completely hypophysectomize a group of rats. They were injected with ovarian follicular hormone and readings made of the changes in electrical potential during the course of the experimentally induced estrous cycles. The animals fell into two groups in regard to their reactions. Some experienced experimental estrus, others did not, but became pseudo-pregnant. At autopsy, it was found in the latter group that small remnants of pituitary had been left. As little as three per cent of the total amount of pituitary tissue was sufficient to give this result, which is an effect of the injected estrogen acting through the remaining three per cent of the pituitary to maintain lutein tissue in the ovaries, a result previously obtained by other investigators by estrogenic treatment of normal animals. In spite of this wide factor of safety, hypo-pituitary effects on the sex function are now easily diagnosed.

In this connection Simmonds' disease, cachexia hypophysea, has a bearing upon the subject of ageing of the female genital system. The most important symptoms are premature ageing, rapid atrophy of the genital organs, regression of the secondary sex characters and loss of hair. This disease is not frequent but its incidence is highest in comparatively young women. It is due to atrophy of the anterior pituitary. It is similar in some respects to "operative" menopause following removal or X-ray treatment of the ovaries.

The converse, hyperpituitary conditions, are readily reproducible experimentally. Precocious puberty has already been cited. Smith and Engle (1927) have induced ovulation of as many as 48 and 63 eggs in the mouse, and Hisaw (1936) 5 eggs at a time in the monkey, by increasing anterior pituitary hormones. This is undoubtedly a factor in multiple births of non-identical twins.

That the thyroid may have a supporting function is shown by the fact that thyroid therapy may frequently be effective in alleviating amenorrhea and sterility, even in cases where basal metabolism may

TABLE 25

A "time table" of outstanding events involving the female reproductive system

Although based on conditions in women, the major sequences have general application to other mammals. As in all time tables, allowances must be made for variables.

Age	Event	Organs involved primarily	Endocrine glands involved	Involutions of organs or parts
Preliminary	Ovogenesis Spermatogenesis	Ovaries Testes	Pituitary	*Many ova*
Pre-natal life 1st day	*Insemination* FERTILIZATION	Ovum—Sperm *New individual;* uterine tubes	Ovary, testis Ovary	*Many sperms* Follicle cells around ovum Polar bodies
10–14 days	Implantation	Uterus (lining)	Corpus luteum	*Zona pellucida*
2–6 weeks	Placenta (formation of)	Chorion (part) Uterus (lining)	Corpus luteum	Chorionic villi except in placenta
3rd month and after 9th month	Sex differentiation Degenerative changes in	Female organs Placenta	Ovaries of embryo (?)	Male accessory sex organs Placenta (villi, blood vessels)
1st week *Post-natal life*	Birth (1) Menses (occasional) (2) "Witches milk" (occasional)	Uterus, vagina Uterus of newborn Mammae of newborn	Placenta Baby escapes from influences of maternal hormones	*Afterbirth* *Uterus* (maternal)
	Atresia of follicles	Ovary	Anterior pituitary (FSH)	Many ova and their follicles
12–16 years	*Adolescence*	Reproductive organs	Ovary (estrogen) Pituitary (FSH)	
13–17 years 14–18 years	*1st menstruation** *1st ovulation*	Uterus Follicle ruptures and becomes 1st corpus luteum	Pituitary (FSH) Pituitary (FSH and LH)	*Uterus* (lining) Atrophy of some other follicles Corpus luteum (afterward)

Life period	Event			
During reproductive life	Cyclic menstruation	Uterus	Ovaries (estrogen alone or combined with progesterone), pituitary	Uterine lining; succession of follicles and corpora lutea
	1st pregnancy	Vagina, ovaries, uterus, tubes	Ovaries, placenta, pituitary (?)	Inhibition of follicles
	1st childbirth	Uterus, vagina		Uterus, corpus luteum (afterward)
	Lactation	Mammary glands	Pituitary (prolactin)	Mammae (afterward)
	Cyclic menses	(1) Spurts of growth in uterus leading to	(2) Periods of function followed by	(3) Minor involutions
	(Long rests in seasonal breeders)	All reproductive organs	Ovaries, pituitary	All genital organs
	Other pregnancies			
Pre-menopausal	Irregularity of menses†	Uterus	Ovaries	Uterus
45–55 years	Menopause, climacteric	Uterus, many organs	Ovaries and supporting endocrine glands	Genital organs; progressive atrophy leading to ultimate *Major involution*
50 years and after	Increased incidence of cancer	Uterus, mammary glands	Ovaries earlier in life; other causes	
Very old age	Atrophic diseases	Genital organs	Ovaries deficient	Senile atrophy of genital organs
65 years	DEATH			

* First few menstrual cycles probably without ovulation.
† Before menopause the last few menstrual cycles are probably anovulatory.

not be low, if conditions are not complicated by other factors (Pratt and Thomas, 1937). It is logical then to suppose that with decreased thyroid activity as old age advances that there may be a decreased endocrine support from this gland for ovarian function.

Adrenal virilism is another instance bearing upon endocrine control of sexual cycles. An adolescent girl or young woman may have irregular menstrual periods or cessation of menses, and begin to develop masculine secondary sex characters with masculine growth and distribution of terminal hair, change of voice and the psychic characteristics. This syndrome may be due to the growth of a tumor of the adrenal gland. Masculine changes usually disappear and menstruation begins rather promptly after the tumor is removed.

The evidence cited clearly places the menopause as a major involution of uterine function, a failure of the lining of the uterus to grow to the point where menstruation will follow. Involutionary changes occur simultaneously in the vagina and mammary glands. A similar condition can be brought on experimentally by removal of ovaries. The amount of hormone necessary to re-establish menstruation is now known and lesser doses are not effective. Therefore, failure of ovarian secretion to reach an adequate level is undoubtedly one of the major factors in menopause. But is the deficiency primarily ovarian, or primarily due to failure of supportive function of digestive organs, pituitary or thyroid?

There is further experimental evidence bearing upon this point. Ovulation usually stops at, or even before, menopause and consequently there are no corpora lutea in the ovary to secrete progesterone. It has already been shown that the corpora lutea are not essential to menstruation. Apparently the follicular hormone is the only necessary ovarian secretion involved. At the time of menopause there is decrease in the amount of estrogenic hormone excreted in the urine. This is also true following operative menopause in young women. There is an increase at this time in the amount of the pituitary secretion which stimulates the ovarian follicles (Albright, 1936). This has been cited as evidence for primary deficiency of ovarian (rather than pituitary) secretion as a cause of menopause. Furthermore, if estrogens are injected, there follows a decrease in excretion of this pituitary hormone and sometimes relief of menopausal symptoms.

Bidder (1932) in a general discussion of senescence favors the interpretation that ageing of an organ is the after result of limitation of size. For instance, "Tumors tend to be limited in size by necrosis of parts far removed from the surface." The limiting factor in central necrosis of tumors is probably inadequate growth of blood vessels. Whether this applies to organs like the placenta, as it undergoes involution, is still problematical. It does not seem to apply to the cyclic involutions of the non-pregnant uterus. From some of the experimental evidence, lack of essential hormones which support growth and function seems a more important factor.

6. ATROPHIC CONDITIONS FAVORABLE TO COMPLICATING DISEASES

One of the most interesting practical considerations concerned with menopause and the involutional conditions which follow or accompany it, is that these conditions often favor complicating infections. Atrophy affects the mammary glands, uterus, tubes, ovaries, vagina and vulva.

The extent to which atrophy of the ovary and uterus may proceed is fully realized when a careful search is made at autopsy or at dissection. The ovaries of a 70 year old woman are found to be nothing but small fibrous folds of tissue and the uterus extremely small and fibrous. Infection of atrophic genital organs may occur after menopause and may become chronic. There are now many reports in the medical literature of cases in which treatment with estrogenic hormone has started growth in these tissues and returned them to a more nearly normal mature condition. This treatment often results in the clearing up of chronic genital diseases, both atrophic and infectious.

To be more specific, the growth effect of estrogens on the vaginal epithelium has been utilized by Lewis (1933) and others in the treatment of chronic gonorrheal vaginitis in children, and by Davis (1935) and others in the treatment of atrophic conditions of post-menopausal life. Under the stimulus of estrogen the thin vaginal epithelium grows to a thick healthy membrane. Glycogen appears in the vaginal epithelial cells. The reaction of the fluid in the vagina changes from an alkaline to an acid reaction which is unfavorable to life of infecting organisms. Treatment for a month or two by local applications of estrogen usually is followed by a cure in all but obstinate cases. The response of the atrophic vagina is readily followed by study of the desquamated cells. Discontinuance of post-menopausal treatment is followed by return to the previous atrophic condition. It seems to the writer that clinical use of estrogens in these cases should begin with the minimal effective dose, which should be less than the threshold for post-climacteric menstruation.

7. HYPERTROPHIC AND NEOPLASTIC DISEASE

Certain hypertrophic diseases seem to occur frequently at the approach of menopause. The ovaries may become cystic, the cysts persisting for a considerable time and sometimes secreting undue amounts of hormone. Such cases may be accompanied by abnormal conditions sometimes involving uterine hemorrhages, and blocked and distended mammary ducts leading to mastitis. These conditions sometimes clear up spontaneously, or it may be necessary to remove the ovaries or to hasten their involution by treatment with X-rays.

Neoplastic diseases such as cancer of the mammary glands and uterus have their highest incidence at or soon after the time of menopause. Macklin (1935) places the incidence of female genital cancer at 20 to 30 per cent of all cancers. This matter was more vividly brought to the writer's attention while attending a football game at which some 72,000 people were present,—perhaps three-eighths of them women. A companion turned from an exciting incident in the game to ask, "Do you realize that one-tenth of all the women present will die of mammary or uterine cancer?" Why the highest incidence should occur around the age of menopause is still a difficult question. Here again, there is some experimental evidence (cited below) bearing upon this point.

The foregoing discussion has developed the thesis that spurts of growth in the genital organs are due to the action of the estrogenic hormone. Female genital cancer is really growth, although an atypical growth, of cells of genital organs.

Rapidly growing and malignant cancer of the mammary gland in certain inbred strains of mice kills the animals in from a month to 6 weeks after the tumor makes its first appearance (Strong, 1936). Studies of the sexual cycles of these animals show a very rapid decrease and disappearance of sexual activity as the mammary cancer grows. The uterus and vagina become extremely atrophic as in old age and as after removal of the ovaries. These atrophic organs of cancerous mice can be induced again to function by injections of ovarian hormones and by implants of anterior pituitary (Allen, et al., 1935). It would seem, therefore, that the uterus and vagina have not lost their reactivity but that the rapidly growing mammary cancer interferes with secretion of essential hormones. This point emphasizes the endocrine relationships of the female genital organs and cancer in these organs.

Very soon after the ovarian hormones were isolated and concentrated, experiments were begun to see if cancer would follow massive doses of estrogenic hormone continued over long periods of time. One of the most interesting experiments in this connection was first contributed by Lacassagne (1932) and confirmed by Burrows (1935) and Gardner, Smith, Allen and Strong (1936) and others. In certain inbred strains of mice over 80 per cent of the females die of mammary cancer before reaching the age of a year and a half (Strong, 1936). The males do not have mammary cancer because the mammary glands in males do not grow. Large amounts of ovarian hormone made the rudimentary mammary glands of the male grow to a size equivalent to those of the female. Many of these males developed mammary cancer and died of it. They were feminized to the point where their mammary tissues developed cancerous growths. It must be recalled that a genetic factor for cancer may be involved in these mice.

It is now known, however, that some structures get their first directional impulses genetically and that then the course of development may be continued or changed by the action of hormones (Danforth, 1938). It is difficult sometimes to determine where the genetic influence stops and the hormonal influence takes over control. Occasionally it is possible to produce genital cancers in strains of mice where such cancers were extremely infrequent before hormonal treatment began.

Other genital tissues than those of the mammary glands react to excessive hormonal stimulation. Recently it has been possible experimentally to produce tumors of the uterus in the guinea pig similar to uterine fibroids so frequent in negroes (Nelson, 1937), and atypical growths of the cervix of the mouse, rat and monkey, which have been diagnosed by pathologists as somewhat similar histologically to human cervical cancer (Gardner, Allen, Smith and Strong, 1938; Perry and Ginzton, 1937; Overholser and Allen, 1935). After accumulating 19 cases of cervical cancer from hundreds of mice subjected to excessive treatment with estrogenic hormones, it has been demonstrated that these cancers are capable of independent growth when transplanted into both male and female hosts (Gardner, Allen, Smith and Strong, 1928).

Cancer is an uncontrolled growth. Just what sets these cells free from the restraint of growth which other tissues of the ageing body feel, is still a question. To quote W. Cramer (1932), "Cancer cells develop and grow in a senescent organism and their continued proliferation is not influenced by the conditions which induce senescence." In the sex hormones, however, there exists a powerful stimulator of growth of genital tissues. Many experiments are in progress to test the question, "Will long continued or abnormally high levels of estrogen produce excessive, atypical, abnormal and perhaps cancerous growths?" Much work must still be done before the final answer is known.

8. A PHILOSOPHY FOR MENOPAUSE

If these hormones are so potent in dominating sexual life, why not turn to them as to "the fountain of youth?" If the primary cause of menopause is deficiency of ovarian follicular hormone, why not supply it at this time as we do thyroid substance to cretins? There seems no logical reason against sex hormone therapy in moderation. Ovarian hormones are not too expensive.

There are still some practical objections, however. Although ovarian hormones are effective by mouth, and several preparations of this sort are available, they are much less effective than by subcutaneous injection, and of course, less easy to take by the latter route for long periods. The pituitary hormones require further chemical study and reduction in cost before they can be used widely and effectively. Again, sex function makes heavy demands upon other bodily functions—demands easily supplied in youth and maturity—but less easily met by the ageing body. The question as to whether sex function experimentally prolonged in ageing people would shorten the expectancy of life is still unanswered.

Therapy with female sex hormones is helpful in some kinds of diseases. It merely substitutes for endocrine functions of the ovaries, and as far as we know, has no beneficial effects on the ovaries themselves. In its present state of development, our conservative physicians advocate short treatment and diminishing doses of hormones,—aiming at alleviation,—at tiding over a difficult climacteric and easing down more gradually to the low sex hormone level of the sixth decade. How many women 10 years after menopause wish to menstruate again or to feel the command of sex urge? Fortunately, smaller doses than needed to restore menstruation may alleviate other symptoms associated with menopause. There may be danger in use of massive doses of these powerful growth stimulants which concentrate on genital tissues. It seems best to be careful until adequate trials in lower animals have clearly defined the risks. There is good evidence that there may be a long interval between the effective stimulus to cancer and its actual appearance, similar to that in the cases of the radium poisoning in watch dial painters and the X-ray burns in early experimenters. Again, conservative physicians point out that other measures are often equally or more effective than hormone therapy and perhaps more sensible from the viewpoint of the whole body.

It seems doubtful that sex hormones flow from "the fountain of youth." Why not think with pleasure (or otherwise) of the days of our youth, living them in retrospect sometimes perhaps, but thankful that some of the powerful, insistent urges of youth leave us free as we age to turn to other things.

9. SUMMARY

The ageing of the female reproductive system involves accentuation of involutionary processes which occur periodically after spurts of growth during normal reproductive life.

Menopause is a "milestone" indicating decrease of ovarian hormone secretion below the level necessary for menstrual function.

Premature ageing of female genital organs, including cessation of menstruation, follows removal of the ovaries or their damage by X-rays.

Therapy with ovarian hormones replaces destroyed or lagging ovarian endocrine function, induces growth of genital organs and restoration of menstrual function.

Some of the basic experimental work with ovarian hormones on which these conclusions rest is cited briefly. Increased hormonal secretion induces growth which leads to short periods of function and which is followed by minor involutions when these hormones ebb. Experimental menstrual cycles show that menses are degenerative processes coming at one point of the hormonal ebb. These are the fundamentals of cyclic sexual and reproductive functions in women.

Specific instances of minor involutions of the genital organs are cited in normal girls, young and adult women.

The visualization of the menstruating surface of the uterus by transplanting small bits to the eyes of monkeys is described and the remarkable regenerative capacity of the uterus is mentioned.

The factor of "safety" or reserve of the ovaries and decrease of this reserve with ageing definitely points to decline of endocrine function as one of the major factors in ageing of the genital system.

Instances of diseased conditions including female genital cancers usually associated with ageing processes are mentioned and experiments described which bear upon endocrine factors partly responsible. The chapter closes with comments on endocrine therapy as applicable at present for normal ageing women.

REFERENCES

ALBRIGHT, F. 1936. Studies on ovarian dysfunction. III. The menopause. Endocrinology, **20**, 24-39.

ALLEN, E. 1927. The menstrual cycle of the monkey, Macacus rhesus: observations on normal animals, the effects of removal of the ovaries and the effects of injections of ovarian and placental extracts into the spayed animals. Contrib. Embryol., Carnegie Inst., Wash., **19**, 1-44.

ALLEN, E., AND DOISY, E. A. 1923. An ovarian hormone: preliminary report on its localization, extraction and partial purification, and action in test animals. J. A. M. A., **81**, 819-821.

ALLEN, E., DIDDLE, A. W., STRONG, L. C., BURFORD, T. H., AND GARDNER, W. U. 1935. The estrous cycles of mice during growth of spontaneous mammary tumors and the effects of ovarian follicular and anterior pituitary hormones. Am. J. Cancer, **25**, 291-300.

ALLEN, E., HISAW, F. L., AND GARDNER, W. U. 1939. The endocrine function of the ovaries. E. Allen (editor), Sex and Internal Secretions, 2nd Edition, Baltimore: Williams & Wilkins.

ALLEN, E., PRATT, J. P., NEWELL, Q. U., AND BLAND, L. J. 1930. Human tubal ova; related early corpora lutea and uterine tubes. Contrib. Embryol., Carnegie Inst., Wash., **22**, 45-76.

ALLEN, E., SMITH, G. M., AND GARDNER, W. U. 1937. Accentuation of the growth effect of theelin on genital tissues of the ovariectomized mouse by arrest of mitosis with colchicine. Am. J. Anat., **61**, 321-341.

ALLEN, W. M., AND CORNER, G. W. 1929. Physiology of the corpus luteum. III. Normal growth and implantation of embryos after very early ablation of the ovaries, under the influence of extracts of the corpus luteum. Am. J. Physiol., **88**, 340-346.

ARAI, H. 1920. On the postnatal development of the ovary (albino rat) with especial reference to the number of ova. Am. J. Anat., **27**, 405-462.

BARTELMEZ, G. W. 1933. Histological studies on the menstruating mucous membrane of the human uterus. No. 443 Contrib. Embryol., Carnegie Inst., Wash., No. 142, 141-186.

BIDDER, G. P. 1932. Senescence. Brit. Med. J., **2**, 583-585.

BURR, H. S., MUSSELMAN, L. K., BARTON, DOROTHY, AND KELLY, NAOMI B. 1937. Bio-electric correlates of human ovulation. Yale J. Biol. and Med., **10**, 155-160.

BURR, H. S., HILL, R. T., AND ALLEN, EDGAR. 1935. Detection of ovulation in the intact rabbit. Proc. Soc. Exper. Biol. and Med., **33**, 109-11.

BURROWS, H. 1935. Pathological changes induced in the mamma by oestrogenic compounds. Brit. J. Surg., **23**, 191-213.

CORNER, G. W. 1923. Ovulation and menstruation in Macacus rhesus. Contrib. Embryol. (No. 75) Carnegie Inst., Wash., **15**, 73-101.

——— 1932-33. The nature of the menstrual cycle. The Harvey Lectures, Baltimore: Williams & Wilkins, pp. 67-89.

COURRIER, R. 1924. Nouvelles recherches sur la folliculine; contribution á l'etude du passage des hormones au travers du placenta. Compt. rend. Acad. d. Sc., **179**, 2192.

CRAMER, W. 1932. Protozoa, senescence and cancer. Brit. Med. J., **2**, 690–691.

DANFORTH, C. H. 1939. Genic and endocrine factors in sex. E. Allen (editor). Sex and Internal Secretions, Baltimore: Williams & Wilkins.

DAVIS, M. E. 1935. The treatment of senile vaginitis with ovarian follicular hormone. Surg. Gynec. & Obst., **61**, 680–686.

DOISY, E. A., VELER, C. D., AND THAYER, S. 1929. Folliculin from urine of pregnant women. Am. J. Physiol., **90**, 329–330.

DORFMAN, R. I., GREULICH, W. W., AND SOLOMON, C. I. 1937. The excretion of androgenic and estrogenic substances in the urine of children. Endocrinology, **21**, 741–743.

ENGLE, E. T. 1938. A menstrual record during the menopause. Human Biology, **9**, 564–566.

FRANK, R. T., GOLDBERGER, M. A., AND SALMON, U. J. 1936. Menopause: symptoms, hormonal status, and treatment. New York State J. Med., **36**, 1363–1371.

FRANK, R. T., GOLDBERGER, M. A., SALMON, U. J., AND FELSHIN, G. 1937. Amenorrhea: its causation and treatment. J. A. M. A., **109**, 1863–1869.

GARDNER, W. U., ALLEN, EDGAR, SMITH, G. M., AND STRONG, L. C. 1938. Carcinoma of the cervix of mice receiving estrogens. J. A. M. A., **110**, 1182–1183.

GARDNER, W. U., SMITH, G. M., ALLEN, E., AND STRONG, L. C. 1936. Cancer of mammary glands induced in male mice receiving estrogenic hormone. Arch. Path., **21**, 265–272.

GARDNER, W. U., AND VAN WAGENEN, G. 1938. Experimental development of the mammary glands of the monkey. Endocrinology, **22**, 164–172.

GOLDING, G. T., AND RAMIREZ, F. T. 1928. Ovarian and placental hormone effects in normal, immature albino rats. Endocrinology, **12**, 804–812.

GOMEZ, E. T., AND C. W. TURNER. 1938. Further evidence for a mammogenic hormone in the anterior pituitary. Proc. Soc. Exp. Biol. and Med., **37**, 607–609.

GREULICH, W. 1937. The relation of the developing apocrine sweat glands to the maturation of the reproductive system in children. Anat. Rec. (Mar.), **67**, (suppl. 3), p. 21.

GRUETER, F., AND STRICKER, P. 1929. Uber die Wirkung eines Hypophysenvorderlappenhormons auf die Auslösung der Milchsekretion. Klin. Wchnschr., **8**, 2322–23.

HALL, B. V. 1936. Variation in acidity and oxidation reduction of rodent uterine fluid. Physiol. Zool., **9**, 471–497.

HAMILTON, J. B., AND WOLFE, J. M. 1938. The effect of male hormone substances upon birth and prenatal development in the rat. Anat. Rec., **70**, 433–440.

HARTMAN, C. G. 1932. Studies in the reproduction of the monkey macacus (pithecus) rhesus, with special reference to menstruation and pregnancy. Contrib. Embryol., No. 134, Carnegie Inst., Wash., Pub. 433, pp. 3–161.

——— 1938. Proceedings Singer-Polignac Colloquium, Les hormones sexuelles, pp. 103–118, Paris, Herman.

HISAW, F. L. 1927. Experimental relaxation of the symphysis pubis of the guinea pig. Anat. Rec., **37**, p. 126.

HISAW, F. L. 1936. (Unpublished.)

LACASSAGNE, A. 1932. Apparition de cancers de la mamelle chez la souris male soumise a des injections de folliculine. Compt. rend. Acad. d. Sc., **195**, 630-632.

LENDRUM, F. C., AND HISAW, F. L. 1936. Cytology of monkey endometrium under influence of follicular and corpus luteum hormones. Proc. Soc. Exper. Biol. & Med., **34**, 394-396.

LEWIS, R. M. 1933. Study of effects of theelin on gonorrheal vaginitis in children. Am. J. Obst. & Gynec., **26**, 593-599.

LEWIS, W. H. 1931. A human tubal egg, unfertilized. Bull. Johns Hopkins Hosp., **48**, 368-372.

LOEB, L. 1907-1908 The experimental production of the maternal part of the placenta in the rabbit. Proc. Soc. Exper. Biol. & Med., **5**, 102-104.

———— 1923. The effect of extirpation of the uterus on the life and function of the corpus luteum in the guinea pig. Proc. Soc. Exper. Biol. & Med., **20**, 441-443.

MACKLIN, M. T. 1938. Familial incidence of cancer. A Symposium on Cancer, 32-45. Madison: The University of Wisconsin Press.

MARKEE, J. E. 1932-1933. Menstruation in ocular endometrial transplants. Anat. Rec., (Mar. 25), **55**, p. 66 (abstract).

NELSON, W. O. 1937. Endometrial and myometrial changes, including fibromyomatous nodules, induced in the uterus of the guinea pig by prolonged administration of oestrogenic hormone. Anat. Rec., **68**, 99-102.

NEWTON, W. H. 1935. Pseudo-parturition in the mouse and the relation of the placenta to postpartum oestrus. J. Physiol., **84**, 196-207.

OVERHOLSER, M. D., AND ALLEN, E. 1935. Atypical growth induced in cervical epithelium of the monkey by prolonged injections of ovarian hormone combined with chronic trauma. Surg. Gynec. and Obst., **60**, 129-136.

PERRY, I., AND GINZTON, L. 1937. The development of tumors in female mice treated with 1:2:5:6 dibenzanthracene and theelin. Am. J. Cancer, **29**, 680-704.

PINCUS, G., SAUNDERS, B. 1937. Unfertilized human tubal ova. Anat. Rec., **69**, 163-169.

PRATT, J. P. 1939. Sex function in man. Chapter XXIV in "Sex and Internal Secretions," E. Allen (editor). Baltimore: Williams & Wilkins.

PRATT, J. P., AND THOMAS, W. L. 1937. The endocrine treatment of menopausal phenomena. J. A. M. A., **109**, 1875-1877.

REBOUL, J., FRIEDGOOD, H. B., AND DAVIS, H. 1937. Electrical detection of ovulation. Am. J. Physiol., **119**, p. 387.

RICHTER, C. P., AND HARTMAN, C. G. 1934. Effect of injection of amniotin on spontaneous activity of gonadectomized rats. Am. J. Physiol., **108**, 136-143.

RIDDLE, O., BATES, R. W., AND DYKSHORN, S. W. 1932. A new hormone of the anterior pituitary. Proc. Soc. Exp. Biol. and Med., **29**, 1211-1212.

ROGERS, P. V. 1937. Changes in electrical potential during the oestrous cycle of normal and experimental rats. Thesis, Yale University.

ROSSLE, R. 1923. Wachstum und Altern zur Physiologie und Pathologie der postfotalen Entwicklung. Munchen: Bergmann, 351 pp.

Rowan, W. 1925. Relation of light to bird migration and developmental changes. Nature, 115, 494–495.

Smith, P. E., and Engle, E. T. 1927. Experimental evidence regarding the role of the anterior pituitary in the development and regulation of the genital system. Am. J. Anat., 40, 159–217.

Snyder, F. F., and Wislocki, G. B. 1931. The effect of the injection of urine from pregnant mammals on ovulation in the rabbit. Bull. Johns Hopkins Hosp., 48, 362–367.

Stockard, C. R. 1931. The physical basis of personality. New York: Norton & Co., 320 pp.

Strong, L. C. 1936. Establishment of "A" strain of inbred mice. J. Heredity, 27, 21–34.

Turner, C. W. 1939. The mammary glands. E. Allen (editor), Sex and Internal Secretions. Baltimore: Williams & Wilkins.

Wang, G. H. 1923. The relation between "spontaneous" activity and oestrus cycle in the white rat. Comp. Psychol. Mon., 2, 1–27.

Warthin, A. S. 1929. Old Age, the major involution. New York: P. B. Hoeber, Inc., 199 pp.

Werner, A. A., and Collier, W. D. 1933. The effect of theelin injections on the castrated woman. J. A. M. A., 100, 633–640.

White, A., Catchpole, H. R., and Long, C. N. H. 1937. A crystalline protein with high lactogenic activity. Science, 86, 82–83.

Wiesner, B. P. 1932. Experimental study of senescence. Brit. Med. J., 2, 585–587.

Willier, B. H., Gallagher, T. F., and Koch, F. C. 1935. The action of male and female sex hormones upon the reproductive glands and ducts of the chick embryo. Anat. Rec., 61 (Suppl.), p. 50.

Zondek, B., and Aschheim, S. 1927. Das Hormon des Hypophysenvorderlappens. I. Testobjekt zum Nachweis des Hormons. Klin. Wchnschr., 6, 248–252.

Zuckerman, S. 1936. Inhibition and induction of uterine bleeding by means of oestrone. Lancet, 2, 9–13.

CHAPTER 15

MALE REPRODUCTIVE SYSTEM

EARL T. ENGLE

New York

Men seldom seek medical advice about their reproductive system as they grow old until they are embarrassed by difficulties of urination and the more intelligent of them fear that they have enlarged prostates. Obstructive prostatic enlargement in varying degrees is found in 4 out of every 10 men after the age of 60. Decline in sexual activity is taken more or less philosophically as a matter of course so that few data are available concerning it. For men no such definite landmarks as menstruation, pregnancy and menopause occur.

The endometrium and vaginal mucosa may be biopsied at any stage of the reproductive cycle; the ovaries are frequently observed at laparotomy. Perhaps 100 women have had their ovaries removed for every man who has been castrated.

The internist, the surgeon and the psychiatrist record observations on the genital physiology and rhythmicity of the female in the course of routine medical examination. Aside from records of paternity, little information about the physiology of the male appears on the medical chart. The gynecologist and obstetrician have become specialists in dealing with the normal as well as the pathological genital system of the female. For attention to the male genital system the only recourse is to the specialists in urology who have gained much knowledge of the pathology and surgery of the genital system, but, in general, have not been interested in reproduction. That is to say, the normal physiology and the wide range of pathological findings in the female genital system are quite well recorded and understood because the woman goes to the doctor, frequently for non-specific complaints, and becomes an object of attention. The man, usually, however, gives no information about the genital system unless there is a specific or suspected involvement of these organs. When there is no specific lesion, nor complaint of sterility the genital physiology and morphology of the male is supposed to be normal.

The changes that may occur in the male genital organs in relation to age are little known. Much of the material presented in this chapter must deal first with the range of normal structural and functional variability at all ages. It is necessary also to restrict the material to be discussed to the genital system and its physiology per se, with little attention to the widely spread psycho-sexual components which are discussed by Hamilton (Chapter 16). That is, the genital system may be discussed solely as a specialized morphological device adapted for reproduction, but the same structures form a part, and possibly a base, of the total sex response. However, it is also clear that, in the adult, sex behavior and sex response may exist in the absence of the gonads or any other morphological units of the genital system. Prepubertal castrates undoubtedly have a total absence of such behavior. Before discussing the testes and prostate, in which ageing is most marked, it is desirable to explain briefly the mechanisms of endocrine integration by which normal functional activity is maintained.

1. ENDOCRINE INTEGRATION[1]

The development of the genital system and the attainment and maintenance of functional adequacy are to a certain degree interrelated with endocrine factors.

The testis is composed of two types of tissue. The seminiferous tubules contain the cells which produce and nourish the developing spermatozoa. In the intertubular spaces are found the blood vessels, lymphatics, loose connective tissue and the specialized interstitial cells, or cells of Leydig. These latter cells are generally accepted as the cells of origin of one or more of the male sex hormones.

Two groups of hormones are involved in the maintenance of the reproductive system.[2] One group consists of those which act only on the gonad, and cause it to function properly, and are known as gonadotropins. These are the gonad stimulating hormones of the anterior pituitary gland. It is not known whether these are the same for both sexes. Two other well known gonadotropic hormones occur in the

---

[1] This brief summary of endocrine-gonad relations merely introduces the problem of hormone balance in maturity and ageing. Further discussion is to be found in "Sex and Internal Secretion," edited by E. Allen, Williams & Wilkins, Baltimore, 1938.

[2] Gonadotropic hormone or gonadotropins are the principles which directly activate the gonads and are frequently called the gonad-stimulating hormones.

Estrogen: a generic name for substances formerly called female sex hormone, so called because of their action in inducing estrus or "heat" in animals.

Androgen: a generic name for substances formerly called male sex hormone, so called because of their action on male animals.

human. One of these is found in the blood and urine of pregnant women and in the human placenta. The other, qualitatively different, is found in the blood or urine of women after the menopause or ovariectomy.

The second group of hormones are the sex hormones which in nature are produced by the gonads in response to the action of gonadotropic hormones on the ovary or the testis. Certain female sex hormones

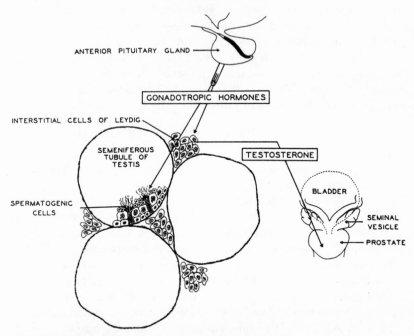

Fig. 84. Diagram showing the action of gonadotropic hormones of the anterior pituitary on the testis. The gonadotropic hormone stimulates the testis, causing it to secrete testosterone, one of the androgens or male sex hormones, which maintains the secretory activity of the accessory glands.

discussed by Allen in the previous chapter are known collectively as estrogens and the male sex hormones as androgens (fig. 84).

Maintenance of genital function in the male depends on the proper balance of gonadotropins, estrogens and androgens.

One gonadotropic factor, frequently referred to as the "luteinizer" because of its action on the ovary, exerts its action on the interstitial cells, causing the production of androgens. Androgens thus produced act on all the other genital organs and probably with other endocrines, on the entire body. Certain experimental evidence indicates that the estrogens also have a rôle in the male genital system, although it is not clear what effects estrogens may cause in the man, nor in what organ they may be produced. As will be shown below, substances identified as estrogens as well as androgens are found in the urine of normal men.

One gonadotropin also acts directly on the seminiferous epithelium, maintaining sperm production and, at least in the rat, certain androgens will maintain sperm production. The experimental evidence on rats indicates that one gonadotropin, (which again because of its action in the female), is called a follicle stimulating hormone acts on the seminiferous tubule, although its effect is enhanced if it is given with the interstital cell stimulator (the luteinizing factor). Either by this means, or experimentally by direct administration of an androgen, the spermatogenic function is maintained.

It is known that the human male by the fifth foetal month, shows an enormous hyperplasia of the interstitial cells, which is maintained until after birth. This hyperplasia undergoes involution after birth, in the same manner as the foetal uterus. The seminiferous tubules, however, do not change appreciably during this period. Experiments with appropriate gonadotropic hormones in rats and monkeys indicate that the quantitative increase of the interstitial cell mass caused by the injection of gonadotropic hormone of human pregnancy is greatest in early life. Thus, a marked interstitial cell hyperplasia can be caused in young animals. It is thought by some that this same hormone which is present in the blood of pregnant women is responsible for the natal hyperplasia as well as for the prenatal descent of the testis. However, this tissue loses its capacity to respond to this gonadotropic hormone by hypertrophy. The interstitial cells of a normal adult rat or monkey may be induced to produce androgens as shown by the growth of accessory organs, but will not show marked hyperplasia.

The interstitial cells of the testis will respond, from or before birth, to the appropriate gonadotropin, but the seminiferous tubules do not show a similar responsiveness at this age. Neither the ovarian follicle nor the testis tubules will respond to the gonadotropins until a much later age.

The present data, while not conclusive, indicate that a period of cellular differentiation and ripening of the tubule is necessary before sperm production can be induced. There is agreement that sperm production in animals cannot be precociously induced by any androgen or gonadotropin (q.v. Engle, 1938a; 1938b; C. Moore, 1936, 1938)

Until the tubule has undergone the necessary development independent of these particular hormones it cannot respond to an otherwise adequate gonad activator. In the human female at least the same loss of reactivity of the ovary is seen at the menopause (Kurzrok and Smith, 1938). It is not known whether or when a similar loss of reactivity is shown by the testis, but in the light of all other data it is to be anticipated.

Both androgens and estrogens are excreted in the urine by both men and women.[3] Small amounts of each have been found in children, both boys and girls (Dorfman, Greulich and Solomon, 1937). Kochakian (1937) found that young men between 21 and 29 excreted 12 to 16 capon units per liter, while 5 men, 50 to 72 years of age, excreted an average of 2 to 3 capon units.

Koch gives as a normal range of androgens in mature men 40-100 I.U. of androgen, and of normal women 30-100 I.U. of androgen (1937); (see also Gallagher et al., 1937, and Kenyon et al., 1937, for further studies of the Koch group).

One of the characteristics of the menopause is the increase in excretion of gonadotropic substance, which is concomitant with decrease of cessation of ovarian function (vide Allen, Chapter 14). That the relationship is a direct one was shown by Fuller Albright who inhibited the excretion of gonadotropins by injections of estrone in women.

---

[3] Until more is learned of the metabolism of the androgens, estrogens, and progestin and their chemical precursors in the body, a certain reserve should be maintained as to the significance of values obtained by urinary assay. There is general agreement that these hormones are produced by the gonads, but estrogenic substance is found in the blood of women after ovariectomy (Fluhmann) and both estrogenic and androgenic substance in the urine after ovariectomy, and in male castrates by Koch (J. Urol., **30**, 393, 1936). Mainly testosterone was extracted from bull's testes which have little or no androsterone in the urine (Koch) while human urine has no testosterone.

The ratio of estrogen-androgen excretion is based on the amount of urinary extract required to produce a standard biological response on a test animal, and compared with the response obtained by crystalline material. The reported values are then expressed in terms of the international unit (I.U.) of crystalline material. An international unit of androsterone is 100 gamma (0.1 milligram) while one I.U. of estrone is 0.1 gamma (0.0001 milligram). Thus Koch's ratio of androgen to estrogen assayed in terms of bird units and rat units is expressed as 1.0 for normal men, and 0.7 for normal women . . . but the comparison should lead to no confusion in saying that a normal male excretes less female sex hormone than male hormone. It may be more in terms of I.U. but greatly less by weight. As used in this comparative sense, the "unit" is merely a convenient abstraction to convey a ratio, and not a statement of actual proportions.

Such a marked increase in production does not appear to be true for men (Saethre). At least, if it does occur in some, its appearance is not so sharply limited to a single decade of life as in women. From the slight evidence of hormone excretion and the abundant clinical experience it is safe to believe that there is no sharp decline in reproductive capacity in relation to chronological age in the male as in the female.

While the reproductive capacity of the woman is in abeyance from the latter part of the fifth decade, the sexual capacity need not be lost. Sexual function in either sex may be seriously restricted in the presence of adequate hormones, or may continue after the removal of the gonads and restriction of sex hormone production (vide infra).

Little data exist regarding copulatory frequency in man at various decades. Pearl's data indicate that this criteria is not so much a function of age as it is an inherent virility which is influenced by social and environmental conditions and by earlier behavior patterns. The greatest amount of sex activity in Pearl's small series of married men was in the decade 20–29, steadily declining thereafter. Of importance, also, is his observation that frequency is greatest among the "farmers" group, less among "merchants and bankers" and least among "professional" men. The decline in activity begins earlier among the "farmers," but the trend of the decline is the same for all groups after 30–39 years.

Pearl's data are meager, and are based on recollection of events in the lives of the individuals studied, but it should be pointed out that for the entire group the variability of sex activity is very high, ". . . men are from 2 to 3 times as variable in this respect as they are in dermal sensitivity, from 3 to 4 times as variable as they are in keenness of sight, from 4 to 5 times as variable as they are in swiftness of blow, and from 8 to 10 times as variable as they are in body weight" (Pearl, 1925).

The ages of men, at birth of their officially accepted children, may afford somewhat more information. These data do not represent the maximum fertility of man at various decades, but indicate actual reproductive performance under existing conditions i.e., age and parity of the partner, and the numerous environmental factors conditioning paternity. These were, in 1934 in the U. S. Birth Registration Area, 2,167,636 births; 3.8 per cent of these births were to fathers 45 to 49 years; 1.4 per cent to fathers aged 50–54; and 0.7 per cent to fathers aged 55 years and over.

A case of "authenticated" fertility in a man aged 94 has been reported by Seymour, Duffy and Koerner (1935). According to the history, this southern white man, after a previous marriage resulting in 16 children, had married a 27-year-old widow. The statement is made that the marriage had taken place "a year or two" before the birth of the child. Examination of the semen showed spermatozoa of average size; only 65 per cent of the customary number were present. Their conformation was entirely normal and their motility was very great.

This case report shows that a man of 94 had presumably adequate sperm to participate in fertilization, and that a child was born to his wife.

2. TESTIS

In the section dealing with ageing in women, it has been made clear that the reproductive function of the woman ceases within a specific age period, though participation in sexual activities need not be affected thereby. In men, however, it is probably that sexual activity decreases or is in abeyance before reproductive potentiality is lost, but adequate facts about the relation of testis structure to sexual capacity are not available. Even in domestic animals sexual activity is not synonymous with fertility. It is generally assumed that the interstitial cells of Leydig secret one or more of the male sex hormones. The facts are better organized when the seminiferous tubules are considered. If no spermatozoa are present, fertility is lost. If spermatozoa are present in the tubules or the epididymis, fertility may be assumed. The recent studies on sperm morphology in relation to male sterility indicate that even an abundance of motile sperm in the ejaculate is no proof of fertility. The percentage of abnormal forms, the short life of the sperm, and other factors, may seriously impair the fertility of the man.

In studies of the morphology of the testis in various life decades, the presence of sperm forming cells and the spermatozoa in the tubules and sperm cells in the epididymis merely indicate that this capacity is present at this age, and that it is an indication of normal endocrine balance. Within these limitations in interpreting the findings resulting from histological study of the human testis, the actual observations may be reported.

The material falls into two general classes. One group of investigators has reported the microscopic condition of the testis obtained at routine autopsy, in relation to age, or to specific conditions of disease. The other group of investigators has studied the testes obtained mainly from surgical castration of psychopathic groups, and compared them with testes from traumatic deaths. Notable among these studies are those of Knud Sand and Okkels (1936), and Rössle (1935). The impressions of the writer are obtained from more than a hundred cases where the entire genital tract has been available for study, the great majority of them from traumatic deaths with adequate histological fixation. A few other specimens, obtained as biopsies from testes of men complaining of sterility, have been illuminating.

1. *The testis tubule.*

One of the functions of the testis is the production of spermatozoa. Normally spermatozoa are produced beginning during puberty. Rarely the testes of mature men may be seen which have no spermatogenic cells, the only cells of the tubule being the sustentacular cells of Sertoli. Similar conditions have been seen in the testes of rats (Smelser), bulls (Lagerlof), and monkeys, which apparently are abnormal in no other manner.

The critical problem for the present report is the time at which spermatogenic function fails or ceases, and if it is related to the problem of ageing. The number of cases is few indeed. Studies of ejaculates are rare. Exner (quoted by Blum, 1936) reported that in 165 cases of men past 60, spermatozoa were present in 68.5 per cent of men aged 60–79, 59.5 per cent at 70–80, and 48 per cent of cases at 80–90.

In our own series more than half of the testes and ducts of man past 70 have abundant spermatozoa (16 cases).

One type of morphological change which occurs with failing spermatogenic action, and may influence it, is in the basement membrane and the capsule of the tubule (tunica propria). Normally this is a delicate basement membrane which is surrounded by laminated collagenous and argyrophile fibers. In all tubules of man or monkey during the ages of sperm formation, this is a thin and delicate membrane if the tubules are in normal spermatogenic condition. The connective tissue of the tunica propria increases in thickness in many individuals, usually with decrease in the size of the tubule. Decreased spermatogenic activity is observed if the capsule is definitely thickened. Transitions from this stage to complete tubular fibrosis and hyalinization are seen. The same condition in localized areas of the human testis can be seen in apparent infarcation of arterial branches. Similar fibrotic changes with "ghost" tubules have been obtained after ligation of spermatic arteries in the monkey.

An interesting feature of the testis of the aged, which probably should be referred to as involutional, was noticed by Simmonds (1910). In many testes with thickened basement membrane, he noted that the spermatogenic cells changed into small round cells resembling those of the undeveloped testis.

The effects of hypophysectomy in adult male monkeys indicate strongly that this process is a true involution (Smith, 1937, 1938). In these animals after removal of the pituitary gland, the spermatogenic cells undergo a prompt *dedifferentiation* and, in the terminal stage, show all of the histological characters of the undifferentiated epithelium of the prepubertal resting testis. In similar instances in the human testis the epithelium does not undergo a lytic degeneration, but appears to have dedifferentiated as in the monkey to an indifferent resting stage.

Simmonds also associated the degeneration of seminiferous epithelium with thickening of the tubular wall, and suggested that the degenerative changes might be a chronic nutritional disturbance as a result of blood vessel change (Simmonds, p. 114). Simmonds reports 80 cases with hyaline transformation and tubular degeneration of the testis, 58 cases of which showed general systematic arteriosclerosis. He saw testis degeneration in men in the forties with cardiovascular disease. However, many instances of hyaline transformation with tubular degeneration are found in the absence of known cardiovascular disease.

An exact causal relationship between the hyaline thickening and seminiferous destruction cannot be established. In both man and monkey the two conditions are associated. As hyaline or collagenous thickening occurs the capillary bed is thrust further from the basement membrane of the epithelium. It is not impossible that the degeneration of seminiferous epithelium is the result of a trophic disturbance affecting the metabolic requirements or respiration of the sperm forming elements.

Other instances of unknown causation where all spermatogenic elements have disappeared, leaving an abundance of normal appearing Sertoli cells on a thin normal basement membrane, appear in younger men as well as the aged man. The effects of avitaminosis, E or A, on the human testis are unknown.

Stieve (1930) and Spangaro (1902) both discuss progressive increase in the elastica content of the tubule wall. Stieve regards the thickening of the wall to be an age change in which the collagenous elements are sacrificed to the elastic fibers. The same changes, according to Stieve, occur in the tunica albuginea and epididymis.

According to Stieve, the tubules in the aged remain the same width when sperm bearing, and have no more involutionary changes than in young men, when there are no complications of medical importance. However, he sees that the tubules of the aged are not round but many angled. This is to be observed in our specimens when the highly refractive basement membrane thickens and throws loops in toward the lumen. This may be a result of increase in elastic fibers and decrease of collagenous fibers in the tubule wall.

One difficulty with statements in the literature is that many reports have been made from material from routine autopsy. Spangaro, for instance, differentiated two forms of senile testis; the normal senile testis which shows no essential change in advancing age; and the atrophic senile testis. This is to say that many testes show no change, but are found in men of an age when senility might well occur. Stieve remarks that the changes recorded by Spangaro as occurring in the atrophic senile testis also may be seen in younger men, when the testis may have been injured by general illness or disease. In our own series of traumatic deaths these changes are frequently seen in individuals who were free of any gross lesions or degenerative disease. Stieve comes to the conclusion, from a study of his accidental deaths, that the testis activity in the aged is not essentially different from that of younger men. He is, however, of the opinion that there are more broken off spermatogenic cells, and a larger proportion of many nucleated protoplasmic clumps in the aged than in younger men. Careful statistical studies of fixed specimens need to be made, as these cells are readily seen in disease, as well as in the semen of younger men of reduced fertility. From a study of many specimens it is difficult to be certain that this is an age change.

Another phenomenon not mentioned by other observers may be seen in many testes, even in traumatic deaths. In these cases spermatozoa may be found in the Sertoli cells, but few mitoses are observed and every evidence of spermatogenic arrest occurs. This is not due to the well known fact that spermatogenic waves occur, and various portions of tubules or testes may be resting while other areas are acting. The state of spermatogenic arrest is uniform in not only one but both testes in these cases.

2. *Interstitial cells (Leydig cells).*

Any statements of the number or volume of interstitial cells are entirely subjective. No counts have been reported in the human.

Attempts to estimate the interstitial cell mass have not been successful. Interstitial cells are found singly or in patches among other
connective tissue cells in the intertubular areas. In juvenile and
atrophic conditions it is frequently impossible to distinguish the resting
interstitial cell from the fibroblast of the areolar tissue.

Recent studies with the gonadotropic hormone from pregnancy urine,
as well as morphological studies, indicate that the large vacuolated interstitial cell may develop rapidly from undifferentiated cells. Whether
these are fibroblasts or resting undifferentiated mesenchymal cells
is unknown. Cejka (1923) relates them to Maximow's polyblast. If
these cells can temporarily be increased in number at the expense
of fibroblasts, it is presumed that they also can undergo dedifferentiation and resume the appearance of a connective tissue cell.

All attempts to relate the number or condition of interstitial cells
to sexual activity in man have revealed nothing. In cases of homo-
sexuality, abnormal sex drive or other psycho-pathological states no
histological or cytological changes were found which were not also
found in the control series of "normal" men (Sand and Okkels, 1936a,
b, c; Rössle, 1935).

Similarly it has been difficult to show any change except pigmentation in the interstitial cells which were associated only with age. Teem
(1935a, b) has examined a large number of testes from routine autopsy
material. The number of interstitial cells was estimated, not counted
nor measured, and a "relative average number" secured. According
to his estimates the relative average number of interstitial cells decreased in the decade 50–59 years.

Stieve reports a case of a man of 68 years of age in which the testis
was removed during the reduction of a hernia. Otherwise healthy, the
man testified that he had not had intercourse for 10 years. Another
was a case of accidental death of a man 74 years old who, up to his
death had had coitus regularly many times per week. In both cases
the histological picture was the same, with active spermatogenesis, and
in at least the latter case, a relatively sparse number of interstitial
cells.

These newer studies with abundance of material obtained from accidental deaths confirm the view expressed by Stieve that there is no
difference except pigmentation in the interstitial cells of the normal
aged individual and of younger men. The range of variability is so
great in the human testis that a large series must be inspected to obtain
the subjective impression of the spread of normality. The technical

difficulties involved are discussed by Sand and Okkels (1936 a) who devised an elaborate system for counting and evaluating the number of interstitial cells in their large series, but abandoned the method as being unsatisfactory.

Stieve has taken exception to the Steinach school who thought that the interstitial cell mass increased with age. This is a misconception, as it also is in cryptorchidism, due to the shrinkage of tubules and therefore the *relatively* greater number of interstitial cells. Oiye (1928) had previously stated specifically that he could determine no change in numbers of interstitial cells in relation to ageing.

3. *Pigment and granules.*

Pigment is a constant finding in the genital tract of the aged male. There may be more than one type of pigment granules but the most constant are the golden brown, round, granules. They occur in the interstitial cells, the efferent tubules of the testis, the smooth muscle of the prostate and the seminal vesicles. In our preparations they are very abundant in the interstitial cells of men beyond 60. In many testes of the aged, the only cells which can definitely be diagnosed as interstitial cells are those which bear pigment. The other cells in the intertubular spaces which do not have pigment may be dedifferentiated interstitial cells or they may be fibroblasts.

In the efferent tubules of many testes of older men, pigment is deposited in the stroma, and can be seen both basally and apically in the epithelium. The presence of much free pigment in the lumina of tubuli efferentia, and its presence in occasional semen spreads, suggest that in this respect the epithelium of the tubuli may serve as real excretory cells. In these cases, pigment is seen in the lumina of the epididymis, but not in the epithelium. Moore has described the increase of pigment in the smooth muscle cells of the aged prostate. Further discussion of this problem may be seen in Stieve (1930) or Oberndorfer (1931).

The crystalloids of Reinke are present in many interstitial cells and are found in most testes. Their function is unknown. Bukofzer (1924) could find no relationship between these structures and age.

It is apparent that the widely spread misconception that a relationship exists between interstitial cells, sex drive, and age is merely another old wives' tale, which in some instances has been proven wrong, in others merely unproven.

3. PROSTATE[4]

The morphology of the prostate at successive life decades has been discussed by R. Moore (1936). His material consisted of 678 prostates secured from consecutive autopsies at the Krankenhaus der Stadt R. Wien, which were prepared in step sections. In this careful study, Moore has given much information about age changes in the prostate which are independent of the pathological changes in it coincident with age.

In general, Moore believes that the "involution proceeds with greater rapidity during the fifth and sixth decades, and that after 60 years the changes are less striking and the velocity greatly decreased . . . on the whole, old age as determined by the morphology of the prostate may be considered definite at 60 years."

In this respect, Moore's studies would indicate that involutional changes occur quite independently in prostate and testis, as in the testis no life decade may be designated as showing definite and equal signs of ageing. Since the function, and to a certain extent, the structure of the prostate depend on the internal secretion of the testis, this matter will be further considered below.

Moore has recorded the increase in collagenous fibers and decrease of smooth muscle in the stroma of the prostate in men over 40, with beginning pigmentation of the smooth muscle cells. A general increase in the size of the acinus, with a lowered number of papillae is characteristic of the pre-senile prostate. With increasing age the dilation of the acini is less marked, and at 80 years more than one-half of the acini are obliterated.

Metaplastic change may occur during the pre-senile period, independent of any inflammatory process. This phenomenon is more frequent in our series in the sixth and seventh decade, but changes have been seen at each decade, one of the most extensive changes being in the prostate of a 19-year-old, killed in an accident.

Hyperplastic cells are described by Moore as being characteristic of the prostate before 60. In opposition to these two types of increased cellular activity, atrophy is an expected feature of the pre-senile prostate.

Moore states that "this atrophy may involve only the epithelial cells

---

[4] The seminal vesicles and other structures which form a part of the male genital system are not discussed here because of lack of data regarding age changes.

or the acinus or a complete structure, or the two types may be combined." Simple acinar atrophy of the epithelium results in a reduction in the size of the cell to a low columnar or cuboidal cell. Atrophy of the acinus usually involves the entire acinus without evident change in the stroma. Sclerotic atrophy is the condition in which there is simultaneous epithelial atrophy and fibroblastic activity. As an end result the collagenous fibers become hyalinized, the epithelium disappears and the sides of the acini meet, leaving a fibrotic or hyalinized scar. Moore points out that this sclerotic atrophy is similar to the involutionary sclerosis similar to that which occurs in the post-menopausal uterus.

Moore states, on the basis of an extensive mathematical analysis of 129 cases, that there is no significant difference in the size of the prostate between 20 and 90 years. Teem however who measured the prostate, from 734 consecutive autopsies, was led to state that "the prostate gland gradually and progressively increases in size from birth to old age. The most abrupt increase in size occurs between the 20th and 30th years· thereafter the gland gradually increases in size until somewhere between the 60th and 70th years when there is another sharp increase in size" (Teem, 1935a).

Moore further attempted to estimate the age of the individual by a microscopic examination of the prostate of 62 cases. His accuracy was high if the patient was less than 74 years old. Moore considers that if "an alteration of structure proceeds at a predictable rate in 85 per cent of individuals, it cannot be called a disease but must be regarded as physiological and inevitable."

The age changes in the prostate which Moore regards as "physiological and inevitable" are listed by him as follows:

(a) Slight irregularity in the height of the epithelium begins between 40 and 45 years.

(b) Lobular atrophy begins between 45 and 50 years.

(c) The glandular epithelium loses its secretory activity between 50 and 60 years.

(d) Sclerotic atrophy first appears between 60 and 65 years.

(e) Atrophy of smooth muscle and relative or absolute increase of the fibrous tissue of the stroma is first apparent between 60 and 70 years.

(f) Laminated corpora amylacea increase in number and size after 65 years.

In his study Moore has seen fit to list all changes in relation to the years of life, and in so doing has perhaps placed undue emphasis on the morphological similarities of all men who reach a certain age. No such definite structural relationship to the age of the patient has been seen in the testis and Stieve has emphasized the lack of such relationship.

Moore does show that in the years 41 to 50 there are 31 per cent and 51 to 60 there are 17 per cent of the men who show a "delayed senility" of from 10 to 20 years. Even with his experienced judgment in estimating the age of the individual from the structure of the prostate, there is a greater error of estimation, particularly at ages above 75. Since Moore made these estimates on only 62 glands out of his entire series, it appears that much more work needs to be done before it can be stated that the degree of normality or involution of the prostate is closely related to the chronological age of the individual. It should also be kept in mind that most, if not all, of these men died in the hospital from diseases such as syphilis, rheumatic heart, multiple sclerosis, diabetes, etc., and do not represent the structure which might be found in sound men.

Benign hypertrophy of the prostate may not be an age change but it is a definite pathological problem occurring in older men. Accurate data are not avilable to show the incidence of prostatic enlargement causing obstruction at each decade. Such enlargement is said to occur in 4 out of every 10 men who pass the age of 60.

Some confusion exists in the literature as to the terms used to describe prostatic change. When an author states that a gland has been histologically diagnosed as benign prostatic hypertrophy or, better, as a fibro-adenoma, it is given a definite classification. When the gland is merely examined, weighed, or measured, without histological examination, and found larger than some approved normal, it is called an enlarged prostate. It is probably that many of the enlarged prostates reported in autopsy series may be instances of benign hypertrophy, but many may be and doubtless are, simply large prostates which are histologically normal and have at no time caused any obstruction in the patient.

The lore about prostatic hypertrophy is nearly as extensive and conflicting as that about menstruation. It has been said that men who have lead celibate lives are especially subject to this disorder; that the rake and the roué are especially susceptible; that gonorrheal infection is an inciting factor; that men who have had gonorrhea are invariably protected against prostatic hypertrophy. That the cause of benign hypertrophy is due to a decrease of sexual activity in men after

40, with resulting congestion of the prostate with its own secretory products, has been expressed by Hirsch (1931).

Walker (1922) believed that the incidence of benign hypertrophy varied with the racial or geographical component. He classifies frequency of hypertrophy thus, Caucasian, Semitic, Arabic, Indian, Mongoloid and Negroid. Hirsch states that the opinion of American urologists is that this condition is rare in the Negroes.

Actual data have been recently presented regarding the Negro, who is, again popularly, assumed to lead an active and unrestrained sexual life. Smith and Jaffe, (1932), have shown that of 1093 autopsies in Cook County Hospital in Chicago, 757 were White and 336 Negro. Hypertrophied or enlarged prostates were found in 153 cases, 111 (14.6 per cent) White and 42 (12.5 per cent) colored; 65 per cent of the Negroes died before the fifth decade, while only 40 per cent of the Whites died before this age. The authors conclude that there is no racial difference.

Material collected in a different manner presents the same conclusion. Derbes, Leche and Hooker (1937) studied hospital admissions in New Orleans from 1927 through 1936, and analysed the cases admitted for prostatic hypertrophy. The Whites represented 0.78 per cent of total White admissions, and Negroes 1.02 per cent of total Negro admissions. The average of the Negro prostatic was 62 years, and of the White 67 years. Thus, according to these writers, the Negro is at least as susceptible as the White, and becomes afflicted five years earlier.

Recently Chang and Char (1936) have presented evidence that prostatic hypertrophy among Chinese has a lower incidence than has been found among the White and Negro races. Hospital admissions in Peiping from 1921–1935 inclusive were studied. Their own data are presented in numbers of cases and ratios. When these figures are reduced to percentages, however, it is believed that the differences are not significant. On admissions of males above 50 the incidence of prostatic hypertrophy from their data was 3.2 per cent among Chinese and 3.8 per cent among foreigners.

On 1900 consecutive autopsies of males over 40 years, in the same hospital, 6.6 per cent of Chinese had benign hypertrophy and 47.2 per cent of the foreigners. The most frequent age for the Chinese was the decade 51–60, and for foreigners 61–70. The number of foreigners was small, and the authors point out that the death rate in China is so great that masses of men in the lower economic levels die before reaching the age of prostatic obstruction.

Moore's series of 304 prostates taken during routine autopsies of men 21–90 years of age showed histological evidence of hypertrophy in 47.7 per cent. In all men 61 years or older, the incidence on microscopic diagnosis was 68.8 per cent. This figure indicates only the histological changes found, but there is no way of knowing what proportion of these men suffered from hypertrophy of such a nature as would cause urinary obstruction.

The etiology of prostatic hypertrophy is unknown. The prevailing tendency to seek a hormonal causation for many disorders has found adherents to the current speculation that prostatic hypertrophy is induced or permitted to develop by one or more of the sex hormones.

It has long been known that the prostate grows under the influence of the male sex hormones, that castration produces atrophy, and that stimulation of the testes of young animals with gonadotropic hormones causes growth of the prostate. In man benign hypertrophy of the prostate occurs at a time when it has been supposed the production of male sex hormones has been reduced.

Teem (1935a) who estimated the number of interstitial cells of the testis and attempted to relate them to the size of the prostate, believed that after the age of 69 the average relative number of interstitial cells decreases more rapidly among subjects who have hypertrophied (enlarged) glands than among those who have normal glands. However good spermatogenesis bears no relation to prostatic hypertrophy.

In the latter part of the last century White and others presented cases to show that castration in man improved the condition of hypertrophied prostate, and relieved the urinary obstruction. The mortality in these early cases was surprisingly high for so simple an operation. The matter was dropped within a few years, with the improvement of general surgical techniques for prostatectomy. Recently, however, Deming et al. (1935) presented one case of a man, 51 years old, with acute urinary obstruction caused by prostatic hypertrophy. Due to the critical condition of the patient, prostatectomy was inadvisable. A bilateral castration was performed, and a month later, during which therapeutic and supportive measures were given, the urinary obstruction was NOT relieved, and apparently Deming believes there was no atrophy of the prostate. In discussion of the paper (p. 396) Kretschmer spoke of "the fact that patients who have been castrated . . . subsequently develop atrophy." Unfortunately, the present reviewer has been unable to find any such cases reported in the literature.

Other experimental attacks on the endocrinological relationships of prostatic hypertrophy have been reviewed recently by Zuckerman (1936), who believes that prostatic enlargement is due to a lack of proper balance between the circulating androgens and estrogens. In some older individuals, according to this view, estrogenic substances become dominant. That estrogenic substances do cause marked epithelial metaplasia in the prostate of rodents and monkeys is well accepted.

Experimental evidence presented by Freud (1933) and by Korenchevesky (1936) shows that estrogen-androgen treatments change the epithelial and fibromuscular relations of the prostate of rodents. Endocrine treatment will cause growth of the prostate, metaplasia of the epithelium and certain degrees of round cell infiltration, but no genuine experimentally produced fibroadenoma of the prostate which is similar to the human pathological condition has, to the writer's knowledge, been produced. The Lower-McCullagh hypothesis of prostatic hypertrophy presumes two testicular hormones, one the prostate stimulating substance "androtin," produced presumably by the interstitial cells, and another opposing substance "inhibin," a hypothetical substance of the seminiferous tubule.

Many studies to analyse the excretion of estrogens or androgens are unconvincing due to technical imperfections, or inadequate control groups.

Much more work will be done before the possible relationships of endocrines to prostatic hypertrophy can be visualized.

When discussing views which are new and recent, such as the endocrine effect on organs, and estrone as the causative factor of cervical carcinoma, or prostatic hypertrophy, it should be clearly borne in mind that the capacity of the organ to respond is as important as the stimulating agent. In a sense the fibroadenoma of the prostate and fibromyoma of the uterus may be an expression of age changes in the tissue. The reason may lie entirely within the tissue itself, or the tissue may be able to respond in this manner to a stimulating agent only at this time of life, that is, after certain alterations in the tissue which are directly related to age. This is believed to be the case in infantile or juvenile organs (Engle, 1938 a).

The histological features of prostatic atrophy, or senile involution, are similar to castration effects. Atrophy is much less frequent than is hypertrophy. In Teem's series of 504 specimens from the Mayo Clinic, diagnosed according to size, not histological condition, there were 189 glands which were called hypertrophic and only 14 atrophic. The matter of prostatic atrophy may prove to be of especial interest due to Moore's observations (1935). In his series of 304 specimens, carcinoma of the prostate occurred in 16.7 per cent. Rich (1935) found an incidence of 14 per cent of 292 consecutive autopsies. He studied only a single section of the gland, however. In reviewing these data Hugh Young (1936) suggests that it may be said that carcinoma of the prostate is more frequent than carcinoma in any other organ of the male.

Carcinoma and prostatic hypertrophy may occur together in the same gland, but Moore and Young both regard these lesions as two distinct diseases which occur independently. Carcinoma, according to Moore, "is intimately associated with senile atrophy and is derived from epithelial cells which have previously undergone atrophy."

4. CASTRATION AND IMPOTENCE

Atrophy of the prostate and seminal vesicles occurs after castration in all mammals, including man. The microscopic changes of castration atrophy of the human have been described for one case by Moore (1936). It has been mentioned above that Teem found among 504 prostates only 14 (2.7 per cent) which he classified as atrophic according to size only, without histological diagnosis. Two of these occurred in the second decade, so were probably merely small, not necessarily atrophic. Three were found in the sixth, and 6 in the seventh decade. Moore set standards for histological determination of senile or castrate involution, or atrophy. The morphological changes in senile involution are the same as in castration, except that in the latter the process is uniform. The senile involution or atrophy of the prostate appears to depend on the absence of an internal secretion of the testis. Teems believes this secretion to be elaborated by the tubules instead of the interstitial cells, because of one case of prostatic atrophy (judged by size) in a man of 67 with masses of interstitial cells, but completely fibrosed tubules.

The low cuboidal epithelium of the prostatic acini appears incapable of secretion and the disappearance of smooth muscle fibers speaks for a loss of capacity to excrete the secretion. The senile involution of the prostate is quite similar to the uterine endometrium after the menopause.

The prostate and seminal vesicles of senile involution are unable to elaborate a normal amount of secretion, and the reproductive potential of these cases would be severely reduced. The evidence from human castrates would indicate that capacity to participate in sex acts was not completely in abeyance. It was pointed out above that in the woman after a true menopause reproductive function was lost but sexual function might be unchanged.

In this relation, as in other aspects of the male genital tract, there is relatively little valid data to be discussed.

The report of war injury cases made by Lange (1934) is the most extensive study of the sexual aspects of castration in man, in which it is indicated that if a man has previously been married, and is not older than 25–30 years at operation, about one-half continue to have libido and potency.

In his series of 125 cases of men castrated under the German law for criminal sex offenders, Rössle (1935) states that, in their experience, libido, in the emasculated criminal is weakened in approximately half of their cases. It is not the purpose of this section to deal with the sex offender, but it is clear from the results of application of the law in Denmark that an adequate parole system, with social and psychiatric control, reduces recidivism to a very low degree. The details of post-operative follow up in Germany are unknown to the reviewer.

Seven other cases of men who were castrated after sexual maturity (30–51 years of age) have been reported by Hammond (1934), in which copulation had continued after castration, in one case as long as 17 years after operation.

Peirson (1932) reported the case of a married man of 38 with two children who had a bilateral embryonal carcinoma. This case also continued to have intercourse twice weekly as before operation. Another case was reported by Oberhoffer and there are doubtless more.

The evidence suggests then that in men in whom the psychic and neuro-motor behavior patterns of sexual activity have been established, complete loss of the testes does not necessarily prevent participation in sexual activity.

The problem of castration has little to do with the problem of ageing. Sexual impotence, however, is a concomitant of the ageing process. Actual data do not exist; it is merely assumed that impotence occurs more frequently after the fifth decade although it is not infrequent in younger men. The psychological factors are dealt with in chapter 16. It is the purpose of this chapter only to suggest that the integration of the complex psychosexual process does not depend entirely on the presence of the testes or the male sex hormones.

Atrophy of gonads and the accessory organs will prevent reproduction, or even ejaculation, but not necessarily the other phases of sexual participation by man.

5. SUMMARY

A review of the morphological and functional changes in the male genital system which may be referred to as the ageing process presents several difficulties, the major one being a lack of precise published data.

The hormonal regulation of genital function does not cease abruptly in the male as it does in the female. However, in senescence as in puberty, the capacity of the organ to respond to an adequate stimulus, is probably more important than the loss of the hormonal activation. It remains to be shown that the involution of the genital system in age is due primarily to an endocrine deficiency. The normal variation in individuals in relation to life decades is apparently very great. The present data available on hormone assays are not abundant but indicate a general decrease in output of the sex hormones with increasing age. The appearance of the gonadotropic hormone which is so constant in the menopausal woman is far less uniform in the man, and is not so clearly related to life decades.

The morphology of the seminiferous tubules of the testis serves as an indicator of endocrine adequacy. If sperm are not being formed in the tubules in males beyond puberty it may be that lacking a history of injury or disease the reason for failure is primarily endocrine. The influence of other factors, such as toxins, genetic constitution, vascular conditions and the autonomic nervous system, as in anxiety states, on the inhibition of sperm production are strongly suspected. On the positive side, if sperm are being formed, endocrine stability is demonstrated. Thus, when spermatozoa are being formed in men of the sixties and seventies, as they are in at least half of the specimens examined, it is difficult to believe in a seriously decreased hormone level. The same statement would stand if it were shown that some of these cases with good sperm were sexually impotent.

There are morphological changes in the testes which are preponderantly associated with older age levels. These involve the thickening of the basement membrane of the seminiferous epithelium and the surrounding tunica propria. These changes may be due to disturbed vascular conditions but this has not been clearly demonstrated.

The interstitial cells of the testes very probably secrete at least a part of the androgen complex but no work has finally correlated their number or cytological condition with age, behavior, state of the seminiferous cells or with the condition of the accessory glands.

The careful work of Moore led him to conclude that "old age as considered by the morphology of the prostate may be considered definite at 60 years." This statement is further modified by Moore that there is an increasing amount of discrepancy in the morphology of the prostate in people 74 and over.

There are, however, a series of structural changes in the human prostate which may be seen, not in specific individuals at precise ages, but in the mass of men past 60.

Benign prostatic hypertrophy may well be an age change which is frequent. Its cause is unknown, but a large number of theories and fallacies have been advanced, of which the current one is, naturally, endocrine unbalance.

Emphasis has been placed in this chapter on the idea that the sex hormones are required for reproduction in both sexes. The degree to which they influence sex response and behavior deserves further analysis. In this field the lore of common opinion is more generally disseminated than are the results of investigators.

The problem of the relation of male impotence to age is so complex, and the sexual life of older men is so complicated by changes, both in the inner physiological environment and the external social surroundings, that little can be said at the present. In the present review, the problem has been briefly stated, and then left in the hands of the theorists. It is a matter for sincere thanks that the endocrinologists have not as yet done their worst in this field of human therapy.

In summary then, it has been stated that while the ageing process leaves its effect on the genital system of the male, it is not so uniform in its expression by chronological years as in the woman. The changes reflected in the structure of the ageing prostate appear to be more pronounced than in the testes, and more generally applicable to men of definite decades of life. The areas where age might affect the physiological and psycho-sexual aspects of men have been inadequately explored.

REFERENCES

BINGEL, A. 1935. Untersuchungen über die Ausscheidung von Keimdrüsenhormon in Urin. Klin. Wchnschr., **14**, 1827–1829.

BLUM, V. 1936. Das Problem des männlichen Klimakteriums. Wien, Klin. Wchnschr., II, 1133–1139.

Bukofzer, E. 1924. Uber das Verhalten der Krystalle und Krystalloide im Hoden bei den verschiedenen Erkrankungen und Altersstuffen. Virchow's Arch., **248**, 427–449.

Chang, H. L., and Char, G. Y. 1936. Benign hypertrophy of the prostate. Chinese Med. J., **50**, 1707–1722.

Deming, C. L., Jenkins, R. H., and van Wagenen, B. 1935. Some endocrinological relationships of prostatic hypertrophy. J. Urol., **33**, 388–399.

Derbes, V. Se. P., Leche, S. M., and Hooker, C. W. 1937. The incidence of benign prostatic hypertrophy among the whites and negroes in New Orleans. J. Urol., **38**, 383–388.

Dorfman, R. I., Greulich, W. W., and Solomon, C. I. 1937. The excretion of androgenic substances in the urine of children. Endocrinology **21**, 741–743.

Engle, E. T. 1938a. The relation of the anterior pituitary gland to problems of puberty and of menstruation, The Pituitary Gland, Monograph of the Society for Research in Nervous and Mental Disease, Baltimore: Williams & Wilkins, **15**, 298–320.

Engle, E. T. 1938b. Sex and Internal Secretions, Edited by E. Allen, Baltimore: Williams & Wilkins; 1939.

Freud, J. 1933. Conditions of hypertrophy of seminal vesicles in rats. Bioch. J., **27**, 1438–1450.

Gallagher, T. F., Peterson, D. H., Dorfman, R. I., Kenyon, A. T., and Koch, F. C. 1937. The daily urinary excretion of estrogenic and androgenic substances by normal men and women. J. Clin. Invest., **16**, 695–703.

Hammond, T. E. 1934. The function of the testes after puberty. Brit. J. Urol., **6**, 128–141.

Hirsch, E. W. 1931. The sexual factor in prostatic hypertrophy. Am. J. Surg., **13**, 34–36.

Kenyon, A. T., Gallagher, T. F., Peterson, D. H., Dorfman, R. I., and Koch, F. C. 1937. The urinary excretion of androgenic and estrogenic substances in certain endocrine states. Studies in hypogonadism, gynecomastia and virilism. J. Clin. Invest., **16**, 705–717.

Koch, F. C. 1937. Male sex hormones. Physiol. Rev., **17**, 153–238.

Kochakian, C. 1937. Excretion of male sex hormones. Endocrinology, **21**, 60–66.

Korenchevsky, V. 1936. Biological properties of testosterone. Nature (London), 137, 494.

Kurzrok, R., and Smith, P. E. 1938. The menopause: The Pituitary Gland, Monograph of the Society for Research in Nervous and Mental Disease, Baltimore: Williams & Wilkins, **17**, 340–349.

Lagerlöf, Nils 1934. Morphologische Untersuchungen über Veränderungen im Spermabild und in den Hoden bei Bullen mit verminderter oder aufgehobener Fertilität. Acta Path. et Microbiol. Scandinav. Supp. **19**, 1.

Lange, Johannes 1934. Die Folgen der Entmannung Erwachsener an der Hand der Kriegserfahrung dargestellt. Leipzig. Thieme, Arbeit u. Gesundheit, H. 24.

MOORE, CARL 1936. Responses of immature rat testes to gonadotropic agents. Am. J. Anat., **59**, 63–88.

——— 1939. Sex and Internal Secretions, Edited by E. Allen, Baltimore: Williams & Wilkins.

MOORE, ROBERT A. 1935. The morphology of small prostatic carcinoma. J. Urol., **33**, 224–234.

——— 1936. The evolution and involution of the prostate gland. Am. J. Path. **12**, 599–624.

OBERHOFFER, E. 1916. The influence of castration on libido. Am. J. Urol., **12**, 58–60.

OBERNDORFER, S. 1931. Die inneren männlichen Geschlechtsorgane. In Henke Lubarsch Handbuch der Speziellen Path. Anat., **6, 3**, 427–891.

OIYE, TAKEO 1928. Statische und histologische Hodenstudien. Mitt. ü. allg. Path. u. Path. Anat. **4**, 393–424.

PEARL, RAYMOND 1925. Biology of population growth. New York: A. A. Knopf; 260 pp.

PIERSON, E. L., JR. 1932. Case of bilateral tumors of testicle with some notes on effect of castration of adult male. J. Urol., **28**, 353–363.

RICH, A. R. 1935. On frequency of occurrence of occult carcinoma of prostate. J. Urol., **33**, 215–223.

RÖSSLE, R. 1935. Ueber die Hoden von Sittlichkeitsverbrechern. Virchow's Archiv., **296**, 69–81.

SAND, KNUD, AND OKKELS, HARALD 1936a. Histopathologie du testicule et sexualité anormale. Rapport quantitatif entre les divers composants du testicule. C. r. soc. biol. **123**, 187–193.

——— 1936b. Histopathologie du testicule et sexualité anormale. Variabilité du tissu testiculaire chez l'homme. *Ibid*, 184–187.

——— 1936c. L'Histopathologie du testicule humain chez des individus à sexualité anormale. *Ibid*, 339–344.

SEYMOUR, F. I., DUFFY, C., AND KOERNER, A. 1935. A case of authenticated fertility in a man aged 94. J. Am. Med. Assn., **105**, 1423–1424.

SIMMONDS, M. 1910. Ueber Fibrosis testis. Virchow's Archiv, **201**, 108–135.

SMELSER, G. K. 1935 Spontaneous sterility in the male rat. Anat. Rec. **64**, Supp. No. 1, p. 53.

SMITH, K. J., AND JAFFÉ, R. H. 1932. Comparative frequency of prostatic hypertrophy in white and colored races. Urol. and Cutan. Rev., **36**, 661–662.

SMITH, P. E. 1938. Comparative effects of hypophysectomy and therapy on the testes of monkeys and rats. Presented before Singer-Polignac Fondation, Paris; **3**: 201–216.

SMITH, P. E. 1938. Sex and Internal Secretions, Edited by E. Allen. Baltimore: Williams & Wilkins; 1939.

SPANGARO, S. 1902. Ueber die Histologischen Veränderungen des Hodens, Nebenhodens und Samenleiters von Geburt an bis zum Greisenalter. . . . Anat. Hefte, **18**, 593–771.

STIEVE, H. 1930. Männliche Genitalorgane. In von Möllendorf, Handbuch der Mikro. Anat. der Menschen VII/2, II.

TEEM, M. V. 1935a. Relation of the interstitial cells of the testis to prostatic hypertrophy. Proc. Staff Meet., Mayo Clin., **10**, 246–255.

———— 1935b. The relation of the interstitial cells of the testis to prostatic hypertrophy. J. Urol., **34**, 692–713.

———— 1936. The size and weight of normal and of pathological prostate gland. Arch. Path., **22**, 817–822.

WALKER, K. M. 1922. Nature and cause of old-age enlargement of the prostate. Brit. Med. J., **1**, 297–301.

YOUNG, HUGH 1935. Recent work on prevalence of carcinoma of prostate. Tr. Am. A. Genito-Urin. Surgeons, **28**, 317–329.

ZUCKERMAN, S. 1936. The endocrine control of the prostate. Proc. Roy. Soc. Med., **29**, 1557–1568.

CHAPTER 16

CHANGES IN PERSONALITY AND PSYCHOSEXUAL PHENOMENA WITH AGE

G. V. HAMILTON

Santa Barbara, California

The majority of clinical psychiatrists now recognize four major turning-points in a life span which extends into old age. These are (1) termination of infancy; (2) termination of childhood and beginning of adolescence; (3) transition from adolescence to maturity; (4) period of change from mature to ageing personality.

1. TERMINATION OF PSYCHOLOGICAL INFANCY AND BEGINNING OF CHILDHOOD ABOUT END OF FIRST HALF-DECADE

The individual now begins to repress various primary impulses or at least to retard their expression in awareness and behavior to permit their socialized redirection (sublimation). Associated with this change are (*a*) marked increase of preoccupation with ego satisfactions, (*b*) corresponding reduction of interest in purely sensual satisfactions (oral, anal, urethral and autoerotic genital stimulation, (*c*) steadily increasing concern with social interests and less with familial, (*d*) growing preoccupation with external reality in general, (*e*) an often critically accentuated sense of adequacy in relation to the environment and its demands, (*f*) a corresponding reduction of the very marked anaclitic tendency of infancy and (*g*) definite increase of masculinity in boys. Traits listed as masculine by Terman and Miles (1936) also now appear in at least a suggestive number of girls, but from a psychiatric point of view the so-called "castration complex" enters here as a complicating factor, since there are marked individual differences in modes of response to it.

From a psychiatric standpoint the most important feature of the shift from infancy to childhood lies in the psychosexual field. No unprejudiced clinician who has made fairly extensive first-hand observations of infants and children can doubt the contention that there is normally a marked preoccupation with sexual matters during the last year or year-and-a-half of infancy (i.e., from about the age of $3\frac{1}{2}$ to 5). It is also believed that under favorable conditions the attainment of childhood is usually marked by an abatement or even a lapse of this infantile interest. Such an abatement or lapse, when it occurs, typically continues until pubescence appears. That environmental influences may keep sexual curiosity alive after the termination of infancy is suggested by the findings of my marital research (1929), which involved intensive studies of 100 men and 100 women. Forty-four of these men and 23 of the women stated categorically that their interest in sexual matters underwent no remembered period of lapse.

Levy-Suhl's (1934) statement that the end of infancy is associated with (a) reduction of the functional activity of the sex glands in both sexes, (b) reduction in the size of the ovaries in girls and (c) termination of an abortive pubescence in both sexes is of considerable interest in this connection. A comparable change begins during the shift from maturity to the ageing period in at least a considerable percentage of persons. And yet, here, as in the infancy-childhood period of change, we also find a considerable percentage of persons whose interest in sexual matters seems to continue unabated.[1]

Freud's (1927) contention that the beginning of childhood is marked by the establishment of a definite functional control (the superego of psychoanalytic terminology) which is roughly definable as an unconsciously acting conscience, finds ample support, in my opinion, in the findings of clinical psychiatry. Since this buried conscience, or superego, not only influences the regulation of sexual impulses but affects the dynamic structure of the total personality, any changes it may undergo during involution will be of interest to us here, especially if they suggest a reversal of the normal growth trends of the infancy-childhood transition period. We know that the infant of $3\frac{1}{2}$, 4 or $4\frac{1}{2}$ years who has not been unduly repressed from without is notoriously free in his expressions of sexual curiosity and desire, quite regardless of social and biological deterrents which appear to be effective a little later, when childhood is fully established. This is important because in the period of involution, but excluding senile dementia cases, the clinical psychiatrist encounters a surprising number of ageing persons, especially men, whose consciously experienced sexual impulses take

---

[1] Although the strivings, conflicts and repressions referable to the oedipus complex are the most important phenomena of the childhood-infancy period of change, a discussion of them would not be directly relevant to the intention of this chapter. The achievement of genitality, the acceptance of maleness by the boy and of femaleness by the girl, which enter inseparably into the oedipus complex and the mechanisms responsible for its disappearance from consciousness, have been omitted from the above outline for the same reason.

socially and biologically forbidden directions. In most of them, fortunately, such impulses do not come to direct expression in behavior, but I am not infrequently asked to examine otherwise normal and responsible ageing persons who are suspected or accused of sexual exhibitionism, more aggressive sexual offenses against little girls, or homosexual invitations to boys.

Farther on, in the proper contexts, further consideration will be given to psychosexual phenomena and other modes of personality function in ageing persons which suggest that psychosomatic involution involves a tendency toward regression to infantile levels. We shall then have an opportunity to examine more closely the traditional assumption that ageing tends to be a reversal of the infancy-to-childhood shift.

2. END OF CHILDHOOD AND BEGINNING ADOLESCENCE DURING SECOND DECADE

This period of change in the personality shows marked individual differences, but the findings from clinical and more objective methods of observation suggest that, underlying these manifestations, there are similarities of psychodynamic process about which we can safely generalize. Thus we find in the pubescent boy and girl more or less critically arising impulses towards rebellion against parental guidance, a phenomenon which suggests an effort on the part of the ego to reject the superego imposed upon it during the infancy-childhood period in favor of one derived from social contacts. The relative indifference to sexual matters observed during childhood is now replaced by a brief period of homosexual interest, which in the absence of seduction by older persons or highly sophisticated contemporaries, seldom goes beyond a few shy and perfunctory attempts to effect genital contact. Sentimental chumships in both sexes and a scornful attitude toward the heterosexual preoccupations of slightly older boys and girls are commonly observed.

With the disappearance of this brief and apparently defensive flash of homosexual interest comes the resumption of masturbation, which has usually been abandoned at or shortly before the onset of childhood. Other common developments observed at the beginning of adolescence are marked exacerbation of self-consciousness and of feelings of inferiority, over-sensitiveness to social opinion and the quest of social approval relating to dress, attitudes toward matters involving personal relationship, etc. Anything like a complete account of this second major turning-point in the development of the personality would carry us far beyond the scope of the present communication, but it is not irrelevant to the purpose of this prefatory survey to define three general urges which seem to underlie much of pubescent attitude and behavior. These are (a) a blind, unconscious urge to effect a final shift of sexual interest from the parent of the opposite sex or brothers or sisters to extra-family heterosexual love objects; (b) a vaguely conscious urge to reject the superego acquired during the infancy-childhood period in favor of one which will reflect newly acquired social standards and tolerate the instinctual demands created by oncoming sexual maturity, and (c) a fairly conscious and deliberately expressed urge to acquire a status in the group which will satisfy critically accentuated or newly arising ego demands.

Perhaps the most important point of similarity between the situation confronting the individual during adolescence and that which he must meet during the ageing period is the one involving physiological changes which affect gonadal and inter-related endocrine functions. Although in the first instance there is an increase in such functions and in the second a decrease, a variable degree of psychical disorientation is observable in both. The adolescent, like the ageing person, feels inadequate and inferior when he is called upon to meet the inner and outer realities of his life with a changed physiological equipment.

Highly selective factors determine, of course, the kinds of human material with which the psychiatrist in private practice deals, but it is a suggestive circumstance that the vague, uneasy, perplexed sense of personal disorientation which I so commonly find among adolescent patients is also typical of those in whom the ageing process is obviously under way. Known or safely inferable physiological changes almost certainly play a determining rôle in the production of this symptom in adolescents and ageing persons, but there is another factor to be considered which can best be defined in terms of psychical-level function. I refer to a reduction[2] of the repressive strength of the ego which is so typical of the adolescents and the ageing persons of my clinical studies that I suspect it to be fairly typical of the two periods of life under consideration. Dysbiological and socially unallowable impulses which

[2] I am indebted to Franz Alexander's (1932) discussion of "strong" and "weak" egos for clues to quantitative evaluations of the ego as the functional system within the total personality to which repression is allocated. My fundamental indebtedness here is, of course, to Freud (1927), to whose original definitions of ego, id and superego functions, modern psychiatry owes its major orientations.

are automatically and habitually repressed during childhood and maturity tend to break through to awareness or (in seriously unstable persons) even to behavior, in adolescents and in ageing persons. In the former group this phenomenon is symptomatic of a total growth phase, whilst in the ageing group it is a regressive manifestation.

3. TRANSITION ADOLESCENCE TO MATURITY LATE IN SECOND AND DURING THIRD DECADES

There now gradually arise a more coherent, more stable attitude toward vocational problems, decreasing self-consciousness, increasing self-confidence and a less slavish acceptance of socially sanctioned attitudes and practices. The range of gregarious interests, which tended to be limited to contemporaries during adolescence, is now extended to include persons a decade or more older. In young adults who have grown up in fairly favorable environmental settings and who are not seriously burdened by adverse constitutional factors there is a definite trend toward altruization of impulses. Stable mating becomes possible.

The period of life that intervenes between the end of adolescence and the beginning of senescence is normally one during which relatively adequate modes of response to the environment can function at a habit level. This is possible because the personality is now served by a fairly stabilized physiological equipment. All this makes for a greater sense of adequacy. In psychiatric terms, the personality now tends to function with reference to reality more habitually and consistently than it did during infancy, childhood and adolescence. Conversely, daydreaming and other unrealistic responses are much less in evidence. Later, when ageing begins, we find at every turn manifestations of regression from this high level of effective adjustment to external reality. Promoters of fraudulent oil and mining companies give tacit recognition to this fact by choosing ageing persons for their victims.

We may assume that normal personality maturation involves a lessening of the triangular conflicts ascribed to the separate claims (a) of the various primary impulses, the incidence of which is presumed to be a species characteristic and which, in their original aim, follow only the pleasure principle; (b) of the ego which maintains contacts with the environment through its perceptual system and adjusts the total organism to it in terms of the reality principle, and (c) of the superego, which is the representative, within the psyche, of parental and social tabus and commands.

The lessening of this conflict that coincides with the passage from adolescence to maturity makes for a stabilization of personality functioning, but this statement is subject to an important qualification which must be taken into account when we seek to evaluate changes in the ageing personality: even in reasonably well adjusted persons one finds evidence that at least some of the conflicts, carried over from the infancy-childhood transition period and accentuated during adolescence, remain unresolved throughout maturity. These chronically unresolved conflicts are likely to undergo further reactivation at some time during the ageing process. When they then come to recognizable expressions in attitude and behavior it is a misleading half-truth to state that such expressions are direct consequences of physiological changes. This point will be elaborated farther on.

4. PERSONALITY CHANGES FROM FULLY MATURED
TO AGEING STRUCTURE

It is reasonable to assume that the shift from physiological maturity to physiological old age marks the beginning of changes in the general configuration of the personality. Nevertheless, when we undertake to state what, specifically, are the differences between a mature and an ageing personality a doubt arises as to what prolonged, intensive studies of an adequate number of cases might disclose.[3] At this point I wish to examine separately various traditional assumptions as to what typically occurs as one advances from middle-age toward the end of a fairly long life span.

The adage that an old dog can't be taught new tricks, that educability declines with the passing of youth and reaches a vanishing point by the time ageing begins, cannot now pass unchallenged. In recent years various students of educational psychology have attempted to estimate the changes in ability to learn that typically occur from youth onward. No close agreement is found among the resultant findings and opinions, but they suggest, in the main, that the occasional university student of fifty, sixty or even seventy years may not be a freakishly exceptional case. Thorndike and his research associates, Bregman, Tilton and Woodyard (1928) found that a decline in learning ability begins shortly after the end of the second decade, but that at fifty and beyond there is still retained a considerable capacity for acquiring

[3] There is an urgent need for collection of data on psychosexual ageing in large samples of the population. A method similar in principle to that used in my marital research could be developed for this purpose.

new knowledge and skills. Fan's (1935) studies of his fellow Chinese led him to a general conclusion that, although youth is the most favorable period for learning, opportunity is a more important factor than age. Ruch (1934) found that the learning scores of persons of sixty and beyond were much inferior to those of adolescents but only slightly inferior to the scores of a group whose ages ranged from 34 to 59. He also observed that liberalism or conservatism, as well as chronological age, are factors of importance. In a study of the growth and decline of intelligence, Jones and Conrad (1933) found that at 55 the decline in this function brings the individual down to the 14 year level. W. R. Miles' (1933a) experiments with 2,000 persons ranging in age from 20 to 95 led him to the conclusion that enlargement of interests and improved judgment can compensate for decrease of manual skill. In another presentation (1933b) of his researches he states that comparison and judgment decline very slightly.

A striking example of the educability of ageing persons is found in their intellectual reactions to psychotherapy. This requires, in the end, a great deal of explanation of the individual to himself in terms of the findings and explanatory formulations of psychoanalytic psychology. These are admittedly difficult to grasp, both because they deal with highly complex psychodynamic processes and because an understanding of them calls for the acquisition of new and initially uncongenial habits of thought. As Kaufman (1937) has recently pointed out, Freud discouraged efforts to psychoanalyze persons "near and above the fifties" because, among other reasons, "old people are no longer educable." Jelliffe as quoted by Kaufman (1937) takes a less discouraging view of the matter and the experiences of both of these psychiatrists make them optimistic as to the possibility of psychoanalyzing ageing persons. My own experience with patients in the sixth and seventh decades of life who have been accepted for psychoanalytic treatment has convinced me that they do not, in fact, lack educability. In the end their grasp of the necessary explanations is as good as that of the younger patients, although the greater resistance of the ageing person is nearly always a retarding factor. And yet it so happens that my seventh decade patients have responded more rapidly than the sixth decade ones. This, of course, may have no other significance than that the vocational and other preoccupations of the older group were less distracting.

Thorndike (1928) published in tabular form some suggestive facts about 91 men of science and 80 men of affairs, all of whom lived to the age of 70 or beyond. The *opera magna* of 22 of the 91 scientists and of 19 of the 80 men of affairs were done after the age of 60 had been reached. Six of the 22 scientists thus listed achieved their *opera magna* after the age of 80 had been reached. There is yet to be determined the rôle played by interest, opportunity and a continuing sense of adequacy, or the opposites of these factors, in determining the intellectual capacity of the individual during the involutional period.

Marked impairment of memory for recent events is so commonly observed in extreme old age that we might seem to be on fairly safe ground in assuming that this difficulty is present to an appreciable degree during the earlier phases of ageing. It is likely that the majority of persons who are in the seventh decade would admit that their memory defect may have a more complex determination than a purely somatic one. At any rate, we must take into account the fact that external circumstances and more subtly operative subjective factors often make for a marked change in the preoccupations of ageing persons. The patronizingly protective attitude of younger adults toward elderly ones, the steadily increasing physical debility that goes with ageing and the common expectation that after sixty the individual's practical usefulness is nearing its end, make for a sense of inadequacy and a consequent withdrawal of attention from various details of present external realities. It may be, then, that since memory is importantly a function of attention, many ageing persons are more forgetful of recent events than need be.

Various facts of clinical experience tend to support a guess that the memory impairments of ageing persons may be in part a psychogenic phenomenon and one that is not wholly irreversible. Therapeutic work with persons in the seventh decade includes among its aims the reduction of discomforts and disabilities by bringing about a more extroversive attitude toward the current realities of everyday life and a more self-confident approach to its problems. It is a suggestive finding that this usually effects a distinct improvement of memory for recent events. This is especially apparent when the psychoanalytic method is used: the therapeutists's explanations must be kept consistent one with another over a period of many months, but the patient of sixty-five, no less than the one of thirty-five, may be expected to remember them in detail and to point out any real or apparent inconsistencies. Again, a night's dreaming is usually elaborated from material derived from the experiences of the immediately preceding day: the free associations of elderly patients who are undergoing psychoanalysis typically disclose a clear and detailed memory for such events.

In spite of the many notable exceptions to be found among men and women in public life, the popular impression that elderly persons tend to be more conservative, more reactionary, more intolerant of changes in manners, morals, religion and politics than are their juniors, is probably correct. Since this tendency is an initial obstacle one regularly encounters in attempting to psychoanalyze ageing persons, a discussion of the psychical factors involved in its determination is relevant to the general aim of this chapter.

A successful psychoanalysis ultimately requires a realization on the patient's part that many of his symptoms are unconsciously elaborated defenses against certain of his own impulses which are primarily antisocial or even perverse. The proposition that one is subject to such impulses and that they are currently coming to expression, albeit in distorted and unrecognizable forms, in one's symptoms, attitudes and behavior, at first seems like a denial of one's habitually held ideals and self-estimates. The therapeutist must induce a more tolerant, less conservative attitude toward such unfamiliar and initially repugnant formulations, and to do this he must discover and disclose to the patient whatever may underlie the obstructing intolerance and conservatism. The following account of what my seventh decade patients and I have found in our efforts to accomplish this leads us into fairly deep water, but unless our discussion of the ageing personality is to be held to a very superficial level it cannot be avoided.

It is a trite enough observation that the feelings of inferiority and of general inadequacy experienced by ageing persons are in part simply a reaction to (a) declining physical vigor, (b) loss of occupation, (c) the calendar and (d) the traditional assumption as to what old age inevitably involves. Feeling inferior and inadequate as social beings, they find a sense of security and support in long established beliefs and practices in so far as these affect the environment with which they must interact. To put it in another way, the ageing person is likely to have an emotional need of finding the world as unchanging and predictable as the infant finds his completely subsidizing world to be.

The next step in our explanation of the conservatism and intolerance that is so often a trait of the ageing personality brings us back to a point brought out in the discussion of the shift from childhood to adolescence. It is stated there that in ageing persons, as in adolescents, there is discoverable a lessening of the repressive strength of the ego, that in consequence unallowable impulses which have been habitually repressed tend to break through to awareness and behavior.

It is impossible in a single chapter to list and describe the consciously arising impulses of a socially dangerous type that torment the ageing persons of a psychiatrist's experience.   They range in social importance from biologically normal but unconventional sexual urges to fantasies of heterosexual and homosexual attacks upon children.   When, as occasionally occurs, such impulses come to expression in overt behavior, the police and public prosecutors are often puzzled to find that the offender is an undemented, currently law-abiding person.   Thus three ageing men whom I have recently studied for our local district attorney's office were conventional minded, rather idealistic citizens whose sexual offenses against children seemed as inexplicable to the offenders as they did to their neighbors.   None of these men presented any other symptom of oncoming senile dementia, and none had hitherto shown any symptoms of sexual perversity.   If we regard the ego as a sort of normally efficient brake upon impulses, it is a fairly apt metaphor to say that in these ageing men the necessary braking system failed at critical moments.   To extend the metaphor to include the more fortunate ageing persons who consciously apply the brakes, we may say that this latter and numerically much more important group is like the motorist whose uncertain brakes make him timidly careful of hilly roads.   In terms of generally accepted psychodynamic formulations, the ageing person whose ego has suffered a reduction of its repressive function has need of being conservative, and intolerant of trends toward the liberalization of existing social sanctions.   A commonplace illustration comes to mind here: the acute discomfort most of my ageing patients experienced during the period when girls and women began to shorten their skirts, roll down their stocking-tops and smoke cigarettes.

The self-deprecation and sense of guilt as well as the easily aroused anxiety of many ageing persons are in part a function of their general feeling of inadequacy, but they find a more specific determinant in the lessened repressive strength under discussion.   Even before the dystonic impulses sufficiently escape repression to enter consciousness the ageing person will disclose in his dreams and symptoms an underlying anxiety lest this happen.   The often objectively groundless self-deprecations, vague feelings of guilt and anxiety of such persons are conscious reactions to unconsciously apprehended dangers from impulses and desires within.

The increasing childishness observed in many persons from the inception of the ageing process illustrates the operation of a reactive tendency first isolated by me (1916) in a comparative study of mammalian responses to chronically baffling situations. I found that, at least from the rodent level upward in the phyletic scale, the organism tends to fall back upon its initial mode of response when it encounters a sufficiently severe and prolonged frustration. Freud's (1920) somewhat later and wholly independent discovery of this tendency (the *repetition tendency* of psychoanalysis) disclosed to psychology its enormous importance as a determinant of human behavior. When it is manifested as a falling back upon modes of functioning characteristic of earlier periods of life we have what is known as regression. The physical disabilities, the reduction of ego repressive strength and the environmental handicaps that confront the ageing person conform to the type of frustration that activated, under experimental conditions, the repetition tendency in the human and animal subjects of my research. From a psychoanalytic standpoint these frustrating developments are activators of the most primitive of all human tendencies, viz., the repetition one.

Regression as a repetition phenomenon so inextricably ties in with the psychosexual changes incident to ageing that the two can be most conveniently dealt with together. The first of the problems to be considered is the possibility that the most directly operative factor involved in ageing is the reduction of gonadal and allied endocrine functions involved in somatic involution. The fact that every woman who lives to be old sooner or later ceases to menstruate and loses her fertility and that in many cases marked disturbances of personality functions are observed during the menopause, lends some support to this possibility.[4] The decline in sexual potency experienced by men during the ageing period suggests that comparable glandular changes occur in them.[5] The traditional assumption that they, as well as women, typically experience a climacteric is also to be considered. A brief recapitulation of material obtained during my (1925) clinical survey will be given here for such suggestive value as it may have in a study of the psychosexual phenomena of ageing.

This survey enabled me to study 200 nervous cases in a community which had never included a neuropsychiatrist among the medical men who served it. Due care was taken to avoid distortingly selective factors, so that at the end of the survey I felt justified in assuming that these 200 cases were a fair sample of the nervous disorders one might expect to find in a middle western town of 30,000 population

[4] Cf. chapter on Female Reproductive Tract by Ed. Allen.
[5] Cf. chapter on Male Reproductive Tract by E. T. Engle.

and in the nearby villages and farms. Seventy-three of the patients were men and 127 were women.

Study of 200 nervous cases according to age indicates that the incidence of nervousness is not significantly higher during the fifth and sixth decades, during which there is usually a marked decline in sexual potency, than it is during the third and fourth decades.

Decade	*Number of cases*
First	3
Second	6
Third	39
Fourth	41
Fifth	44
Sixth	43
Seventh	11
Eighth	9
Ninth	4

Twenty-seven or 21 per cent of the 127 nervous women of my clinical survey, were in the fifth decade. Twelve of these 27 women were in the menopause when they presented themselves for study and treatment. Thus we find that less than one-half of them (44 per cent) could ascribe their nervousness to the menopause.

Seventeen or 23 per cent of the 73 nervous men were in the fifth decade, a finding which suggests either (a) that the menopause is an over-rated factor in the traditional explanation of nervousness in women in their forties, since the relative incidence of nervousness among men in their forties was even slightly higher than among the women; or (b) that critical glandular changes provocative of nervousness may be as common among fifth-decade men as they are among women.

When we come to sixth decade cases we find that 28, or 22 per cent of the women fell within this period, and that only 5 or 18 per cent of these were in the menopause. In other words, during a decade when the menopause was of relatively infrequent occurrence, as many nervous women were encountered as in the fifth decade, when the menopause is most likely to occur.

Fifteen, or 21 per cent of the men were in the sixth decade. When this finding is appraised in the light of those given in the above three paragraphs considerable doubt arises as to what direct causative value should be ascribed to known endocrine changes in women, and inferred corresponding changes in men, when we seek to account for disturbances of personality functions during the fifth and sixth decades.

If we exclude the disappearance of the menstrual function and of fertility in women, there are almost no undebatable generalizations which can be made concerning a possible climacteric in either sex which critically punctuates their psychosexual lives. We are on equally uncertain ground when we attempt to generalize concerning personality changes associated with the menopause in women and with the decline in sexual drive and potency which most men seem to experience after they reach the fifth decade. Havelock Ellis (1933), who prefers the term "critical age" to "male climacteric," makes an interesting statement in this connection.

"The biological foundation (of the critical age in males) is genital decadence with changed neuroendocrine reactions. Kenneth Walker would place the age of this change at about 55 or 60, Rankin between 57 and 63, Max Marcuse between 45 and 55 and even at 40. *In many cases, I would say, such a period occurs even near the age of 38.*"

I have italicized the last sentence of this quotation because, in my own experience, both as a clinician and as an investigator, the men who have come to me for relief from failing sexual potency have been, with rare exceptions, between the ages of 37 and 40. These cases are of course highly selected by the very fact of clinical practice and do not offer a safe basis for wider generalization.

When we turn to a study of the psychosexual and associated personality phenomena presented by women who have passed the menopause and by men of a comparable age we find certain facts of clinical observation which tend to complicate rather than to simplify the task confronting the student of ageing. This statement is amplified in the summary of some of my own material that directly follows:

1. Many women find that, with the subsidence of the menopause, there comes a withdrawal of interest from environmental concerns, a dreary sense of unsatisfaction, preoccupation with gastrointestinal and other bodily functions which may pass over into a more or less serious morbid melancholy and anxiety, sexual frigidity, a generally egoistic outlook upon life and a resultant unsympathetic, selfish, querulous attitude toward persons with whom they formerly sustained a more wholesome relationship. They are easily offended, feel slighted when there is no adequate objective ground for this reaction, develop a host of petty grievances, expend a good deal of emotion on self-pity and look for scapegoats onto whom they can project their inner self-dissatisfactions.

A comparable phase is encountered in men in the sixth, seventh or

even as late as the eighth decade. I have had more extensive opportunities for studying these manifestations in women than in men
because the latter much less readily turn to psychiatrists for relief
from minor discomforts than do women.

2. In recent years I have found that reactive depressions occurring
among men and women in their fifties or sixties are usually amenable
to psychoanalytic treatment. Such a patient ordinarily presents no
history of previous depressions, a circumstance of considerable importance, since otherwise one might suspect the disorder to be a recurrent manic-depressive cycle. A reactive depression in an elderly
patient usually seems to have been precipitated by situations which
might easily discourage and depress any normal person. Thus we find
among apparent precipitants the death or defection of a spouse or of
a blood relative or close friend who had been an important source of
habitually experienced satisfactions, vocational and economic reverses
and intractable physical discomforts and disabilities.

The typical case is acutely and almost continuously unhappy, self-
centered, uninterested in everything that lacks a direct and obvious
bearing on his or her own welfare, pessimistic as to the future and
disinclined to engage in any but the most necessary physical or mental
activities. Mild gastrointestinal disorders usually enter into the
picture and assume an undue importance in the patient's scheme of
things. Heavy, uneasy sensations referable to the epigastrium seem
to occupy the foreground of consciousness in many cases. Dizziness,
a sense of the heart pounding in the ears and a demonstrable rapidity
of heart action are also common. In the psychosexual field we usually
find frigidity as well as impotency.

Although these patients often speak deprecatingly of their past
and present capacities, performances and attitudes, they do not typically
manifest the tendency to develop the grotesquely self-accusatory ideas
of a true melancholia. A dreary sense of futility, failure and old-age
infirmity, and not the aggressive self-hatred of melancholia, characterize a reactive depression after fifty.

It seems to me a suggestive fact that these changes, which one often
encounters in a lesser degree of intensity among elderly persons who
are acquaintances and not patients, are therapeutically remediable.
This point, in so far as it relates to the psychosexual phenomena involved, calls for further elaboration.

3. The sexual impotency and frigidity observed in women who
either sharply introvert after the menopause without falling into a

reactive depression or who develop this disorder, is not, in my experience, a terminal age change. It may disappear during a psychoanalysis and be replaced by sexual fantasies, conscious sexual desire, masturbation and erotic dreams culminating in the orgasm. In such cases Bartholin's glands secrete freely during periods of sexual excitement and the breasts again become responsive. In some of my cases in the seventh decade and at least in one eighth-decade woman there occurred waves of increased sexual tension which came with a periodicity suggestive of the lunar cycle in younger women. Such a reawakening of sexual desire and capacity for the orgasm may occur after five, ten, or as in the case of a woman in her eighth decade, twenty-two years of complete frigidity.

In psychoanalyzed cases the sexual reawakening was marked by concurrent personality changes which represented a sharp reversal of the post-menopause shift from normally extroverted to maladaptively introverted modes of functioning.

I have observed a comparable development in elderly men who have been psychoanalyzed by methods adapted to their needs. Patients who have reported a total absence of sexual desire and of erections over periods of time ranging from five to fifteen years have responded to purely psychotherapeutic (psychoanalytic) treatment by experiencing erections, sexual desire and occasional nocturnal emissions with erotic dreams. Masturbation is resumed if circumstances make copulation difficult or inexpedient. The men, like the women, present an associated reversal of introversive trends when impotency and frigidity are thus replaced by a fair degree of sexual drive and ability to function.[6]

I wish to give at this point a provisional list of various factors that seem to me, in light of our present knowledge, to play more or less important rôles in determining the psychosexual changes of the ageing period:

Havelock Ellis's (1933) findings and my own suggest that at some time during the latter half of the fourth decade of life there is a sufficient recession of gonadal function[7] to render the individual male

---

[6] The psychiatrists's explanations of the mechanisms involved in the psychosexual changes incident to ageing are necessarily working hypotheses which it has not yet been possible to subject to rigid test. Moreover the observations themselves regarding both the decline in functioning and the therapeutic improvement are largely based upon the patient's statements, and cannot be measured.

[7] Cf. Raymond Pearl's Biology of Population of Growth, chapter 6. He found a marked falling off in frequency of coitus after the 30–39 year period of life.

liable to a sexually inhibiting fear that his reduced potency may mean a complete loss of it. Most males escape a serious and persistent psychical impotency during the late thirties, but there is much clinical evidence to support the opinion that from then onward both conscious and unconscious reactions to a physiologically conditioned decline of potency introduce a psychical factor of definite importance.

1. This factor (potency fear) is of less importance in women who have not yet reached the menopause, largely because their rôle in the sex act is a relatively passive one. The alleged (and perhaps actually existing) temporary increase of the sexual drive experienced by women during the menopause may delay the appearance of the potency-fear factor in them, but in my own experience as a clinician I find that it is definitely in evidence from the end of the menopause until general somatic involution is far advanced.

2. A growing sense of sexual unattractiveness, often very marked in women but also present in men, introduces another, quite obvious factor.

3. A more general sense of inadequacy and a consequent repression of inner strivings which seem to the ageing person to be difficult or impossible to satisfy is also a factor which makes for frigidity and impotency. Fear of their children's opinions and a tendency of the latter to take over the management of their ageing parents' lives often increase the importance of this factor.

4. In most individuals the ego is so conditioned early in life that it tends to respond to the sexual impulses as dangerous. During maturity this tendency is overbalanced by the sheer strength of the sexual drive, but the physiological reduction of gonadal function involved in ageing turns the balance in favor of sexual repression.

5. Studies of elderly persons suggest that a gradual reduction of the ego's repressive strength may be typical of the ageing process. It is definitely my impression, derived from clinical studies, that in most persons this reduction has among its consequences an increase of pre-existing unconscious feelings of guilt and of anxiety lest the ego's enfeebled repressive strength may not be sufficient to cope with sexual impulses pushing upward from the id. Objectively considered, neither the feelings of guilt nor the anxiety are justified in the great majority of ageing persons since the ego, in spite of its enfeeblement, usually retains sufficient repressive strength to insure continued control of such impulses. Nevertheless, the guilt and anxiety incite the ageing ego to block or at least to retard the expression of sexual impulses in

consciousness and behavior. All this makes for a reduction or even an absence of desire and of potency. These processes, it must be remembered, occur at unconscious levels of psychical function. It is true, of course, as Kardiner (1937) has pointed out in some detail, that elderly persons also experience anxiety in reaction to environmental situations which incite feelings of inferiority and inadequacy, especially when a strong control is exercised over their lives by their children. It is usually possible to distinguish between anxiety of this origin and that which is primarily a reaction to instinctual demands.

6. A possible factor involved in the lessening of sexual desire and potency after ageing begins was disclosed during my (1929) marital research, the results of which are given in earlier publications. The persons studied were, for the most part, young adults. Among the questions asked the subjects of the research was one which referred to the initial reaction to a realization that the parents probably engaged in sexual intercourse. Most of the answers suggested that, whatever the reaction may have been, no clear memory of it could be restored to consciousness, but 26 per cent of the men and 29 per cent of the women stated categorically that they were more or less seriously distressed when the thought first came to them that their parents indulged in this act. More important still to our present inquiry was the attitude of most of the young people of my research toward any sexual desires or activities that might be experienced by persons a generation or more older than themselves: it was one of repulsion. They felt, even when they held beliefs to the contrary, that it was undignified and unaesthetic for ageing persons to have a personal interest in sex.

This attitude, which I found to be so common among young adults, is not infrequently carried over into the ageing period. Many persons of both sexes who have reached their fifties and a still larger number who have passed their sixtieth year vaguely feel that it is time they were done with sex as a personal issue. This feeling, which is often contradicted by the elderly persons' intellectual convictions in the matter, and which may not come clearly into consciousness, must at least have a dampening effect upon potency as well as upon desire.

Earlier in the present discussion reference was made to regressive tendencies of the ageing period as repetition phenomena. Their further discussion was deferred until we could examine the more outstanding facts and theories concerning the psychosexual changes of elderly years because regression is largely a part of such changes. Regression from more mature to less mature modes of response to the sexual urge can and typically does occur when impulses related to the sexual function are seriously and persistently frustrated from within. If inner freedom to strive toward satisfactions derived from genital contact with persons of the opposite sex is lost, if the individual unconsciously blocks awareness of such striving, there is a tendency to fall back upon the major satisfactions of infancy.   These are, in inverse order of their development from birth onward, (a) autoerotic genital (masturbatory), (b) urethral, (c) anal and (d) oral.   To these should be added the less definitely localized satisfactions derived from bodily stimulation which have no essential reference to an external love object.

It is reasonably certain that the majority of white, educated Americans of both sexes, both married and unmarried, practice at least occasional masturbation during each decade of their lives.   Its occurrence at any age after the termination of psychological infancy is a regressive phenomenon in the sense that it represents a reversal of the normal growth trend away from autoerotic toward heteroerotic modes of sexual functioning.   Since ageing involves a decline of gonadal and related endocrine functions, one might expect to find a corresponding decrease in the frequency of masturbation from decade to decade as the individual advances from middle life toward the end of his life span.   This expectation has been denied by my clinical experience.   I find that masturbation or genital manipulation without orgasm is of more frequent occurrence among seventh-decade patients than it is among those who are in the fifth or sixth decades of life.   I do not refer to the masturbatory flairs occasionally observed in elderly men whose prostatic difficulties are held responsible for such manifestations, but to the fact that women, even more than men, show a definite tendency to increase their masturbation during the seventh decade.   The first explanatory formulation that comes to mind is that ageing involves an increasing tendency toward psychosexual regression which more than offsets the decline in gonadal function during the period of life in question.   This possibility which, in light of such facts as are available, seems to me to be a likely one, raises a question as to what factors enter into the determination of psychosexual regression at any age.   My clinical studies of ageing persons have led me to suspect that frustration is in itself a highly important factor here. The ageing person typically encounters both environmental and internally arising obstacles to a satisfying sexual life which he finds increasingly more difficult to overcome as he advances in years.   Habits and attitudes carried over from youth and middle age, supplemented by whatever may remain of a physiologically conditioned drive, tend to continue an undercurrent of feeling that a life devoid of sexual satisfactions or future possibilities for what has been missed is intolerably bleak and empty. It is this feeling, I suspect, that impels the ageing person to fall back upon masturbation as a replacing satisfaction.

Probably most psychiatrists, especially those who are also psychoanalysts, would regard the foregoing discussion as an elaboration of an obvious fact of clinical observation. In our therapeutic work most of us now take it for granted that frustration of any major craving tends to favor regression from more mature to less mature modes of personality functioning. Whether such frustration is due to environmental conditions, interfering psychical processes or endocrine and other somatic changes, the individual who feels incapable of overcoming them tends to establish a greater dependence upon the easily available satisfactions that are in the foreground of infantile experience than is considered normal to adult life. I have wished to clarify and stress this point here because such a simply conceived and defined factor as frustration could be easily overlooked in a symposium devoted to a consideration of ageing from many different angles.

The importance of the frustration factor as a determinant of psychosexual regression in younger persons was brought out during my marital research (1929). Seventy-nine of the 100 men and 58 of the 100 women of this research admitted at least occasional postmarital masturbation. Forty-nine of these men and 31 of the women attributed its occurrence wholly or in part to spousal absence; 12 men and 11 women to spousal unwillingness or lack of desire; 14 men and 4 women to spousal illness, and 6 men and 22 women to their own sexual maladjustments, although they longed for sexual satisfaction with the opposite sex.

Manifestations of regressive self-stimulation among ageing persons include not only masturbation but also an increasing tendency to be preoccupied with bodily sensations in general. Mildly pleasant as well as mildly unpleasant sensations which are barely if at all attended to during early adult life easily attain focal importance in attention after ageing begins. The mildly hypochondrical tendencies of still healthy ageing persons is another example of regressive autoeroticism.

The incidence of prostatic difficulties among men after the seventh decade is reached makes it difficult to estimate the relative importance of primarily physical and regressive psychical factors in accounting for their increased frequency of urination. It is a suggestive circumstance that this symptom is frequently observed in seventh decade women, even when there is no physical disorder to account for it. Psychoanalytic studies of such cases have led me to believe that their increased frequency of urination is in part a resultant of the same conditions to which, in the foregoing discussion, their masturbation is attributed, viz., frustration of primarily heteroerotic desires. One of the findings of my marital research gives some support to this opinion: Among the sexually excitable young married women who were incapable of achieving the orgasm were several who volunteered the information that they were at times subject to a mild degree of urinary incontinence.

There is an old saying to the effect that young men boast of the satisfying sexual experiences they have had, whilst old men boast of the regularity and copiousness of their bowel movements. There can be no doubt that the anal concern of infancy, which was first called to our attention by Freud, (1905), tends to recur during the involutional period of life. When the colon is functioning normally and excretion is adequate as to frequency and amount of discharge, the younger adult typically gives no thought to the matter when the urge to evacuate is not actually present, but this is not true of ageing persons. With them it is more typically an important part of the day's routine, to be contemplated with pleasure in both prospect and retrospect when the function is normal. Before the ultimately constipating effects of laxatives were generally known by the public the unnecessary use of such drugs by elderly persons was the rule rather than the exception. "Doctor," a healthy old man is quoted as having said to this family physician, "Hunyadi is my favorite beverage."

Gastroenterologists have given increasing recognition to psychiatric explanations of colon disturbances in recent years. In younger adults this type of ailment is so commonly associated with self-frustrating psychosexual maladjustments, and it lends itself so readily to psychotherapeutic treatment, that there can be no reasonable doubt as to the existence of a causal connection between the two. In elderly years, when physiological and environmental as well as psychical factors tend to narrow the range and intensity of sexual satisfactions, increased preoccupation with anal functions may fairly be regarded as a compensatory regression.

The old adage that after middle age one tends to dig his grave with his teeth reflects the importance of oral pleasures during the involutional period. Eating, along with excreting and sleeping, often become the chief satisfactions of life with persons whose somatic involution is not yet sufficiently advanced to justify such an infantile mode of existence. In psychoanalytic theory, the garrulity of old age, as well as the increased preoccupation with eating, is looked upon as a manifestation of regressive oral eroticism.

Freud (1927) classifies all the phenomena of human life at a psychical level of function under two major headings: *Eros* and *Thanatos*. The use of the first of these two terms reflects his opinion that the general urge to live expresses itself in primarily erotic strivings and their derivatives. The opposite urge to abandon life, according to this view, ranges in its modes of expression from the normally recurring desire to sleep to deliberate suicide. The Buddhist's Nirvana, which is represented as a state of bliss in which there is total lack of desire without complete extinction, is an expression of *Thanatos*—the death craving of psychoanalysis—modified by *Eros*, the craving to live. Such a state of being is actually achieved by the very young infant at frequent intervals, and regressive longings for it are an increasing experience as involution advances. From birth until the end of psychological infancy, behavior and, presumably, desire, show a general trend toward life as a commitment to the environment and its demands, although at first the most frequently asserted need is the one met by complete physical and mental quiescence. As infancy advances there appear, in the order given, phases of development during which oral, anal, urethral and autoerotic genital stimulation attain the importance of major satisfactions. During senescence this trend is reversed until, in very old but undemented people, the death craving as such is placidly admitted to consciousness.

5. DISCUSSION

The clinical psychiatrist studies organic function at psychical levels of manifestation in an effort to correct dysfunction. In other words, in his rôle as psychotherapeutist he is constantly testing certain types of function with reference to their modifiability. If the individual under treatment has reached a period of life at which various irreversible processes of somatic involution[8] may reasonably be assumed to be under way, the clinician is confronted by a problem which is

[8] Cerebral changes responsible for senile dementia and other types of old-age disorders which involve gross mental incompetency have been deliberately excluded from the present discussion. The majority of persons who die in the eighth or ninth decades of life escape these calamaties. Somatic involution is a much more uniformly distributed process with them.

the central theme of this chapter. He must ask himself if the accompanying changes in psychosexual and other modes of personality function are likewise and in the same degree irreversible. There is also to be considered a question as to the degree, if any, in which the somatic and the personality changes of old age are interactive processes. The clinician asks, for example, if, as we see in our culture, the partial or complete sexual impotency and frigidity, the sense of inferiority, lack of initiative and increasingly anaclitic (literally, "leaning-up-against") tendencies; the avoidance of social contacts; the self-deprecation, sense of guilt and easily aroused anxiety; the ultra-conservatism and the general implasticity of attitude so commonly observed in elderly patients, are inescapable resultants of primarily somatic changes at infra-psychical levels of function. Any marked correction of such symptoms by therapeutic methods would suggest, of course, that they may be modifiable or even, in a measure, escapable reactions to (1) the increasing physical disabilities of advancing years, (2) environmental changes due to social recognition of such disabilities and (3) birthdays. The occurrence of a reasonably marked and prolonged reduction of physical disabilities directly following a corresponding correction of psychosexual and personality changes, ordinarily regarded as inescapable concomitants of elderly years, would suggest that ageing is so importantly an interactive process that not only psychiatrists but society in general may well revise certain traditional attitudes and opinions.

It has been the object of the present chapter to examine the problems just defined in light of some illustrative material drawn from intensive clinical studies of ageing persons.[9] In order to facilitate an evaluation of this material there was included a review of certain commonly accepted generalizations concerning the development and involution of the human personality.

6. SUMMARY

Assuming that the processes of somatic involution are, in the main, irreversible, a question arises as to whether the psychosexual phenomena and personality changes observed among ageing persons are likewise irreversible. There is also a question as to the degree in which psychical and somatic involutional phenomena may be interactive processes.

[9] Since data on non-clinical cases and experimental findings are limited, this discussion was necessarily based upon the relatively few cases available for study clinically.

Evaluations of the psychosexual phenomena and personality changes observed in ageing persons cannot be adequately made without reference to all of the four major turning points recognizable in a total life span which includes a period of involution. These are:

(1) The termination of psychological infancy and the beginning of childhood.

(2) The termination of childhood and the beginning of adolescence.

(3) The transition from adolescence to maturity.

(4) The period during which the personality changes from a matured to an ageing structure.

The findings of psychopathology show that most of the somatically conditioned changes or newly established trends in modes of personality function which mark the first, second and third of these turning points are reversible processes. This appears to be also true of the fourth turning point.

Clinical studies of ageing persons suggest that, before extreme old age is reached, lack of educability, impairment of memory for recent events and marked increase of intolerance and conservatism are escapable developments.

The traditional assumption that men and women typically experience a climacteric which marks a critical decline in sexual potency and desire remains a debatable one. Clinical observations disclose the fact that these symptoms can appear as psychical reactions to physiologically conditioned reduction of sexual potency.

Detailed studies of psychosexual and related forms of regression in ageing persons disclose the importance of frustration as a factor involved in the appearance of such phenomena. Disabilities of a primarily somatic nature, social and other environmental handicaps and unconscious psychical interferences carried over from earlier life make for frustration of adult types of sexual impulses which still arise in elderly persons, and tend to throw them back upon the autoerotic and pregenital satisfactions of infancy.

REFERENCES

ALEXANDER, FRANZ 1932. The medical value of psychoanalysis. New York: W. W. Norton and Co., 247 pp.

ELLIS, HAVELOCK 1933. The psychology of sex. New York: Ray Long and Richard Smith, 377 pp.

FAN, T. T. 1935. A consensus of adults' opinion of learning. Chung Hwa Educ. Rev., **23**, 161–180.

FREUD, S. 1905. Drei Abhandlungen zur Sexualtheorie. Vienna: Franz Deuticke, 79 pp.

FREUD, S. 1920. Jenseits der Lustprinzips. Vienna: Int. Psa. Verlag, 60 pp.
———— 1927. The ego and the id. London: The Hogarth Press, 88 pp.

HAMILTON, G. V. 1916. A study of perseverance reactions in primates and rodents. Behavior Monographs, **3**, 1–65.
———— 1925. Introduction to objective psychopathology. St. Louis: The C. V. Mosby Co., 354 pp.
———— 1929. A research in marriage. New York: Albert and Charles Boni, 570 pp.

JONES, H. E., AND CONRAD, H. S. 1933. The growth and decline of intelligence: A study of homogeneous group between the ages of ten and sixty. Genet Psychol. Monog., **13**, 223–298.

KARDINER, A. 1937. Psychological factors in old age. New York: Family Welfare Association of America, 50 pp. Mental hygiene in old age, pp. 14–26 in a symposium.

KAUFMAN, M. R. 1937. Psychoanalysis in late-life depressions. Psa. Quart., **6**, 308–325.

LEVY-SUHL, MAX 1934. The early infantile sexuality of man as compared with the sexual maturity of other mammals. Int. Psa., **25**, 59–65.

MILES, W. R. 1933a. The maintenance of our mental abilities. Scient. Mo., **34**, 549–552.
———— 1933b. Age and human ability. Psychol. Rev., **40**, 99–123.

RUCH, F. L. 1934. Differentiative effects of age upon human learning. J. Genet. Psychol., **11**, 261–286.

TERMAN, L. M., AND MILES, C. C. 1936. Sex and personality: Studies in masculinity and feminity. New York: McGraw-Hill, 600 pp.

THORNDIKE, E. L., BREGMAN, E. O., TILTON, J. W., AND WOODYARD, E. 1928. Adult learning. New York: The Macmillan Co., 335 pp.

Chapter 17

AGEING OF THE NERVOUS SYSTEM

MACDONALD CRITCHLEY

London, England

A study of the neurological features of old age debility possesses in addition to its intrinsic value as a contribution to human biology, the prospect of throwing light upon the nature of ageing processes in general. Despite the volume of work, the pathogenicity of old age remains a subject of controversy. On the one hand there is the view of such writers as Marinesco who regard ageing as an inevitable and essentially physiological process. This view contrasts with that of Cicero, Allbutt, Metchnikoff, and others who believe that old age is a disease in itself. As an eloquent exposition of the former idea we may first of all quote Warthin (1928):

"The senescent process is potent from the very beginning, involution is a biologic entity equally important with evolution . . . its processes are as physiologic as those of growth. . . . It is, therefore, inherent in the cell itself, an intrinsic, inherent, inherited quality of the germ plasm, and no slur or stigma of pathology should be cast upon this process. . . . Senescence is due primarily to the gradually weakening energy charge set in action by the moment of fertilisation."

The contrary conception may be expressed in the words of Tilney (1928):

"No evidence thus far adduced is sufficient to convince us that there is such a thing as a strictly old brain. The brain in aged people may present certain morbid changes, but these are in their turn incident to many pathological assaults upon the tissues sustained during life which, in some individuals more, in others less, are in all alike the consequence of infections, intoxications, or other morbid influences. . . . All of this is a strong argument in favour of the theory which holds old age in the brain, as in other organs, to be the result of life's successive and cumulative intoxications," and later . . . "According to this view, old age has a pathological background. It arises from definite conditions which may be combated or corrected."

Although the evidence adduced from the neurology of old age is scanty and incomplete there are certain facts available. In order to avoid the pitfalls of unjustifiable speculation, it will be advisable

483

therefore to set down what is actually known concerning the nervous system in aged persons. One should perhaps deal first with the pathological data, before passing to the more equivocal evidence obtained at the bedside.

A certain amount of anatomical knowledge has accumulated dealing with the involutional changes which develop in the nervous system. Much of the data, it is true, is more of historical than scientific value. We have in mind such evidence as William Harvey's examination (1635) of the brain of Thomas Parr who died at the age of 154; James Keill's record (1700–1720 of John Bayles who succumbed at 130 years; the clinico-pathological dossier dealing with the centenarian Dr. Holyoke (1829); Berruti's description of the brain of a 104 year old subject (1857); Prof. Rolleston's study (1922) of John Pratt, aged 107 (1884); and the reports of Sir George Humphry (1889) and Prof. Cunningham (1889) on the brains of persons aged 103 and 106 respectively.

In addition, we have certain more detailed neuropathological studies of the senile nervous system, based usually upon isolated cases. The authors of such papers include Constantini (1911), on the brain of a man of 105; Marinesco and Minéa (1921 and 1935), whose studies concerned the brain of a female aged 105; Kuczynski and Kopolowa (1925), who based their work on a subject aged 118, and Askanazy (1929) who studied the neuropathology of a woman who died at 101. Most recent and most interesting of all is the careful report by Schükrü-Aksel on the brain of the Turk Zaro Aga, who featured in the circuses as "the oldest man in the world" and eventually died at the age of at least 130 years. (According to Zaro Aga's claim his age at death should have been 156 years.)

Furthermore, we have drived information from a number of carefully drawn-up reports on the brains of various eminent men dying at a ripe age. Among such studies of Eliteghirnen we recall Louis and Chambardel's investigation of the brain of Anatole France who died at the age of nearly 85; Mauer and Weimann's description of the brain of Ernst Haeckel who attained 86 years. The brains of Mommsen the historian (aged 87) and Bunsen the chemist (aged 89) were also examined minutely. Spitzka made a close anthropometric research into the brains of six distinguished American savants, at the same time referring to similar studies of 137 outstanding personages, many of whom had lived to a great age. We also remind ourselves of Hindze's work in the U.S.S.R. on the arterial patterns in the brains of various aged Russian scientists; and also of the monograph by von Economo—

practically his last publication—entitled "Wie sollen wir die Elite-gehirnen verarbeiten?"

Lastly we have a number of theses devoted to the pathology of the senile brain, by such writers as A. Léri (1906), Marinesco (1927), Critchley (1929), and in particular, Gellerstedt (1933). To these must be added the more numerous and detailed studies of senile dementia by Alzheimer (1910), Simchowicz (1924), Marinesco, Perusini, Rizzo, Uyematsu (1923), Grünthal (1927) and many others.

1. GROSS CHANGES

Skull. Patchy or widespread atrophy is an unusual finding. More common is the interesting condition of hyperostosis of the inner table of the skull. This appearance, which is almost confined to the female sex, may develop in middle age and increase with advancing years. Its pathogenesis is obscure and it is not even certain whether any clinical features typically accompany this change. Perhaps more common is a diffuse thickening of a calvarium, a manifestation which is' not sex-linked. According to Augier the process is a duplex one; cerebral atrophy tends to produce a cranial hypertrophy which is followed by a senile erosion, more especially of the external table of the skull. With advancing years, also, the diploë becomes increasingly vascular.

Meninges. These are almost always thickened and often adherent. The Pacchionian bodies may be hypertrophied. Patches of calcification or even of ossification may appear in the pachy- or lepto-meninges, including the falx.

Cerebrum. A general atrophy, visible to the naked eye is commonly present. This change may be most marked on the frontal and occipital poles as well as over the outer aspect of the frontal lobes. Loss of brain-weight naturally follows but, without applying the technique of Reichardt, one cannot directly connect volumetric with gravimetric reduction. Cross-section of the brain reveals that the white matter is even more atrophied than the gray. The color of the gray matter, both central and cortical, is abnormally deep. As a rule, the lateral ventricles are widened and their walls may be marked with various corrugations or granular excrescences. The meninges may be detachable with ease from the cerebral cortex, though at times the opposite is true. In the latter case, a worm-eaten appearance (état vermoulu) becomes demonstrable over the surface of the brain, after the coverings have been stripped.

2. MICROSCOPIC CHANGES

Changes in the nerve cells comprise first a numerical atrophy—most marked in the 3rd cortical laminae and most conspicuous in the frontal region. Often the cell-outfall occurs in strips, suggesting some relationship with vascular dysfunction. Some degree of atrophy is, however, universally diffused and the cellular elements of the basal ganglia, thalamus, regio subthalamica, cerebellum, and brainstem are also reduced in number. Surviving neurones are usually relatively small in size. Most important, however, is the excess of pigmentary elements whether due to lipochrome or lipofuchsin surcharge, or to infiltration with fat or with ferruginous deposits. These changes are widespread though least obvious in the vegetative centres of the hypothalamus. Important alterations may affect the intracellular network of fibrils which become thickened and, in silver-staining preparations, excessively impregnated. The fibres collect into coarse bundles; later the cell-body itself may disappear, leaving behind a mere skeleton of tangled, densely-stained coils (= Alzheimer's fibrillary change). This finding is most conspicuous in the allocortex of the temporal lobe. The Purkinje cells may display upon the proximal portion of their axons a spindle-shaped swelling with a surrounding retiform structure and sometimes with internal vacuolation ("torpedoes").

Proliferative together with regressive changes in the neuroglia are always present. The former constitute the widespread glial overgrowth which is to some extent responsible for the état criblé in the base of the cerebrum. The latter, which comprise lipoidal changes and a mucocytic degeneration of the oligodendroglia, have been regarded by Gellerstedt as outside the limits of the normal senium. Hortega cells are also increased in number, and appear as small rod cells.

The senile brain is also characterized by depositions of various kinds throughout both gray and white matter. Corpora amylacea may be numerous, lying usually outside the nerve-cells, especially around the blood vessels, under the pia and ependyma, the external medullary layer of the cornu ammonis, and the fimbria. There may be deposits of free iron especially in the perivascular spaces within the globus pallidus. Most important however are the so-called "senile plaques." These consist in annular or stellate argentophil formations scattered throughout the cerebral cortex, especially in the deeper layers of the occipital, frontal, and temporal regions. Occasionally they are visible in the brain-stem also. Their structure is complex but altered microglia cells and fibres are important constituents, and substances chemically related to amyloid are demonstrable. Although "senile plaques" are commonly present in aged brains, especially when demential changes had existed during life, they are not absolutely pathognomonic of senility, being very occasionally encountered in young brains and in cases of Alzheimer's disease of early onset.

Changes in the blood vessels of an involutional type, such as hyaline infiltration, thickening of the media and intima, and splitting of the internal elastic lamina are usually present. Quite distinct from these are the changes of an arteriosclerotic nature, which though outside the pure picture of senile alterations, are very commonly coexistent.

Senile cerebellar changes have been particularly studied by Anglade and Calmette, Sommer and Spiegel, and others. The alterations are mainly comparable to those occurring in the cerebrum differing mainly in the presence of "torpedoes" and the absence of senile plaques.

The pathology of the senile spinal cord has been described chiefly by Leyden, Nonne, Sander, Fluegel, Critchley, and more recently by Stern. According to the last, there are two kinds of lesion within the gray matter, namely, focal outfalls of ganglion cells of vascular origin, and pigmentary atrophy of the ventral horn cells of a systemic character. These changes are most marked in the upper cervical segments. The vegetative cells of the lateral horns are notably free from pigmentary atrophy. Degeneration of the myelin sheaths may occur in patches, but systemic lesions are not seen. Neuroglial fibres are increased, particularly in certain regions such as the ventral horns, the zone surrounding the central canal, Clarke's column, and a sector within the dorsal columns. This glial proliferation bears no relation to the parenchymatous changes and is not of vascular origin.

We may also bear in mind the occasional appearance of lateral and central fissuring which, according to Fries, may develop within the senile spinal cord. This "senile syringomyelia" is probably due more to vascular insufficiency than to true old age changes.

3. CLINICAL CHANGES

We may now pass from anatomical to clinical evidence. At once we encounter considerable technical difficulties in our research, despite the wealth of our clinical resources. The physician who sets out to study the neurology of old age should at the start face up to the very particular difficulties which lie before him. In the first place he will have to bear constantly in mind that the pathological changes of senility, which we may now regard as well-established data, are diffuse processes, involving usually the whole of the peripheral and central nervous systems. Clinical manifestations will therefore be widespread, and pure syndromes, due to isolated lesions, will be rare. Secondly, the investigator will find the frontiers between healthy and abnormal old-age—between senescence and senility—so ill-defined as to be scarcely recognizable. Often it becomes merely a matter of personal opinion whether a particular symptom or physical sign is to be regarded as normal or pathological. Thirdly, he will find that the psychological state of many of his aged subjects will preclude accurate objective study by rendering the patient inaccessible to subjective testing. Add to this fact the handicaps of defective vision and of hearing, and the difficulties of sensory examination become obvious. Fourthly, he must realize that extraneural senile changes may mimic or mask neurological signs. Thus a disorder of gait, an abnormal attitude or stance, a defect in motility, may result from senile affections of the joints, skeleton or muscles themselves rather than from nervous disease. Lastly it is necessary to emphasize that the same criteria of normality do not obtain in the clinical examination of the nervous system in elderly as opposed to younger subjects. Certain findings which would be considered "abnormal" in the average adult are so usual as to be "normal" in an old person, in the same way that the physical norms are obviously different in the infant and in the adult. We may therefore start by seeking to establish a set of clinical constants or standards. Without embarking upon any detailed discussion of these "normal" old age changes, one may merely refer to them under the heads of changes in sensation, in reflexes and in motility.

A progressive defect of vibratory sensibility is very common, evidenced first in the distal portions of the extremities. Impairment of superficial sensibility to tactile and painful stimuli is a rather less common finding, though again most obvious distally. Special senses also share in this increasing blunting of perception. Presbyopia, loss of hearing for high tones, enfeebled sexual libido, and impaired keenness of gustatory and olfactory sensibility are well-known, and are considered elsewhere in detail.

Reflex activities are likewise altered in a large proportion of "healthy" senescents. This becomes apparent at a relatively early age in the pupillary reactions, where sluggish contraction to light typically occurs coupled with some degree of miosis. Equally characteristic is a sluggishness or even absence of the ankle jerks. The plantar reflexes are often equivocal in old age and not very infrequently an extensor reponse appears without any other manifestation of pyramidal affection. The abdominal responses of course usually cease to be obtainable at a considerably earlier age, as the result of laxity of the muscles concerned.

Changes in motility comprise first a general atrophy of the musculature. "Focal" atrophies, though not uncommon, must be regarded as manifestations of a distinctly pathological order. Restricted range of ocular movement, as witnessed by loss of conjugate upward deviation and defective convergence, are perhaps the sole examples of a paretic character. On the other hand, a slight but generalized poverty of movement, is characteristic and is usually associated with slowness of movement, an attitude of flexion and a mild state of hypertonus or—better perhaps—difficulty in relaxation. What is popularly termed the usual "inelasticity of the aged" is to be ascribed in part to these motility-disorders.

Against the background of these "normal" findings, certain morbid neurological syndromes may stand out. There is no necessity to narrate the various nervous disorders which may happen to appear at any unusually late age or which the victim may bear with him into the closing years of his life. Neither need we discuss the more obvious cerebro-vascular syndromes which may arise. It is desirable to focus one's attention upon the neurological disorders peculiar to the senium.

Senile paraplegia. Some measure of weakness of the legs is very common in the aged. The term "senile paraplegia" is a purely descriptive one and gives no hint of the diverse changes which may be responsible. Actually it is possible for a senile weakness of the legs to result from lesions in the paracentral lobule of the cerebral cortex; or from multiple or diffuse subcortical changes; or from an affection of the spinal cord. Lastly, in the so-called "senile myosclerosis" the loss of power is due to a fibrosis permeating the muscles of the lower limbs. In practice, of course, changes may be developing simultaneously throughout the central nervous system at all levels, so that "pure" cases of cortical, subcortical or spinal paraplegia are rare in the aged.

Senile cerebellar syndromes are far from common. Here again one should, strictly speaking, exclude all instances of cerebellar vascular disease. There is however a fairly well-defined clinico-pathological syndrome which, appearing in the sixth or seventh decade, slowly progresses. Numerous terms have been suggested for this affection— such as delayed cortical cerebellar atrophy—but simple "senile cerebellar atrophy" is perhaps adequate. The disorder is an interesting one in that the Purkinje cells are affected in an almost selective manner. It is unnecessary to discuss here the possible kinship between this disorder and the rarer olivo-ponto-cerebellar atrophy. Finally in referring to senile cerebellar affections one must recall those unusual instances of heredo-cerebellar ataxy where symptoms develop at a comparatively late age (Sanger Brown, 1892; Neff, 1894-95).

Senile amyostatic syndromes are perhaps the commonest among nervous disorders of late life. We have already mentioned that even in cases of "healthy" old age, some degree of hypokinesis, bradykinesis and hypertonus must be conceded as "normal." Frequently however this syndrome is so marked as obviously to transcend physiological bounds—particularly when associated with obvious mental deterioration. One may be content merely to mention the various components of the amyostatic syndrome: the marche à petits pas typical of the aged and the arteriopath alike; the hypertonus (originally noted by Foerster (1909) as arteriosclerotic rigidity;) the impassive features, fixed and bowed stance, and infrequent movement; the slight reduction of motor power with a more obvious slowness in movement; the various psycho-motor changes, such as catatonia (catalepsy), counterpull (Gegenhalten of Kleist, 1922), ideational or ideomotor apraxia, palipraxia, tonic innervation, forced grasping and groping, etc. The amyostatic syndrome obviously suggests an affection of the pallidal or "old" motor system but closer clinical analysis suggests that dysfunction at all levels of the nervous system must participate. As a special instance of this syndrome we may mention the not uncommon though little known Jakob's disease, where severe pallidal symptoms develop upon the background of a senile dementia.

Hyperkinetic phenomena are comparatively rare in the aged. Although senile tremor is a well-known and even a conventional mark of the aged it is actually somewhat of a rarity. Its manifestations vary and features at times "cerebellar" at other times "striatal" may be demonstrated. Reasons have been given elsewhere for believing that senile tremor often bears hereditary characteristics, and that it merely represents a late variety of the so-called "idiopathic" "essential" or "familial" tremor. Senile chorea is a much rarer disorder and is one which is easily confounded with the commoner Huntington's disease or with the apoplectic choreas. Tortipelvis, senile dystonia and senile athetosis are among the curiosities of neurology. Psychomotor spontaneous movements of a restless and often bizarre nature are concomitants of a demential state and are analogous with the similar movements occurring in schizophrenics and defectives.

Senile psychoses. The psychological characteristics of the healthy senium have already been considered in another section of this work. Between these changes and the first symptoms of a frank senile psychosis there is the subtlest gradation. That is not to say, however, that senile dementia differs from the pattern of thought processes in the healthy aged, merely in degree.

If we limit our attention to the psychoses which are approximately specific for advanced life, we must consider senile dementia; arteriosclerotic dementia, and the presenile dementias (Alzheimer's disease, Pick's disease and presbyophrenia).

As a definition of senile dementia, it is difficult to better the one proffered by the American Psychological Association:

"A well-defined type of psychosis which as a rule develops gradually, and is characterised by the following symptoms: impairment of retention (forgetfulness) and general failure of memory, more marked for recent experiences; defects in orientation and a general reduction of mental capacity; the attention, concentration, and thinking processes are interferred with; there is a selfcentering of interests; often irritability and stubborn opposition; tendency to reminiscences and fabrications. Accompanying this deterioration there may occur paranoid trends, depression, confused states, etc. Certain clinical forms should, therefore, be specified but these often overlap."

These clinical forms are usually described as the confusional, maniacal, melancholic, and paranoid subtypes.

The arteriosclerotic dementias are quite distinct entities, whether considered from the point of view of aetiology, pathology, or symptomatology. They are not necessarily associated with advanced age and may occur in unmistakable form in early adult life. Since however arteriosclerosis frequently complicates the pathology of the senile brain, it would not be surprising if the clinical picture of senile dementia was not often rendered complex by the addition of symptoms usually regarded as characteristic of cerebrovascular disease. This conception of mixed senile and arteriosclerotic psychoses raises many problems which have been strangely neglected. We do not know, for instance, if the mental symptoms of arteriosclerosis differ according to whether they develop in youth, maturity or old age. Does the presence of long-standing cerebrovascular disease in any way facilitate involutional changes, as suggested by Kraepelin? These are but instances of the many open questions in the psychiatric study of old age.

The pre-senile psychoses proper are rare. Two of them, namely Pick's disease and Alzheimer's disease, are fairly well-defined, at least from the point of view of pathology. Whether presbyophrenia deserves to be regarded as an entity is very doubtful. Owing to the confusion which has attended its use in diagnosis, the lack of a specific anatomical picture, and the probable identity with other types of mental disease in the elderly, it would be better to jettison this term altogether. Gillespie has attempted to isolate another psychosis which he speaks of as "simple pre-senile dementia," but here again the claim seems based upon too slender evidence.

The clinical story is very alike in both Alzheimer's and Pick's disease. In both there is a fairly rapidly progressive dementia, starting usually in the sixth decade. Both are associated with focal neurological manifestations, such as paralyses, defects of an aphasic, agnostic, or aprexic character, and epileptiform seizures.

To the morbid anatomist, however, the two psychoses are very different. In Pick's disease there occur circumscribed and symmetrical areas of cortical atrophy. Alzheimer fibrillary changes, arteriosclerotic lesions, and senile plaques do not occur. The areas of cortical atrophy are mysterious in that they do not correspond with particular vascular territories, nor with Flechsig's zones of myelination. No convincing correspondence with cytoarchitectonic areas can be made out, though Kaplinsky sought to show that the youngest regions of the cortex are most liable to be affected.

The nature of this psychosis remains obscure. Pick originally suspected it to be a variant of cerebral arteriosclerosis, but following Stertz, we now realize that this is not the case. A localized premature involutional process has been mentioned, and also a hypothetical disorder of iron metabolism. Perhaps the most plausible suggestion is that of a late heredo-degeneration, for Pick's disease is now known to assume at times familial characteristics.

In Alzheimer's presenile psychosis, the pathological features resemble those of senile dementia, but differ—not only in their early occurrence— but in their diffuseness and their intensity. Here again, the nature of the disease remains inscrutable. Grünthal (1926) mentions two views: (1) that this psychosis may be the expression of a dementia accompanying a premature senility, and (2) that it may be the result of an exogenous toxi-infection. The former view, while compatible with the anatomical findings, does not explain why the changes are so severe nor why they appear so early.

4. DISCUSSION

Having surveyed the evidence upon the ageing of the nervous system collected from pathological and clinical sources, one may turn to the examination of a number of obscure problems which naturally emerge. Bearing constantly in mind that the neurological aspect forms merely a small facet on the polyhedral subject of the nature of old age, one may isolate three chief topics for discussion, viz.: (1) the relationship between nervous involution and arteriosclerosis; (2) localized processes of ageing within the nervous system and (3) premature and precocious senility.

Relationship with cerebral arteriosclerosis. Obviously there is a very intimate association between the clinical phenomena of senility and those of cerebrospinal arteriosclerosis, as well as between the pathological features of the two conditions. Thus certain disorders, for example the so-called "senile epilepsy" and some of the cases of senile paraplegia, are dependent much more closely upon vascular changes than upon a purely involutional decay. Can it be that all senile processes, clinical as well as pathological, are ultimately caused by vascular insufficiency whether from capillary fibrosis or from sclerosis of the larger vessels? Such, of course, is the popular idea as voiced by the dictum of Cazali that "a man is as old as his arteries."

On the other hand we have the possibility that the connection is coincidental rather than causal.

This latter view is supported by the fact that senility and arteriosclerosis may both occur prematurely in which case they usually manifest themselves in more or less pure form. For instance, in the rare cases of juvenile hyperpiesis with or without sclerotic vascular changes, no clinical signs are present which could strictly be considered as "senile." Whether the cerebrum in such cases exhibits marks of senility, e.g. senile plaques, cellular atrophy, Alzheimer tangles, etc., is not yet known for certain. Conversely the cases of premature or precocious senility do not necessarily include the signs or lesions of cerebral arteriosclerosis.

It may be argued, too, that hyperpiesis (and to a lesser extent arteriosclerosis) is a presenile rather than a senile affection. Both being progressive in nature they are unlikely to be compatible with an extreme old age. In this way it can be argued that the very aged, by reason of their survival, must be singularly immune from severe cerebrovascular changes. This idea is perhaps supported somewhat by the common observation of a relatively low blood pressure in extremely old subjects.

Obviously however the discussion is more of academic than practical importance, by reason of the common association of advancing years and cerebral arteriosclerosis.

Localized and premature involution within the nervous system. An interesting and striking phenomenon in neuropathology is at times encountered in changes of an involutional nature confined chiefly to certain anatomo-physiological systems. Such changes may develop either in late age or at an unusually early age. For discussion among the former group such affections as paralysis agitans, Pick's disease and delayed cerebellar atrophy may be enumerated. Although in none of these disorders do senile plaques occur, there is nevertheless a cellular outfall with changes in the neuronic relics such as one encounters in senile brains, more diffusely distributed. The similarity is striking enough to make it tempting to regard these affections as localized expression of neuronic ageing. One cannot, as yet, pursue the argument beyond this stage, for we are still ignorant of any histological features which we can consider pathognomonic of senility. Senile plaques are, of course, our most approximate criteria of old age, but neither in cerebellar atrophy nor in Parkinson's disease would one expect to encounter such features in the particular region of the nervous system concerned.

Neurologists have also been led at times to regard certain progressive systemic affections of the nervous system as examples of an involutional change commencing at a precocious age and remaining delimited in its scope. Amyotrophic lateral sclerosis and Friedrich's ataxia are among the instances that have been quoted. The term "abiotrophy" was suggested by Sir William Gowers to include such affections within the conception of a premature neuronic decay. Once again it is necessary to recall that the pathological process bears only an incomplete similarity to that of senility, in so far as only the neuronic degeneration and the glial overgrowth are common to both.

Obviously identity of these pathological changes with those of a premature and localized process of senility remains unproven. Herein however lies a suggestive line for further study. The unequivocal existence of senile changes limited to certain regions of the nervous system, would strongly support hypotheses as to the "pathological" nature of old age.

Premature and precocious old age. Light may perhaps be thrown upon the major problem as to the nature of old age in general, by way of a study of those rare instances of involution occurring exceptionally early. Knowledge of the causes and nature of a premature appearance of senility may contribute to the understanding of the opposite phenomenon, a healthy and deferred old age.

By "premature ageing" we refer to involutional changes established in middle life. When senile appearances develop in childhood or youth we speak of "precocious senility" or "senium praecox."

The nature and varieties of such conditions are fully discussed elsewhere. One may perhaps pause to emphasize some of the complexities of the question and also to indicate where a neurological approach might assist.

Among the "premature" cases we can recognize factors of two kinds. In the first place we realize the importance of such aetiological factors as race and heredity, both being a constitutional or physiological order. Conversely we recall that morbid processes may play a rôle in determining prematurity. As Sir Clifford Allbutt has said: "in medicine we do not count the ages of people by the revolutions of the earth around the sun, but we measure them by the revolutions of their own morbid processes."

But if premature senility is clearly a process which is partly physiological and partly pathological, precocious old age bears almost entirely the imprint of a morbid state. The evidence of Simmond's disease (and its probable identity with Hastings Gilford's progeria) indicates abundantly that all the characteristics of extreme age can be reproduced in early life by a morbid affection of the pituitary body.

One should bear clearly in mind however that the problems of senium praecox are still largely unsolved. Nothing is known of the neurohistology of the brain in such cases—whether senile plaques, Alzheimer's fibrils and other hallmarks of senility are present. We know little of the reactions of such a patient towards his environment—whether his metabolism, his mentation, his resistance or vulnerability towards disease are those of a young or an old person. It seems clear that senium praecox can be simulated by such disorders as congenital ectodermal defect, or cutaneous geromorphism (Souques and Charcot). Whether the nervous derivatives of the epiblast also share in this change is unknown. In the same way we believe that precocious mesoblastic decay can occur as an isolated phenomenon, as witnessed by fragilitas ossium, blue sclerotics and possibly even some types of myscular dystrophy.

Possibly the analogies between old age and senium praecox are more apparent than real. Closer study shows that there are various traits of infantilism in all such cases. The patient with precocious senility is not so much one who has passed through the arches of the years with undue rapidity as one who has in some ways failed to "grow up"—or rather has skipped a decade or so. Mental testing supports this statement, as also careful study of the skeleton. Thus Keith (1913) has shown that the bones of a patient dying from progeria at 19 years, showed abnormalities some of which were typical of an infantilism while others were those of a premature development.

5. SUMMARY

A description is given of the morbid anatomy and histology of the nervous system in old age.

The neurology of old age is also discussed from a clinical angle. Mention is made of the peculiar difficulties inherent in such a research and the almost inextricable association of senile with arteriosclerotic syndromes. The mental disorders occurring in the elderly and the aged are also described.

Special attention is given to the possibility of involutional changes being localized to certain neuronic systems and appearing therein at an exceptionally early age. The problems of senium praecox and premature old age are also discussed.

The ageing of the nervous system takes place independently of degenerative changes of the cerebrospinal blood vessels. Although both types of change are commonly present in association, there is probably no direct causal relationship between arteriosclerotic and cerebral involution.

Clinical and pathological study of the nervous system in senility suggests that ageing is not entirely a simple physiological process nor yet an exclusively pathological state. It is to be infered that both features are operative though their relationship cannot as yet be determined. The pre-senile psychoses and the phenomena of precocious and premature senility offer suggestive avenues for research in this connection.

REFERENCES

ALZHEIMER, A. 1910. Beiträge zur Kenntnis der pathologischen Neuroglia und ihren Beziehungen zu den Abbauvorgängen im Nervengewebe. Nissl's Arbeiten, **3**, 401–562.

ANGLADE, M., AND CALMETTES, A. J. B. 1907. Sur le cervelet senile. Nouv. Icon. de la Salp., **20**, 357–364.

D'ANTONA, L. 1928. Sulle amiotrofia mielopatiche dell'eta senile. Riv. di Neurol., **1**, 1–20.

ASKANAZY, M. 1929. L'anatomie des gens qui depassent cent ans. Rev. med. de la Suisse rom., **49**, 769–772.

AUGIER, M. 1932. Crane et Cerveau chez le Vieillard. L'Anthropologie, **42**, 315–322.

BERRUTI, L. 1857. Abstract in Constatt's Jahresbericht, **16**, (2) p. 46 only.

BOUMAN, L. 1928. Die Axonschwellungen der Purkinjeschen Zellen inbesondere bei Dementia Senilis, Zeit. f. d. g. Neur. u. Psych., **113**, 379–425.

BRAUNMÜHL, A. VON 1928. Zur Histopathologie der Oliven, unter besonderer Berücksichtigung seniler Veränderungen. Zeit. f. d. g. Neur. u. Psych., **112**, 213–232.

———— 1932. Kolloidchemische Betrachtungsweise seniler u. präseniler-Gewebsveränderungen. Z. Neur., **142**, 1–54.

BROWN, S. 1892. On hereditary ataxia, with a series of 21 cases. Brain, **15**, 250–282.

CANSTATT, C. 1839. Die Krankheiten des höheren Alters, und ihre Heilung. F. Enke. 2 vols. 268 pp., 419 pp.

CHARCOT, J. M. 1868. Clinical Lecture on Senile and Chronic Diseases. Translated by William S. Tuke. New Sydenham Soc., **95**, xvi, 307.

CHIARI, H. 1912. Zur Kenntnis der "senilen" grubigen Atrophie an der Aussenfläche des Schädels. Virchows Archiv, **210**, 425–433.

CONSTANTINI, F. 1911. Un senile "normale" di 105 anni. Rev. Sperm. di Fren., **37**, 510–536.

CRITCHLEY, M. 1929. Nature and significance of senile plaques. J. Neurol. and Psychopath., **10**, 124–139.

———— 1931. Goulstonian lectures on the neurology of old age. Lancet, **1**, 1119–1127; 1221–1230; and 1331–1336.

———— 1932. "Neurologische Betrachtungen über das Greisenalter." Deut. med. Woch., **58**, (ii), 1476–1477.

———— 1936a. Art. "Alzheimer's Disease." Butterworth & Co., London: Brit. Encycl. Med. Practice, **1**, 354–358.

———— 1936b. Art. "Idiopathic (Family) Tremor." Practitioners Library of Med. & Surg., **9**, 990–991.

CRITCHLEY, M., GILLESPIE, R. D., AND HILL, T. R. 1932–3 B. Discussion on the mental and physical symptoms of the presenile dementias. Proc. Royal Soc. Med., **26**, 1077–1091.

DE GIACOMO, UMBERTO, AND GAMBINA, F. 1930. I Sintomi extra-piramidali delle cerebropatie senili, Cervello, **9**, 53–84.

DEMANGE, E. 1886. Étude clinique et anatomopathologique sur la Vieillesse. Paris: Germer, Bailliere et Cie., 162 pp.

DURAND-FARDEL, M. 1854. Traite clinique et pratique des Maladies des Vieillards. Paris: Germer-Bailliere et Cie., 876 pp.

EASTON, J. 1799. Human Longevity. Salisbury: J. Easton, 292 pp.

ELLIS, M. S. 1920–21. Norms for Some Structural Changes in the Human Cerebellum from Birth to Old Age. J. Comp. Neurol. & Psychol., **32**, 1–33.

FLUEGEL, F. E. 1927. Quelques recherches anatomiques sur la degenerescence senile de la moelle epiniere. Rev. Neurol. **34**, (i), 618–623.

FOERSTER, O. 1909. Die arteriosklerotische Muskelstarre. Allg. Zeit. f. Psych., **66**, 902–918.

FREEMAN, W. 1936. "The senile and presenile scleroses." Reprinted from Bloomer: Practitioners' Library of Medicine and Surgery, **9**, 869–880.

FREUND, C. S., AND ROTTER, R. 1927. Extrapyramidale Bewegungsstörungen im höheren Alter. Archiv. f. Psych., **81**, 751–754.

——— 1928. Über extrapyramidale Erkrankungen des höheren Alters mit einem Beitrag zur Pathogenese seniler Parenchymveränderungen. Zeit. f. d. g. Neur. u. Psych., **115**, 198–271.

FRIES, E. 1906. "Syringomyelia in old age." (Die Syringomyelie in Senium.) Arbeit a. d. neurolog. Inst. a. d. Wien. Universitat, **13**, 170–193.

GEIST, L. 1860. Klinik der Greisenkrankheiten. F. Enke., 191 + 650 pp. (2 vols. combined in 1st vol. pub. in 1857.)

GELLERSTEDT, N. 1933. Zur Kenntnis der Hirnveränderungen bei der normalen Altersinvolution. Upsala Lakareforenings, **38**, 193–408.

GILFORD, HASTINGS 1904. Ateleiosis and Progeria. Brit. Med. J., **2**, 914–918.

GPÜNTHAL, E. 1926. Alzheimer's Disease; histopathologic and clinical study. Zeit. f. d. g. Neur. u. Psych., **101**, 128–157.

——— 1927. Klinisch-anatomisch vergleichende Untersuchungen über den Greisenblödsinn. Zeit. f. d. g. Neur. u. Psych., **111**, 763–818.

HACKEL, W. M. 1928. Über den Bau und die Altersveränderungen der Gehirnarterien. Virchows Archiv, **266**, 630–639.

HARVEY, W. 1635. "Works." London: New Sydenham Society 1847, p. 589.

HOLYOKE, E. A. 1829. Memoir of E. H. Holyoke, M.D., Boston: Med. Communicat. Mass. Med. Soc., **4**, 185–260.

HUMPHRY, G. M. 1889. Old Age. Cambridge. Macmillan & Bowes, i–xii, 1–218.

——— 1890. Senile Hypertrophy and Atrophy of the Skull. Med.-Chir. Trans., **73**, 327–336.

KEILL, J. 1700-20. Anatomical account of Bayles, supposed to have been 130 years old. Philos. Trans., (abridged) **5**, part i, 351–354.

KEITH, A. 1913. Progeria and Ateliosis. Lancet, **1**, 305–313.

KLEIST, K. 1922. Die psychomotorischen Störungen und ihr Verhältniss zu den Motilitätsstörungen bei Erkrankungen der Stammganglien. Monatssch. f. Psych. u. Neur., **52**, 253–302.

KUCZYNSKI, H., AND KOPOLOWA, K. 1925. Von den körperlichen Veränderungen bei höchsten Alter. Krankheitsforschung, **1**, 85–163.

LADAME, C., ET MOREL, F. 1931. Contribution a la topographie des lesions histol. du cerveau senile. Schweiz. Arch. Neur., **27**, 301–310.

LEJONNE, AND LHERMITTE, J. 1906. Les Paraplegies par retraction chez les Viellards. Nouv. Icon. de la Salp., **19**, 255–275.

LERI, A. 1906. Le Cerveau Senile. Lille: Le Bigot Freres, 120 pp.

LHERMITTE, J., AND KLARFELD, B. 1911. Etude anatomo-pathologique de certaines lesions atrophiques du cortex cerebral du vieillard. L'Encephale, **6**, (2), 412–421 and Rev. Neurol., **22**, 74–76.

LHERMITTE, J., AND NICOLAS, M. 1925. Les amyotrophies de la main chez le vieillard, L'Encephale, **20**, 701-712.

LHERMITTE, J., AND DE MASSARY, J. 1930. L'Amyotrophies thenarienne non-evolutive du vieillard. Rev. Neurol., **27**, 1202-1207.

LHERMITTE, J. 1907. Etude sur les Paraplegies des vieillards. Paris: Maretheux, 250 pp.

———— 1928. La myosclerose retractile des vieillards. L'Encephale, **23**, 89-115.

———— 1922. Les Syndromes anatomo-cliniques du corpus strie, chez le vieillard. Rev. Neurol., **29**, 406-432.

MACLACHLAN, D. 1863. A Practical Treatise on the Diseases and Infirmities of Advanced Life, London: Churchill & Sons, 718 pp.

MARIE, P., AND FOIX, C. 1912. L'Atrophie isolee non-progressive des petits muscles de la main. Nouv. Icon de la Salp., **25**, 353-363, 427-453.

MARINESCO, G. 1927. Etudes sur le mecanisme histo-biochemique de la vieillesse et du "rajeunissement." Berlin u. Köln: A. Marcus & E. Weber's Verlag. Verhandl. des I. Internat. Kongr. f. Sexualforschung, **1**, 117-177.

MINEA, J. 1921. Contributions a l'etude de lesions des cehles nerveuses dans la senilite. Arch. de Neurol., **1**, (2), 55-65.

MÖBIUS, P. J. 1883. Notiz über das Verhalten der Pupille bei alten Leuten. Centralbl. f. Nervenh., **6**, 337-340.

———— 1883. Notiz uber das Verschwinden der Kniephanomens bei alten Leuten. Centralbl. f. Nervenh., **6**, 217-219.

NASCHER, I. L. 1916. Geriatrics. 2nd edit. Philadelphia: P. Blakiston's Son & Co., 527 pp.

NEFF, I. H. 1894-95. A report of 13 cases of Ataxia in adults with hereditary history. Am. J. Insanity, **51**, 365-373.

NONNE, M. 1899. Rückenmarksuntersuchungen in Fällen von perniciöser Anämie, von Sepsis und von Senium, nebst Bemerkungen über Marchi-Veränderungen bei akut verlaufenden Rückenmarks-processen. Deut. Zeit. f. Nervenh., **14**, 192-241.

OSEKI, M. 1924. Über die Veränderungen des Striatums im normalen Senium. Arb. a d. neurol. Inst. Wien. Univ., **26**, 339-364.

PEARSON, G. H. J. 1928. Effect of Age on Vibratory Sensibility. Archiv. Neurol. and Psych., **20**, 482-496.

PETREN, K. 1900-01. Über den Zusammenhang zwischen anatomisch bedingter u. functioneller Gangstörung im Greisenalter. Arch. f. Psych., **33**, 818-871; **34**, 444-489.

RAUZIER, G. 1909. Traite des Maladies des Vieillards. Paris: J. B. Bailliere & Sons, 692 pp.

ROLLESTON, G. 1884. Notes on post-mortem examination of a man supposed to have been 106 years old. Scientific Papers and Addresses, Oxford, **1**, 141-154.

ROLLESTON, H. D. 1932. Some medical aspects of old age. London. Macmillan & Co. Revised and enlarged edition pp. 205.

SAIGO, Y. 1907. Über die Altersveränderungen der Ganglien-zellen. Virchows Archiv, **190**, 124-134.

SANDER, M. 1900. Untersuchungen über die Altersveränderungen im Rücken-
mark. Deut. Zeit. f. Nervenh., **17**, 369–396.

SAUNDBY, R. 1913. Old Age, its Care and Treatment. London: E. Arnold,
312 pp.

SCHACHTER, M., COHEN, E., AND NEDLER, D. 1934. "Contribution a l'etude
Neuro-clinique des Vieillards." Rev. Medicale de l'Est., **62**, 79–85.

SCHLESINGER, H. 1930. Klinik u. Therapie der Alterskrankheiten. Leipzig:
Thieme, 132 pp.

SCHÜKRÜ-AKSEL, I. 1937. Uber das Gehirn des "ältesten Mannes der Welt"
(Zaro Aga). Arch. f. Psychiat. u. Nervenkrank., **106**, 260–266.

SCHUSTER, P. 1924. Die im höheren Lebensalter vorkommenden Kleinhirner-
krankungen usw. Zeit. f. d. g. Neur. u. Psych., **91**, 531–550.

SCHWALBE, J. 1909. Lehrbuch der Greisenkrankheiten. Stuttgart: Ferdinard
Enke., 914 pp.

SIMCHOWICZ, T. 1924. Sur la significance des plaques seniles et sur la formule
senile de l'ecorce cerebrale. Rev. Neurol., **31**, (1) 221–227.

SOUQUES, A., AND CHARCOT, J. M. 1891. Geromorphisme cutanee, Nouv. Icon.
de la Salp., **4**, 169–176.

STIEF, A. 1924. Beiträge zur Histopathologie der senilen Demenz, mit besonderer Berücksichtigung der extrapyramidalen Bewegungsstörungen.
Zeit. f. d. g. Neur. u. Psych., **91**, 579–616.

STERLING, M. V. 1929. Le Syndrome dystonique de la vieillesse. Rev. Neurol.,
36, 937–941.

STERN, K. 1936. Beitrag zur Histopathologie des senilen Rückenmarks.
Zeit. f. d. g. Neur. u. Psych., **155**, 543–554.

TILNEY, F. 1928. The ageing of the human brain. Bull. N. Y. Acad. Med., **4**,
1125–1143.

UYEMATSU, S. 1923. On the pathology of the senile psychoses. J. Nerv. &
Ment. Dis., **57**, 1–25; 131–156 and 237–260.

WARTHIN, A. S. 1929. Old Age. New York: Paul B. Hoeber, Inc., pp. 199.

WEBER, F. PARKES: 1929. A Note on Combined Congenital Ectodermal Defects. Brit. J. Child. Dis., **26**, 270–275.

ZALKA, E. v. 1928. Altersveränderungen des Plexus Choroideus. Virchows
Archiv., **267**, 379–412.

CHAPTER 18

THE EYE

JONAS S. FRIEDENWALD

Baltimore

The complex anatomical structure of the eye and its adnexa include within its small extent examples of almost all the tissue types found in the rest of the body. In addition, the eye contains avascular structures,—the cornea, lens, and vitreous, that are not duplicated elsewhere. The number and variety of senile changes to be found in this small organ is, therefore, very great. The older literature with its emphasis on the morphological aspects of senescence is very abundant in regard to the eye. The Surgeon-General's catalogue lists five monographs on this subject published between 1895 and 1905. More modern studies concerning the chemical and physico-chemical senescent changes in the ocular tissues are less extensive. An excellent review of these latter studies is to be found in the book by Krause (1934).

The interpretation of changes commonly found in the ocular tissues of the aged is fraught with the same difficulties that have been confronted in every chapter of this book. Are these changes brought about by the unavoidable processes inherent in the mere existence of these tissues over a prolonged period of time; are these changes in the ocular tissues produced indirectly by the senescence or disease of other perhaps remote organs; are they produced by the prolonged and cumulative effects of subliminal insults inflicted by the imperfect environment in which we live, or finally, are they the evidence of disease processes which happen to occur most frequently in the aged but which are, themselves, not directly related to the passage of time? These questions are, for the most part unanswerable on the basis of the present data and may, indeed, be essentially unanswerable. For the purposes of the present discussion, changes which occur commonly or universally in the aged will be regarded as senescent changes. Changes which are, themselves, of infrequent incidence but which occur exclusively or almost exclusively in the aged will be regarded as diseases unless they can clearly be shown to represent merely an exaggerated and extreme form of some more usual senile change. It must be admitted that we are here assuming that the senescent process is not strictly dependent upon the calendar age and, furthermore, that the degree of senescence of a particular organ or tissue is not strictly dependent upon the degree of senescence of the body as a whole. Such assumptions are, however, implicit in any attempt to study the process of ageing in individual organs, since without these assumptions the only relevant data would be the calendar age and final length of life of the individual.

1. LIFE SPAN

Total loss of function of the eye, i.e., blindness, may be taken as equivalent to death of the organ. It should be possible, therefore, to compute by methods similar to those illustrated by Dublin in Chapter 6 the life span and average life expectancy of this organ. Such computations for the organism as a whole are based on the age specific mortality rates. To make an equivalent computation with regard to the duration of vision one would require a knowledge of the number of people annually becoming blind in each age group. Such data are not directly available at present, though it is to be hoped that statistics which will necessarily be collected in connection with the blind pension service will some day be available for this analysis. The best that can be done at the present time is to take the census data as to the proportion of blind in each age group of the population. This is probably an underestimate of the true amount of blindness, first because the census probably represents an under count in this respect, and second, because the average length of life of the blind is probably somewhat less than that of the rest of the population. Figure 85 presents the data gathered in the 1910 census. Since only 2.5 per cent of persons over 85 years of age are blind, it is necessary to plot the curves logarithmically in order that survival of vision and survival of life should appear on the same chart.

The two curves have many points of similarity. There is an initial rapid fall corresponding to the high infantile death rate and the high incidence of congenital and juvenile blindness. This fall is almost completed at age 2 years in the life table diagram but reaches a corresponding point only at 12 years in the sight diagram. Following this there is a gently sloping plateau that extends through the 15th year for life, the 25th year for sight. Following this plateau both curves fall at a slowly increasing rate. At extreme old age the life table diagram flattens out. This final segment of the curve is not represented in the sight diagram, but it is plain that the number of survivors with vision could not reach zero at an age younger than 120 or 130 years.

Though the vast majority of persons live their whole lives without becoming blind, it is not to be assumed that their visual efficiency remains unimpaired with advancing age. The relation of visual acuity to age was first studied by Donders (1864). Several other writers (Boerma and Walther, 1893; Boussuge, 1904) have at various times made similar analyses on groups of old people. The results of a few of these investigators are shown in figure 86. In some of these studies the effort was made to exclude "disease" from the statistical group. The marked differences between the findings of the different observers

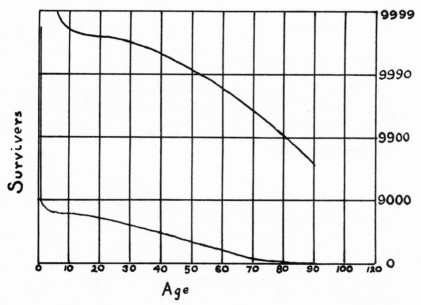

FIG. 85. The lower curve shows the survivors at each age of a group of 10,000 simultaneously conceived. The upper curve shows the survivers with vision in the same group assuming that none died. Based on data of U. S. Census 1910.

may be due in part to a different definition as to what is disease and in part to actual differences in the population studied. It is to be noted, however, that all these investigators agree in finding a steady fall in visual acuity as age progresses.

It has been shown that the extent of the visual field is less in the aged (Ferree and Rand, 1930); that the speed of dark adaptation is decreased and the minimal threshold of light perception raised (Ferree and Rand, 1934a); that aged eyes suffer a greater proportionate loss of visual acuity in dim illumination; and it is probable that the critical speed of flicker is also reduced in the aged (Ferree and Rand, 1934b). These studies have not, however, been sufficiently extensive to make possible a statistical analysis as to the average age of onset and average rate of progress of the decline of these functions. It is nevertheless clear that in respect of all the measurable visual functions the eyes of otherwise healthy old persons are slightly less efficient than those of the

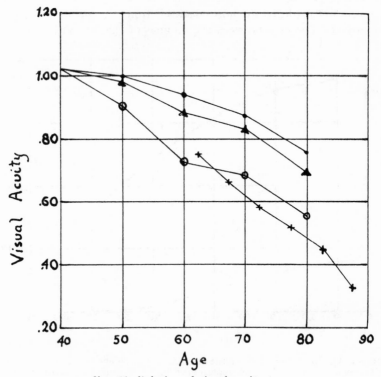

Fig. 86. Relation of visual acuity to age

young. The characteristic changes in refraction and reduction of the amplitude of accommodation with age will be discussed below.

2. OCULAR DISEASES OF THE AGED

Aside from changes in the eye directly resulting from sclerotic changes in the local blood vessels, there are several diseases which are responsible for so large a share of the blindness of the aged that their relation to the senescent process requires some discussion. The most important of these are cataract and glaucoma.

The lens is, histologically such a simple structure that its possible response to injury is limited almost exclusively to cataract formation. It is no wonder, therefore, that a multiplicity of possible causes of this condition have been discovered. However, if we set aside those instances of cataract which are clearly due to injury, metabolic disease, congenital defect, etc., and consider only "idiopathic" forms of the disease we are confronted with a phenomenon clearly related to advancing years. In spite of numerous efforts it has not, as yet, been possible to discover in exactly what way the senescent process causes this local manifestation. A certain degree of hereditary predisposition is clear for cataracts frequently appear in the eyes of siblings at nearly the same age. While most patients with cataracts show obvious evidence of general arteriosclerosis, it is by no means established that the degree of arteriosclerosis of patients with cataracts is in general in excess of that found in other persons of the same age. Nevertheless, the possibility remains that sclerotic changes in the vessels upon which the lens depends for its nutrition, may be excessive in cases of cataract. Attempts to correlate senile cataract with some disturbance in the blood chemistry have been unavailing. It has been argued by some that the cumulative effect of many years exposure to sun light, especially if that light contains an undue amount of ultra violet may be responsible for the trouble,—and it is pointed out in this connection that cataract is much more frequent in India than in the western world. In this country, however, the states of Colorado and Wyoming which stand near the top of the list for intensity of the ultra violet component of sunlight, stand near the bottom in the incidence of cataract. Current studies on the possible relation of vitamin defect to the etiology of cataract have not exhausted the field but, as yet, have contributed nothing of significance to our understanding of senile cataract.

It may be pointed out that the lens is dependent for its nutrition upon the capillaries of the ciliary processes and that, with advancing age the interstitial tissue surrounding these capillaries becomes denser and frequently shows hyalin degeneration (Kerschbaumer, 1888). In addition, the capsule of the lens becomes thicker, denser, and less permeable with age (Friedenwald, 1930). The possible influence of these phenomena on the metabolism of the lens is obvious, but it has not been shown that these changes occur in excessive degree in cases which develop cataracts.

The diseases of which increased intraocular pressure is the chief symptom are multifarious, but if cases due to congenital malformation, and cases secondary to injury or inflammation of the eye are excluded, and only "primary" glaucoma is considered we are confronted with a disease whose incidence is almost exclusively in the age period beyond middle life. The disease occurs in two forms: acute congestive and chronic non-congestive glaucoma.

Acute congestive glaucoma has been shown to result from a vasomotor crisis in the ciliary body with congestion of the capillaries in the ciliary processes, and serous and fibrinous extravasations from these vessels. No explanation is available as to why this should occur more frequently in persons of advancing years. Indeed, similar vasomotor disturbances in other organs appear to be more common in the younger age groups. There is no evidence of excessive local or general arteriosclerosis in these cases, nor is this disease associated with arteriolar sclerosis and malignant hypertension. It must be pointed out that acute congestive glaucoma occurs most commonly between 45 and 65 whereas the non-congestive forms of this disease has a somewhat later age incidence.

Chronic non-congestive glaucoma apparently results from a decreasing efficiency of the mechanism normally responsible for the reabsorption of the intraocular fluid. Sclerosis and hyalin degeneration of the tissues surrounding Schlemm's canal are commonly seen in the advanced stages of this disease but are generally absent at its onset. It has been suggested that the outflow channels may be plugged by granules of melanin pigment which, as we shall see below, are discharged into the anterior chamber from the ageing iris, but this has not been confirmed by histological study of cases examined in the early stages of the disease. There is no evidence that the degree of general arteriosclerosis is excessive in cases of glaucoma, but the possibility remains that excessive arteriosclerosis of the local vessels may be important, and indeed some evidence in favor of this hypothesis has been advanced (Friedenwald, 1936).

3. SENILE CHANGES IN OCULAR TISSUES

1. *Orbit and ocular adnexa.*

A diminution of orbital fat leading to enophthalmus is responsible for one of the most characteristic physiognomic features of senescence. No evidence has been brought forward indicating a weakening of the extraocular muscles in the aged, but the amplitude of convergence is generally less in old individuals, and there is often an increasing degree of exophoria. A slight drooping of the upper lid is very common, but this appears to be due to a lengthening of the tendon of the levator muscle rather than to weakness of the muscle. The eyelids of the aged are thin, lacking in subcutaneous fat, and show a marked loss of elasticity. If the lids of a young person are pulled away from the eye and then suddenly released they snap back into place often with an audible click. In the aged they sink more slowly into place and often do not return to their normal position without the intervention of muscular contraction. In extreme degrees of this condition the lower lid hangs permanently away from the eyeball and becomes everted. This progressive loss of tone in the lids usually begins in the sixth decade of life. There is no loss of function in the lachrymal gland attributable to age, but histological examination reveals an increase in the interstitial fibrous tissue of this organ in the aged.

2. *Conjunctiva.*

The conjunctiva is exposed to numerous and repeated traumata throughout life. This is especially true in persons whose occupations or habits of life includes much exposure to the wind and weather. We may, therefore, roughly assume that those affections, such as pterygium, which occur commonly in aged persons of outdoor occupations are due to the effects of trauma, while those that occur with equal frequency in persons who lead a sheltered life are, for the purposes of this discussion considered as senile manifestations. The conjunctiva of the aged is thin and friable. Hyalinization of the sub-epithelial connective tissue is common. There is frequently a dilatation of the conjunctival veins. Calcareous concretions in the serous glands of the palpebral conjunctiva is very common. One of the most striking differences between the conjunctiva of the aged and the young is the loss of lymphoid tissue, and more particularly the loss of the propensity of this tissue to hypertrophy (follicular conjunctivitis) under the influence of mild irritants.

3. *Cornea.*

The cornea tends to lose somewhat of its luster and transparency with advancing age. The former is attributable to the accumulation of minor irregularities in the epithelial surface. The latter is poorly understood, since we have no adequate explanation of the transparency of the tissue in the young. The corneal fibers tend to become slightly thicker with age, the water content of the tissue is somewhat reduced. According to Bürger and Schlomka (1928) the water content of bovine corneal tissue decreases from 85.4 per cent at age 7 days to 81.3 per cent at age 14.1 years.

In almost all elderly persons, and in a few young individuals a ring of opacification develops close to the corneal margin. An interesting statistical study on the age incidence of the corneal arcus has been published by Hinnen (1921). Histological examination reveals a lipoid infiltration,—cholesterol esters and neutral fats,—in the affected tissue. The clinically visible arcus is, however, only a small part of the lipoid infiltration of the ocular tissues in these cases. Bowman's and Descemet's membranes in the cornea are even more intensely infiltrated than the corneal stroma. Lipoid infiltration of the sclera goes hand

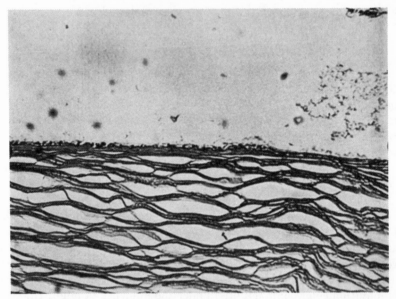

FIG. 87. Henle Warts in Decemet's Membrane. Patient aged 70

in hand with the arcus. Perivascular lipoidal changes in the iris, subepithelial lipoid infiltration in the ciliary body, lipoid infiltration of Bruch's membrane are all part of the same symptom complex. The relation of these phenomena to senescence is not clear. Experimentally the whole complex can be reproduced in rabbits by feeding large doses of cholesterol (Versé, 1916) and is accompanied in these animals by the deposition of atheromatous plaques in the arteries. Current opinion is inclined, therefore, to attribute both the ocular lipoid infiltration and the atheromatous plaques to some disturbance of the lipoid metabolism. Instances of juvenile arcus can, at times, be accounted for on the basis of hypercholesterolæmia due to biliary obstruction or nephrosis, but the cholesterolæmia of hypothyroidism does not appear to be associated with these lesions.

In addition to the lipoid infiltrations, local globular thickenings of Descemet's membrane are seen with great regularity in the aged. These were first described by Henle and are known as Henle warts (fig. 87). They are generally limited to the periphery of the cornea but occasionally cover the whole posterior surface of the cornea like dew drops, and may than cause slight decrease in visual acuity. In a small proportion of individuals in whom this wide spread distribution of Henle warts occurs, there develops a change in corneal permeability with resultant chronic oedema of the cornea and the formation of blisters on the corneal surface (epithelial dystrophy of the cornea),—a condition which leads eventually to blindness. A shallow circular groove at the corneal margin is seen in the aged, presumably due to an atrophy of the tissues in this region.

4. *Iris.*

The color of the eyes fades in the aged. The pupil is small and reacts feebly. The histological basis for these changes has been carefully studied by Fuchs (1884) and Seefelder (1909). The collagen

fibers of the iris, especially in its anterior layers become denser and thus cast a veil over the deeper lying pigment. Along with this the complex pattern of crypts and trabeculae on the iris surface becomes flattened out and obscured. Similar increase in the collagen fibers about the blood vessels, often with hyalin degeneration, is found. The sphincter pupillae undergoes fibrosis and hyalinization. A peculiar feature which occurs very regularly after the sixth decade (Hinnen, 1921) is a loss of pigment from the pigment epithelium on the posterior surface of the iris. This begins in small spots at the pupillary margin which subsequently grow and coalesce giving the iris finally a moth eaten appearance. Much of the pigment is discharged into the anterior chamber and can be seen deposited on the posterior surface of the cornea and on the trabeculae at the filtration angle. The pattern of the pigment atrophy does not correspond to the anatomical units in the iris vascular supply and is, therefore, not readily attributable to local arteriosclerosis. Except for the loss of pigment the epithelial cells appear quite normal.

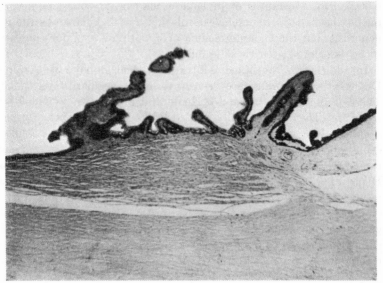

A

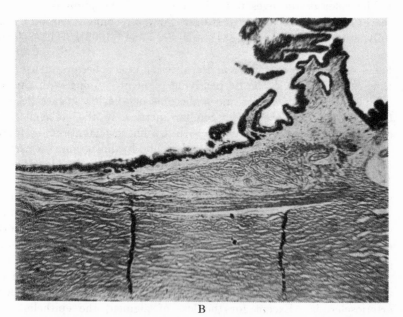

B

FIG. 88. Age changes in the ciliary body

5. *Ciliary body.*

The histological changes in the ciliary body with advancing age have been described exhaustively by Kirschbaumer (1888) and Herbert (1923). The increasing fibrosis, lipoid infiltration, and hyalinization of the ciliary processes with advancing age have already been noted. The ciliary muscle likewise shows an increase in its interstitial fibrous tissue and the muscle fibers in the aged are thinner and more dense than in the young (fig. 88). There is, however, no marked decrease in muscular power, as has been shown by very detailed studies of van der Hoeve and Flieringa (1924). They have made it quite clear that

TABLE 26

Relation of the amount of protein to the age of the lens

From Jess (1913)

Age of lens	Weight of lens	Total protein	Soluble protein
	grams	*per cent*	*per cent*
5 weeks	0.9309	32.33	24.95
1.5 years	1.8522	34.5	19.93
4 years	2.0508	34.24	19.41
6 years	2.5416	36.0	17.62
12 years	2.6720	35.59	17.69
16 years	2.6788	35.5	16.10

the declining range of accommodation is to be attributed to changes in the lens, not in the ciliary muscle.

6. *Lens.*

The lens is an epithelial structure surrounded by a homogenous glassy capsule. No blood vessels enter the lens and its metabolic exchange is, therefore, dependent upon the nutritive characteristics of the surrounding aqueous fluid and the permeability of the lens capsule. Throughout life new lens fibers are continuously being proliferated by the growth and elongation of the epithelial cells at the lens equator. New fibers are laid down on top of older ones, and the life history of the lens fiber can be studied by observing the differences between successive layers of fibers. Those at the center of the lens were produced during the early months of intrauterine life, those at the periphery are embryonal even in an aged individual.

These cells begin their differentiation as flat hexagonal epithelium, gradually elongating, they assume the form of a tall thin fiber still

hexagonal in cross section. The length of individual fibers composed
of a single cell attains, at a maximum several millimeters. The cell
or fiber during its period of growth is surrounded by a membrane containing lipoid. The cytoplasm is a homogenous material of very high
protein content. During the period of growth the nucleus remains
apparently unchanged but with cessation of growth of the fiber, the
nucleus disappears. Subsequently the cell membrane also disappears
and the cytoplasm, losing water, becomes dense, rigid, almost horny
in character. Chemically these changes are characterized by an increase in the amount of insoluble protein, phospho-lipids and cholesterol,

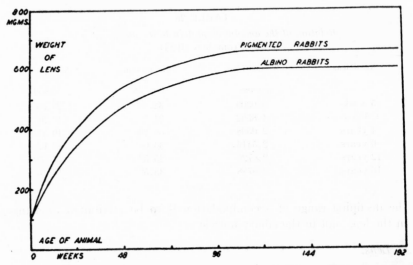

Fig. 89. The weight of the lens of pigmented and albino rabbits at various
ages (Krause).

and calcium, and a relative increase of sodium as compared to potassium, together with a loss of water and of glutathione (nitroprusside
reaction).

It is apparent that one cannot speak unambiguously of an aged
lens, for the lens contains from birth to old age parts which are embryonal in character and parts which are old. The difference between
an old and a young lens is, therefore, a difference in the relative proportion of young and old tissue within it, and senescence for the lens
represents essentially the accumulation of a larger and larger proportion
of inert dessicated tissue in its center. While the lens grows con-

tinuously throughout life the growth rate is not constant but becomes slower and slower as age advances, never reaching zero, however, unless the tissue dies in cataract formation (fig. 89).

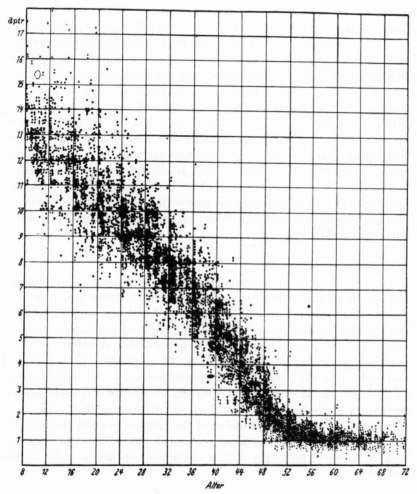

Fig. 90. Range of accommodation in 4000 cases (Duane)

Since the young portion near the surface of the lens is soft and deformable while the older portion nearer the center is rigid, the cortex alone takes part in the act of accommodation, and as the cortex occupies progressively a smaller fraction of the whole volume of the lens, the amplitude of accommodative change decreases. This decrease begins at birth and proceeds with remarkable uniformity as age progresses (fig. 90). Such differences as are found between different individuals of the same age are largely dependent on the different amounts of muscular effort at accommodation which the individuals can be induced to make, for the fluctuations in successive tests on the same individual are nearly as great as the fluctuations between different individuals. Bernstein (1932) has studied statistically the variations in accommodative power of different individuals of the same age with variations in their subsequent length of life and has found a positive correlation between accommodative power and longevity. It would be highly desirable to have these studies amplified on a large and more modern body of material. If Bernstein's findings are confirmed, the measurement of accommodative power may attain the position of a useful index of the degree of senescence of the individual. Nevertheless the question will still remain open as to whether the variations measured represent variations in deformability of the lens or variations in muscular effort of the subject.

7. Vitreous.

The vitreous is an inert non-living tissue. It consists of an insoluble framework arranged in more or less concentric sheets and a mucoid fluid. No change in the fluid has been noted with age but the insoluble framework increases in amount, the sheets becoming more and more closely packed in the periphery. It is apparent, therefore, that we are dealing here again with a process of accumulation of non-vital material. The older sheets in the central portion of the vitreous tend, as time goes on, to show irregular regions of collapse and agglutination so that an increasing number of floating vitreous opacities is the rule. The increased density and number of the lamellae close to the retina is responsible for one of the most prominent ophthalmoscopic changes seen in the aged, namely a dulling of the lustrous sheen of the retinal surface.

8. Retina.

Changes in retinal function with age have already been discussed. In the periphery of the retina near the ciliary body degenerative changes appear quite regularly in otherwise healthy eyes in the fifth decade (fig. 91). When ocular disease is present these changes may appear

much earlier.   They consist in the disappearance of the middle nuclear
layer and its replacement by fluid spaces which on section appear round
or oval but actually form an interlacing pattern of tunnels or channels.
The fluid contains a basophilic material which gives the histological
reactions of mucin.   The distribution of these atrophic changes does

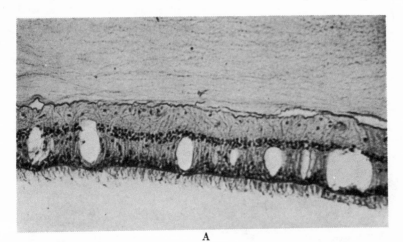

A

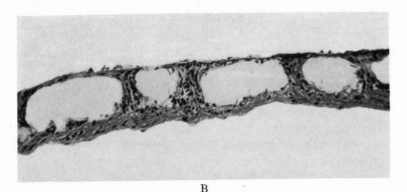

B

FIG. 91. Beginning and advanced cystic degeneration of the retina

not correspond to any anatomical unit of the retinal vascular tree and
it is difficult, therefore, to attribute them to local arteriosclerosis.
Nevertheless, it must be pointed out that the zone of atrophy is that
farthest from the parent arterial supply of the retina, and lesions of
this type are not found in dogs,—animals notoriously free from arterio-

sclerosis. As age proceeds the cystic degeneration extends progressively farther back toward the posterior pole but it rarely reaches behind the equator of the eye. It seems reasonable to attribute the progressive narrowing of the visual field in the aged to this change.

The remainder of the retina is thinner and denser in the aged than in the young, apparently due to a loss of water. A variety of senile atrophic and degenerative changes especially in the macular region of the retina should be enumerated among the diseases of the aged, but they all appear to be the consequences of local arteriosclerosis and will not be discussed further.

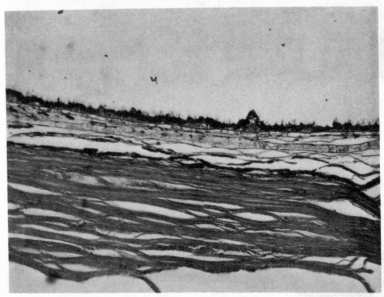

Fig. 92. Nodular thickenings of Bruch's membrane. Patient aged 70

9. *Choroid.*

The arteries of the choroid, like those of the spleen, show marked thickening and hyalinization of their media beginning in middle life even without any evidence of generalized arteriolar sclerosis (Wood, 1915). The nature of this change and its relation or lack of relation to the histologically similar changes in the vessels of other organs in cases of malignant hypertension constitute an interesting problem, the solution of which must wait on a better understanding of the pathogenesis of arteriolar sclerosis. In addition to this puzzling phenomenon there is an increase in the interstitial fibrillar tissue of the choroid with advancing years (Kerschbaumer, 1892). Bruch's membrane, which lies between the choroid and the pigment epithelium of the retina becomes thicker with age and partakes of the lipoid infiltration described above in connection with the lipoid arcus of the cornea. This membrane is strikingly similar to Descemet's membrane on the inner surface of the cornea, and like it shows localized nodular thickenings in the aged analogous to the warts of Henle (fig. 92).

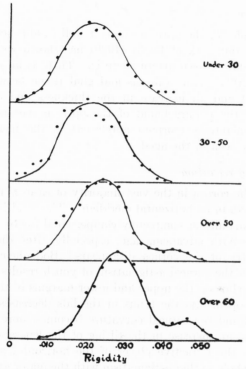

FIG. 93. Frequency distribution of ocular rigidity in different age groups (Friedenwald).

10. Sclera.

The sclera of the aged is thinner and denser than that of the young and shows a loss of water. In a recent study Friedenwald (1937) has developed a method for the measurement of the distensibility, or its reciprocal the rigidity, of the eyeball in the living individual. The application of this measurement to otherwise normal eyes of varying ages revealed an increasing ocular rigidity which first appears in the sixth decade of life (fig. 93). The function which is measured includes not only the elasticity of the sclera but also the pliability of the cornea and the compressibility of the intraocular vascular bed, but the elasticity of the sclera appears to be the most important factor in the measurement. Since the sclera is composed of relatively undifferentiated fibrous tissue the measurement of its elasticity may be useful as an index of the ageing of the connective tissue of the body as a whole. Further studies along these lines are indicated.

11. *Optic nerve.*

Senile atrophy of the optic nerve is a well established clinical phenomenon but the work of Fuchs (1920) has shown very clearly that this is the result of local arteriosclerosis. There is an increase in the interstitial fibrillar tissue (fibrous and glial tissue between the nerve fiber bundles) and an increase in the thickness and density of the trabeculae of the pia-arachnoid of the optic nerve sheath (fig. 94). Basophilic concretions (corpora amylacea) in the meningeal sheath are commonly seen in the aged.

12. *Changes of refraction.*

In youth the cornea in the vast majority of cases is more curved in its vertical than in its horizontal meridian. The resulting astigmatism is as a rule partially or completely compensated for by a slight tilting of the lens. With advancing age, especially after the fifth decade, this asymmetry of the cornea disappears. Bodenheimer (1937) has suggested that the corneal astigmatism of youth results from the pressure of the eyelids on the upper and lower margins of the cornea when the eyes are open. As the tonus in the lids decreases this influence is diminished and the corneal curvature becomes more spherical. At the same time an increase in the tilting of the lens about its vertical axis increases the refractive power of the horizontal meridian of the eyeball as a whole so that astigmatism with the major axis horizontal is the rule in the aged while astigmatism with the major axis vertical is the rule in youth.

With the growth of lens the anterior surface of this organ approaches more closely to the posterior surface of the cornea (fig. 95). Consequently the anterior chamber becomes shallower with age (Rosengren, 1930) and the optical nodal points of the lens move forward. This results in an increase in the effective dioptric power of the lens and hence a slight tendency toward myopia. With the progressive growth and increased density of the lens nucleus, the refractive power of this

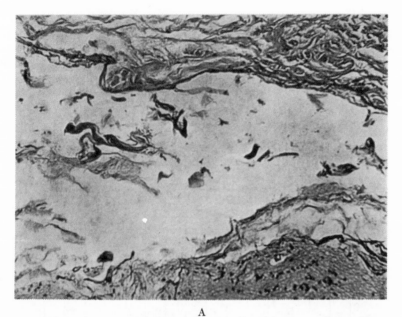

A

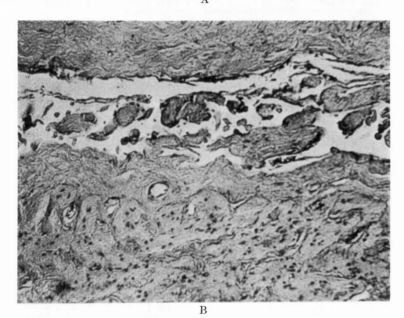

B

Fig. 94. Increase in thickness and density of trabeculae of pia arachnoid of optic nerve sheath with age,—A. young, B. old.

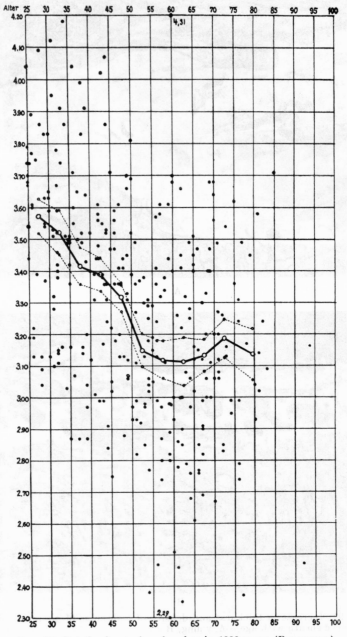

FIG. 95. Depth of anterior chamber in 1000 cases (Rosengren)

portion of the lens is increased adding to the myopic tendency. These two phenomena together account for the short sight of the aged which, if it follows normal presbyopia often gives the individual a false sense rejuvenation since he finds himself at an advanced age once more able to read without glasses. The phenomenon has been referred to as "second sight." Changes in accommodation have been discussed above.

4. SUMMARY

By comparing the expectancy of sight with the expectancy of life it is clearly demonstrable that the normal life span of the eye as a functioning organ exceeds that of the body as a whole. There is, however, a steady decrease of the average efficiency of all measurable visual functions with advancing age even in otherwise healthy eyes. The characteristic senile morphological and chemical changes of the ocular tissues may be summarized as increased density, loss of water, increased interstitial fibrillar tissue, accumulation in some portions of the organ of an increased amount of inert material, loss of fat and of elasticity, together with isolated examples of some rather bizarre forms of tissue atrophy. In relation to the eye, as in relation to other organs, the dominant and at present insoluble problem of senescence is as to whether these changes represent inherent tendencies of mortal flesh, or whether they represent the cumulative effects of potentially avoidable disease or of potentially avoidable subclinical damage produced by a non-ideal environment.

REFERENCES

BERNSTEIN, F. 1932. Alterssichtigkeit und Lebenserwartung. Forsch. u. Fortschr., **8**, 272–273.

BODENHEIMER, E. 1937. Personal communication.

BOERMA, K. AND WALTHER, D. 1893. Untersuchungen über die Abnahme der Sehschärfe im Alter. Arch. f. Ophth., **39**, pt. 2, 71–82.

BOUSSUGE, P. 1904. De l'oeil senile. Lyon: Lyon University Press, 30 pp.

BÜRGER, M., AND SCHLOMKA, M. 1928. Beiträge zur physiologischen Chemie des Alterns der Gewebe. III. Mitt. Untersuchungen an der Rinderhaut. Ztschr. f. d. ges. exp. Med., **61**, 465–476.

DONDERS, F. C. 1864. Accommodation and refraction of the eye. London: New Sydenham Soc., 635 pp.

FERREE, C. E., AND RAND, G. 1930. Study of factors which cause individual differences in size of form field. Am. J. Psychol., **42**, 63–71.

——— 1934a. Critical values for the light minimum and for the amount and rapidity of dark adaptation. Brit. J. Ophthal., **18**, 673–687.

——— 1934b. The effect of increase of intensity of light on the visual acuity of presbyopia and non-presbyopic eyes. Trans. Illuminat. Eng. Soc., **29**, 296–313.

FRIEDENWALD, J. S. 1930. Permeability of lens capsule, with special reference to etiology of senile cataract. Arch. of Ophth., **3**, 182–193.
——— 1936. Circulation of aqueous: Mechanism of Schlemm's canal. Arch. of Ophth., **16**, 65–77.
——— 1937. Theory and practice of tonometry. Am. J. Ophth., **20**, 985–1024.
FUCHS, E. 1884. Anatomische miscellen. Arch. f. Ophth., **30**, pt. 3, 123–156.
——— 1920. Über senile Veränderungen des Sehnerve. Deutsch. Ophth. Gesell., 182–185.
HERBERT, H. 1923. The pectinate ligament in its relation to chronic glaucoma. Brit. J. Ophth., **7**, 469–477.
HINNEN, E. 1921. Die Altersveränderungen des vorderen Bulbusabschnittes von 924 gesunden Augen, nach Untersuchungen am Spaltlampenmikroskop. Ztschr. f. Augenheilk., **45**, 129–142.
JESS, A. 1913. Beiträge zur Kenntnis der Chemie der normalen und der pathologischen veränderten Linse des Auges. Ztschr. f. Biol., **61**, 92–142.
KERSCHBAUMER, R. 1888. Ueber Altersveränderungen der Uvea. Arch. f. Ophth., **34**, pt. 4, 16–34.
——— 1892. Ueber Altersveränderungen der Uvea. Arch. f. Ophth., **38**, pt. 1, 127–148.
KRAUSE, A. C. 1934. The biochemistry of the eye. Baltimore: Johns Hopkins Press, 264 pp.
ROSENGREN, B. 1930. Studien über die Tiefe der vorderen Augenkammer mit besonderer Hinsicht auf ihr Verhalten beim primären Glaukom; eine Untersuchung mit dem Lindstedtschen Apparat; die Kammertiefe des normalen Auges. Acta Ophth., **8**, 99–136.
SEEFELDER, R. 1909. Zur pathologischen Anatomie der Hyalinen Degeneration des Pupillarrandes. Ztschr. f. Augenheilk., **21**, 289–294.
U. S. BUREAU OF THE CENSUS FOR 1910. 1917. The blind in the United States.
VAN DER HOEVE, J., AND FLIERINGA, H. J. 1924. Accommodation. Brit. J. Ophth., **8**, 97–106.
VERSÉ, M. 1916. Über die Blut-und-Augenrevänderungen bei experimenteller Cholesterinämie. Münch. Med. Wochnschr., **63**, 1074–1076.
WOOD, C. G. R. 1915. Choroidal sclerosis. Ophthalmoscope, **13**, 374–376.

Chapter 19

THE EAR

STACY R. GUILD

Baltimore

1. HEARING

Since ancient times, probably, impaired hearing has been recognized as one of the common afflictions of the aged. That a decline in acuity of hearing with ageing should be regarded as normal has been stated in medical works for the past two or three centuries, also that the impairment is greater for sounds of high pitch than for those of low pitch. So long as tests of hearing were made only with whispered and conversational voice, tuning forks, watches, acumeters, etc., it was impossible to state in more than qualitative terms the differences in amount of impairment for different tonal regions. Since the development of electrically generated sources of sound, audiometers, it has been possible to compare the differences more accurately. However, even yet the line between normal and more than normal impairment for the age cannot be sharply drawn. The distinction would be easy if the normal could be defined as the best for each age. No investigator of hearing has used this criterion of normal. Instead, each has used an arbitrary, and a different, standard to separate the cases to be included in "normal variation" from those to be regarded as complicated by local or by systemic disorders not due to age.

Quantitative measurements of a difference in hearing associated with age were first reported by Zwaardemaker, in 1891. His tests with a Galton whistle showed a gradual regression of the upper limit of hearing, beginning already in adolescence. The figures given in his second paper on the subject, in 1893, are: an average of the tone of e^7 for young children and a^6 for "advanced age." In terms of frequencies these tones are, respectively, about 20,500 and 13,500 double vibrations per second. An upper limit of hearing below g^6 (about 12,300) Zwaardemaker regarded as outside the range of normal even for old age. Bezold (1892), using a different basis of selection of material, found less change of the upper limit than did Zwaardemaker, and expressed doubt as to the value of the latter's "law of presbyacusia." Struycken, in 1913, using a different instrument, the monochord known by his name, to measure the upper limit, confirmed Zwaardemaker's conclusion that there is regression with ageing. The idea is now generally accepted.

The gradual raising of the *lower* limit of hearing, reported by Cuperus, through Zwaardemaker, in 1893, as a second law of presbyacusia, has failed to secure general acceptance as a part of the clinical picture of uncomplicated ageing of the organ of hearing. Richter (1894) concluded that in addition to regression of the upper limit, ageing in itself causes an impairment that can be detected by all tests of hearing and for all tonal regions. His conclusion that the decline is of about equal amount for all tones was not in agreement with that of Bezold (1893), and has not been supported by later work.

Bunch (1929, 1931) and Bunch and Raiford (1931) correlated age with the records of hearing acuity obtained by testing patients with an audiometer that produces tones with the frequencies of from 32 to 16,384 double vibrations per second. The intervals between tones are half-octaves, except for the highest octave, in which two intermediate tones (frequencies of 10,321 and 13,004) are produced. The patients whose records were used for the studies of the effect of age on hearing had no complaints of ear trouble. Figure 96 shows the averages of the thresholds for tones transmitted to the ear by air conduction; the data are based on 693 patients, grouped by decades of chronological age. The examinations were not made in a sound-proof room, therefore the proper reference line is the average for the younger group instead of the line on the chart marked "zero loss" or "normal hearing." Their observations show, on the average, with each decade a progressive loss in the acuity of hearing for all tones. For the tones with frequencies up to and including 512 double vibrations per second (an octave above the fundamental of the note *middle c* of the musical scale) the total impairment with ageing is but very slight. For tones above this frequency, however, the higher the tone the greater is the average degree of impairment in each older age-group.

Bunch and Raiford also noted that in each age-group white males have, on the average, a somewhat greater impairment for all tones above a frequency of 2048 double vibrations per second than do white females. Ciocco's (1932) study of a yet larger material than was available to Bunch and Raiford, and by a different method—incidence of types of audiograms instead of averages for groups, confirmed their conclusions both with respect to the tonal regions affected by ageing and to the differences between the sexes at each age.

The normal amount of impairment for the higher tones in people

over fifty is sufficient to be of significance in the understanding of conversation and to make impossible a "balanced" hearing of the full
harmonic content of music. The latter effect is but seldom noticed by
the individual, or at least seldom causes complaint, probably for the
reason that the impairment develops so slowly that the suppression of
perception of the higher overtones is not realized. Although the high
pitched elements of speech are but poorly, if at all, heard by an old
person with hearing normal for the age, he seldom has difficulty under-

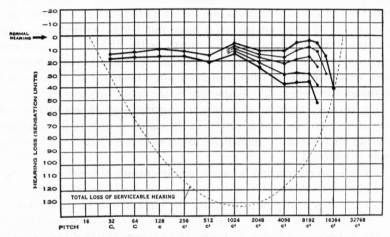

FIG. 96. Shows the data of Bunch and Raiford's chart 10, transferred to a
standard audiogram form. The upper line is the average of the audiograms of
161 adults between the ages of 20 and 29 years, the lower line the average for 50
people over 60 years of age. The intermediate lines, from above downwards on
the chart, are the averages, respectively, for people in the fourth, fifth and sixth
decades of life. For tones below the frequency of 1024 double vibrations per
second (*high c* of the musical scale) the average impairment with increasing age
is so slight that separate lines can be given on the chart only for the youngest
and the oldest groups. It is of interest to note, however, that the actual averages
for each of the low tones show a slight progression in impairment for each decade.
The significant impairments are for the high tones.

standing the meaning of phrases and sentences in conversation with one
other person. But most elderly people do have difficulty understanding
conversation when several people are speaking at the same time, as
at a party. This difficulty is not peculiar to elderly people, it is a
complaint frequently made by younger people who have impaired
hearing for high tones. The characteristics by which one voice is
distinguished from another are mostly the differences in the relative
intensities of the several overtones of the fundamental frequencies of

speech sounds. The difficulty a normal elderly person has in understanding conversation in a group is in large part an inability to distinguish in the mixture of sounds the voice to which he wishes to listen, rather than an inability to hear the voice at all.

A condition that may be termed premature ageing is encountered in hearing. For example, a 45-year-old person may have an impairment of hearing for high tones equal to the normal for 75 years of age. Whether or not the hearing of such individuals continues to decline in later years is not known. The question raised cannot be answered until such time as accurate examinations of acuity of hearing have been made periodically throughout life on a large number of individuals. Quite possibly those people who in the fourth or the fifth decade have more impairment of hearing for high tones than is normal for the age are the ones whose cochleae, when obtained after death at later ages, have histologically demonstrable atrophy in the basal turn (see below).

The reverse condition of premature ageing is also encountered occasionally. Some individuals even in the eighth decade of life have good hearing for tones with frequencies up to as high as 10,000 double vibrations per second.

There is no correlation between average acuity of hearing at any age and chronic systemic diseases (Bunch, 1931, and Ciocco, 1932).

A decline in acuity of hearing for the highest tone of the audiometer is already evident in early adult life. For a series of 80 medical students, average age about 23 years, the average threshold intensity for the tone with a frequency of 16,384 double vibrations per second was definitely greater than the intensity at which most children of 10 to 15 years of age can hear this tone. This fact is in good agreement with Zwaardemaker's observation of a slight lowering of the upper limit of hearing for the Galton whistle in adolescents as compared to younger children.

1. *Hearing by Bone Conduction.*

Thus far the discussion has been entirely of hearing by air conduction of the sound to the ear. The acuity of hearing by the less commonly utilized means of transmission of sound waves to the inner ear—transmission through the bones of the skull, also declines with advancing age. The amount of the decline is not as well established as it is for hearing by air conduction. Usually the ability to hear by bone conduction is examined for only one or two tones, and these of relatively low frequency, 128, 256, 435 or 512 double vibrations per second.

Usually, also, these tests are made with tuning forks, with which the measurements of thresholds are only of qualitative value in comparative studies of groups.

It has been known to otologists for a long time that some allowance for age should be made in the interpretation of the significance of a clinical finding of impaired hearing by bone conduction. Politzer wrote, in his widely used textbook, in 1882: "As is well known, the power of the perception through the cranial bones is diminshed in old age to a varying degree." The reports of tuning fork tests by Bezold (1893), Richter (1894), Sporleder (1899) and Ziffer (1908) are all confirmatory of this general idea. Struycken (1913) reported that the upper limit of hearing by bone conduction, as tested with the monochord, regresses with age more or less parallel to the upper limit by air conduction, the upper limit by bone conduction being usually slightly the higher. Unpublished observations in our laboratory at Baltimore are in agreement with those of Struycken.

Ciocco (1935), for 907 patients who had good hearing by air conduction, as tested with the audiometer, for the tone with a frequency of 512 double vibrations per second, divided the records as to acuity of hearing of this tone by bone conduction into three groups: normal, slightly shortened and shortened. Only those who heard the tuning fork by bone conduction less than half the normal time were included in the latter group. His conclusion is: "The incidence of those with 'shortened' bone conduction increases with advancing age; the differences between groups [decades of age] are large and are statistically significant." Until similar, or better, studies have been made of the hearing by bone conduction of other tones also, one is not justified in generalizing the most interesting conclusion, from the point of view of the physiology of ageing, that is reached by Ciocco; namely, that the decline in acuity of hearing by bone conduction is greater than by air conduction.

2. Anatomical Changes.

The literature on the anatomical changes associated with the ageing decline in hearing is extensive. The most recent is a monograph, published in the summer of 1937, by Fieandt and Saxen of Helsingfors. A detailed review of the publications on the subject would not be profitable in the present study, because (1) most of the accounts are based on histologic studies of temporal bones from people whose hearing either had not been examined at all or only by tests so incomplete that the relation to normal hearing for the age cannot be determined, and (2) artefacts due to histologic preparation or to postmortem autolysis have often been mistaken for true lesions.

There is general agreement that the most common lesion of the inner ear in elderly people is simple atrophy, of greater or lesser degree and extent, of the nerve or of the nerve and endorgan in the basal turn of the cochlea. As Alexander (1913, 1924), Mayer (1920), Wittmaack (1907, 1916), Steurer (1926), Lederer (1926), Fieandt and Saxen (1937), and others have pointed out, histologically these atrophies are indistinguishable from those which at younger ages are attributed to the effects of toxins, to hereditary factors or to unexplained degeneration. Similar lesions have by several authors been attributed to the effect of circulatory disturbances, especially to arteriosclerosis. This is the explanation usually advanced for the frequent occurrence of atrophy in the inner ears of old people. The evidence in favor of this plausible argument is not convincing, because (1) but rarely have any vascular lesions been observed in the inner ear itself, (2) the degree of atrophy frequently does not parallel the severity of the systemic vascular disease, and (3) it offers no explanation of the localization of the atrophy, which usually is limited to the basal turn of the cochlea and is of greater degree in the lower than in the upper part of this turn.

Crowe, Guild and Polvogt (1934), on the basis of a detailed study of serial sections of 79 temporal bones from patients whose hearing had been carefully examined during their last illnesses, were able to correlate atrophies in the basal turn of the cochlea with impaired hearing for high tones more definitely than had previous investigators. In ears which had a gradually increasing degree of impairment for the successively higher tones the typical lesion is a partial atrophy of the nerve of the basal turn, the atrophy is of greater degree toward the lower end. In ears with which all tones were well heard up to, for example, a frequency of 2048 double vibrations per second, and all higher tones, if heard at all, had a severe impairment of threshold, the typical lesion is total atrophy of part or all of the endorgan in the lower half of the basal turn, in addition to atrophy of the nerve to this region. The latter type of lesion is almost entirely limited to males; this probably explains the sex difference in hearing impairment for high tones noted by Bunch and Raiford and by Ciocco (see above).

But, and for the present study this exception is very important, in most of the ears which had no more than the normal impairment of hearing for the age, or even for a later age, on the basis of Bunch and

Raiford's averages, the writer and his colleagues found no atrophies of greater extent, or other lesions, than are also present in many ears with good hearing for all tones. Had not a "control" group of ears been studied as carefully as the ones with impaired hearing there might seem to be an explanation, histologically, in the inner ears of these patients. As it is, the ones with normal hearing for the age form the largest part of the "unexplained" group of their study.

In the sections of the temporal bones from 28 people over 60 years of age Mayer (1920) observed one or both of two types of changes from the normal appearance of the basilar membrane of the basal turn, calcification and hyalinization. On the basis of these observations he advanced the theory that impaired hearing for high tones in old age is in part due to an increased rigidity of the basilar membrane. The observations by Crowe, Guild and Polvogt do not confirm Mayer's theory. In their material the histologic changes in the basilar membrane described by Mayer vary greatly in extent, are not peculiar to the older ages, and when present do not seem to be related to the degree of hearing impairment.

No one has studied the auditory pathways and centers of the central nervous system from the point of view of changes associated with the ageing decline in hearing; it is quite possible that the structural changes responsible for the normal degree of impairment are in this part of the complete organ of hearing. It is also quite possible that the real lesions of ageing of the auditory apparatus are in the exceedingly complex, though minute in size, endorgan of the cochlea; the finer details of the organ of Corti are not revealed by the usual histologic technique.

Even though, as noted above, the histologic evidence is not convincing, circulatory changes cannot be ruled out as the primary cause of the normal impairment of hearing associated with age. The effect may be merely a depression of sensitivity, due to a partial anoxemia of the endorgan or of centers in the nervous system, without the production of organic lesions. One bit of evidence that favors this theoretical possibility is in a recent German report (Hartmann, 1936, seen in abstract only) of tests of aviators in a low-pressure chamber. The upper limit of hearing, as tested with a monochord, became impaired when atmospheric pressure was markedly reduced, and the hearing returned to normal (for the individual) when the oxygen content of the air was increased without changing the total reduction of atmospheric pressure. Furstenberg's (1937) observations on the hearing of young adults with essential hypertension are susceptible of the same interpretation—

partial anoxemia. Before treatment of the hypertensive condition by section of the splanchnic nerves many of his patients had a greater impairment of hearing for high tones than a few weeks or months later, when circulatory conditions had improved after operation. The examinations were made with an audiometer.

The osseous tissue of the ear probably becomes more brittle with advancing age, as does other bone in the body. The minute spontaneous fractures in different parts of the otic capsule, reported by Mayer (1930, 1931), and in the osseous trabeculae of the floor of the aditus ad antrum (Guild, 1936) are of very common occurrence in elderly people. Whatever the mechanical force directly responsible for these physiologic fractures may prove to be, the frequency with which they are present is evidence that the bone becomes more brittle with ageing. In all probability the structural change here is the same as in other bones, an increase in the proportion of inorganic content with respect to fibrils, but so far as the writer is aware the temporal bone has not been examined from this point of view. It is a common laboratory experience that with the same batch of stains the sections of temporal bones from old individuals have a "flat" appearance that is in marked contrast to the "brilliant" differentiations of colors imparted to the sections from young individuals.   Nuclei of osteocytes usually remain unstained in the sections from old individuals, so that the lacunae of the bone appear to be empty.

Guild (1936) reported positive association between spontaneous, or physiologic, fracture of all of the osseous trabeculae of the floor of the aditus ad antrum and impaired hearing by bone conduction, and suggested that sound waves transmitted through these trabeculae reach the fluids of the inner ear from the direction best for effective stimulation of the cochlear endorgan, the organ of Corti. Such fractures are most frequently present in older individuals; this fact may be the anatomical explanation of Ciocco's observation (see above) that in older people there is often, for the same tone (512 double vibrations per second) more impairment of hearing by bone conduction than by air conduction.

3. The Middle Ear.

The ligaments of the ossicular articulations, in contrast to those of most joints of the body, consist largely of the elastic type of connective tissue.   There is but very little elastic tissue in the tympanic membrane. On the other hand, there is much elastic tissue in the sheath of the tendon of the tensor tympani muscle, in the ligament around which the tensor tendon turns and in the bands which join the tendon proper. It is conceivable that alterations in the properties of the elastic tissue could impair the efficiency of the ossicular chain as a transmitter of sound waves to the inner ear and thus be in part responsible for the ageing decline in hearing. However, changes in the elastic tissue of the middle ear have not been reported, and in the small number of specimens the writer has stained specially for elastic tissue no differences have been detected in ears from individuals of different ages.

4. *The External Ear.*

So far as the writer is aware no special studies have been made of the ageing of the external ear. Probably the skin of the external canal and the pinna participates in the changes that occur elsewhere in skin with ageing. The hairs in the outer part of the canal frequently become coarser in later life, especially in males. There is no reason to suspect that the impairment of hearing normal to later life is caused by changes in the external ear.

2. VESTIBULAR APPARATUS

The effect of ageing upon the functions, either dynamic or static, of the vestibular parts of the ear is unknown. Phylogenetically these structures antedate the cochlear. Semicircular canals, utriculus and sacculus are present in all vertebrates from fishes to man. Only in mammals is the auditory part of the inner ear similar to that of man; even the so-called cochlea of birds and reptiles is anatomically very different. Therefore the absence of reports of an ageing effect in the vestibular apparatus may plausibly be interpreted to mean that, due to its relatively primitive status, there is no decline in functional performance with increasing age of the individual. On the other hand, the actual meaning may well be that the functional tests employed fail to reveal the impairment due to ageing.

The methods commonly used for clinical examination of the vestibular parts of the ear—caloric and rotation tests, with observations of the induced nystagmus, past-pointing, etc.—are crude in comparison to the tests made of hearing. The stimulations applied to the endorgans of the vestibular apparatus are far greater than anything which may be termed physiologic. The methods that have been proposed for testing the *thresholds* of response of vestibular reflexes are too time-consuming for routine use with patients, therefore they have been used by any one investigator only on small numbers of people. So far as the writer is aware differences related to age have not even been sought in these special investigations with the less crude methods of functional examination of the vestibular apparatus.

The possibility exists that the general "slowing down" of motor functions with advancing age is in part due to an ageing of the vestibular apparatus itself or of the synapses of its numerous connections.

Histologically there is no typical difference in the appearance of the vestibular structures in ears from old and from young individuals.

3. SUMMARY

Impaired hearing for high pitched sounds occurs so frequently in old people that it must be regarded as the normal condition. The average acuity of hearing for high tones (from *high c* of the musical scale upwards) decreases with each decade of life, the higher the tone the more is the average impairment. Hearing for extremely high tones is lost entirely, as a rule.

The majority of elderly people have nearly as good hearing for tones below *high c* as do younger people. Therefore more than a slight impairment of hearing for low tones, by air conduction, cannot be regarded as the normal condition. By bone conduction of the sound, however, marked impairment occurs so often in old people that it should be regarded as normal.

The line cannot be sharply drawn between impaired hearing due to ageing alone and that due to ageing plus other factors: the clinical picture is simply that of a slight to moderate degree of so-called "nerve deafness." This type of impaired hearing is not limited to old age.

The more severe impairments of hearing for high tones, when low tones are well heard, can usually be correlated with simple atrophy of the nerve, or of the nerve and endorgan, in the basal turn of the cochlea. The cause of the atrophy is not known. Proof is lacking that ageing of itself causes any organic lesions of the inner, middle or external ear.

There is no correlation between chronic systemic diseases and the average impairment of hearing at any age or between systemic diseases and the amount of atrophy in the cochlea.

Absence of reports of an ageing decline in the functions of the vestibular apparatus may mean merely that the methods of testing are too crude to reveal small differences.

REFERENCES

ALEXANDER, G. 1913. Die Anatomie und Klinik der nichteitrigen Labyrinth-erkrankungen. Arch. f. Ohrenh., **92**, 227–249; **93**, 138–162.

ALEXANDER, G. 1924. Pathologische Anatomie der nervösen Anteile des Gehörorgans. (Chapter in) Alexander-Marburg Handbuch der Neurologie des Ohres. Berlin and Vienna: Urban & Schwarzenberg, 1, 701–818.

BEZOLD, F. 1892. Einige weitere Mittheilungen über die continuirliche Tonreihe, inbesondere über die physiologische obere und untere Tongrenze. Ztschr. f. Ohrenh., 23, 254–267.

———— 1893. Untersuchungen über das durchschnittliche Hörvermögen im Alter. Ztschr. f. Ohrenh., 24, 1–24.

BUNCH, C. C. 1929. Age variations in auditory acuity. Arch. Otolaryng., 9, 625–636.

———— 1931. Further observations on age variations in auditory acuity. Arch. Otolaryng., 13, 170–180.

BUNCH, C. C., AND RAIFORD, T. S. 1931. Race and sex variations in auditory acuity. Arch. Otolaryng., 13, 423–434.

CIOCCO, A. 1932. Observations on hearing of 1,980 individuals: a biometric study. Laryngoscope, 42, 837–856.

———— 1935. Disproportionate shortening of bone conduction: a statistical and clinical study. Acta oto-laryng., 22, 529–539.

CROWE, S. J., GUILD, S. R., AND POLVOGT, L. M. 1934. Observations on the pathology of high-tone deafness. Bull. Johns Hopkins Hosp., 54, 315–380.

CUPERUS, N. J. 1893. Ueber das presbyakusische Gesetz an der unteren Grenze unseres Gehörs. Arch. f. Ohren., 35, 299–303.

FIEANDT, H. VON, AND SAXEN, A. 1937. Pathologie und Klinik der Altersschwerhörigkeit. Acta oto-laryng., Suppl. 23, 1–102.

FURSTENBERG, A. C. 1937. Transient or variable nerve deafness from circulatory effects. Paper presented at meeting of American Otological Society, May 27, 1937. In press, Tr. Am. Otol. Soc.

GUILD, S. R. 1936. Hearing by bone conduction: the pathways of transmission of sound. Ann. Otol., Rhin. & Laryng., 45, 736–755.

HARTMANN, H. 1936. Die obere Hörgrenze bei Sauerstoffmangel. Luftf. med., 1, 192–202. (Seen only in abstract, in Zentralbl. f. Hals-, Nasen- u. Ohrenh., 1937, 27, 699.)

LEDERER, L. 1926. Die Altersveränderungen am Gehörorgan. (Section in) Denker-Kahler Handbuch der Hals-Nasen-Ohren-Heilkunde, Berlin: J. Springer and Munich: J. F. Bergmann, 6, 705–709.

MAYER, O. 1920. Das anatomische Substrat der Altersschwerhörigkeit. Arch. f. Ohren-, Nasen-u. Kehlkopfh., 105, 1–13.

———— 1930. Über die Entstehung der Spontanfrakturen der Labyrinthkapsel und ihre Bedeutung für die Otosklerose. Ztschr. f. Hals-, Nasen- u. Ohrenh., 26, 261–279.

———— 1931. Die Ursache der Knochenbildung bei der Otosklerose. Acta oto-laryng., 15, 35–73.

POLITZER, A. 1882. Lehrbuch der Ohrenheilkunde für practische Aerzte und Studirende. Stuttgart: F. Enke, 2 vols., paged consecutively, 878 pp.

RICHTER, G. 1894. Vergleichende Hörprüfungen an Individuen verschiedener Altersklassen. Arch. f. Ohrenh., 36, 150–169, 241–270.

SPORLEDER 1899. Ueber funktionelle Prüfungsresultate und über Sections-ergebnisse in höheren Alter. Arch. f. Ohrenh., **47**, 234–235.

STEURER, O. 1926. Die atrophischen, dystrophischen und degenerativen Erkrankungen des inneren Ohres. (Chapter in) Henke-Lubarsch Hand-buch der speziellen pathologischen Anatomie und Histologie. Berlin: J. Springer, Vol. 12, Gehörorgan, pp. 445–489.

STRUYCKEN, H. J. L. 1913. Tabellen über die obere Hörgrenze bei patholog-ischen Verhältnissen. Beitr. z. Anat., Physiol., Path. u. Therap. d. Ohres, **6**, 289–301.

WITTMAACK, K. 1907. Weitere Beiträge zur Kenntnis der degenerativen Neuritis und Atrophie des Hörnerven. Ztschr. f. Ohrenh., **53**, 1–36.

———— 1916. Über die pathologisch-anatomischen und pathologisch-physi-ologischen Grundlagen der nichteitrigen Erkrankungsprozesse des in-neren Ohres und des Hörnerven. Arch. f. Ohren-, Nasen-, u. Kehlkopfh., **99**, 71–136.

ZIFFER, H. 1908. Ueber die Veränderungen des Gehörorgans im vorgeschrit-tenen Alter. Monatschr. f. Ohrenh., **42**, 63–74.

ZWAARDEMAKER, H. 1891. Der Verlust an hohen Tönen mit zunehmenden Alter; ein neues Gesetz. Arch f. Ohrenh., **32**, 53–56.

———— 1893. Das presbyacusische Gesetz. Ztschr. f. Ohrenh., **24**, 280–287.

Chapter 20

PSYCHOLOGICAL ASPECTS OF AGEING

WALTER R. MILES

New Haven

Physiological age changes have been recognized throughout man's history. The physical facts of birth, growth, maturity, senescence, and death have been accepted and commented upon by science, literature and philosophy. Psychological life changes have been, until recently, often less realistically regarded and less accurately measured. Perhaps in consequence, as the pendulum swings from the mystical view of an ageless soul to a scientific study of a developing, maturing and finally declining personality, there is a tendency to over-emphasize the physical analogy. It is natural that this should be so for two reasons. The first results from the fact that the physical structure of man is more amenable to exact observation and measurement, and that the closer the psychological structure is to the physiological, the more precisely demonstrable are his functions. The second results from too enthusiastic acceptance of a mind body unity, in which the recognition that there can be no mind that is not a part, or a function of a part, of a body, has led to the unguarded assumption of a one-to-one correlation between the products as well as the functions of the mind and the body. Individual emotion in the sense of defensive, self-agrandizement of the aged on the one hand, has been added to by the emotion of a hero or ancestor worship on the part of one group of immature youth, while on the other the self-depreciative attitude of older people has been intensified through a so-called "Oslerism" or age liquidation plan sometimes cloaked as benign euthanasia on the part of another young group. Thus the total problem is complicated through the existence of partisan positions.

Psychological interest in a scientific view of the normal changes during adulthood has naturally followed an earlier study of normal development in childhood. The study of the psychological life beginning as it does with the adequate function of the central nervous system of the unborn child may now be followed by observation and measurement through infancy, childhood and adolescence to young maturity, and from the beginning of adulthood to the end of the psychological existence with the final complete cessation of function of the intricate organism that conditions it.

Studies carried on during the last decade have begun to fill in some of the unexplored regions of the mental life-age area in maturity. Outlines of high- and low-land have been sketched, valuable mental ores revealed, and the fertility in mental soil discovered in the mid-country has been found to extend onward toward the distant boundaries, in certain instances beyond the region where estimation of soil consistency would suggest this possibility. Most significant perhaps in the study of psychological ageing is the discovery of a consistent tendency in reference to the hierarchy of mental functions. Closest to the age trend of decrement of physiological processes are the psycho-physiological, the motor functions of activity and those of sensory perceptions. As function becomes more complex psychologically, and less dependent upon gross bodily organization, the decrement appears less significant until in the highest processes of interpretation and imagination unconstricted by limitation of speed and amount, measurable performance continues with relatively little decline in quality or persistence to the very end of the normal life span. Thus Emerson's dictum is vindicated that the essence of age is intellect.

Mythical heroes are reported to have been free from the disabilities of old age, but ordinary mortals have not discovered any effective antidote for the "incurable disease" associated with longevity. In mythical heavens a single generation held the stage forever, and the number of players was definitely restricted to a small, static circle of familiar characters, a projection of ego-centered, tribally limited, wishful thinking. The realistic biological process of development and replacement brings change and thereby opportunity for selective improvement, or the reverse, and permits the participation of almost limitless numbers, as series follow series. Age characteristics are essential elements of the process. Youth contributes physical vigor, enthusiasm and the spirit of adventure; by tradition it is free to follow fresh impulse unhampered. Age contributes mental experience, evaluation in historical terms, and the spirit of caution. Seasoned by effort and conscious of consequences, it is more or less wisely selective in process. A congenial mutually dependent and mutually appreciative relationship of joint responsibility in terms of actual capacity and contribution develops in balanced social communities. The young are vigorous but not impatient, the old are wise but not dogmatic.

The growth of youth to attain its full strength in maturity has been minutely studied and the physical and psychological elements of its contribution to a balanced culture have often been measured and described in scientific terms. A brief summary of the measured psychological traits of normal maturity and old age is presented in the following pages. The arrangement follows a designed pattern beginning with those traits nearest the anatomical end of the psychophysiological scale, and proceeding thence toward the affective and more psychological side of the same scale. The often sought elixir of youth is probably of little use in prolonging the life of the body, but it may symbolize an effort to meet advancing age with a subjective, compensatory, emotional set. The hardy mature can probably dispense with it under normally favorable conditions. A few strengthening draughts may prove of positive therapeutic value at certain periods when the sudden personal recognition of age change comes with sharp urgency. But the nourishment of appropriate physical and mental work seasoned with equally appropriate recreation and social and cultural activity, proves by test to be more definitely sustaining and contributory to physical and mental longevity.

1. AGE AND ACTIVITY[1]

Anatomical changes, coincident with age, have always been observable, not only from the point of view of physicians and other professionally trained students of man, but also by society in general. Middle aged and elderly people have usually accounted it an achievement of great personal significance if they could succeed in looking younger than would be expected for their actual chronological age. Certain of the anatomical signs of increasing age in adults display themselves whether or not the individual is sensitive or unconcerned about their appearance, and increasing accentuation. Time unmistakably leaves patterns of furrows and wrinkles, capillary changes, scars and discolorations on the plastic facial surface. Changes occur in the appearance of the eyeballs and in the conformation of the tissue surrounding the eye, in wear, discoloration and loss of the teeth, in the pigment of the hair and in its distribution. These alterations are familiar, but so slowly do they take place, and so much more do we attend to the less changing personality that they may long escape subjective comment and even conscious notice. Since the human face conveys more you-

---

[1] For one of the best recent bibliographies on senescence see under Age in the Surgeon-General's Catalogue, Fourth Series, Vol. 1, Washington. D. C. 1936, pages 158–162.

ness or me-ness, to use Myerson's apt phrase, than other parts of the anatomy, every individual expresses his personality through the anatomical age mask which life experience has modelled. The psychological impression of the personality persists through the changing aspects which maturity brings, and even into old age, although skin, posture, gait, voice and other expressions follow a course of alteration, intercorrelated and closely adhering to the curve of life age.

Young men as a group can be expected to show greater strength, swiftness, precision of movement and steadiness of motor control than is generally characteristic of old men, and in an earlier period there was often a tendency to think of young, middle-aged and old as forming three rather sharply differentiated groups. Recent researches in the measurement of adult activity fail to display clear-cut age-ability classifications. They reveal instead quite regular curves of change throughout the life span with the evidence of much overlapping of scores or ratings of capacity in succeeding decades (Miles, 1933). Examinations of motility made in the psychological laboratory by apparatus simple enough to be applied to all ambulatory types of people and yet sufficiently accurate in timing and other characteristics to be dependable, yield results for the major part of the life span illustrating these tendencies.[2]

Figures 97 and 98 trace curves of average performance from decade to decade for sample populations. No two of the series of curves are identical, but together they show clearly the relation between rate of speed in work and life age. Furthermore, they demonstrate no sudden alteration at any period, but rather a gradual rise of speed capacities in childhood and youth, followed by slow decline of the same functions in maturity. Simple digital extension-flexion speed shows the least alteration of either rise or decline of efficiency. In this activity, capacity reaches a maximal point relatively early and the drop in speed is comparatively small. In rotary motility (timed dexterity in a rotary motion) younger and older ages show definitely less speed than middle adulthood, the deceleration from the 5th to the 8th decade following a regular course, in which men in their 80's have come to be 50 to 60 per cent slower than the 20-year group. The curve for manual reach and grasp, exhibiting performance of a function requiring quick-

[2] Many of the data cited in the present chapter are from the Stanford Later Maturity Research, conducted in the Department of Psychology, Stanford University, under the direction of the writer and made possible by grants from the Carnegie Corporation of New York.

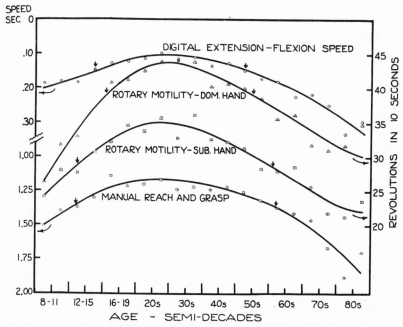

FIG. 97. Normal changes in manual motility with age (Miles, 1931)

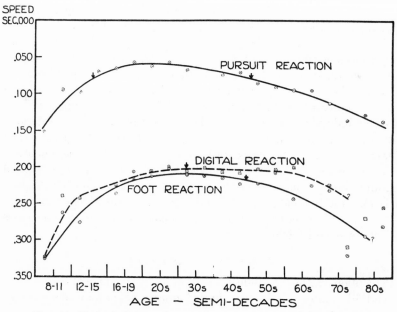

FIG. 98. Normal changes in reaction time with age (Miles, 1931)

ness and accuracy of hand and arm, shows a fairly rapid improvement in coördination ability from 8 to 18, then quite a change, first of improvement, later of decrement, until age 50, followed thereafter by somewhat more marked decline, that is regular but not precipitous. If we state the results here in terms of the correlation between speed and age for the period from 20 to 95 years, the coefficient is $-.53 \pm 0.03$, a value which expresses the considerable influence of age upon psychomotor activity. Similar coefficients are found for the other activity performance scores in this period.

Because of the importance of the age-efficiency problem in industry it is perhaps well to point out the extent of overlapping in the score distribution from age to age. The curves discussed above illustrate averages and do not show how wide is the range of success and failure in each age group. Analysis of the original score-data show in contrast to the apparent overpowering influence of years, a considerable percentage of ratings by older persons equal to or exceeding the mean performance of others two decades younger. Of the 331 men whose results are plotted here, 52 are 70 years of age or older, and of these the fastest third are able to perform at a level whose average is slightly higher than the mean range of the 60-year-old group (see short arrow on the curve) or, at the younger end of the curve, of the 14-year-old group (see arrow). Vertical arrows on the other curves make further comparison of the fastest third of the older men readily available.

The reaction time curves of Figure 2 give further evidence that psychomotor activity in various types of performance follows always a life-span course of rise and fall, and that the average change from one period to the next is not sudden but gradual. The graphs as shown here are representative age averages. They are not averages for the self-same individuals measured as they passed from decade to decade. Individual curves would, of course, vary more than these smoothed averages, and no person need feel compelled to follow the smoothed path of decrement traced here. Single life curves have yet to be worked out, and observation leads me to guess that beside a tendency to wide variation in individuals, we shall find a general trend of lessened decrement in practiced skills when these are maintained through the years with interest and fidelity.

2. PERCEPTION AND AGE

Perception, although rightly classed as psychological experience, depends like motor activity on a limited number of anatomical structures and a similarly small, or relatively small, group of physiological functions. The sensory endings must perform their part before the cortical elaboration can take place, and the psychological concomitants be realized. The situation is roughly the reverse in temporal order of that in motor activity which although dependent upon mental process in its patterning and direction, is nevertheless more obviously dependent on the physical effector mechanisms, and therefore largely subject to age changes in the form of muscular decrement or specific disability. Both motor and perceptual activity tend to include a speed element, and having within themselves this essence of promptness, ordinarily a desirable feature, neither of them can escape the speed tax levied by involutional changes on the bodily functions.

Sensation as stimulus to activity response has been commonly observed to exhibit in old age a gradual diminution of acuity. Visceral and cutaneous sensations show age changes which are almost universally noticed in some of the more special senses. Critchley (1931) referring to observations of Rolleston, points out "how often severe thoracic or abdominal disease exists in the aged without pain; an extensive pneumonia or peritonitis can be entirely unsuspected; gall stones and renal calculi may be passed without the ordinary colic." It has also been found that in many aged persons "minor surgical operations and dental extractions can be carried out with but little pain and discomfort. The catastrophe of coronary thrombosis can take place with none of the agonizing symptoms found in younger individuals."

The diminution or loss of sensation in the lower extremities with increasing age has been clinically observed many times. When the sensitivity of the muscles or joints is examined by applying to them a vibrating tuning-fork or other rapidly oscillating instrument the measurement is called "vibratory sensibility." Pearson (1928) reported the relation of age to vibratory sensibility when measured by a small 128 v.d. tuning fork agitated in a standard manner. The base of the fork was held against various boney points and the time was taken with a stop-watch until the subject said he could no longer feel the fork vibrating. The time values ranged from just above zero to about 20 seconds. If we combine the results for right and left sides obtained by Pearson for 7 examination points on the body including ulna, radius, olecranon, internal malleolus, external malleolus, tibia and patella, the total average measures are probably quite dependable. Counting the results for the second decade as 100 per cent, the succeeding later decades show respectively 87, 81, 79, 54 and finally 53 per cent for the 7th decade. The results are further substantiated by the increasing number of people showing absence of vibratory sensation in each succeeding decade after the 3rd.

It has been thought that a probable basis for this decrease in vibratory sensibility with age was a change in the posterior columns of the spinal cord. Corbin and Gardner (1937) working on this hypothesis counted the number of myelinated fibers in the 8th and 9th thoracic dorsal and ventral roots in 34 human cadavers ranging in age from 1 day to 89 years. The curves of their decade averages resemble those shown in Figures 97 and 98 of this chapter. If we take the average for the 4 nerve roots found for the 10 to 29 year group and designate this value as 100 per cent, then the myelinated nerve fiber count for the age group 40 to 59 shows 80 per cent, 60 to 79, 71 per cent, and the one case of 89 years of age, 68 per cent. These findings appear important and, I believe, represent results along a line of investigation that needs to be further pursued for the better understanding of changing sensitivity and experience in old people.

Recently the relation of the taste sense to age has been examined by Arey et al. (1935) who made an anatomical taste-bud census on 38 human cadavers of persons 20 to 70 years of age, and 13 others from individuals 74 to 85 years of age comparing their results with those of Heiderick (1906) for ages 0 to 20 years.   From birth to 20 years of age the average number of taste-buds per papillae remains surprisingly constant numbering about 245. During maturity and early old age the mean value is about 208 and it declines to an average of 88 for the age period from 74 to 85 years. Taste-buds were also counted in the trench wall surrounding the papillae with relatively similar results. "The mean number of taste-buds on the trench wall is 10 for the first post-natal year, rises to 18 in the next two years, and attains the value of 74 between the fourth and 20th years. The mean drops to 48 in maturity and early old age, and decreases to 13 (and probably less) in extreme old age." Functional taste studies in relation to age are needed for comparison with the foregoing anatomical findings.

The higher senses, particularly hearing and vision (Chapters 18 and 19), are noteworthy in showing progressive age changes similar to those just reviewed. The change in visual accommodation range has been considered one of the most reliable and at the same time one of the most easily measurable indexes of physiological age in adults. Presbyopia as a psychological phenomenon is easily observed and before the era of corrective refraction must often have created a condition of frustration experienced by many older persons in a more or less pronounced way, although the actual physiological change came on slowly. Opthalmological science has now in large part met the difficulty of blurred near vision by well fitted eye-glasses.

Although vastly helped by properly fitted glasses, old eyes cannot on the average keep up with younger ones. For concrete proof we may turn to a research conducted by Bronson Price (1931), reviewing briefly some of the findings. A group of subjects ranging in age from 6 to 89 were examined by means of a battery of six varieties of perception-test materials all parts of which were presented to view for standard exposure intervals (0.1 sec.) by means of the Weaver tachistoscope. The observer, when fully ready, could by pressing a key cause the tachistoscope window to open, exposing a printed card for a standard interval. Immediately after viewing each card the person examined made note of what had been seen, recording at leisure all the details he had gathered. Subjects wore their glasses, if they were in the habit of doing so for reading, and great care was exercised through instructions and preliminary trials that optimal adjustment to the apparatus was secured. Letters, numbers, short sentences, colors, groups of lines and common expressions faultily written made up the printed material. Each card was exposed only once and for all subjects tested the exposure time was the same; the score was the number of items correctly seen and recorded. The average results for the 684 persons studied are shown in table 27, where the entries after the age of 20, are combined as averages for age semi-decades. These results, like those for psychomotor performance, show characteristic rise and decline with age. The rise in childhood and early adolescence is rapid. A plateau extends from 7 to 29, and beyond this age is followed by a gradual, uninterrupted decline in average score. The performance ability for 39 individuals 70–74 years old equals that of 17 children 8–9 years old. These results appear particularly significant, since they show the relatively large residual age change in visual efficiency which medical science cannot overcome. They point to the peripheral and perhaps also central organic changes in perceptual speed for which spectacles are of no avail.

Experience and experiment show that perception is not as prompt in the old as in the young, and that its span is shorter. But it must also be said that industry has found that neither speed of activity nor speed of perception are adequate criteria for work and worker value. Persistence in effort and practice with materials used compensates to no small extent for speed in older workers by producing a more even work rate and product. Interest and skill are basic in such compensation and they tend in paths other than the simple automatic ones to counterbalance the decline in perceptive ability with its correlate of decrease in work rate.

TABLE 27

Influence of age on visual perception span and speed

(Group results from Price for a total of 684 males and females)

Age groups	Number of cases	Mean scores	S.D.'s
6–7	3	59.2	18.7
8–9	17	75.0	18.5
10–11	12	90.8	18.5
12–13	38	103.0	13.9
14–15	24	106.1	15.9
16–17	24	115.0	17.9
18–19	18	111.7	16.0
20–24	41	109.9	14.3
25–29	39	111.2	19.3
30–34	45	102.8	16.7
35–39	43	106.6	18.7
40–44	45	105.0	17.7
45–49	44	103.4	19.8
50–54	60	99.5	21.9
55–59	53	88.6	21.5
60–64	52	90.2	19.8
65–69	52	82.5	20.8
70–74	39	75.0	20.5
75–79	23	68.0	22.9
80–84	10	52.0	16.8
85–89	2	55.0	10.0

3. AGE AND INDIVIDUAL DIFFERENCES IN PERFORMANCE

We have seen how age and performance scores, whether measured as amount or as rate of speed in the work, correlate regularly with age in adulthood. Attention has been drawn in passing to the fact that averages conceal deviations in individual achievement. With respect to activity it was noted that individuals might vary widely in their old-age performance curves from an average course dependent on general trends in groups. With reference to perception it has been possible to refer only briefly to the important matter of quality versus quantity of output, and of contrasting characteristics in the work of old and young, care and conservation of materials for the former, speed and quick grasp for the latter.

The wide range of individual achievements at every age should be emphasized. At the same time the persistence of high and low levels of performance of certain groups throughout the mature years should also be mentioned together with its important corollary in deviation

TABLE 28

Individual differences in performance ability within different age groups of men

Measured capacities	Number of subjects and age groups			
	C (49) 18–29	D (79) 30–49	E (111) 50–69	F (54) 70–89
Visual acuteness	10.2†	19.0‡	21.6§	0.0¶
Motility:				
Rotary speed	24.5	25.3	23.6	3.7
Reach precision	14.3	20.3	31.8	1.9
Hand promptness	57.8	54.8	64.8	24.1
Foot promptness	31.1	37.0	39.2	6.9
Immediate memory	9.5	8.3	12.2	0.0
Judgment for position	28.6	16.7	42.0	35.7
"Good judgment" (Otis Speed Test of Intelligence)	6.1	26.6	19.0	11.8

* Taken from W. R. Miles, Abilities of Older Men, Person. J., 1933, 11, 352–357.

† Per cent of C who just equal or are poorer than the mean of E.

‡ Per cent of D who just equal or are poorer than the mean of E.

§ Per cent of E who just equal or are better than the average mean for C and D combined.

¶ Per cent of F who just equal or are better than the average mean for C and D combined.

from the norm of the individual work curves of certain older persons The range at every adult age of every kind of performance measure is far wider than the difference between means of the most and the least effective age periods of adult life. In consequence, the amount of overlapping in the individual scores for different age groups is worthy of profound consideration. Generalization concerning the effects of age should certainly not be based upon averages alone. Presented in a simplified form in table 28 are illustrative percentage comparisons showing the proportion of selected age groups that reach or exceed the average performance score of other younger or older groups in certain measured functions. The data conform to expectation in terms of experience and observation, in indicating that there are younger individuals whose work is poorer than the average of the older, and older individuals who exceed the younger averages in their individual performance.

In the basically physiological function of visual acuteness the failure of all persons 70–89 to equal the average of younger adults is noteworthy. Equally striking and more important psychologically is the high percentage of persons past middle life who exceed the average of the younger group in promptness of response with the most highly trained bodily servant of the mind, the hand. Comparisons are included for other than activity and sensory measures, two of them quite dependent on physiological speed, a third on the more psychological function of judgment. As in the case of visual acuteness versus hand promptness, so when speed of immediate memory is compared with judgment for proportion, the more basically physiological function of rate of response shows greater age decrement, while the more psychological function of mental experience holds off the negative age influence. Speed of intelligence, combining both elements, takes an intermediate position. In a later section will appear for comparison the lesser age decrement in scores of intelligence when the speed factor is eliminated.

It seems probable that the appearance of higher and lower scores at the different age periods signifies, for the individuals so rating, trends that will appear when measurements of them are repeated again and again at successive life stages. A few repeated test performances substantiate this impression derived from the observation of human beings as younger and older adult workers. The individual of above average performance in younger years tends to be the superior older adult; and less than average performance tends also to persist in a given individual with the years. Exceptions occur largely in terms of greater or less practice and experience, and these exceptions may be the stimulus to endeavor on the part of those who wish to develop skill with age, offsetting through wisdom based on continued intelligent exercise the necessary decrement in the function of physical receptors and affectors.

Summarizing the findings in table 28 we may say that there is no function reported in which age decrement does not appear when scores are viewed in terms of statistical averages. On the other hand, wide overlapping is a prominent feature of the results. We can hardly feel convinced that the total range of human capacities has been more than briefly sampled in the measurements so far made. And the habit of continued use as exemplified in the hand response may play no small part in the total picture. The measures available still too regularly confuse the more basically physiological with the more intrinsically psychological functions and adequate interpretation based on adequate understanding is difficult to achieve at every point.

4. INFLUENCE OF AGE ON SPEED AND ACCURACY OF LEARNING AND MEMORY

Forgetting, like remembering, may be benign or baneful, but in general the ability to recall experience is subjectively regarded as favorable, and its opposite is held to constitute a handicap of considerable consequence to the individual. When forgetting is benign as in the repression of painful experience it may pass unnoticed, but at the conscious level distortion or memory loss of "important" mental or pleasant experience images may seem almost like an inner mutany. Many if not all failures in memory seem to call either privately or socially for notice on the behavior balance sheet. "Why did I forget that?" This question may be repeated as the years accumulate and the answers show as wide a range as personality adjustment itself exhibits.

Within the last decade and a half psychologists, turning from investigations of children and college students, have begun seriously to work on the learning and memory abilities of middle-aged and older adults. The volume of studies by Thorndike and his associates on "Adult Learning" (1928) is one of the most important publications in this field. It has claimed wide attention for the generalization that "nobody under 45 should restrain himself from trying to learn anything because of a belief or fear that he is too old to be able to learn it." Further we read that "teachers of adults 25 to 45 should expect them to learn at nearly the same rate and in nearly the same manner as they would have learned the same thing at 15 or 20."

These reassuring statements are based on the learning by adults of materials in which they were interested, which they wished to learn, and which were usually associated with or developed from earlier interests. In terms of speed and accuracy of immediate recall, decline does occur with age and it must therefore be in some psychological factors other than the perception of the material and its reproduction by the muscular system that compensatory adjustment and organization takes place when achievement in learning suffers no decrement with age.

Learning speed and accuracy in two motor tasks and three verbal tasks was investigated by Ruch (1934) in one of the Stanford studies with 40 subjects in each of three groups, ages 12 to 17, 35 to 58, and 60 to 82. The first motor-learning task was performed under the guidance of direct vision while the second, which required the use of mirror vision was more complicated. The correlation coefficients of the learning scores with age for these two performances were found to be as follows:

	Adolescents (12-17)	Middle Aged (35-58)	Old (60-82)
Direct vision learning	$+.196 \pm .102$	$-.316 \pm .096$	$-.505 \pm .080$
Mirror-vision learning	$+.350 \pm .094$	$-.460 \pm .084$	$-.592 \pm .068$

Improvement with age indicated by the plus appears as usual in the adolescents, decrement is characteristic of the two adult groups, and especially of the elder. The more complicated problem put a premium on increasing maturity in adolescents, and penalized the majority of older adults. These results suggested and supported Ruch's hypothesis that decrement in speed and accuracy of learning is particularly prominent for middle-aged and older persons when the required work involves reorganizing parts or wholes of established habit-systems in new combinations. This evidence is of course in line with the tendency for habit systems to become effectively stable at the expense of adaptability.

Under the usual circumstances of life the assets of experience having been appropriately invested adequate and relatively smooth working balances are achieved for the tasks involved in the days work, whatever it may be. That a balance of this kind may hold out even to extreme old age has been shown in the lives of distinguished men who have reached advanced years, especially statesmen and philosophers. Emerson's description of John Adams at the time of his son's inauguration to the Presidency of the United States well describes and illustrates mental capacity and experience admirably organized in old age. Other less eminent but as well preserved aged survivors exemplify similar ability in relative degree. Thus it could be said of a gentleman of 106, "He had his memory and other mental faculties particularly perfect to the last, being enabled to discourse about the ordinary affairs of his business, and the common concerns of life, without any hindrance arising from want of recollection or incapacity to form a just opinion on the subject submitted to his consideration."

5. INTELLIGENCE AND AGE

Usually a striking agreement holds between intelligence scores and years of life age from the earliest testable period up to mid or late adolescence and the coefficient of correlation expected for this period is near 80. In maturity, performance in tests of intelligence in which speed is a primary factor follows a curve predictable on the basis of results described for motor, and sensory response and learning in terms of speed and accuracy. This was shown during the World War when the Army Alpha test was administered to 15,385 army officers, although at that time the homogeneity of the age groups was questioned. More recently and with a group of 547 persons between 24 and 60 years of age carefully selected for homogeneity from decade to decade the same tendency has been found for score on Army Alpha to decrease with age (Jones and Conrad, 1933). In a population of 2000 probably equally representative in successive age periods the scores on a short form of the Otis test are found to decrease gradually from age to age from early to late maturity (Miles, C. C., 1935). The decline is slight in the 20's and 30's, somewhat steeper in the 40's, 50's, and 60's, falling rather rapidly from 70 onward to 90.

The drop in intelligence-speed score from age 18 to age 85 in one population was 24 points, 62 per cent of the young adult average. In mental age months this amounts to 70 (5 years, 10 months), in Otis IQ points it is 36. "The correlation between age and score from the age of 20 to 95 years is approximately $-.50 \pm .02$ and the difference between the average scores in the 'twenties' and in the 'eighties'—is 9.9 S.D. diff" (Miles and Miles, 1932). When the ratings of the same adults were compared, as scored before and after a two-year interval (Miles, C. C., 1934), it was found that the decrements associated with increasing age were actually larger than those predicted from the average curve where the scores of different people made up the values at successive points. This latter finding not only strengthens the significance of the earlier results, but perhaps also suggests that survival may be actually associated with more adequate mental as well as more enduring physical equipment.

Speed of response is, as observed above, dependent to no small extent on the physiological equipment available for psychological perception and response. Hence it is with interest, but without surprise that we learn that when the speed factor is eliminated the coefficient of age-score correlation for intelligence during the span of adult maturity drops from an average of .4 or .5 in various more or less homogeneous groups to .3 or less for a single somewhat heterogeneous population. It is difficult to isolate physiological factors other than speed from test performance, and to date no results are available in which decline in general intelligence test scores does not appear. This should not surprise us in view of the fact that older people have observedly a slower psychology in adjusting their mental-physical work to a tempo appropriate to the organization of wider and especially of unfamiliar experience. This being the case, they are at a disadvantage in test performance in which they have generally had less practice than young people; and probably also their attitudes and motivations are less comfortably regimented for what seems to them, more than it does apparently to younger people, an artificial method for rating essential capacity.

Expression of age decrement in terms of the correlation between age and intelligence score does not sufficiently emphasize the overlap in performance of older and younger groups. In figure 99 the extent of similarity between the abilities of younger and older is presented in graphic form. Here two superimposed figures show the percentage-distribution of test scores on hard intelligence items solved without time restriction by 130 individuals in the age range 50 to 64 and 700 in the range from 20 to 34 years. The base line indicates the IQ range equivalents while the ordinates represent the percentage of each group at the various positions on the IQ scale. It is obvious that the average performance of the younger is superior to that of the older group, but equally noteworthy is the relatively large percentage of the older people who are able to score in each of the higher brackets. In the upper IQ range, 130–144, the older group shows 4.6 per cent of its total number in comparison with 3.3 per cent of the younger people, a positive difference attributable to biological-survival selection or to chance heterogeneity in the groups compared, perhaps to both.

In terms of economic contribution and social leadership the presence of even a small increment at the upper end of the distribution may balance the higher percentage values of the older group in the lower IQ categories. But aside from this consideration we are impressed in viewing this comparison of test ability in younger and older that we are here viewing the indices of mental production of human populations that are only moderately different from each other in total intellectual ability when measured in as fair a manner as we can at present apply, and it is clear that on the basis of his chronological age alone it is scarcely possible to predict an individual's intelligence score to a degree much better than chance. The persistence from decade to decade of score differences in terms of occupation or education points to a contrast among individuals, and in groups, of greater importance industrially and socially than the demonstrated age differences. Formulations regarding his life goals and evaluations of the extent to which an

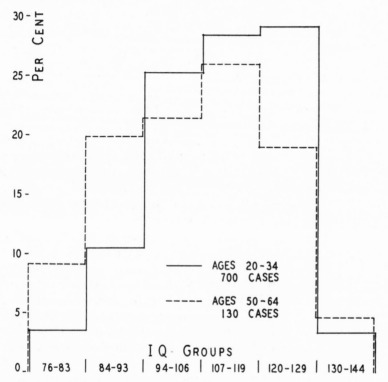

FIG. 99. Percentage distribution of intelligence test scores for younger and older adults.

individual has organized his energy for reaching these objectives would probably serve us at present as better bases for intelligence test score prediction and intellectual classification than the more definitely measurable datum of age.

In another study it has been found that intellectual persistence, a non-speed factor in test performance, does not show age decrement in a group of 400 subjects aged 20 to 95. Speed test performance tends as we have seen to correlate negatively with age. The coefficients fall generally between −.3 and −.5, depending on the age range and the type of test. Power test scores of intelligence yield coefficients of correlation with age that are considerably smaller (−.1 to −.3). If the correlation is computed between age and power test scores, with the element common to the latter and the speed test factored out, the correlation is not negative but positive and possibly statistically significant (+.14 ±.05). In these results we seem to see the well known trend of physiological decline in terms of speed and bodily energy offset by a psychological gain in intellectual practice and persistence.

In the power intelligence test itself items of different types show different degrees of age decrement in score. Thus for the Otis 75 item intelligence test administered without limit as to time the correlations between age and partial scores for 400 adults follow a rising scale of values from the mathematical, depending on solutions of more or less difficult problems little related to ordinary experience, to the verbal elements, even the most difficult of which are relatively familiar. The values of the coefficients are as follows: number relations, −.26; arithmetical problems, −.24; proverbs, −.16; analogies, −.10; logical selection, −.09; vocabulary, −.04; synonym-antonym, +.01. The language functions best withstand physiological decrepitude, and perhaps this is well for it is doubtless through them that the factors of experience and the accumulations of culture may best be preserved and handed on.

Galton's early study of the ability to make spatial estimates should be mentioned here. His results computed by Ruger and Stoessiger in terms of the degree of error of judgment of some 3800 individuals in three different untimed judgment tests resulted in correlations with coefficients on the positive side, but all of them close to zero (+.058 ±.011; +.071 ±.011; +.033 ±.011).

In the test results for performance not necessitating quickness in reaction but depending essentially on comprehension, reasoning and judgment, in matters where experience may contribute to the goodness of response, older adults appear most nearly to maintain their characteristic mature scoring level as long as they continue to maintain mental practice and intellectual interest. Performance in these tasks thus seems to register in addition to native capacity certain other psychological values: the preserving effectiveness of practice and the actual increment of knowledge accumulated through the years under favorable conditions of persistent exercise. Perhaps to no small extent is scorable achievement in tasks of this kind maintained on a basis of earlier repetitive exercise even when adaptive performance in unfamiliar tasks has suffered decrement. Work of a skilled or familiar character is thus less diminished in effectiveness by motor and sensory decrepitude.

Many more complex and more specialized tests are needed to reveal the breadth and the limits of the mental powers of age in terms of familiarity and skill and of the possible degree of accumulated and organized knowledge that may tend to hold performance near peak level in the fields of human profession and occupation that are open to more and to less able adults. In individuals of active mind, wide and varied interests, and persistent endeavor, well-formed and practiced mental habits plus the knowledge increment may tend to compensate in later age for the quickness in comprehension and action that typify early maturity. In attempting the measurement of the mental activities and performances that are least subject to old age decrement and in seeking to define the extent of mental increment through experience, we approach the psychological limit of the psycho-physiological scale of human capacity and achievement.

6. AGE AND INTERESTS

Just as the individual tends to have a habitat so also he identifies himself with various classes and types of materials and with certain varieties of behavior and groups of ideas. He is not equally attracted to all, nor is he generally entirely negative toward any kinds of interests and relationships that attract other human beings. Definite polarization appears early and around it the pattern of individuality evolves. To predict this pattern in detail would be impossible, but weighted probabilities are recognized as distinguishable. Sex, family, education and environment all contend powerfully and successfully not only for space concessions but also with respect to exhibit materials. Occupation, theoretically the major-domo of the household of interests and attitudes, may hold its position throughout life without leave of absence or change in management but age the silent partner exerts its influence, slowly, persistently modifying the general pattern and scheme of the individual economy.

Psychologists and educators largely under the influence and leadership of Hall, became so occupied with the interests and attitudes of children that those of adults were for a long time scientifically ignored. Then came vocational guidance, adult education and personality psychology, with explicit interest in problems of maturity. In his later years even Hall himself (1923) contributed to the new field of research. The most comprehensive study of change of interests with age is that of Strong (1931) made in connection with the Stanford Later Maturity Research. From his large material on interests and occupations accumulated during a period of years Strong analyzed 2340 records of men from 20 to 60 years of age. Each record consisted of responses to 420 items, mainly in terms of likes and dislikes of familiar subjects, personalities and work situations. The individuals whose records were appraised were drawn from eight occupations: engineering, law, insurance, the ministry, medicine, education, writing, and Y. M. C. A. work. The records were classified into four decade divisions in terms of the ages of the individuals, resulting in respective populations of 604, 759, 581, and 396.

Strong's results indicate that as age increases interests definitely change. Thus interest in physical activities, exploring, aviation, auto-driving, become less with age, while interest in home, art galleries, detective stories, or contributing to charities, increases. Interest cannot on the basis of this study be said to narrow with age as there is not significant difference in the number of items or item groups liked or disliked in the four successive periods. Nor does interest shift uniformly; for apparently about 50 per cent of the total change takes place between 25 and 35, perhaps 20 per cent between 35 and 45, and the remaining 30 per cent between 45 and 55, and there is little or no change from 55 to 65. Of course it is not possible to determine from these data to what extent interests characteristic of a certain age group were always typical of that particular group whatever its age; i.e., whether the changes are largely cultural and not really true age changes. The internal evidence in terms of the very nature of the changes is probably the best evidence that culture in this sense is not chiefly responsible for the results obtained.

Aside from a decline of interest in physical skills of a daring or semi-dangerous nature, a conspicuous age shift is registered with respect to items which suggest interference with established habits. Other changes are as follows: the desire for occupational variety decreases; linguistic interest as such declines, but interest in reading increases with age; liking for amusements declines in general except where a distinctly cultural element is involved. "Older men also prefer, more than younger men do, those amusements pursued largely alone in contrast to ones involving others. There is no question that older men are less interested in people associated with them whether in business or amusement." Strong comments here that each age group necessarily grows up in its own special social environment and this tends toward an age segregation. Whether the eight occupational groups are viewed in combination or separately, the same age tendencies appear. And yet the typical occupational trends persist and continue to be differentiable all along the line. Strong declares, "The differences between these groups (average inter-correlation .009) far outweigh the differences between age groups or the changes common to all eight occupations." A useful interest maturity scale has been a material result of this large analytical study by Strong.

One cannot leave the topic of attitudes and interests without referring again to Hall (1923) who generalized characteristically from his questionnaire material. Two opposing tendencies he concluded are present, one which leads toward a narrowing of interests to those which are local and quite personal to the ageing one, and another, a broadening view not only inclusive of local affairs but reaching to the state, the nation and world. Hall holds this latter breadth of view to be more typical in recent times, conditioned somewhat by the World War and by the political enfranchisement of women. He notes further a broad interest of the old which he calls an educational instinct to tell the word how to be and to do better. This interest in the betterment of mankind he concludes, springs as pure and unselfish as any which social man develops, even though it contains a large element of self-identification with what seem, to the active young, the more conservative attitudes and ideals of the past.

7. DRIVE AND MOTIVATION IN RELATION TO AGE

The folk-saying that human desire waxes and wanes from early to late maturity and in extreme old age fades away, cannot yet be substantiated in terms of an accurately plotted curve. Measurement of the sum of all activity in all the varied occupations and pursuits in which human beings engage would no doubt give a good single index of human drive and motivation for accomplishment. But no exact record of his kind is available, and so appraisals must be made indirectly on the basis of broad statistics and descriptive evaluations. The sum of occupational activity or intent may be guessed at in age terms from the well-arranged tables of the 1930 U. S. census. The figures appear in our table 29 showing for each population-age-group the per cent of U. S. males classified as gainfully occupied, and also the per cent that each age group is of the total number of employed males over 10 years of age.[3] The persistence of work-desire, work habit or work need is shown in the persistence of the indices of 95 or over to the middle 50's in 93 as the index for the late 50's, and succeeding semi-decade per cents as follows: in the 60's, 87 and 76, in the early 70's, 57, and for the period beyond 74 years, 32 per cent. The constancy of the values from the middle 20's to the middle 50's may, I think, be taken as an

TABLE 29

Prolongation of human motivation as indicated by the percentages of adult males who are gainfully occupied in different age groups*

Age groups	Gainfully occupied	Worker distribution
years	per cent	per cent
25–29	97.0	12.4
30–34	97.6	11.7
35–39	97.7	12.0
40–44	97.6	10.6
45–49	97.2	9.4
50–54	95.7	7.9
55–59	93.0	5.9
60–64	86.8	4.4
65–69	75.7	2.8
70–74	57.5	1.5
75 and over	32.3	0.8

* Reproduced from Fifteenth Census of United States, 1930, Population, Vol. 5, Washington, 1933, p. 115.

In Government publications the comparable data from the United States Census of 1920 have been given in terms of three age range groups instead of the eleven used here. The three are 25 to 44 years, 45 to 64 years and 65 years and over, and their respective percentages for gainfully employed males are 97.2, 93.8, and 60.1. In the 1910 Census only two groups are used to cover this life period: 21 to 44 years, and 45 years and over. Persons ten years old and over who usually work at a gainful occupation even though temporarily unemployed at the time of the census are counted as "gainful workers."

indication of the relatively stable level of motivation, whether socially or psychologically conditioned, that continues through the three decades of more vigorous maturity. For the older ages the percentages are progressively smaller, but it is a testimony to the enduring strength of

[3] In the 1930 Census persons ten years old and over who *usually work at a gainful occupation* even though temporarily unemployed when the census data were gathered were counted as "gainful workers".

human drive, or human habit, that three-fourths of the men in the age period from 65 to 69, more than half of the 70 to 74-year-olds, and a third of the men 75 years old or older were recorded as gainful workers at the time this roll-call was taken. And this is not a special characteristic of the 1930 census, for other years show the same trends and similar figures.

The relation between age and the strength of drive can only be estimated descriptively. Psychologists and psychiatrists assess individual drive from a careful clinical study of the individual and review of his life history, with analysis of the occupational and other activities viewed in terms of organization and goals. Students of personality speak of drive as ranging in intensity from "very strong and persistent" to "very weak and intermittent." Motivation is rated at one extreme as "near zero," while of the individual whose behavior reveals an excess of drive it may be said that he is "too highly motivated for his own best good." Either extreme of the scale includes many who are doubtless psychopathic. Most people agree that the number of those who actually work themselves to death is probably small in proportion to the fairly large group of persons with little ambition. Health and constitution are involved here in a typical individual or familial way rather than in age terms and it seems probable that some index of drive may be ultimately worked out that will, like the measures of intelligence, remain fairly constant in relative position within the age group from decade to decade.

Society generally expects that young adults will be vigorously activated by strong internal pressures without having as well-defined or stable goals as older people and that the labor turnover will therefore be large in the younger years. Middle-aged adults are expected to have chosen their objectives and to be able to use their drives with economic advantage and effectiveness in achievement even if the gross activity measured in purely physical terms begins, for them, to decline. Adults between middle life and old age are not infrequently characterized as "letting up in pressure," a condition which may point to some realization of discomfiture from physiological age decrement or may simply involve a better organization of time and energy in terms of experience. Most probably we have here a change of emphasis in terms of the relative scale of motivation urgencies. Many people in later maturity have reached some of the specific goals toward which they organized and drove their earlier life activities. In these cases when life and vitality are prolonged, the objectives already reached are gradually replaced by others. In less vigorous old folk incentive may simply wane or striving be followed by appropriate satisfaction in accomplishment.

Accident proneness gives a negative measure of the intelligent caution and foresight, which are attributes of the wisely, if not of the too strongly motivated. Marbe's age-accident data indicate in which age classes proneness to accident is most and in which it is least to be expected. He quotes the following age-accident-incidence statistics from the records of a military accident insurance company.

Cases	Ages	Incidence
998	16–21	1.94
990	22–26	1.68
1,012	27–58	1.28

The results are not he says due to older men having less hazardous tasks but rather to a certain characteristic foolhardiness and failure to recognize danger on the part of the younger groups.

The sex drive is known to wax and wane in intensity with the years, and within each age group its strength varies widely in individual terms. Custom based upon a probable psycho-physiological foundation has established the rule of approximately equal ages for man and wife and wide deviation from this convention usually constitutes a challenge to both cultural and psycho-biological laws. Terman and Butten-wieser's studies of married compatibility indicate that socio-sexual adjustment has many individual factors beside this one of age-similarity. Hamilton's review in chapter 17 includes further discussion of the age-sex topic.

Motivation and drive, whether expressed in occupation or in impulse, probably tend to follow in constitution-endowment terms as certain an age course as do other psycho-physiological functions of man. In normal individuals there is generally a fair balance between desire and capacity for both work and play, and in terms of this balance society has built up a convention of expectation and a standard for approval and disapproval. Appropriate expenditure of effort with appropriate recreational accompaniment is the general rule for the old as it is for the young. Social censure is felt and usually expressed for excess as for lack in the expression of motivation in mental and physical effort. If in youth, drive, motivational direction, and work output are not balanced by recreational activity, a word of warning seems in order, for all work and no play has the reputation of producing personality dullness. If in middle life, the drive-motivation deviation is markedly on the negative side, social censure in one form or another is likely to be expressed unless invalidism is proved. In late age, great activity is not expected and if in this period a man works with effectiveness and distinction in a field of vital concern, society points him out with distinct pride, and the sense of his achievement becomes a matter of general group satisfaction. From these patterned attitudes it is clear that our culture has assumed a normative relationship between motivation-drive and age, and that in the frame of these relationships it has set up recognized taboos as well as special privileges. Psychologists favor a wide margin in attitude toward the age-motivation relationship for they are impressed with the great range of individual differences at every life stage.

8. AGE AND CERTAIN PERSONALITY TRAITS OF ADULTS

The contrast between younger and older adults with respect to personality traits has always been a favored subject of discussion and debate. With youth we associate enthusiasm, self-confidence, frankness, and sometimes officiousness; with age, caution, frugality, sentimentality, and persistence. Actually every thoughtful person knows that any generalized traits such as these cannot be strictly applicable as universal age attributes. When we come to deal with personality we find the same tendency, as with other psychological characteristics, for a wide overlap between different age groups.

In the Stanford Maturity study a group of some 300 men and women have been studied with respect to the traits measured by the well-known Bernreuter Personality Inventory. Adequately validated in terms of their appropriate measurement of individuals known to exhibit the traits measured, the scales of this inventory have proved useful to clinical psychologists in studying traits of individuals called by the general designations of neurotic, self-sufficient, introvert and dominant. In group studies of younger adults their use has revealed interesting psycho-cultural behavior tendencies. In the maturity study also, interesting results, both negative and positive, and both in need of validation from much larger groups, have been secured from the responses of 154 men and 174 women drawn from a representative mixed city population.

The findings show first of all a negative age result expressed in terms of a surprising degree of constancy in response of younger and older. For the subjects studied, who sample the grade-school, high school, college and professionally trained populations, the age-trait correlations are small, showing little dependence on age of the behavior tendencies measured. The score for the neurotic trend, an indicator of ambivalence, instability, and insecurity in general attitude, self-estimated, shows only one significant, positive correlation out of eight obtained. The situation is similar for "self-sufficiency," the self-estimate of independence in social pursuits and intellectual activities, and for the trait of "introversion" which is designed to tap the tendency to introspective function and preoccupation in the individual mental life. "Dominance," the index, again self-estimated, of tendencies to determine and direct activities and persons rather than to be directed by or submissive to them, like the other three traits shows no significant correlation with age for the women, but a slight and statistically significant negative correlation for the men of this particular population, especially exemplified in the men of better than average education. For the 154 men studied the coefficient of correlation between age and "dominance" is $-.174\pm.048$.

It may be recalled that the heaviest dominance items in the 125 that make up the Bernreuter questionnaire are those that emphasize extrovert, aggressive, vigorous activities: soliciting funds for a cause, organizing clubs or groups, taking the responsibility for introducing people and enlivening their associations. The negative traits emphasize shyness, diffidence, self-distrust, the sense of inferiority and lack of self-confidence. Negative correlation with age in adult men of a single trait constellation of the Bernreuter series, emphasizes especially the need for further investigation with larger groups. Is the tendency suggested a characteristic of the particular population studied and not a trend differentiating older and younger? Is it largely a social adjustment phenomenon, or do we see here a complex of behavior expressions rooted in physiological conditions? Perhaps if the tendency proves to be typical, a psychological explanation, combining the social and the physiological, is the correct one.

Data from the information questionnaire responses of two men in their 70's, both college educated and both having approximately equal intelligence scores, illustrate a contrast between persons of this age group whose "dominance" ratings show a large contrast. Both men are members of a group studied intensively with reference to abilities and traits.

A man of age 70, married, has four children, and three grandchildren. His health is equal to that of his father at the same age. His health and energy are better than his brothers' and sisters'. His build is average, members of his family stock have average life expectation. His health is frail, his energy average; he has a cardiac weakness. Both health and energy seem to him poorer than five years ago; he has no occupation, he was formerly a clergyman. If he were to choose again he would wish to follow the same profession. His responsibilities are now less; he lives on a pension. He says he has no interests, no objectives and no skills. His abilities to do and to manage are much less than five years ago. Eyesight, ability to read and hearing are about the same as five years ago; but ability to walk and memory for recent events are poorer. In his own estimation, he is happier now than five years ago. This man's "dominance" rating is 8 per cent, a very low score on a scale in which 50 per cent is the general average.

Another man in the 70's who reports equal or similar education is also married, has five children and five grandchildren all in good health. He has better health and energy than his father at the same age, or than his brothers and sisters. He is average in build. The family life span is average. His occupation now is as secretary of a club. Formerly he was a salesman. If he could choose again he would be a physician. His objectives are to eat, sleep and be merry. He has fewer responsibilities than he had five years ago. His eyesight, steadiness of hands, and ability to read are the same. His ability to work and to administer affairs, and his memory for recent events, are in his estimation a little poorer than they were five years ago. His general happiness is greater than it was. This man's dominance rating of 61 per cent is relatively high for his age.

Certain items in these two sketches would reveal the approximate age of the men even if it were not definitely stated. But the contrast in personality type could be found in almost any group at any age, and neither personality can be said to typify the 70's. Both men have superior higher school education, above average intelligence, admirable persistence in mental work, as shown in a test performance. Yet they differ markedly in the responses that make up the dominance rating and obviously also in other respects that are no doubt basic to these responses: physical vigor and life interest. One is full of energy and fond of what life has to offer; the other is frail and his state of mind is revealed when he says that he has no occupation, no interests, no objectives. One still has wishes for what his life might have been in even more effective terms; the other is content with the past as it was. The psychological factor of retirement may be involved here, but the essential contrast seems to be a matter of the pattern of life expression and this in turn to depend on a physiological factor of life energy. The demand and the challenge of work still to be done and the sense of interest and physical energy to do it may serve to prolong psychological effectiveness.

9. AGE AND DISTINGUISHED ACHIEVEMENT

In recent times attention has been drawn by many, but by none more picturesquely than by Osler, to the undesirability of the dominance of older men in the world of action and ideas, a dominance which he believed might often tend to delay human progress. "The sum of human achievement in action," in science, in art, in literature was, said he, almost entirely the work of men under 40. In emphasizing the desirability of encouraging younger men to "show what is in them" Osler saw a definite place for those of greater years as helpful sympathetic critics to "determine whether the thoughts which the young men are bringing to the light are false idols or true and noble births." This statement of the limitedly useful rôle of men over 40 with the added formula of the "uselessness of men above 60" has played its stimulating part in arousing both younger and older to discussion and defense.

Younger men have, fortunately, perhaps in part as a result of the attitude of which Osler's words were one expression, now more nearly come into their own. On the other hand, and of no doubt equal psychological importance, recognition has become more general of the valuable part that can be played by men and women over 40, and in many instances by those over 60 and 70. The old can carry a necessary burden of administration, conservation and completion, which if left to younger people would essentially hamper their independence and freedom for the development of new work and new ideas. And who shall say which function is the more valuable or the more essential? If society is to preserve its culture as a basis for further evolution, the maintenance and servicing functions, generally the part of older people, are probably as necessary as the new building and devising of the young. Planning can no doubt be most effective when the needs and insights of all groups are thoughtfully considered. In youth and young manhood skills are developed and objectives defined; in middle life comes the peak of original, active achievement, in the later years, the verifying of hypotheses, the continued testing of the new materials and formulations, and the teaching activity that preserves the accumulated values. "When enthusiasm and experience are most evenly balanced" said

Beard, productivity is maximal. But life is not simply a matter of major productivity, and society must provide for the periods of preparation and of after-care as well as for the moment of production of the great work. Nor is the peak age for great achievement identical in all fields, or as restricted to a single age group as Osler and some others have suggested. Intellectual productivity of the higher orders follows the same psycho-physiological pattern that underlies all human action.

When production depends largely on physiological activity, the "great work" like lesser achievements in these same fields comes earlier; when it depends on psychological factors to a relatively greater extent, the unique system or formulation tends like other products of mature experience and generalized judgment to appear later. Dorland's data based on the masterpieces of some 400 eminent persons are illuminating in this respect. The average age for the master work of his chemists and physicists is 41; inventors, poets, dramatists and playwrights, 44; novelists, 46; explorers and warriors, 47; actors and musical composers, 48; artists and divines, 50; reformers and essayists, 51; physicians and surgeons and statesman, 52; philosophers, 54; astronomers and mathematicians, satirists and humorists, 56; historians, 57; jurists and naturalists, 58.

These group averages, arranged simply to illustrate high intellectual productivity in relation to age illustrate equally well the psycho-physiological age trend present in all human activity. The peak of physiological maturity is reached earlier, the psychological maximum at a somewhat later age. And thus among the greatest and most original thinkers this tendency appears as well exemplified as among average folk. With them also when achievement depends primarily on original, active, doing and thinking it can and probably must come relatively earlier, when grasp and interweaving of vast accumulations of knowledge and experience are involved it comes later.

Evidence that great achievement is not limited nor its appearance predictable in terms of specific life age accumulates from various sources. Fulton, in bringing together some eighty-seven most important works in the history of physiology finds the age of authorship of 76 dated productions among these to have been the work of men under age 40 to the extent of 45 per cent, of men over 40, 55 per cent. Lehman analyzing lists of "best books" compiled by bibliographers and librarians on the basis of popular appreciation and of the critical judgment of specialists, found the age range from 35 to 45 statistically most favorable for creative writing. But production was by no means lim-

ited to this period.   Approaching the matter from a somewhat different
point of view, the same investigator ascertained the ages of production
of 100 chemists each credited with but a single contribution in his field.
These results show 41 per cent of the productions before the age of 40,
34 past 40 years of age, 19 past 50, 5 beyond 55 and one at the age of 69.

Life curves plotted in terms of achievements show the tendencies for
age correlation in terms of active performance in earlier maturity followed generally by a slight gradual diminution in later years.   They
show the appearance of experiential products at later ages than the more
actively conditioned types of work.   And finally at every age they display individual deviations from the means in terms of curves that
deviate irregularly or, more often, regularly but persistently above or
below the general averages.   Among the deviates on the plus side have
been men like Henry Dandolo, elevated to be Doge of Venice when he
was past 70, and continuing his leadership beyond the age of 80, at this
late age commanding the Venetian fleet which stormed and captured
Constantinople.   An unsuccessful candidate for the imperial throne of
the new Latin Empire which he had largely brought into being, he,
rather than the younger emperor, was called upon and again led his
troops successfully in support of the empire before his death at the age
of 85.   Leadership like this involving mental capacity for administration and physical energy for the management of men is rarely the
function of the aged.   Men like Dandolo show that age alone exercises
no absolute veto; that unusual achievement and high distinction are
essentially individual and not age characteristics.

10.   SUBJECTIVITY OF TIME AND MENTAL LONGEVITY

The past, the present, and the future are all well represented in our
individual subjective lives.   As a rule we are clearly aware of what
happened a day or an hour ago, and recognize the intervening time
distance in comparison to more immediate or present happenings.   We
can also easily distinguish these occurrences from what we plan or anticipate for the next hour, or the day as it appears ahead of us.   When
we want to do so, we can lay out much of our experience in series of time
plots, organized chronologically in regular year or decade cycles.   Space-
plotting of experience may be carried out with even greater accuracy,
since we are more likely to remember *where* things happened than we
are to recall *when* they occurred.   But even though we can perform this
time- and space-sorting within our individual experiences, the distribution seems somehow artificial, and we have the feeling that the rich-

ness and the value of the experiences are not basically dependent on the time and space elements, but rather that the experience as a personal possession, or perhaps as a personality projection, transcends time and position, making these appear to be no more than incidental features.

In a normal state of mental health and adjustment man can scarcely do other than think of himself as superior in value and in importance to physical objects, and particularly to those pieces of domestic or industrial equipment, the inanimate paraphernalia which are scattered about him in his environment. Only rarely when under great emotional stress or in a definitely psychotic state does a human being think or speak of himself as less than the dust. Yet many of the material objects normally viewed by man as inferior to himself have a long history, and a definite prospect of enduring throughout the ages. How natural then that, feeling superior to these things, man should allow his sense of basic importance and his confidence in the continuity of his own personality to irradiate, with the result that he develops the compelling illusion of himself being as long-to-continue as anything he sees or touches, and indeed endowed with a quality more permanent than matter. Because the tremendous self-experience is uniquely self-limited it is easier to think of other people than of one's self as mortal, and one can therefore more readily note in them than in one's self the changes that come with increasing age. The individual mind of man has a feeling of personal superiority with respect to his own place in the universe, and, regarding time as his slave to be commanded rather than obeyed, is generally able to feel free from the hampering sense of temporal and spatial limits. This psychological declaration of independence from time is no doubt protective and, for most of our life activities, a useful type of adjustment. It is a psychological weapon for wresting a charter to life.

Man's persistent need for a philosophical formula is no more urgent than are the more homely and practical demands of his immediate psycho-physiological existence. A great part of the satisfaction of maturing and ageing depends on learning and practicing the art of mental strategy by which we placate time and marshal our ultimately scattering and weakening, but, we may hope, to the last still dependable, veteran forces within the safest psychological strongholds. Thoughtful personal experience can teach one to find comfortable and even more or less impregnable positions where as the years go on the joy of living may be experienced. Through the busy years of early and middle maturity little conscious thought may be given to the problem of psycho-physical self-preservation which is actually engaging the efforts of the organized personality. Living and working successfully require a planfulness which takes intelligent account of age change, but in the middle years effective organization in these terms may occur almost unnoticed. There are those who like to define that which they believe has most contributed to success in meeting the later years. Of the many formulas proposed for longevity that of the centenarian, Fontenelle, Dean of the French Academy, probably expressed psychological attitude as much as physical fact in attributing his own long life to the simple and pleasant prescription of a good course of strawberry eating every season. Eugen Kahn has wisely observed, "Joy in living owes its existence and its continuance first of all to attitudes and conditions which have their origins in the personality itself. It is obvious that there is no joy in living as such; that is, no joy in living outside of some connection with a personality both in the narrower and in the wider sense of this term." For purposes of a practical psychology we are all faced with the common and important task of adjusting ourselves, our goals and our views to the normal psychological changes which occur during adulthood, so that as experiencing personalities we may assure ourselves of the continuance of abundant joy in living. The physiological life curve begins to turn slowly downward soon after it has reached its maximum. But experience, a psychological aspect of life endowment through which growth continues in maturity, may be widened and deepened through intelligent effort and planful organization. And so I think we may say on the basis of factual observation, and without being charged with wishful thinking, that through appropriate training and practice and the effort to prolong mobility and plasticity in the earlier years, effective mental control may be achieved, knowledge accumulated, and wisdom increased thus extending mental longevity.

11. SUMMARY

From generation to generation young and old have regarded ageing from their characteristically diverse points of view. Against the purely physiological measuring standards, active enthusiastic youth has tended to check off middle or late age at or near the zero end in what has seemed to the remote and inexperienced surveyor a condition approaching inertia and impotence. In terms of an index of wisdom and influence, more admiring or more envious human engineers, even though young, have occasionally extolled, probably to an exaggerated degree, the high attainments of aged experience. And age has in its turn viewed on the one hand the deficiencies, and on the other, the intrinsic positive capacities of youth, now with superior disregard, again with tolerant benevolence, or even with appreciative encouragement, according as the choice of reference points and axes was made in the experiential, the informational, or the alert, adaptive planes.

Medical and biological sciences, and especially their more materialistic generalizers, have from one side of the field of human observation recognized the grim fact of recession in maturity: after the vigorous positive growth in youth comes, in the course of time, a gradual negative process of physically conditioned mental decay. They may quote Shakespeare's lines: "And so from hour to hour we ripe and ripe, And then from hour to hour we rot and rot, And thereby hangs a tale." But it should be remembered that Shakespeare put these words in the mouth of a fool.

Far on another side of the wide field of human thought, philosophy, and especially religious philosophy, has voiced its affirmation of the positive aspects of age in the challenging invitation of Browning's sage: "Grow old along with me; The best is yet to be, The last for which the first was made." Is this mere euphoria and wishful thinking? It seems in our time to fall to the lot of the psychologist among others to make the attempt to combine the accumulation of the insights of the ages with the results of modern scientific experimental observation and so to arrive at a more balanced interpretation. It is the present endeavor to find a way through the misleading camouflage of pessimism or of excessive enthusiasm to the underlying facts of human behavior and experience. Three propositions seem to embody the principal results of this endeavor.

First of all briefly stated, perhaps too briefly, the psychological factors of ageing include and depend upon a completely demonstrated physiological regression. "We must all be born again atom by atom from hour to hour, or perish all at once beyond repair," said Holmes, but in this process of renewal that which dies bulks always as just more than its replacement. Anatomical and physical changes show from younger to older adulthood a moderate but continuous loss on the balance sheet of the somatic destruction-repair ledger. Bodily strength, swiftness, and exactness of gross motion tend to fail as the years pass. In every act, simple or complex, in which these factors are involved, function necessarily becomes less successful with advancing age. In spite of favorable conditions of health, food, interests or experience, age de-

crement ultimately becomes inescapable in achievement and performance of every human kind. When other factors are equal, the loss is
probably proportional to the extent to which a given activity involves
the physical mechanisms and the functions of the various bodily systems expressing strength, speed and precision.

To the demonstrated proposition of decline with age of physical
power and activity an important corollary may be appropriately ap-
pended. In certain functions decrement is not wholly undesirable.
Thus decrease in sensitivity to pain in late adult life is without doubt a
definite asset. Perhaps of social as well as personal adaptive value is
the waning of the sex drive as the pressure of economic responsibility
conflicts with the procreative urge. And of social merit is probably
the decrement in individual ambition for personal achievement which
permits or even encourages a rise in effectiveness of the next generation.
Emerson summarizes the affective assets of age: "At fifty years, 't is
said, afflicted citizens lose their sick-headaches." And further: " 't is
certain that graver headaches and heartaches are lulled once for all, as
we come up with certain goals of time. The passions have answered
their purpose: that slight but dread overweight, with which, in each
instance, Nature secures the execution of her aim, drops off. To keep
man in the planet, she impresses the terror of death. To perfect the
commissariat, she implants in each a certain rapacity to get the supply,
and a little oversupply, of his wants. To insure the existence of the
race, she reinforces the sexual instinct, at the risk of disorder, grief, and
pain. To secure strength, she plants cruel hunger and thirst, which
so easily overdo their office, and invite disease. But these temporary
stays and shifts for the protection of the young animal are shed as fast
as they can be replaced by nobler resources." The effectiveness and
comfort of later maturity are probably definitely augmented by the
shedding process which in its turn is definitely a by-product of physiological regression.

To our first proposition, that physiological decrement is the demonstrated basis of an essentially biological interpretation of psychological
ageing, the second equally important proposition may immediately
be added. This one depends upon the acceptance of a series of facts
long intuitively perceived and now experimentally demonstrated which
show that the range, at every age, of individual differences in capacity
and achievement is many times larger than the year-to-year age decrement. The overlapping of one age range with the next is very great,
and only the averages of measurements on very large groups of individ-

uals give significantly diverse measures from year to year, or even from decade to decade. In individual cases it may therefore occur that the essential characteristics of youth in strength, speed and precision are found to be relatively preserved even in great age; and also that the relative lack of these same qualities appears even in youth. Relative position on the human rating scales within each achievement and performance range tends to be maintained under conditions of health from one age to another. A superior individual will even in old age exceed the average of the young, and the less able youth will not tend to become the more able sexagenarian. The years of a man's age give no reliable measure of his probable capacity; for achievement is far from correlating one-to-one either positively or negatively with length of life. Success and failure in psychophysiological work are functions of individual personality. Certain fundamental tendencies in them tend to persist throughout the life span, or alter from age to age in characteristic ways.

The last of the three propositions whose demonstrations seems to me to emerge from recent experimental work is this: the more the behavior product involves experience and considered judgment, the more resistent it is to the psychophysiological age deterioration. The accumulation of information and the exercise of the intellectual functions, together with the controlled organization of emotional attitudes, make possible the development of human wisdom. This is the characteristic prerogative and contribution of well preserved age.

Only through the gradual and constantly organized and integrated process of accumulating information does knowledge come. Interest and motivation persisting year after year are essential for this process. Professional and practical techniques and skills can reach seasoned exercise only through long periods of practice. Where physical stamina and energetic alertness are of relatively greater account for production than is considered practice, youth will probably always exceed, but in the exercise of the higher mental processes, in comprehension, in reasoning and in judgment, age alone can develop, through year after year of practice, the qualities of a broad philosophical objectivity. Increasing years offer opportunity for increasing effectiveness in life organization. Personal goals become better defined, one's own abilities better understood, the emotional stresses of frustration and disappointment are met with less expense to the personality. The intellectual traits depend for their effectiveness upon the stability of the emotional elements. Intellectual persistence is not wholly dependent upon physical energy;

it springs in large part from interest, motivation and social habits. In a society which dictates retirement at sixty, and tends to push its elders from the fields of active life, older people face a double difficulty: involutional changes that are physiologically intrinsic, and social mores that are psychologically extrinsic.

Effectiveness in later maturity can be increased by the recognition of the physical decrement and through organized effort in psychological compensation. Social adjustment of younger and older in a complex society that best functions when all ages are fitted into the scheme can occur more adequately when individual differences, rather than age differences, are more fully stressed. The happiness and comfort of the old involves the recognition of their potential contribution of wisdom. Progress, economic, scientific or artistic, depends chiefly upon the activity of the young and the middle-aged. But the old, especially, can improve the opportunities and further the projects of the young.

There is no critical age line beyond which psychological production ceases. Again, it is the individual personality and not the age that sets the final limit. "Faust" was completed by a poet of eighty. Corot, at 77, is reported to have said: "If the Lord lets me live two years longer I think I can paint something beautiful." This spirit of persistent idealism is timeless: it knows no age.

REFERENCES

AREY, L. B., TREMAINE, M. J., AND MONZINGO, F. L. 1935. The numerical and topographical relations of taste buds to human circumvallate papillae throughout the life span. Anat. Rec., **64**, 9-25.

BAILEY, T. 1857. Records of Longevity. London: Darton, 399 pp.

BÜHLER, C. 1933. Der menschliche Lebenslauf als psychologisches Problem. Leipzig: Hirzel, 328 pp.

CORBIN, K. B., AND GARDNER, E. D. 1937. Decrease in number of myelinated fibers in human spinal roots with age. Anat. Rec., **68**, 63-74.

CRITCHLEY, M. 1931. The neurology of old age. The Lancet, **1**, 1119-1127, 1221-1230, 1331-1337.

FULTON, J. F. 1930. Selected Readings in the History of Physiology. Springfield: Thomas, see pp. VIII and IX.

HALL, G. S. 1923. Senescence: The Last Half of Life. New York: Appleton, 525 pp.

HEIDERICH, F. 1906. Die Zahl und die Dimension der Geschmacksknospen der Papilla Vallata des Menschen in den verschiedenen Lebensaltern. Nachr. v. d. kön. Gesell, d. Wiss. z. Göttingen. Math.-physik. K., **1**, 54-64.

HOLLINGWORTH, H. L. 1927. Mental Growth and Decline. New York: Appleton, 396 pp.

JONES, H. E., AND CONRAD, H. S. 1933. The growth and decline of intelligence. Genetic Psychol. Monog., **13,** 298 pp.

LEHMAN, H. C. 1936. The creative years in science and literature. Science, **43,** 151-162.

———— 1937. The creative years: "best books". Scientific Mo., **45,** 65-75.

LORGE, I. 1936. The influence of the test upon the nature of mental decline as a function of age. J. Educ. Psychol., **27,** 100-110.

MILES, C. C. 1934. The influence of speed and age on intelligence scores of adults. J. Gen. Psychol., **10,** 208-210.

———— 1935. Sex in social psychology. In a Handbook of Social Psychology, Ed. by C. Murchison, Worcester, Mass.: Clark Univ. Press, Chapt. 16, 596-682.

MILES, C. C., AND MILES, W. R. 1932. The correlation of intelligence scores and chronological age from early to late maturity. Am. J. Psychol., **44,** 44-78.

MILES, W. R. 1931. Measures of certain abilities throughout the life span. Proc. Nat. Acad. Sci., **17,** 627-633.

———— 1933. Age and human ability. Psychol. Rev., **40,** 99-123.

———— 1935. Age in human society. In a Handbook of Social Psychology, Ed. by C. Murchison, Worcester, Mass.: Clark Univ. Press, Chapt. 15, 596-682. (Contains selected bibliography of psychological references.)

PEARSON, G. H. J. 1928. Effect of age on vibratory sensibility. Arch. Neur. and Psych., **20,** 482-496.

PRICE, B. 1931. A perceptual test for comparing the performance of age groups: preliminary report. Psychol. Bull., **28,** 584-585.

RUCH, F. L. 1934. The differentiative effects of age upon human learning. J. Gen. Psychol. **11,** 261-286.

STRONG, E. K., JR. 1931. Changes of Interests with Age. Stanford University, Calif.: Stanford Univ. Press, 235 pp.

TERMAN, L. M., AND BUTTENWIESER, P. 1935. Personality factors in marital compatibility. J. Soc. Psychol. **6,** 143-171; 267-289.

THORNDIKE, E. L., BREGMAN, E. O., TILTON, J. W., AND WOODYARD, E. 1928. Adult Learning. New York: Macmillan, 335 pp.

CHAPTER 21

CHEMICAL ASPECTS OF AGEING

C. M. McCAY

Ithaca

"Thou canst help time to furrow me with age, but stop no wrinkle." — *Richard II.*

"Eine einzige Zahl hat mehr wahren un bleibenden Wert als eine kostbare Bibliothek voll Hypothesen."—*Robt. Mayer.*

The goal of the biochemist in the study of ageing is to define the process in terms of quantitative chemical changes. The differences between the bodies of a youth and a man of eighty are evident even to the casual observer. These extremes interest the biochemist but his service should be initiated long before the final alterations of the declining years have taken place. He must ultimately detect these changes and define them in terms of quantitative biochemistry nearer the time of their beginning. Here alone lies some hope of reversing reactions which day by day introduce the changes that finally result in senility.

The paucity of biochemical data defining these age changes is due in part to the slow rate at which transformations take place. In no case has a biochemist had the patience to determine such values as the chemical balance of an animal body during a whole life cycle. Perhaps available techniques are still inadequate to detect the continual changes that proceed in the body day by day.

There is no doubt that the life span can be modified considerably by such factors as nutrition and living regime. The biochemist cannot hope to confine his attention to one set of conditions and term this a normal state of ageing. It is more probable that he will have to state that certain chemical changes take place in the animal body under certain defined conditions of diet and living. Then he can hope to select those variables that lead to the slowest rates of change in approaching senile degeneration.

In studying age changes the biochemist is first confronted with the problem of experimental animals. Such animals should have relatively short life spans. They need to be large enough to afford analytical samples that will yield accurate values by modern methods. If nutritional variables are to be considered in the hope of retarding human senility the chosen species should consume foodstuffs similar to those of man. The white rat is probably the most useful animal for such biochemical studies today. In addition to this species, chickens and sheep probably afford excellent opportunities in the study of senescence.

The food of this animal is similar to that of man. The organs of its body are large enough for analyses. Its mean life span is about two years. Large numbers can be maintained at a modest cost. The nutrition is well defined.

Many other species from insects to man have been employed in the past. Some data have been obtained from analyzing the organs and bodies of dogs, swine, rabbits and other domesticated animals. For the most part, however, these species tend to live too long to permit rapid progress in such research. Insects have some advantages for fundamental studies but their nutrition is poorly defined and their bodies are too small for analytical studies upon organs.

1. GROWTH RATE, LIFE SPAN, AND CHEMICAL COMPOSITION

"These eyes, that see thee now well coloured, shall see thee withered"—
Henry VI.

In the middle ages, the monk, Roger Bacon, stated that there were two limits to the length of life of a species. The first of these depended upon the conditions of living such as available foodstuffs and other factors of environment. In the case of man, these variables were thought to be subject to modification and the life span thus subject to extension. However, Bacon, believed that the span could not be protracted indefinitely but that every species had a limit set by the Lord, which could not be exceeded. Bacon's concepts seem valid today, because all are aware of the great difference in the life span of animal species. Thus the rat is very old at three years, while an old horse may be nearly thirty.

The possible life span of a given species will probably always remain unknown, however. This fact is of interest to the biochemist in the first place because he can be assured of reasonable success in extending the life span by the control of such variables as those of nutrition. In the second place, he may look for different changes in the body of an experimental animal such as a rat that passes through its life cycle in two years compared to a period twice this long. Thus it was found in the laboratory at Cornell in the case of rats with life spans that had been extended to nearly four years, that the bones were so fragile that they were crushed by the scalpel in the process of dissecting away the muscles (McCay et al., 1935). On the other hand, rats that died within the period of two to three years, which is usually termed "normal" retain very firm bones that are difficult to crush. Some of the bones of those with the extended life spans were mere shells that floated in water, while the normal bone of a rat that dies at the end of two years always sinks. The end stages were different here although one case may have been the terminal picture of forces acting over a longer period of time. The alternative to consider is a possible modification of the rate and final state as a result of manipulating the nutrition to extend the life span. This may also be an illustration of the tendency of different organs to age at different rates. Thus the bones may seldom degenerate to the point of terminating the life of an animal because some other organ such as the heart tends to break down first.

2. GROWTH RATE AND LIFE SPAN

"Withered, grotesque, immeasurably old."—*Wordsworth*

The relation of the rate of growth to the total span of life has been debated since the time of Aristotle. More than a hundred years ago Edmonds (1832) devoted a book to the thesis that alternate periods of hardship and prosperity afforded one of the secrets to a long life. He claimed that adversity in youth tended to retard the rate of maturing and estimated that an increase of a year in the duration of infancy tended to increase adult life by seven times this amount.

In early considerations of the effect of growth rate upon total life span, deductions were based upon data from different species. Such relationships were reviewed by Bunge (1903), Flourens (1855), and Lusk (1928). Until modern times little attention has been given to the problem of individual variation within a given species. However, the problem has tended to come to the front due to the discovery of vitamins and the effects of these agents in controlling growth rates.

Several experimental attempts have been made to determine if slower growing animals have longer life spans. Robertson and Ray (1920) kept a group of mice from birth until they died of old age. They determined their rates of growth and total life span. Finally they concluded that those which grew the more rapidly lived the longer. Any such group of animals probably includes diseased individuals. These tend to grow at a slower rate and to die prematurely. Inasmuch as it is impossible to evaluate the extent of disease in such an experimental group, the effect of these members upon the composite growth curve and the total life span cannot be determined. At the same time the conclusions that are drawn from such experiments tend to be dominated by data from this fraction. *For this reason the relationship between growth rate and life span cannot be determined upon a heterogeneous group of animals permitted to grow at the maximum rate of which they are capable.*

Since the time of Robertson other workers have attempted to draw conclusions from groups of rats treated in a similar manner. No valid deduction concerning the relationship between the rate of growth and life span can be drawn from such experiments.

For this same reason it is doubtful if this question can be answered in the case of human beings. One cannot attack the problem even if he has growth rates and life span data upon the same group of people.

If the same animal could live twice, it might be forced to grow slowly during one life and rapidly in another. The answer would then be known. Since this is impossible, the nearest approach is to select two groups of animals at the time of weaning. If these groups are made as nearly equal as possible, they should contain approximately the same number of diseased individuals and this short lived fraction will not dominate the outcome. If one of these groups is obliged to grow slowly and another allowed to grow normally, the answer can be obtained.

Such an experiment has been reported with rats (McCay and Crowell, 1934). One group was allowed to grow to maturity at a normal rate. Two groups were retarded by reducing the energy of the diet to a level adequate for maintenance but insufficient to permit growth. One group was thus held for more than 700 days and another in excess of 900 days without being allowed to grow to maturity. When they were finally given adequate calories and permitted to grow, they did so although they had already exceeded the mean length of life of this species which is about 600 days. Members of both retarded groups were alive when those that grew to maturity at the normal rate had all died. This indicated that the life span was flexible and that the possibility of its extension was unknown as well as that the retarded animals tended to outlive those that matured normally.

Since this early study which was completed in 1934, a new one has been made in the Nutrition Laboratory at Cornell. In the earlier study the rats were fed varying amounts of a diet that was complete in all such factors as vitamins, proteins and minerals even when eaten in the small amounts allowed the retarded animals. This procedure was open to the criticism that the larger animals that grew normally and consumed more of the diet were obliged to excrete more waste products such as nitrogen and salt while the retarded ones were smaller and hence ate less and threw a smaller burden upon their kidneys.

A second experiment was therefore designed in which the same amount of protein, minerals and vitamins was fed to each individual, but the animals that were allowed to mature normally were given all the calories they wished in the form of a mixture of sugar and lard. In this second study 106 rats were divided into two groups at the time of weaning. One of these groups contained 33 members. These were allowed to grow to maturity normally. The last one of this group died at the extreme age of 965 days. The accompanying photograph (fig. 100) shows the last two members of this group that lived.

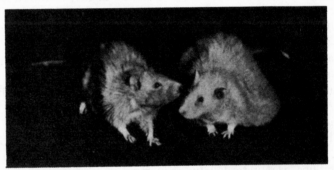

Fig. 100. The last two survivors from the group of 33 rats that were allowed to grow normally in the second retarded growth study. The animal with the tumor was the one that finally lived to be the oldest in this group.

The remainder of the 106 rats numbering 73, were retarded in growth for 300 days. During this period 35 died due to two accidents in losing control of the room temperature, but 38 were still alive at 300 days. These were distributed into four groups, two containing 10 each and two nine each. The first of these groups was fed adequately and thus completed its growth starting at 300 days. The other three were retarded for 500, 700 and 1,000 days. The growth curves are illustrated in the background of figure 101 in which a representative of each group lies in front of its growth curve.

At the time of the death of the last member of the control group, there were still 18 animals alive distributed among the various retarded ones. Only three were alive, however, in the group that matured after 300 days. Even these appeared old in contrast to the group held for 1,000 days (figs. 102 and 103).

Such experiments in retardation are of interest because they show that the total life span can be greatly extended, by control of the growth rate by means of the diet. This is only one of the many possi-

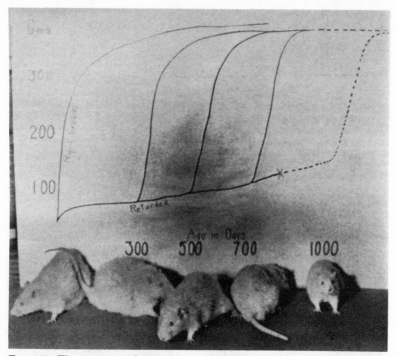

FIG. 101. These rats are almost the same age, about 800 days. The background of growth curves shows the age at which each matured. The "young" one on the extreme right is still awaiting its opportunity to complete its growth. Although the rat on the left represented a group twice as large as any of the others at the start of the experiment, it and all other members of this "normal" group were dead at the end of 965 days while some members of each of the retarded groups were still alive.

bilities in altering the regime. Such changes must modify the course of the biochemical changes involved in ageing.

The factors within the body of the animal that grows normally and that terminate its life must be profoundly modified in the retarded ones. To date few differences have been detected although the aortas of all retarded animals that have died in the second year of the experiment have been calcified while only half of those dying during the same period in the normal growth group have proved to be similarly calcified. This calcification of the aorta as well as of the heart and kid-

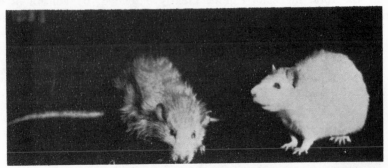

FIG. 102. The old rat on the left from the last survivor of the normal group. The tumor of the previous picture receded before death. The "young" rat on the right is the same age and represents one of the retarded animals that was still waiting to become a thousand days of age before growing to maturity. Today Shakespeare could not say "Thou canst help time to furrow me with age, But stop no wrinkle (Comedy of Errors)."

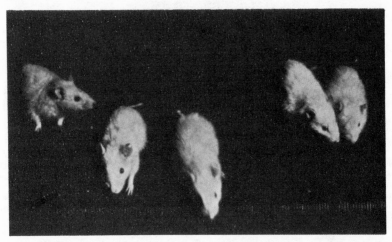

FIG. 103. Half grown retarded rats at the age of 890 days. Although these rats had already exceeded the span of life of a normal rat by about fifty per cent, they had never been allowed enough calories to permit them to grow to maturity.

neys of rats used in studies of retarded growth has been discussed by Hummel and Barnes (1938). A new method of attack upon the problems of arteriosclerosis is therefore suggested but only adds a paradox to the life span problems because the retarded animals prolong their lives in spite of this condition. Some other link in the chain of reactions within the body of the rat must break before the one related to calcification (fig. 104).

The small number of animals permits no conclusions concerning the incidence of spontaneous tumors but the longer the growth of the animal is retarded the later the tumors seem to arise.

There is a considerable body of literature supporting the thesis that the life span is extended by slower growth. Ingle (1933) working with Cladocera effected an increase in life span by retarding the growth rate.

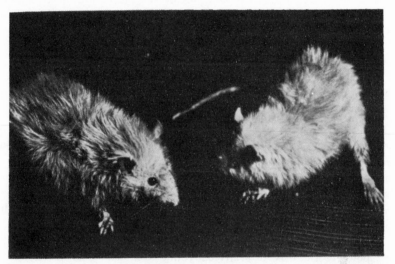

Fig. 104. Rats from a retarded growth experiment after they had attained an age of 1320 days, equal to about 132 years for man. "He is deformed, crooked, old and sere ill-faced, worse bodied."

In the case of insects, many workers have shown the modifications induced in the various stages of the life cycle by retarding one stage. The studies of Kellogg and Bell (1903) with silk worms are typical of insects. Northrup (1917) showed a similar effect in the case of drosophila.

The effect of retardation of growth upon the ultimate size of the body as well as the chemical composition has been much debated. In the case of rats that have been retarded for very long periods, the body seems to be unable to attain the same size that would have been considered normal. In other species most of the evidence also indicates that retardation produces an animal of somewhat smaller size (McCay, Crowell and Maynard, 1935).

Retardation seems to affect the reproductive powers of female animals. Rats seem able to breed at a later date after retardation. In case they are subjected to alternate periods of growth and retardation, the females exhibit normal oestrous cycles during growth and abnormal ones during the retarded periods (Asdell and Crowell, 1935).

If both sexes of rats are retarded for long periods and then allowed to grow the male tends to attain a larger size than the female. Both tend to live about the same length of time suggesting that the slower growth rate may be one explanation for the longer life of the female of the species under normal conditions (McCay, Crowell and Maynard, 1935).

3. NUTRITION AND LIFE SPAN

"Consequently to preserve life is to use meates and drinks according to the age of the person. For the dyet of youth is not convenient for old age nor contrariwise."—*Thomas Cogan. The Haven of Health 1596.*

Since very early times authors have stressed the importance of diet in preserving the animal body against the encroachments of old age. The past hundred years have produced an embryo science of nutrition. Hundreds of workers give their entire time to advancing this science today. However, almost all attention has been devoted to the study of the nutritional requirements of growing animals to the neglect of the adult.

The reason for this emphasis upon the growing stage is due in the first place to the ease of studying young animals. The diseases that appear in old age may have started but are unobserved in the young. In the second place, the growing body is a seat of very rapid chemical changes. As a result the effects of different diets become evident very quickly. In the adult, however, body stores have been built within such organs as the liver and the animal is no longer growing so its needs are less. Therefore, it requires long protracted efforts to produce dietary effects in the mature. Many of the current concepts concerning the nutrition of mature animals are questionable because they are derived from reasoning by analogy, from young, immature animals. Hence the decisions regarding the diets of adults usually represent compromises between food habits established by long usage and modern evidence based upon experiments with developing animals.

Human experience has long shown the value of temperance in the consumption of food. Luigi Cornaro (1464–1566) stressed this in the series of essays written in the late years of his life. Francis Bacon stated, "It seems to be approved by experience, that a spare diet, and almost a pythagorical,—such as is either prescribed by the strict rules of a monastical life, or practiced by hermits, which have necessity and poverty for their rule,—rendereth a man long-lived." Such statements as these comprise the content of many of the works written about diets for the aged. Usually they share the book with some pet theory that the author desires to promote.

In modern times a beginning has been made in relating nutrition to the life span. Osborne and mendel (1915) were fully aware of the problems involved and discussed them frequently in the course of their growth studies. They even made one attempt to keep retarded animals

TABLE 30

Life span and protein level fed rats

(Slonaker)

Protein level	Males				Females			
	Weight		Age		Weight		Age	
	Mean	P.E.	Mean	P.E.	Mean	P.E.	Mean	P.E.
per cent	*grams*	*grams*	*days*	*days*	*grams*	*grams*	*days*	*days*
10	192	1.8	700	3.7	159	1.0	762	7.2
14	222	1.4	767	5.9	185	1.2	848	7.0
18	191	1.4	760	7.2	198	2.2	810	6.2
22	202	1.7	675	5.7	167	2.2	766	7.4
26	214	1.6	650	3.0	158	1.2	730	7.3

until the end of life, but they lost them prematurely from disease. Slonaker (1912) attempted to determine the effect of vegetarian and omnivorous diets upon the length of life of rats. He found the vegetarian rats tended to die much sooner. This early attempt needs to be repeated since advances in the past twenty-five years have probably made it possible to select a vegetarian diet that would give very different results. This early work of Slonaker is of special interest because of the long life of some of his animals.

In a later study, Slonaker (1931) studied the life activities of rats fed different levels of meat in the diet. His results, in terms of life span, are summarized in table 30.

These data seem to indicate an optimum of protein near the 14 per cent level. Due to the methods of preparing the diets, however, it is possible that these differences may have been the result of factors other than the protein. Dried meat was used to vary the protein levels and in each case this replaced varying amounts of a mixture of plant foods. The results might have been different if casein had been used to replace starch in the diets.

This study of Slonaker illustrates one useful technique. The animals are paired at the time of weaning to make groups as equal as possible. They are then fed a given diet throughout the remainder of their lives. Such factors as reproduction, activity and the development of diseases are then determined. This method is useful if the diet is adequate for all special periods, but may give fallacious results if the diet fails

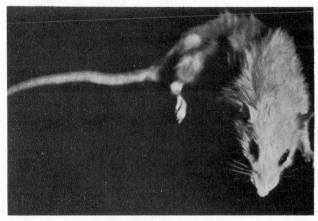

Fig. 105. Extreme old age. This was the last survivor in an experiment to determine the effect of the level of protein ingested upon the span of life.

to satisfy requirements during special periods, such as growth, gestation and lactation. Thus a protein level of 10 per cent may prove adequate for an adult not involved in reproduction and fail for a growing animal or it may be sufficient for a normal male and fail for a lactating female. Dietary drains during crucial periods may thus weaken the body of the female and shorten the life span or lead to the development of special diseases.

For the above reasons nutrition students need to employ additional techniques that satisfy the requirements of animals during special periods. Groups of animals that are to remain unbred can be reared to adults with an adequate allowance of protein for growth. During the adult stage protein levels can be compared. Such studies have been in progress in the laboratory at Cornell for the past five years, but the results in regard to the effect of the protein level in the diet of the adult upon the total life span still remain an unsolved problem.

Likewise, studies are needed in which animals are brought to maturity upon different levels of protein and then maintained under the same conditions for the remainder of life. Protein is cited as a current example, but all the dietary constituents need to be studied in this manner. The same statements that have been made about protein might be made about sodium chloride, or calcium or vitamin A as well as numerous other substances.

Sherman and Campbell (1924) have compared the effects of two different diets upon the life activities of large groups of rats. They have found that a diet that may be sufficient to permit growth and and reproduction, such as a mixture of wheat and dried whole milk in a ratio of 5:1 with one per cent of salt, can be improved by increasing the milk to one-third of the mixture. By such improvement they found the number of young produced and the length of life of the animals were both increased. From their experiments it is evident that one diet is inadequate compared to the other if we consider an adequate diet as one that permits the optimum in life activities. This optimum needs to be measured in several different terms, such as length of life, freedom from disease, and reproductive activities.

In an extension of this early work Sherman, Campbell and Rice (1937) supplemented the diet of wheat and milk (5:1) with calcium carbonate, butter fat and dried skimmed milk. The first two were employed both as single additions and in combination.

The rate of growth was improved by the addition of calcium or dried skimmed milk. These supplements also produced a more efficient utilization of feedstuff as measured in terms of body weight produced from a thousand Cals. The addition of skimmed milk also produced slightly more rapid growth in the early age period and slightly larger animals in the end.

In the case of the females the period of producing young was longer and larger numbers of young were born and reared upon the diets supplemented with calcium or butterfat. Slightly earlier maturity resulted from feeding skimmed milk or calcium. Eleven per cent of the females were sterile upon the original diet and 20 per cent failed to rear young. All supplements improved this condition.

The following values show the mean length of life in days found upon adding the various supplements:

Diet enrichment	None	Calcium	Butter fat	Calcium and butter fat	Skimmed milk
Males..............................	658	703	667	689	681
Females...........................	723	746	818	739	754

Observations made in the course of these studies indicated that the animals receiving the supplement of skimmed milk were superior in firmness of body and condition of the fur coat during youth and early adult life. The addition of butter fat to the diet seemed to give a softer hair, while those fed calcium supplements seemed to retain their youthful appearance longer.

None of the large number of rats used in the above experiment, as far as reported, lived to the ripe old age of those in Slonaker's early experiments nor did any have a length of life comparable to the oldest in the retarded growth experiment made at Cornell. It is possible, but unlikely, that breeding is a factor here. It seems more likely that factors such as growth rate are able to overbalance minor dietary improvements.

Sherman's data indicate a useful type of experiment in which a given dietary is improved from the point of view of the entire life activities instead of from a single consideration such as growth rate. In past problems of nutrition, it is possible that growth rate has been accepted too readily as a proof of a better diet. In the future it may prove desirable to develop slower growth rates with improved life span activities such as reproduction and length of active middle life.

In the second study of Sherman and coworkers there was no general correlation between growth rate and life span. They found the life span was greater in the animals whose early growth rate had been slowed by the supplement of butter. On the other hand, the life spans were also greater for the other supplements that had resulted in an accelerated growth rate. Such experiments are dealing with deficiencies and the results are probably too complex to permit conclusions concerning the interplay of the two factors of growth and life span.

Chen (1935) attempted to study the effect of beef proteins upon the length of life. He concluded that beef protein tended to shorten the life span. However, his diets were poorly designed and the number of animals too small to permit true conclusions.

Orr and associates (1935) attempted to compare a diet typical of that eaten by the Scotch people with a similar one supplemented with milk and vegetables. In terms of life performance, the supplemented diet proved much superior from the point of view of growth rate, life span and reproduction. The results are similar to those of Sherman, probably due to the same reason, namely, an inadequate diet at the beginning. This experiment also permits no conclusions concerning the relationship between growth rate and life span because the animals were probably suffering throughout life from manifold deficiencies which not only slowed the growth rate, but foreshortened the life. If growth rate and life span are to be studied as especially related factors, the lowered rate of growth can be produced better by a single deficiency which is made good after the animals attain adult size.

In one of a series of articles dealing with the practical problems of middle age, Comrie (1935) has discussed the diet. He advances little beyond the concepts of Cornaro. However, he states it in modern terms advising the man doing hard work to eat about 3000 Cals. and the working woman to eat 2500 Cals. These are too much for those engaged in sedentary occupations. Comrie notes that men usually overeat in regard to meat and women in regard to pastries and feels that both tendencies need curbing.

Evidence to show specific dietary effects upon the course of development of degenerative diseases in man is difficult to obtain. Langstroth (1929) has presented clinical evidence of the beneficial effects of diets richer in vitamins and poorer in purified foodstuffs. Such evidence is open to many criticisms, but probably is the best available today.

The needs of the adult for protein remain uncertain even today. At the end of the nineteenth century, a few dominant personalities nearly convinced the civilized nations that a high intake of protein was desirable. They fixed the amount to be ingested daily as 100 grams or more. Shortly after the turn of the century, however, this level was severely criticized by Hindhede (1913), Fletcher, Chittenden and others. The present generation, especially in America, has tended to consume more milk proteins but at the same time they have also inclined toward diets rich in vegetables. A few experiments by individuals have attempted to stem this tide in favor of diets richer in meat. Thus a few persons have lived upon diets rich in meat for a period of a year or two. However, their conclusions that such diets are satisfactory for long continued use cannot be accepted without question,

because their experiments represent too short fractions of the total
life span and also because too few individuals have been involved to
permit generalizations.

The attack upon the protein problem can probably be made to
best advantage today by long period studies with omnivorous animals
such as rats and dogs. After sufficient clear cut evidence has been
gained from such experiments there is no reason that demonstrations
cannot be made with groups of people. No one can state today the
amount of protein that an adult should consume.

Protein level in the diet is reflected quite readily in the weight of
the kidneys and the blood urea level. McKay et al. (1928) fed middle-
aged rats upon three levels of protein. These were placed upon the
diets at 346 days of age and killed at 400 days. The diets contained
18, 31, and 67 per cent protein. Each group of rats consumed about
the same number of Calories per area of body surface. The rapid
response of the blood urea and kidney weight was evident even in this
period of 54 days.

The effect of protein upon these middle-aged rats was much less
than upon young growing ones. This result was explained later.

This enlargement of the kidneys is a response to the blood composition and is the result of both *hyperplasia and hypertrophy* of the kidneys. The kidneys of adult rats respond in even one week to a high
protein level in the diet. After removing one kidney from rats Smith
and Moise (1927a) found the other to be 5 per cent enlarged after 3
days and 48 per cent after 150 days. This increase is proportional to
the protein level in the diet. The dry material of the kidney increases
showing that water was not responsible for the enlargement.

Later McKay and McKay (1930) took account of the higher ingestion
of protein by young rats and thus explained the more marked effects
upon the kidneys of young than upon old ones. For this same reason
McKay concluded a diet with 1 per cent cystine may be toxic to growing
rats and not very injurious to the kidneys of adults.

Rats over 60 days of age excrete more albumin if fed a high protein
diet. At 350 days of age rats fed Sherman's A and B diets usually
have intact kidneys, but at 500 days of age on these same diets spontaneous focal lesions become common (Smith and Moise, 1927).

Renal enlargement is not produced in rats by feeding urea in amounts
equal to protein so the cause of the enlargement is somewhat obscure
(McKay et al., 1927).

In the course of studies at Cornell in which rats have been fed high and low protein levels, the leucocytes of the blood as well as the urea levels have tended to run high upon the higher protein levels. The effects of continuous high levels of nonprotein nitrogen and blood leucocytes during the last half or any considerable fraction of the life span of an animal, are unknown. However, in old age one might expect different developments in animals that have had their kidneys and blood so modified for long periods although the final picture in terms of chemical pathology cannot be anticipated.

The kidneys of rats fed high protein diets throughout life were studied by Blatherwick and Medlar (1937). In a diet made rich in protein by including seventy-five per cent liver, the mean life span for both sexes was only 506 days. There was marked injury of the kidneys, especially in nephrectomized animals. Female rats were more refractory to the production of nephritis than male ones. The addition of dessicated thyroid to the diet of the females that had been nephrectomized favored the development of nephritis. A diet containing seventy-five per cent of casein also injured the kidneys but the action seemed slower than in the case of similar liver diets.

No injury was found in diets containing twenty per cent of liver or casein. These latter are of special interest since they represent more nearly diets that may be eaten by man. Unpublished data from the Animal Nutrition Laboratory at Cornell indicate that rats fed low protein diets after middle age tend to live longer than those fed high protein ones. It has also been found that diets containing liver tend to extend the life span in comparison to casein diets. This probably indicates that there are essentials in liver that exert a favorable effect and thus tend to overbalance the increased kidney injury found by Blatherwick and Medlar.

These life span studies of Blatherwick and Medlar (1937) are also interesting inasmuch as they found diets containing five per cent of irradiated yeast developed marked calcification of the kidneys and aortas as well as renal calculi in a hundred per cent of these animals. The mean life span of the rats used in all their studies was relatively short, however, but no explanation seems available.

4. METABOLISM

Metabolism in old age was reviewed by Robertson in 1907. Few advances have been made since that date. In fact more critical consideration eliminates some of this earlier material.

One of the most extensive studies that have been made was that of

Fenger (1904) upon a woman who lived for a period of 15 years upon a very frugal diet. At the age of 61 this woman started the regime outlined.

No. 1. 1889–1892—Daily, 1 egg, 1 liter oat meal soup, 2 liters of skimmed milk, 45 cc. of red wine and 8 grams sugar.

No. 2. 1892–1894—Daily, 2 eggs, 1 liter oat meal soup, 2 liters skimmed milk, 45 cc. of red wine and 8 grams sugar.

No. 3. 1894–1900—Daily, 3 eggs, 0.5 liter of soup, 2 liters skimmed milk, 45 cc. red wine, 8 grams sugar, 60 grams of plum and raspberry juice.

No. 4. 1900–1903—Daily, 3 eggs, 0.5 liter of barley soup, 1.5 liter of sweet milk (whole), 0.5 liter buttermilk, 45 cc. red wine, 8 grams sugar and 60 grams of plum and raspberry juice.

This diet served to maintain the body weight which fluctuated between 42 and 45 kg. This diet allowed, in the case of No. 1, about 1.95 grams protein, 0.53 gram fat, 3.7 grams of carbohydrates per kg. In No. 4 the following were allowed: protein, 2.3; fat, 1.94; carbohydrate, 3.6.

The Calories per kg. in the four periods ran 25, 26, 26.4, and 32–35. Per day the calorie allowance varied from 1125 to 1600.

The ability to utilize food in the case of Fenger's subject did not seem to change with age.

One of the interesting balances was that for salt. The intake was estimated at 1.5 grams per day. About half of this was excreted in the feces. The night urine was about 50 per cent richer in salt than the day.

Protein was well digested and absorbed. At the age of 73 this woman was still in good health.

Chemical balances were also run by Koch (1911) upon five men ranging in age from 54 to 79 years. These men were living in the almshouse of Helsingfors, Finland. These men were fed simple diets of meat, potatoes and vegetables. They consumed an average of 556 grams of dry stuff, 2453 grams of water, 106 grams protein, 55 grams of fat and 34 grams of ash.

They excreted feces daily of the following composition.

	grams
Dry matter	41–62
Protein	12–18
Fat	3–5
CHO	17–31
Ash	6–10

Of the food consumed, they utilized an average of 86 per cent of the protein, 92 per cent of the fat, 94 per cent of the carbohydrate, and 92 per cent of the Calories.

To compare with these were Forster's (1877) values shown in table 31. These were diets allowed poor, old people in various almshouses.

These data all indicate there is no marked alteration in the ability of the old body to utilize foods. However, gastric acidity seems to show an age relationship (Vanzant et al., 1932). The incidence of achlorhydria increases steadily from youth to old age. At the age of 60 about a quarter of both sexes showed no free acid. Normally free gastric acidity increases rapidly from childhood to 20 years. At puberty the mean value for boys rises above that for girls.

In men there is a drop in free acidity after the age of about 40, but in women the level tends to be maintained quite constant until

TABLE 31

Diets consumed by old people

(Forster)

	Protein	Fat	Carbo-hydrate	Calories
1. Munich women......................	79	49	266	1,871
2. Munich men and women.............	92	45	332	2,157
3. Brandenburg.......................	98	28	561	2,962
4. Scchwerin (Schwerin)...............	92	40	502	2,772
5. London............................	70	32	341	1,983

60 years of age. In both sexes the combined acidity tends to remain constant from youth to old age. There is little evidence for progressive senile atrophy of the gastric mucosa.

The ability of the senile body to digest and absorb food in spite of such changes indicates a considerable margin of safety in the mechanisms for food assimilation.

Mühlmann (1927) observed the marked decrease in excretion of S and N in the course of human ageing. However, his values fluctuated widely since he appears to have made no attempt to control the food ingested. He believed that the body lost in its ability to assimilate protein as age progressed and thus less S appeared in the urine and more in the feces.

The oxidized form of the sulfur in the urine tends to decrease with age according to Mühlmann (1932-3). However, only a few old individuals were included in his series and no control was made nor record kept of food ingested.

The decline in basal metabolism in old age has been recognized for nearly a hundred years. One of the best of the earlier studies was that of Sonden and Tigerstedt (1895). They showed the decline in carbon dioxide excretion with age. Their subjects ranged in years from seven to eighty-four. They calculated this decrease in terms of body surface. They also ran the carbon and nitrogen in the urine of their subjects and followed the decline of these elements in old age.

In modern times the problem of the changes in basal metabolism with ageing has been given much attention by Benedict and Root (1934). Their data indicate clearly the wide fluctuations from extrapolated curves that must be expected. Perhaps they also indicate that basal metabolism is a valuable measurement of true senescence.

TABLE 32

Basal metabolism of Japanese in old age

(Kise and Ochi, 1934)

Age	Man	Woman
	calories per sq. m. per hour	*calories per sq. m. per hour*
50–59	36.05	34.02
60–69	34.91	33.15
70–79	33.16	31.90
80 and over	32.06	30.42

Benedict (1935) finds the normal heat production in women over sixty-five is about 1000 Calories per 24 hours irrespective of weight or age. In a series of measurements upon women between the ages of 66 and 88, the total heat productions per 24 hours varied from 799 to 1549 Cals.

Ninety-four elderly Japanese were studied by Kise and Ochi (1934). Of these 44 were males. All were over 50 and one over 90 years of age. Their values are summarized in table 32. They compared their values with those for Japanese between the ages of 20 and 50. The means were:

	20–50 yrs.	*50 yrs. +*
Male	37.3 ± 0.18	34.46 ± 0.25
Female	33.8 ± 0.30	32.62 ± 0.24

In terms of Calories per square meter of body surface per hour the basal metabolism drops steadily in the case of man until the age of about eighteen. After this there is a slow but steady decline according to DuBois (1936). The basal metabolsim is higher for the male throughout life. During the middle third of life the downward trend of the curve for the female is slight compared to that of the male. The rate of decline for women is shown clearly in McKay's (1928) data (table 33).

DuBois (p. 169) (1936) has summarized the available data for people over sixty. As one would expect there is great variability due to the degree of senescence. Thus the Japanese found one man, age 93, with a figure of 34.1 Cals. per sq. m., and a woman, age 75, with a value of 26.5.

The basal metabolism of eight women ranging in age from 77 to 106 years and for 14 men ranging from 74 to 92 was measured by Matson and Hitchcock (1934–35). No correlation was found between the basal metabolism and degree of senescence.

TABLE 33

Decline of basal metabolism with age in women

(McKay, 1928)

Average 35 to 40 years.....................	33.8 calories per sq. m. per hour
40 to 50 years.....................	33.4 calories per sq. m. per hour
50 to 60 years.....................	31.0 calories per sq. m. per hour

Those data may be considered to represent the final stages in the life cycle. They show the ends of the curves which have been traced upon a few subjects by Benedict (1928) who even noted the decline with advancing age during the period of middle life.

In the case of adult dogs Kunde and Norlund (1927) could find no change in basal metabolism with advancing age. They state: "the basal metabolism of 4 fully grown adult dogs, housed in the laboratory from 2 to 12 years, shows no decline as a result of the advanced age, when living under conditions of moderate amounts of daily exercise and a high protein diet"

The basal metabolism of about a hundred rats was followed by Benedict and Sherman (1937) from middle age until death. The total heat production of the same individuals tended to decrease very slightly with age and the body weight also decreased leaving the authors rather perplexed in interpreting results. On the basis of weight alone the old rats had a higher basal metabolism when compared with middle aged rats. The body temperature tended to decrease by about 2°C.

in rats more than 800 days of age. One has no means of evaluating the effect of disease in these old rats that were studied.

The decline of basal metabolism with the weight of years is evident. The variability of values indicate clearly that senescence is much more than a matter of time, however. As the body fails, the basal metabolism decreases with the other powers.

5. CHANGES IN BODY COMPOSITION

"And now I wax old, seke, sory and cold, as muk upon mold, I widder away."—*Towneley Mysteries*.

Since very early times ageing has been associated with withering. Leeuwenhoek (1632–1723) and Spallanzani (1729–99) were both fascinated by the production of suspended animation in rotifers by dehydration. To them hydration seemed one of the keys to the secrets of life (Milne-Edwards, 1862).

Modern science has confirmed the early views that senescence is characterized by losses of water from various parts of the body. Today this is a well established phenomenon because it is one of the most marked changes and because the determination is a simple measurement.

In one of the earliest of modern studies von Bezold (1857) employed mice, bats, birds, frogs, goldfish and even crustacea. He determined both ash and dry matter in animals of different ages. In the case of higher animals he found development into the adult was associated with a decrease in body water and an increase in ash.

The percentage of water in the brain and spinal cord of rats of different ages was determined by Donaldson (1918). From data in the literature he compared the dehydration of the brain of man and rat in the course of ageing.

The brain of an animal loses water throughout life. Donaldson and Hatai (1931) compared these water losses in the different parts of the rat brain. There is a very rapid loss until the animal is 30–50 days of age. From this period until 500 days of age, the decline is very slow. The olfactory bulbs tend to maintain a water content of 83 per cent, the cerebellum one of 79 per cent, while the brain stem of the adult averages 72–75 per cent. The oldest rats included in this study were only 530 days of age. This is only the mean life span for a male and these rats can hardly be considered old by modern standards.

Maurice (1910) followed the changes in the moisture and phosphorus compounds in the brains and organs of dogs ranging in age from one day to eight years. His data indicate the trend in the loss of water as the nervous system grows older. More astounding, however, are the relatively large increases in lipid materials or at least substances soluble in alcohol and ether.

Maurice also found rather extensive changes in the phosphorus compounds. In his analyses he determined "inorganic" phosphorus by measuring the amount set free by proteolytic digestion of the tissue with acidified pepsin. This digestion was made after the lipid had been extracted. His "nucleid" fraction was the portion that failed to dissolve after enzyme digestion and the values were obtained by subtracting the soluble phosphorus plus the lipid phosphorus from the total.

Part of Maurice's data are summarized in table 34. These data indicate a tendency for the total phosphorus of the dry matter to decrease with age while the lipid phosphorus increases. This study should be repeated with modern analytical procedures and species other than the dog.

The bodies of animals at birth are all relatively rich in water. In the course of the early period of life and rapid growth all tissues tend to have more solids and less water. Part of these solids is fat. While numerous studies have been made of these water changes, relatively little attention has been paid to fat. Lowry (1913) followed the changes in the dry matter of organs as rats matured. Unfortunately, his values for year old rats are based upon analyses of only two individuals.

The relatively high per cent of the dry matter of the animal body that is stored in the muscles in old age is suggestive, but two rats can hardly be representative.

The loss of water in ageing tissue is well illustrated by Lowry's data (table 35).

Lowry also assembled a table showing how man dehydrates as he matures. Such data are difficult in comparison, however, because they cannot be reduced to a fat-free basis in the course of old age.

In a carefully controlled series of experiments Hurst (1933) determined the entire fat and water in the bodies of rats ranging in age from 1 to 112 days of age. Some of his data are shown in table 36.

The female tends to deposit a little more body fat than the male

TABLE 34

Changes in the P distribution with age in the dog

(Maurice)

Age group	P in dry matter				Alcohol-ether extract, per cent dry matter	H$_2$O
	Total	Lipid	Nucleic	Inorganic		
Cerebrum						
						per cent
1–15 days	1.87	0.53	0.13	1.21	31.4	89.7
4 wks.– 4 mos.	1.63	0.67	0.07	0.88	43.0	83.2
6 mos.–13 mos.	1.55	0.62	0.10	0.83	46.7	80.1
2 yrs. – 8 yrs.	1.52	0.76	0.08	0.69	55.4	77.8
Cerebellum						
1–15 days	1.92	0.57	0.08	1.28	34.2	88.2
4 wks.– 4 mos.	1.75	0.70	0.09	0.96	47.8	80.9
6 mos.–13 mos.	1.64	0.66	0.10	0.88	52.4	77.8
2 yrs. – 8 yrs.	1.58	0.72	0.10	0.76	56.8	75.5
Encephalon						
1–15 days	1.89	0.54	0.12	1.23	31.8	89.7
4 wks.– 4 mos.	1.65	0.68	0.08	0.90	43.7	83.2
6 mos.–13 mos.	1.56	0.63	0.10	0.84	47.7	79.9
2 yrs. – 8 yrs.	1.54	0.75	0.08	0.71	55.6	77.4
Medulla						
1–15 days	1.74	0.73	0.07	0.93	42.2	84.8
4 wks.– 4 mos.	1.79	0.80	0.10	0.89	61.7	74.4
6 mos.–13 mos.	1.68	0.84	0.08	0.75	68.3	71.7
2 yrs. – 8 yrs.	1.70	0.92	0.11	0.71	71.0	67.9
Nerves						
4 wks.– 4 mos.	0.99	0.43	0.07	0.49	43.5	70.3
6 mos.–13 mos.	0.72	0.33	0.06	0.32	57.9	56.1
2 yrs. – 8 yrs.	0.60	0.28	1.06	0.26	59.6	48.7
Spleen						
1–15 days	1.70	0.23	0.15	1.32	21.2	79.7
4 wks.– 4 mos.	1.61	0.27	0.13	1.21	19.0	78.9
6 mos.–15 mos.	1.32	0.22	0.09	1.01	18.1	78.0
2 yrs. – 8 yrs.	1.09	0.23	0.12	0.74	16.3	76.8
Liver						
1–15 days	1.18					77.1
4 wks.– 4 mos.	1.21					73.0
6 mos.–15 mos.	1.21					70.3
2 yrs. – 8 yrs.	1.03					67.9

during the period of growth.   Both sexes tend to lose water from their bodies at about the same rate.   This is a true dehydration and not an apparent effect from lipid deposition in the body.

TABLE 35

Increase in percentage of dry matter in tissues of the rat with age

(Lowry)

	Age		
	Birth	20 days	1 year
Skin...........................	12.3	41.1	
Skeleton......................	18.1	33.3	52.6
Muscles.......................	10.7	22.6	25.2 (10 weeks)
Viscera.......................	15.2	19.1	25.6 (5 months)
Eyeballs......................	7.4	14.4	20.1
Heart.........................	13.8	18.0	22.4
Lungs.........................	15.9	18.9	
Liver.........................	19.4	24.3	26
Spleen........................	14.3	17.2	22.6
Kidneys.......................	13.3	17.2	22.9

TABLE 36

Water and fat in the bodies of rats of different ages

(Hurst)

Number of specimens	Sex	Age	Fat in fresh body		Moisture in the fat-free body	
			Mean	P.E.	Mean	P.E.
		days	per cent	per cent	per cent	per cent
6	Male	1	3.0	0.32	85.6	0.40
6	Female	1	3.5	0.15	87.1	0.60
6	Male	10	5.6	0.51	80.9	0.26
6	Female	10	7.4	0.24	80.3	0.51
6	Male	21	5.9	0.19	79.4	0.19
6	Female	21	8.2	0.32	78.3	0.13
6	Male	42	4.4	0.16	76.2	0.23
6	Female	42	4.6	0.08	76.5	0.16
6	Male	112	6.1	0.18	72.9	0.59
6	Female	112	9.2	0.21	72.3	0.23

Even such organs as the eyes share with the body in the general dehydration that characterizes ageing.

The effect of age upon the changes in moisture of the lens and cornea of the eye are shown in the data of Bürger and Schlomka (1928). These eyes used were taken from cattle of different ages.

The effect of age upon the composition of cattle was determined by Moulton (1923). He found calculations must be reduced to a fat free basis since animals tend to fatten with age. In cattle the increase in body phosphorus, ash and nitrogen is rapid for a period of five months, then it gradually decreases until the animal is 50 months of age. No data were presented beyond this period. Moulton summarized the earlier studies and concluded that mammals in general show a decrease in water content and an increase in protein and ash until chemical maturity is reached.

TABLE 37

Dry matter in lens and cornea of cattle eyes

(Bürger and Schlomka, 1928)

Lens		Cornea	
Age	Dry matter	Age	Dry matter
	per cent		per cent
0.32	31.5	0.95	14.6
2.3	34.4	1.25	15.4
7.6	35.1	5.45	17.4
12.2	35.8	15.05	18.7
15.5	36.6		

Animals relatively mature at birth have a lower water content. Mammals reach chemical maturity at different ages but these are a fairly constant relative part of the total life cycle.

From a study of limited data Murray (1922) concluded that the composition of the bodies of animals varied little when reduced to a fat free basis. He estimated the composition as follows:

	Ash	Protein	Water
Young growing animals	4	20	76
Adults	6	22	72

The animal body may vary in fat up to 60 per cent. Swine seem able to store more body fat than Herbivora.

The dehydration which accompanies ageing of colloids has led Marinesco (1913) to postulate that colloidal phenomena may account for changes in the animal body. He believes that at certain ages, variable with the species, colloidal particles within the body tend to reunite and then cover their surfaces with lipid material. Thus he attempts to account for the granulations of nervous tissue in certain old animals. In old age he visualizes a denser gel with a slower rate of diffusion for crystalloids.

The progressive dehydration of cells provides the basis for the colloidal theory of ageing. Ruzicka (1922) claims that older cells have a pH nearer the isoelectric point than younger ones. He believes ageing represents passage from a highly to a less dispersed state. The evidence behind Ruzicka's theories is not very convincing. In fact there is considerable conflicting evidence concerning such factors as the change in hydrogen ion concentration of the blood in the course of ageing.

The analogy between ageing in the animal body and in colloidal solutions has been discussed recently by Wells (1933) who shows that in many ways they are similar phenomena.

6. DEHYDRATION

"But the natural moisture which is daily wasted may, by diet and a right course of moderating ones living, be restored."—*The Cure of Old Age—Roger Bacon.*

Everyone recognizes that the phenomenon of dehydration must be related to the substances of the body that control the movements of water between tissues. If we are ever to become as optimistic as Bacon and be convinced that the dehydration of age can be reversed, it is probable that we will effect this reversal through our knowledge of composition of some governing constituents, such as sodium chloride. To date the phenomena stand unrelated, but a beginning has been made in studying changes in the composition of the body as senescence approaches.

7. OTHER CHEMICAL CHANGES IN THE BODY

"One of them is fat and grows old; God help the while!"—*Henry IV.*

In any consideration of the chemical changes in the animal body as the result or cause of the ageing process, two probable sources of error must be kept in mind. In the first place, available data usually cover only the first half of life and we are thus obliged or perhaps tempted to extrapolate into the period of ageing. In the second place, the small amount of available data has been assembled from chemical analyses of lower animals like the rat. Reasoning by analogy we tend to consider these data as applying to man.

In spite of the fact that laboratories teaching human anatomy are overstocked with material that could be used for studying the chemical composition of the body in the last stages of life, the biochemist has neglected his opportunities. We know little even concerning the chemistry of the bones during the last third of life. Workers have been content to study animals until middle life, leaving the field with the inference that the body composition tends to remain static after this period.

An attempt to apply recent analytical methods to the study of age changes was made by Ehrenberg (1925). He analyzed the bodies of mice, the livers, brains and kidneys of rabbits, and the livers and brains of men of different ages. He determined such organic compounds as arginin, histidin, and cystin. He also determined the P and N extracted by alcohol and ether. His data show no real age trends, probably due to variability of individuals and insufficient numbers in the various age groups.

The body fat of the newly born child differs in composition from that of the adult. In early studies, Langer (1881) found the fatty acids of the newly born to melt at 51 degrees and those of an adult at 38 degrees. He also found the fat of the child contained butyric and caproic acids which in the adult he could not detect.   The differences he found were:

	Child	Adult
Oleic acid	67.7%	89.8%
Palmitic acid	29.0%	8.2%
Stearic acid	3.3%	2.0%

In the early months in the life of a child Jaeckle (1902) found the body fat to have a much higher content of fatty acids than in later life. In a newly born child he found the I. No. varied from 39 to 49 while in an adult it had a mean value of 65.   This change, however, took place during the first 12 months of life.

His values are the reverse of those of Ssadikow (1928). Perhaps modern life in Leningrad and that of a third of a century ago in Pasen account for these differences.

At birth Ssadikow (1928) found body fat with an I. No. of 80, while at 35 days of age the value was only 56.   A similar value was observed in a 12-year-old cat.

Fehling also found the rabbit embryo of 20 to 30 days of age had 2 to 4.9 per cent fat, while at birth this increased to 6.5 and in the adult averaged 7.8.

On a dry basis Thomas (1911) discovered great species differences in the body fat at birth and at different ages.

Cholesterol as well as fat seems to show age relationships although an ever present possibility continues to haunt the worker, namely, that these sterol changes are specific pathological ones.

The cholesterol and Ca both increase in the aorta of a horse as it grows older. Bürger (1928) quotes these values from the study by Keunhof.

TABLE 38

Cholesterol and calcium in aorta of horse

(Bürger from Keunhof)

	Age		
	1-5 years	10-25 years	Over 25 years
Cholesterol, mgm. per cent..............	130.5	215	230
Calcium, mgm. per cent............... .	10.5	20	25

TABLE 39

Cholesterol and calcium in the aortas of cattle

(Gerritzen)

Mean age	Dry matter	Cholesterol		Calcium	
		Fresh	Dry	Fresh	Dry
	per cent	*mgm. per cent*	*mgm. per cent*	*mgm. per cent*	*mgm. per cent*
9.5 days	26.6	124.9	482.4	10.3	40.0
30 days	25.9	108.8	401.4	10.1	37.8
2.5 years	26.3	102.3	368.7	11.8	44.8
8 years	26.0	101.7	416.5	12.3	48.0
12.5 years	26.1	110.3	431.7	16.6	55.6

In the lens of cattle eyes the cholesterol also seems to increase with age according to the analyses of Bürger and Schlomka (1928).

Age	Cholesterol, mgm. per cent
0.26	196
3.1	270
4.5	300
7.0	328
12.0	587
13.5	603

The aortas of 73 cattle of various ages were analyzed for cholesterol and calcium by Gerritzen (1932). His values fail to exhibit marked age changes in this species although the regular increase in calcium was marked (table 39).

The skin of man tends to lose both moisture and cholesterol in the process of ageing, although the cholesterol values tend to approach a permanent level after the first few weeks of life. Bürger and Schlomka (1928) dissected skin from dead patients of various ages. The fluctuations in their analytical values are probably due in part to the complications of pathological changes as well as the preparation of the sample. The cholesterol, dry matter, and nitrogen of the skin at various ages are shown in table 40.

Little attention has been given to the other organic constituents of the body. In the course of other studies Bürger (1934) measured the increase of nitrogen in human skin in relation to age. His values probably reflect the changes in water as the skin grows older.

TABLE 40

Changes in skin composition with age

(Bürger and Schlomka, 1928)

Age	Cholesterol content, dry basis	Dry matter	N, dry basis
	per cent	*per cent*	*per cent*
Fetal and newly born	0.87	25.5	14.1
1 month to 1 year	0.43	30.6	15.0
1–9 years		35.6	15.1
10–29 years	0.34	36.4	16.0
30–49 years	0.28	36.7	15.6
50–69 years	0.27	39.8	15.8
70–89 years	0.29	35.0	15.4

The nitrogen of human skin tends to increase with age (Bürger, 1934). Some of his values are the following:

Mean age, years	N, grams per cent
0.92	4.21
6.45	5.38
26.05	5.81
43.25	5.73
59.85	6.27
79.75	5.38

Bürger (1928) also noted the increase in nitrogen in such organs as the lens of the eye. His analyses were made upon the eyes of cattle of different ages. Here again we are probably reflecting the trend toward dehydration as the animal grows older.

Lens

Age	N, per cent
0.05	4.94
1.62	5.51
7.60	5.78
12.2	5.81
15.5	5.89

Iron seems to be deposited in the tissues of old animals. Zondek and Karp (1934) could estimate roughly an animal's age by the iron in such organs as the kidneys. They postulate a definite period in about middle

TABLE 41

Iron in milligrams per kilogram of dried substance

(Zondek and Karp)

	Liver	Kidney	Testis
Young animals:			
Rat..........................	180	140	130
Rabbit........................	170	155	125
Guinea pig....................	145	140	125
Cat...........................	200	125	
Dog...........................	200	150	115
Old animals:			
Rat..........................	About 700	335	280
Rabbit........................	Up to 700	400	260
Guinea pig....................	450	350	280
Cat...........................	Up to 800		
Dog...........................	Up to 600		

life when the iron shifts from the lower to the higher value. This is summarized in their table for several species.

Thus iron seems to play a rôle at the end of life as well as a vital part in the early life of a young animal.

Both sex and age seem to influence the glycogen stored in the liver. Stohr (1932) fasted white rats for 24 to 32 hours and then determined the liver glycogen.

Although his differences seem marked, they were based upon small numbers of rats. Even the old adults seem to be about half the normal weight and no consideration appears to have been devoted to previous nutrition.

The high iron content of the liver of newly born animals that are obliged to live for a considerable period upon milk has long been established. Few other elements have been studied. Krüger (1844) and his students compared the phosphorus and sulphur in the livers of cattle and men of different ages. Seven men and one woman were included in their series. These ranged in age from 23 to 70 years. Two newly born infants were also included. Their data indicate that the sulphur, phosphorus and iron of the liver decrease with change from the newly born to the adult.

These workers also ran an extensive series of analyses of the spleens and livers of cattle.

These results indicate the higher values for liver elements in the newly born infant in comparison with the adult. In the case of cattle, however, only the liver P seemed higher in the foetus.

Sherman and coworkers (1925) have followed the alterations in calcium and phosphorus throughout the life cycle of the rat. The increas in calcium of the body is very rapid during the growth period. This increases from about 0.25 per cent at birth to 1.0 to 1.2 per cent in the bodies of adults. During the period of 280 to 540 days the gain in calcium in the body was very slight. This represents the last half of life in their studies. Females that did not rear young tended to have more body calcium than males, but they did not carry this study beyond middle life to determine if the difference persisted into the period of old age. There was even an increase in the calcium in the body of males from the 8th to the 12th month.

The per cent of calcium in the body of an animal that is retarded in growth tends to exceed the normal, but the total amount is less. Females lose calcium in producing litters, but regain it during the rest period. No data were secured upon these animals during their old age.

Slight decreases in the magnesium content of the testes and brain in the course of ageing were found by Delbet and Breteau (1930). However, their data are very questionable, since it appears that they failed to employ sound analytical methods.

8. AGEING OF THE BLOOD

"Time hath not yet so dried this blood of mine, nor age so eat up my invention."—*Much Ado About Nothing.*

The blood of animals of different ages has been given more attention by the chemist than any other component of the body. Blood can be studied in the course of ageing because samples can be taken without injury to the individual.

The hemoglobin in the blood of man tends to remain relatively constant after the age of 11 although there is, according to Williamson and Ets (1926), some trend toward a decline in the male after the age of 60.

The hemoglobin of rat's blood was measured at twenty day intervals by Williamson and Ets, until their animals were 250 days old. In this species, as in many others, there is a tendency for the hemoglobin to decrease until the young are weaned. After weaning the value increases to a maximum of 15.5 grams per 100 cc. at 5 months of age. After this it tends to remain at about 13.8 gm. until the rat is 250 days old. The latter half of the life span was not studied.

Many studies of the effects of age upon the number of erythrocytes have proved inconclusive. Schwinge (1898) reviewed the older literature and concluded the slight changes found in old age were those related to blood concentration rather than total number of cells.

The conflicting evidence concerning the changes in red cells and hemoglobin of the blood has been presented by Millet (1932). He also presented some new observations. His data were too variable, however, to be conclusive, but the size of erythrocytes in old age seemed to be definitely larger.

The specific gravity of the blood varies with many physiological factors such as exercise and rest (Jones, 1887). At birth it has a very high value of 1.066 for both sexes. This drops rapidly the first two years and then slowly climbs to a maximum of 1.059 in the male at an age of 35 to 45. After this there is a slow decline to a value of 1.054 at the age of 75. The blood of women tends to have a lower specific gravity than that of man. At the end of life, as at birth, both values are equal.

Bürger (1928) finds that there is a progressive lowering of the resistance of erythrocytes to hypotonic solution as a man grows older. He assumes that the blood progressively increases its percentage of old cells as the body ages. These older cells seem to be less resistant.

Blood serum shows an increase in refractive index as an animal grows older. Hatai (1918) studied rats from birth until nearly 600 days of age. An excerpt from his table shows the progressive increase but these findings have never been repeated and confirmed.

Today one is struck by the small size of the adults used in these experiments and the oldest rats were females less than 17 months old.

These facts probably prevent comparison of modern data. Nevertheless the trend is clear.

On the basis of the refractive index Hatai notes three periods in the life cycle (1) from birth to the end of the suckling period; (2) the period of sexual maturity; (3) adult period after 90 days of age. This index is modified after an animal suckles for the first time. After 200 days of age it fluctuates widely. Hatai believed this was a reflection of the diseases that begin at this time. He notes that it is difficult to find sound rats after this age. This observation is suggestive for those concerned with studying the problems of ageing since it affords a tool for differentiating normal and diseased animals during the last half of life.

The refractive index for adult rats and men is about the same. Hatai compiled a table from the data of others showing the progressive increase

TABLE 42

Refractive index of the blood serum of rats

(Hatai)

Body weight	Age	Solids	N_D
	days	*per cent*	
5.1	Newborn	4.1	1.34136
13.8	10	4.7	1.34340
23.7	20	6.3	1.34598
78.9	50	6.7	1.34732
176.5	120	8.0	1.34965
166.4	450	8.8	1.35115

of refractive index of human serum. Many other factors such as fasting, food composition, and sex affect the refractive index of serum.

The total nitrogen in the blood of rats increases with age (Swanson and Smith, 1932). At weaning, this value is 0.81 gram per 100 cc. of plasma, while at 360 days of age it is 1.22 grams.

Wells (1913) followed the change in proteins in rabbits blood between the ages of 21 and 140 days. The increase was progressive during this period but tended to decrease in adults.

According to Toyama (1919), in rats the percentage of total proteins increases rapidly during the suckling period but slowly during puberty. There is little change in the adult, but a slight fall at 385 days. The per cent of albumin increases rapidly for the first thirty days. This falls and then rises again until the end of puberty. The globulin rises steadily until at 255 days the relative amount of it exceeds the albumin.

The per cent of non-protein bodies is quite constant throughout life. The oldest rats used were only 385 days of age, however.

Reiss (1909) ran refractive indices upon the blood of children from $1\frac{1}{2}$ days to 18 years of age. He failed to find the progressive changes of Hatai.

As early as 1844 Bacquerel and Rodier claimed the blood cholesterol increased in old age (after Parhon).

From a very limited number of cases Parhon (1923) claimed some increase as a result of age, but his data were few and variable.

Until rats are about three and a half months of age the blood cholesterol remains below 0.04 per cent. In the adult this may rise to as high as 0.08 per cent according to Roffo (1925), although he found no correlation with age. He also determined the total lipids in the blood of rats between the ages of two and five months. These values varied

TABLE 43

Changes in chicken blood with age

(Baker and Carrel, 1927)

Age	Total lipid	Lipid P	Cholesterol	Protein
	per cent	mgm.	mgm.	per cent
6 months	0.88	5.7	255*	3.5
4–5 years	1.06	7.4	143	4.6

* Three months.

from 0.3 to 0.6 per cent, but showed no correlation with the age of the animal.

The protein, total lipid and lipid phosphorus fractions increase in the blood of ageing chickens, but the cholesterol decreases. The following values were found by Baker and Carrel (1927) in the sera of chickens (table 43).

The lactic acid seems to rise regularly with the age of man although the regular change may be obscured by such factors as urobilinemia. The values of Loiséleur and Morel (1931) show increases of blood lactic acid from 10 to 16 mgm. between the ages of 10 and 60 years.

In old age the mechanisms for handling carbohydrates seem to become less efficient. Marshall (1931) ran glucose tolerance tests upon old men. The level of the blood sugar rose to about 22 per cent after the feeding of 50 grams of glucose. This level is higher than that for normal young men. The threshold level also seemed to be higher because glucose did not appear in the urine in most cases unless this threshold level of about 0.2 per cent was exceeded.

Various curves for the decrease of the blood sugar to normal were found. In a fourth of the cases the "log" type of curve was found. A "diabetic" type occurred in half the cases although the men were usually normal.

The gradual failure of the kidneys in the aged is reflected in the higher level of indoxyl and urea in the blood as well as the slower rate of excretion of such substances as phenolsulphonphthalein, according to Laroche and others (1933).

The uric acid in the blood of 37 individuals varying in age from 71 to 91 years was determined by Currado (1929).

Values ranged from 2.56 to 4.36 mgm. per cent.

The changes in the calcium and various forms of blood phosphorus have been studied in both children and adults by Stearns and Warweg (1933). Unfortunately their studies did not include adults in the last half of life but their curves suggest a constancy or rather a wide individual variability after the first few months of childhood. This does not preclude the possibility of variability in these compounds in old age but suggests they are relatively constant in the adult.

Up to the age of 85 the plasma calcium and the plasma lipids fall within the range characteristic of adult men according to the studies of Page and coworkers (1935).

In rats Watcharn (1933) finds the calcium and magnesium of the serum tend to be quite constant throughout life. Young males, however, of 3 to 4 months have a higher magnesium level in their serum than older ones. This averages 5.4 mgm. per 100 cc., while the value for the others of both sexes averages 4.4 mgm. per 100 cc.

Serum calcium tends to be significantly higher in young rats. No seasonal variations were found for either age or sex.

The serum calcium is more variable in the female rat, while in man the reverse is true according to Boynton and Greisheimer (1930–1) as well as Okey, Stewart and Greenwood (1930).

In the studies of Greisheimer and others (1929) the calcium of the blood sera of both men and women tended to decrease with age. In normal men this fell from a mean of 11.6 mgm. per 100 cc. to one of 10.0 as age progressed. In women the fall was from 11.8 to 9.7. These authors compiled a table summarizing similar data of earlier workers. These data indicated similar changes of about the same magnitude. These findings contrast with those of Page.

The calcium, magnesium and potassium content of muscle and blood of guinea pigs, rabbits, dogs and cats were determined by Cahane (1927). His data indicate that the calcium of both muscles and blood decreases with age, while magnesium and potassium exhibit no regular changes. In man limited evidence indicates the ratio of K/Ca in the blood of people over 60 tends to be higher.

The phosphorus compounds of blood tend to change in their distribution if a growing rabbit or dog is compared to an adult, according to Bomskow and Nissen (1932). The greatest difference is that of the inorganic phosphorus which is known to be higher in growing animals than in adults. Unfortunately these observations did not extend into old age.

The sodium of the blood does not change with age. Ornstein and Vascauteano (1934) found about the same values at all ages and in both sexes.

The exchange of components between the blood and spinal fluid is not affected by age in the case of man (Katzenelbogen, 1935).

9. CHANGES IN THE COMPOSITION OF TEETH AND BONES WITH AGE

"A fair face will wither; a full eye will wax hollow—*Henry V*.

In one of the early textbooks of biochemistry Berzelius (1831) included a section comparing the composition of the teeth of men of different ages. He even included data upon the teeth of an Egyptian mummy. His table showed the carbonates to have fallen from about 10 to one per cent in the case of an old man, while the calcium phosphate remained about the same. This table also shows more organic matter and less ash in the teeth of a day old baby than in those of an adult.

In modern times Wilton (1931) found the changes in the teeth of guinea pigs suffering from scurvy to be similar to those of old age except the former were reversible. This change consists in degeneration of the odontoblasts. The deposition of the calcium in these cases seems to become amorphous and to lose its ability to form calcium compounds with the protoplasm, "Verkalkung und nicht Kolkbindung entsteht." This author terms "verkalkung" just a calcium precipitation, while "kalkbindung" is a directed formation of protein-calcium compounds.

Wilton also believes the bone changes in scurvy and in ageing to be similar except senile changes proceed much further.

Among the early workers von Bibra (1844) devoted much attention to the changes in the composition of bone with age. He compared the composition of the bones of both men and animals. In birds he noted the increase of ash with age. His tables are also interesting because many analyses were run upon individual bones of the body. In regard to age changes von Bibra states, "Hohes Alter selbst ist gewissermassen ein pathologischer Zustand, und ich habe in der That gefunden, dass die Knochen der meisten Greise etwas erweiterte Markkanälchen, mehr Fett und Zugleich etwas weniger anorganische Substanz zeigen, als Knochen, als Knochen von Individuen des Mittleren Alters." The great variability of the ash in human bones prevented von Bibra from drawing definite conclusions. However, he recognized that the ash increased in the bone after birth. His studies included such diverse species as the ox and fox. Thus he sets an example of work in the field of comparative biochemistry that has been too little used in the intervening century.

Even in the time of von Bibra there was considerable literature dealing with the composition of bone. The interest in bone was probably due to the concept that these structures were more resistant to change than the organs of the body and hence represented more certain reflections of the conditions that accompany ageing. The exchange of the constituents of bone is probably more rapid than has generally been realized. Thus Krogh (1937) found that after a single dose of radioactive phosphorus given to an adult rat that 29 per cent of this appeared in the bones in a week. Part of it also appeared in the teeth. In young, growing rats relatively more was taken up and the exchange was more rapid.

Little attention has been given by the chemist to the organic constituents of either bone marrow or the bone itself.

In advanced age it is known that the fat of the bone marrow is replaced by a semi liquid, gray and translucent material, "gelatinous marrow." The bone marrow is said to comprise 3.4 to 5.9 per cent of the human body, although these values seem high (Jaffe, 1936). About half of the marrow is red and half fat. In other words, the red marrow equals the liver in weight.

The gelatinous marrow seems to result from starvation (Saloin, 1928).

Glikin (1907) found lecithin to be very rich in bone marrow at the time of birth. It then drops to a minimum in old age. Glikin extracted bones with ethyl alcohol on the water bath. The bone was ground and the powder extracted in a soxhlet with chloroform. Phosphorus was determined upon this extract. He ran determinations upon the bone marrow of sheep, cattle, horses, swine, as well as upon human beings. He found the lecithin in the fat as shown in table 44.

Bolle (1910) studied the age variations more extensively than Glikin. He came to the same conclusion, that the phospholipids were high in the marrow of the young in comparison to the old. In certain diseases such as paralysis he found very low values of 0.36 to 1.52 per cent. In one case of tuberculosis, however, more than a third of the marrow fat was phospholipid.

TABLE 44

Lecithin in bone fat

(Glikin)

Species	Age	Num- ber of cases	Lecithin as per cent of bone fat	
			Range	Mean
Beef............................	"Old"	4	1.3 – 2.7	2.4
Calf............................		4	2.9 – 6.8	4.2
Horse..........................	2–18 years	6	0.89– 4.25	1.4
Foal		1		2.1
Swine..........................	Old	3	2.3 – 2.4	2.3
Pigs...........................	Young	5	28.1 –47.2	
Sheep..........................	Old	2	1.7 – 2.6	2.1
Sheep..........................	Young	2	3.7 – 6.5	5.1
Dogs...........................	Old	3	2 – 3.7	3.1
Puppies........................		3	9.5 -37.7	
Men............................	34–88 years	6	1.8 – 3.3	2.4
Children.......................	7–24 months	4	13.4 –61.2	

In a cat, one half year old, he found over 6 per cent of the bone fat was P-lipid, while in cats 1 to 5 years of age the values were 1.27 to 2.05 per cent.

Little attention has been paid to bone fats, although Reichart (1870) found that disease tended to alter the quality as well as the amount of these lipids. Thus he observed a melting point of 43°C. for healthy bone fat and 33°C. for that in certain diseases.

Weiske (1889) found the feathers and bones of birds exhibited marked changes with age.

In chickens the water content of fat free bones changed from 77.6 to 34 per cent from hatching to one year of age. In buzzards, the value dropped to 25.6 per cent. Water value of bird bones tended to be higher than those of mammals. In chicken bones the fat tended to sink with age, while in mammal bones it rose from 1.65 to 22.6 per cent.

The organic part of the fat free bone decreased with age in chickens from 74.4 to 42.9 per cent, while the N of the organic bone substance rose from 14.4 to 16 per cent.

The ash rose with age on a dry, fat free basis but remained lower than that of mammals. In chickens it rose from 25.3 to 57 per cent and in buzzards to 63.6 per cent.

The composition of ash in bird bones showed an increase of CO_2 and calcium with a decrease in magnesium as age progressed. The phosphorus did not change, but the fluorine decreased with age.

In the feathers Weiske noted the loss in water with age. The fat was lower than that for bones and varied considerably. The ash of the feathers showed little change with age, although the calcium tended to rise. The large feathers of the tail were richer in calcium than the others.

Mason (1887) could find no increase of ash with age in human bones nor could he confirm Fremy's view that the increase of organic matter with age was responsible for the fragility.

Wildt (1872) studied the composition of the bones of rabbits from birth to over 3 years of age. Some of his data are reproduced in table 45.

A few of the changes in composition of the ash that were found by Wildt are shown in table 46.

Wildt felt there was little change in adult bone in the course of ageing.

Aeby (1872) studied human as well as animal bones to determine age changes. Between the ages of 19 and 86 he could find no relation between composition and age. His values varied between the following ranges:

per cent

Bound water	10.1–14.7
Specific gravity	1.6– 2.1
CO_2 of ash	1.8– 2.9
Organic	30.1–34.8
Ash	65.2–69.8

His analyses were made upon partly dried bone which contained what he defined as bound water.

He observed slight increases in calcium and specific weight of bones as beef cattle grew older.

Lehman found the organic substance of different bones to vary. Thus in a forty-year-old suicide he found in humerus 31.5, radius 33.8, ulna 33.2, femur 28.6, fibula 34.1, tibia 34.1. Von Bibra (1844) noted various bones of both man and rabbit differed in organic matter.

TABLE 45

Age changes in rabbit bones

(Wildt)

Age	Fresh bones before drying			
	H₂O	Fat	Organic less fat "ossein"	Ash
	per cent	*per cent*	*per cent*	*per cent*
Birth	65.7	0.57	13.6	15.6
3 days	60.2	0.55	16.7	17.2
14 days	62.0	1.65	15.1	18.6
1 month	56.1	1.92	16.3	23.4
2 months	51.4	0.54	15.8	30.1
3 months	51.2	1.61	14.8	30.9
4 months	37.3	5.9	18.1	37.2
6 months	26.7	12.3	17.7	41.8
8 months	26.7	17.4	15.4	39.2
1 year	20.9	18.1	15.4	44.4
2 years	24.7	17.0	15.5	41.7
3–4 years	21.4	16.3	16.1	45.0

TABLE 46

Distribution of elements in bone ash of rabbits

(Wildt)

Age	Per cent of ash			
	CO₂	CaO	MgO	P₂O₅
Birth	3.6	52.2	1.4	42.0
3 days	3.8	52.2	1.4	42.1
1 month	4.0	51.9	1.2	42.2
3 months	4.7	52.5	1.0	41.0
8 months	5.5	52.8	0.9	40.0
3-4 years	5.7	52.8	0.8	39.8

They also noted different bones of the same body to vary by about six per cent in calcium phosphate.

In an extensive study of the bones of a normal dog Schrodt also found considerable variation.

Individual bones within the body of an animal seem to vary in their ability to maintain their composition, according to the findings of Aron and Sebauer (1908) in a dog fed a calcium-poor diet and one fed a normal diet.

This raises the question concerning relative changes in different bones of the body in the course of ageing but no data are available.

Among different species of animals without consideration of age, there is considerable variability in the composition of the bones. Thus

TABLE 47

Composition of bones of two different species

(Morgulis)

	Organic without fat	In bones			In bone ash		
		$CaCO_3$	$\frac{Mg_3}{(PO_4)_2}$	$\frac{Ca_3}{(PO_4)_2}$	$CaCO_3$	$\frac{Mg_3}{(PO_4)_2}$	$\frac{Ca_3}{(PO_4)_2}$
Elk (Ceuris alces)............	29.4	7.20	1.59	62.50	10.19	2.55	88.5
Turtle (Testudo).............	37.2	12.05	1.95	49.85	19.16	3.10	79.4

TABLE 48

Increase of Ca with age in the rib bones and aorta of man

(Bürger and Schlomka)

Rib bone (dry)		Aorta (dry)	
Mean age	Ca	Mean age	Ca
years	*mgm. per cent*	*years*	*mgm. per cent*
6.7	145	6.3	53
24.8	250	29.2	147
32.2	446	44.4	947
44.1	618	64.4	1,155
54.6	1,221	76.0	1,638
65.4	1,399		

Morgulis (1922) found such extremes as those of table 47 in the composition of bones from the elk and the turtle.

The studies of Wildt (1872) were extended slightly by Graffenberger (1891). He analyzed two old rabbits of $6\frac{1}{2}$ to $7\frac{1}{2}$ years of age. In the bones of these animals the water had decreased further to 14–17 per cent. He also found more calcium carbonate and less phosphate.

In the rib bones and aorta of man the calcium seems to increase with age at about the same rate according to Bürger and Schlomka (1928).

These same authors found the dry matter in human rib bones to rise from a value of 20 per cent in newly born to 42 per cent in sixty-five year old people (Bürger and Schlomka, 1927).

The rate of growth of an animal may exert some influence upon the composition of the adult bones. Aron (1911) noted, however, in the case of dogs retarded in growth, that the bones continued to grow and maintain their composition. His retarded animals showed a marked deficiency of fat in the bone marrow, but this was probably the result of starvation.

Miss Outhouse (1933) observed that even in middle life the composition of an animal's bones may reflect the rate of growth. A rat that grew slowly tended to have slightly larger bones in relation to its body size when compared with one that grew rapidly. Furthermore, the bones in the slower growing animal tended to have more solids and more ash. Of two adult rats of body weight of 420 grams each, Miss Outhouse found the one that attained this weight in 148 days had 66.7 per cent of dry matter in its bones, while the slowly growing animal that had taken 279 days to attain the same body weight had 69.4 per cent of dry matter.

Her series of studies showed this result consistently into middle life but unfortunately was not extended into the last half of life.

The bones of rats tend to increase in calcium, phosphorus and carbonate as the animal matures. Thus Kramer and Shear (1928) found the following values for the leg bones.

AGE	Ca	P	CO₂
days	*per cent*	*per cent*	*per cent*
5	15.8	7.2	1.6
46	18.8	7.8	2.6
5 months	21.0	8.9	3.6
Adult (??)	24.1	10.3	4.0

These data indicate that the proportion of calcium carbonate is greater in relation to the calcium phosphate as the rat grows older. Unfortunately these studies did not include the last half of the life cycle.

The increase in carbonate has also been observed in the bones of cattle (Neal et al., 1931).

The ratio between the calcium phosphate and carbonate tends to decrease in value as the animal matures. In their studies with dairy cattle Neal and coworkers obtained the ratios of 7.3 for animals 6–12 months of age and 6.6 for adults.

In the course of growth magnesium is deposited in bones at a different rate from the calcium and phosphorus, according to Hammett (1925a).

In fresh bones at several different ages he observed the following amounts of Ca, P and Mg.

The fate of these elements in the course of old age is unknown. Magnesium is especially interesting because of the consumption of this element by some individuals in France in the hopes of retarding senility.

In considering bone ash in the rat Hammett (1925b) finds a tendency toward a fixed composition in the male at 65 days of age and in the female at 100 days.

TABLE 49

Per cent of element in the fresh bones of rats

(Hammett, 1925a)

Age	Sex	Humerus			Femur		
		Ca	Mg	P	Ca	Mg	P
23	♂	6.1	0.16	3.2	4.8	0.13	2.5
	♀	6.4	0.16	3.3	5.2	0.14	2.7
75	♂	12.5	0.30	6.2	11.6	0.27	5.8
	♀	13.4	0.31	6.7	12.4	0.28	6.3
150	♂	16.2	0.37	8.0	15.4	0.34	7.7
	♀	17.0	0.38	8.3	16.2	0.36	8.0

In growing animals bones increase in ash and organic matter with age. Individual bones progress at slightly different rates in these changes. The following data were taken from a table of Hammett (1925c) (table 50). These data also show the ability of the female to build ash into her bones more rapidly. Hammett did not continue his studies into the latter half of the animal's life.

In the body of the rat about 99 per cent of the calcium is in the bones.

If the percentage composition of the ash is considered, the magnesium is found to decrease in the period from 50 to 65 days of age. This change in the bones of females is about two weeks later than that of males and tends to parallel the water changes. In the ash the per cent of Ca rises and that of P falls as the rat grows from 23 to 150 days.

In rats restricted to a diet low in magnesium, the bone tends to become unusually heavy and richer in ash, Ca and P, according to Orent and others (1934). Unfortunately these studies were only made upon rats up to 55 days of age. The part played by Mg in very old bone remains unknown. The rapid mobilization of Mg when there is a deficiency in the blood of young rats, found by Orent and coworkers, suggests useful experiments for the modification of the bone composition in old animals. In one case of an animal upon a magnesium deficient diet the Mg dropped to a value below 0.1 per cent of the dried bone.

In guinea pigs Tribot (1906) found the bones attained their greatest ash content at 150 days of age and then gradually decreased to 555 days after which they remained constant.

TABLE 50

Composition of rat bones at different ages

(Hammett, 1925c)

Age	Sex	Humerus			Femur		
		Ash	Organic matter	H₂O	Ash	Organic matter	H₂O
days							
23	♂	17.1	18.0	65	13.3	18.3	68.4
23	♀	17.5	19.4	63.1	14.3	19.7	66.0
65	♂	31.5	21.0	47.5	28.3	21.7	50.0
65	♀	31.5	21.0	47.6	28.8	21.3	49.9
150	♂	43.4	22.2	34.4	41.3	23.0	35.7
150	♀	45.1	22.8	32.0	43.0	23.5	33.6

The teeth of a rat lose water and gain in ash continually from 23 to 150 days of age, according to Matsuda. These changes were not followed during old age.

10. TISSUE CULTURE AND THE AGEING OF SERUM

"Old, cold, withered and of intolerable entrails."—*Merry Wives of Windsor.*

The growth stimulating principles of serum change with the age of the animal. In the early studies of Carrel (1913), the superiority of extracts of the embryo in promoting the growth rate of connective tissue in vitro, was observed. He found extracts of the organs of old animals were less effective in stimulating growth than those of young ones.

Furthermore, he found fragments of connective tissue from animals of different ages had different properties of growth. "The velocity of growth always varied in inverse ratio to the age of the animal from which the tissue had been extirpated." However, tissue fragments of different dynamic conditions when placed in identical media tended to assume the same rate of proliferation after a few days.

Carrel postulated that the increase of the growth inhibiting action of serum in the course of life determines a decrease in the activity of white cells. This in turn may modify their secretions.

Carrel was unable to get an exact measure of the age of an animal from the rate of tissue growth. However, in comparing the growth rates of heart and liver tissues in plasma taken from chickens 4 months, 2 years and 5 years old, there was more growth in the youngest plasma. This also proved true for the growth of connective tissue in the serum from a kitten one month old in comparison to that from an old cat. The same phenomenon proved true in testing sera from human beings 20 and 45 years old.

In a study of the relative effectiveness of plasma of chickens ranging in age from 6 weeks to 9 years, Carrel and Ebeling (1921) found the tissue tended to live longer in the younger plasma as well as grow more rapidly. The rate of growth tended to decrease more rapidly than the age increased.

Plasma, according to Carrel and Ebeling (1921), seems to contain both a growth promoting and an inhibiting substance. Heating at 65° increases this inhibiting property more in the case of young than in that of old animals due in part to destruction of the growth promoting factor. Even after heating, the inhibiting power of the older serum is the greater. The carbon dioxide precipitate from the serum of a young animal stimulates growth of fibroblasts while that from an old animal has no activating power.

The experiments of Carrel need to be extended by studies with sera of other species and by biochemical isolation of the factors responsible for the reactions he has observed.

Kotsovsky (1931) found old tissues tended to retard growth. He fed tadpoles with powder from the hearts of old and young animals.

Little additional biological evidence is available showing the effects of age upon such properties as the nutritive value of tissue. However, it is well known that the tissues of adult animals may store large amounts of vitamins whereas the growing animal may consume these factors and have little reserve. Therefore, such observations as those of Kotsovsky may represent crude measurements of such stored factors

Certain elements such as aluminum tend to increase in the animal body as it grows old. In the organs of puppies Underhill and Peterman (1929) could find only traces of Al, while in dogs ranging from 5 to 15 years in age they found the following amounts:

Al in milligrams per 100 grams of tissue

Liver	0.74–1.42
Kidney	0 –0.20
Brain	0.22–0.38
Lung	0.42–5.15

One might expect the lungs to accumulate considerable aluminum in the course of breathing dusts of clay.

Such accumulated elements may prove to be the basis for differences observed in biological testing.

11. SUMMARY

Almost nothing is known of the biochemistry of ageing. However definite advances must be recognized in the discoveries that the life span can be greatly extended by manipulating the diet. Our philosophy need no longer anchor us to the concept of a fixed life span. Evidently there are great gaps in our knowledge of the chemical changes with ageing.

Little hope of progress in studying the process of ageing, can exist until special institutes of research are established in which whole groups of specialists will devote their lives to coöperative attempts to solve the intricate problems. The field of nutrition probably affords the most promising line of attack but specialists in this field must work side by side with the physicists, biochemists, bacteriologists, pathologists, physiologists, histologists and psychologists. Thus far Russia seems to be the only nation that has established such institutes. When these coöperative attacks are made upon the basic problem of age-changes it is likely that the by-products will afford entirely new methods of attacking the diseases of old age such as cancer, arteriosclerosis and those of the heart.

REFERENCES

AEBY, C. 1872a. Ueber die Constitution des phosphorsauren Kalkes der Knochen. J. f. pract. Chem., **5,** 308–311.

———— 1872b. Ueber die Nähern Bestandtheile des Knochenphosphates. *Ibid.*, 169–171.

ARON, H. 1911. Wachstum und Ernährung. Biochem. Zeit., **30,** 207–226.

ARON, H. AND SEBAUER, R. 1908. Untersuchungen über die Bedeutung der Kalksalze für den wachsenden Organismus. Biochem. Zeit., **8**, 1–28.

BAKER, L. E. AND CARREL, A. 1927. Effect of age on serum lipoids and proteins. J. Exper. Med., **45**, 305–318.

BENEDICT, F. G. 1928. Age and basal metabolism of adults. Am. J. Physiol., **85**, 650–664.

———— 1935. Old age and basal metabolism. New England J. Med., **212**, 1111–1122.

BENEDICT, F. G. AND ROOT, H. F. 1934. The potentialities of extreme old age. Proc. Nat. Acad. Sci., **20**, 389–393.

BENEDICT, F. G. AND SHERMAN, H. C. 1937. Basal metabolism of rats in relation to old age and exercise during old age. J. Nutrition, **14**, 179–198.

BERZELIUS, J. J. 1831. Thier-Chemie, Dresden: Arnoldischen Buchhandlung 704, pp.

BEZOLD, A. V. 1857. Untersuchungen über die Vertheilung von Wasser, organischer Materie und anorganischen Verbindungen im Thierreiche. Zeit. f. Wiss. Zool., **8**, 487–524.

BIBRA, F. E. VON. 1844. Chemische Untersuchungen über die Knochen und Zähne. Schweinfurt: Morich'schen Buchdruckerei, 435 pp.

BLATHERWICK, N. R. AND MEDLAR, E. M. 1937. Chronic nephritis in rats fed high protein diets. Arch. Internal Med., **59**, 572–596.

BOLLE, A. 1910. Über den Lecithingehalt des Knochenworks Von Mensch und Haustieren. Biochem. Z., **24**, 179–190.

BOMSKOW, C. AND NISSEN, H. 1932. Über die Verteilung der Phosphorfraktionen im Blut des wachsenden Organismus. Ztschr. f. d. ges. exper. Med., **85**, 142–147.

BOYNTON, RUTH E. AND GREISCHEIMER, ESTHER M. 1930–31. Individual variation in serum calcium in normal men and women. Proc. Soc. Exptl. Biol. Med., **28**, 907–913.

BUNGE, G. VON 1903. Wachstumgeschwindigkeit und Lebensdauer der Säugethiere. Pflüger's Arch. ges. Physiol., **95**, 606–608.

BÜRGER, M. 1934. Die chemischen Alternsveränderungen im Organismus und das Problem ihrer hormonalen Beeinflussbarkeit. Verhandl. d. deutsch. Gesellsch. f. in Med. Kong, **46**, 314–333.

BÜRGER, M. AND SCHLOMKA, G. 1927. Beiträge zur physiologischen Chemie des Alterns der Gewebe. Z. exper. Med., **55**, 287–302.

———— 1928a. Beiträge zur physiologischen Chemie des Alterns der Gewebe. Zschr. ges. exp. Med., **63**, 105–116.

———— 1928b. Ergebnisse und Bedeutung chemischer Gewebsuntersuchungen. Klin. Wchnschr., **7**, 1944–1952.

CAHANE, M. 1927. Teneur du tissu musculaire et du sang en calcium magnesium et potassium au point de vue ilikibiologique. C. R. Soc. Biol., **96**, 1168.

CARREL, A. 1913a. Artificial activation of the growth in vitro of connective tissue. J. Exper. Med., **17**, 14–19.

————. 1913b. Mechanism of the growth of connective tissue. *Ibid.* **18**, 287–299.

CARREL, A. AND EBELING, A. H. 1921a Age and multiplication of fibroblasts. J. Exper. Med., **34**, 599–623.

CARREL, A. AND EBELING, A. H. 1921b. Antagonistic growth principles of serum and their relation to old age. *Ibid.* **38**, 419–425.

CHEN, CHAO-YU 1935. Nutrition Bull. Series B, No. 2, Peiping.

COMRIE, J. D. 1935. Diet in middle age. Brit. J. Phys. Med., **9**, 224–226.

CURRADO, C. 1929. L'Uricemia Nell'eta' senile. Boll. d. Soc. Ital. di biol. sper., **4**, 9–13.

DELBET, P. AND BRETEAU, P. 1930. Vieillissement et magnésium. Bull. Acad. Med. Par., **3s**, 103; 256–266.

DONALDSON, H. H. 1910. On the percentage of water in the brain and in the spinal cord of the albino rat. J. Comp. Neur. Psych., **20**, 119–144.

DONALDSON, H. H. AND HATAI, S. 1931. On the weight of the parts of the brain and on the percentage of water in them according to brain weight and to age, in albino and in wild Norway rats. J. Comp. Neurol., **53**, 263–307.

DUBOIS, E. F. 1936. Basal metabolism in health and disease. Philadelphia: Lea & Febiger. 494 pp.

EDMONDS, T. R. 1832. Life tables founded upon the discovery of a numerical law regulating the existence of every human being illustrated by a new theory of the cause producing health and longevity. London: J. Duncan, 38. pp.

EHRENBERG, R. 1925. Chemische Altersuntersuchungen. Biochem. Z., **164**, 175–182.

FENGER, S. 1904. Beiträge zur Kenntniss des Stoffwechsels im Greisenalter. Skand. Arch. Physiol., **16**, 222–248.

FLOURENS, P. 1855. On Human Longevity, London:

FORSTER, J. 1877. In Voits Untersuchungen der Kost., p. 186. Munich (After E. Koch).

GERRITZEN, P. 1932. Beiträge zur physiologischen Chemie des Alterns der Gewebe. Z. ges. exp. Med., **85**, 700–711.

GLIKIN, W. 1907. Über den Lecithingehalt des Knochenmarks bei Tieren und beim Menschen. Biochem. Zeit., **4**, 235–243.

GRAFFENBERGER, L. 1891. Über die Zusammensetzung der Kaninchenknochen in hohen Alter. Landw. Versuchsst., **39**, 115–126.

GREISHEIMER, E. M., JOHNSON, O. H. AND RYAN, M. 1929. The relationship between serum calcium and age. Am. J. M. Sc., **177**, 704–710.

HAMMETT, F. S. 1925a. A biochemical study of bone growth. J. Biol. Chem., **64**, 685–692.

———— 1925b. A biochemical study of bone growth. *Ibid.* **64**, 693–696.

———— 1925c. A biochemical study of bone growth. *Ibid.* **64**, 409–428.

HATAI, S. 1918. The refractive index of the blood serum of the albino rat at different ages. J. Biol. Chem., **35**, 527–552.

HINDEHEHE, M. 1913. Protein and Nutrition. London: Ewart, Seymour & Co., 201 pp.

HUMMEL, KATHARINE P. AND BARNES, L. L. 1938. Calcification of the aorta, heart and kidneys of the albino rat. Am. J. Path., **14**, 121–124.

HURST, R. E. 1933. The variations in the water and lipids in the bodies of rats of different ages. Cornell: Thesis, 45 pp.

INGLE, L. 1933. Effects of environmental conditions on longevity. Science, **78**, 511–513

JAECKLE, H. 1902. Ueber die Zusammensetzung des menschlichen Fettes. Z. f. Physiol. Chem., **36**, 53–84.

JAFFÉ, F. H. 1936. The bone marrow. J. A. M. A., **107**, 124–129.

JONES, E. L. 1887. On the variations of the specific gravity of the blood in health. J. Physiol., **8**, 1–14.

KATZENELBOGEN, S. 1935. The cerebrospinal fluid and its relation to the blood. Baltimore: Johns Hopkins Press, 468 pp.

KUNDE, M. M. AND NORLUND, M. 1927. Inactivity and age as factors influencing the basal metabolic rate of dogs. Am. J. Physiol., **80**, 681–690.

KELLOGG, V. L. AND BELL, R. G. 1903. Variations induced in larval, pupal and imaginal stages of Bombyx Mori by controlled variations in the food supply. Science, **18**, 741–748.

KISE, Y. AND OCHI, T. 1934. Basal metabolism of old people. J. Lab. & Clin. Med., **19**, 1073–1079.

KOCH, ELIZABETH 1911. Ein Beitrag zur Kenntnis des Nahrungsbedarfs bei alten Männern. Skandin. Arch. F. Physiol., **25**, 315–330.

KOTSOVSKY, D. 1931. Allgemeine vergleichende Biologie des Alters. Ergeb. Physiol., **31**, 132–164.

KRAMER, B. AND SHEAR, M. J. 1928. Composition of bone. J. Biol. Chem., **79**, 147–175.

KROGH, A. 1937. Use of Isotopes as indicators in biological research. Science, **85**, 187–191.

KRÜGER, FR. 1894. Ueber den Schwafel- und Phosphorgehalt der Leber- und Milzzellen in verschiedenen Lebensaltern. Ztsch. Biol., **31**, 400–412.

LANGER, L. 1881. Ueber die chemische Zusammensetzung des Menschenfettes in verschiedenen Lebensaltern. Monatsh. f. Chemie, **2**, 382–397; Jahresber. d. Agrikulturchem., **24**, 389.

LANGSTROTH, L. 1929. Relation of the American dietary to degenerative diseases. J. A. M. A., **93**, 1607–1613.

LAROCHE, G., SCHULMAN, E. ET DESBORDES, J. 1933. L'indoxylémie chez les vieillards. C. R. Soc. Biol., **112**, 290–292.

LOISÈLEUR, J. AND MOREL, R. 1931. Influence de l'age et de l'etat fonctionnel du foie sur la lacticémie. C. R. Soc. Biol., **106**, 35–37.

LOWRY, L. G. 1913. Dry substances in the albino rat. Anat. Rec., **7**, 143–168.

LUSK, G. 1928. Science of Nutrition. Philadelphia: W. B. Saunders Co., 844 pp.

MARINESCO, G. 1913. Mecanisme chimicol—colloïdal de la sénilité et mort naturelle. C. R. Soc. Biol., **65**, II, 582–584.

MARSHALL, F. W. 1931. The sugar content of the blood in elderly people. Quart. J. Med., **24**, 257–284.

MASON, W. P. 1887. Per cent content of bones of different ages in ash. Chem. News, **56**, 132; Jahresber. f. Agriculturchem., **30**, 450.

MATSON, JAMES R. AND HITCHCOCK, F. A. 1934–35. Basal metabolism in old age. Am. J. Physiol., **110**, 329–341.

MATSUDA, Y. 1926–27. A biochemical study of tooth growth. J. Biol. Chem., **71**, 437–444.

MAURICE, H. 1910. Variations avec l'age dans le teneur de quelques organes en phosphore total et en divers corps phosphores. Thesis. Friboug, Switzerland: Fragnière Frères, 75 pp.

McCay, C. M. and Crowell, M. F. 1934. Prolonging the life span. Scientific Monthly, **39**, 405–414.

McCay, C. M., Crowell, M. F. and Maynard, L. A. 1935. The effect of retarded growth upon the length of life span and upon the ultimate body size. J. Nutrition, **10**, 63–79.

McKay, E. M. and McKay, L. L. 1930. Age and the effect of unusual diets. J. Biol. Chem., **86**, 765–771.

McKay, L. L., McKay, E. M. and Addis, T. 1927. Influence of age on degree of renal hypertrophy produced by high protein diets. Proc. Soc. Exp. Biol. Med., **24**, 336–337.

———— 1928. Influence of age on the relation of renal weight to the protein intake and the degree of renal hypertrophy produced by high protein diets. Am. J. Physiol., **86**, 466–470.

McKay, Hughina 1932. Basal metabolism of women over thirty-five years of age. Ohio Sta. Bull., No. **497**, p. 145.

Millet, M. M. and Balle, E. 1932. Sur la valeur hemoglobinique des hematies du vieillard. Helvers. Le Sang, **6**, 735–746.

Milne-Edwards, H. 1862. Lecons sur les physiologie. Paris: Librairie de Victor Masson, 535 pp.; Vol. 7, p. 526.

Morgulis, S. 1922. A comparative study of the composition of the femur. J. Biol. Chem., **50**, li–lii.

Moulton, C. R. 1923. Age and chemical development in mammals. J. Biol. Chem., **57**, 79–97.

Mühlmann, M. 1932–33. Über den Einfluss des Alters auf den Stoffwechsel insbesondere auf die Schwefelsäure in Harn. Deut. Arch. f. Klin. Med., **174**, 432–443.

———— 1927. Wachstum, Altern U. Tod. Zeit. f. Gesamte Anat. **27**, Abt. **3**, 1–245.

Murray, J. A. 1922. The chemical composition of animal bodies. J. Agri. Sci., **12**, 103–110.

Neal, W. M., Palmer, L. S., Eckles, C. H. and Gullickson, T. W. 1931. Effect of age and nutrition on the calcium phosphate/calcium carbonate ratio in the bones of cattle. J. Agri. Research, **42**, 115–121.

Northrup, J. H. 1917. The effect of prolongation of the period of growth on the total duration of life. J. Biol. Chem., **32**, 123–126.

Okey, Ruth, Stewart, Jean M., and Greenwood, Mary L. 1930. The calcium and inorganic phosphorus in the blood of normal women at the various stages of the monthly cycle. J. Biol. Chem., **87**, 91–102.

Orent, E. R., Kruse, H. D. and McCollum, E. V. 1934. Studies of magnesium deficiency in animals. J. Biol. Chem., **106**, 573–593.

Ornstein, I. and Vascauteano, E. 1934. Sur la teneur du sérum sanguin en sodium, au point de vue ilikibiologique. C. R. Soc. Biol., **115**, 1335–1336.

Orr, J. B., Thomson, W. and Garry, R. C. 1935. A long term experiment with rats on a human dietary. J. Hyg., **35**, 476–497.

Osborne, T. B. and Mendel, L. B. 1915. The resumption of growth after long continued failure to grow. J. Biol. Chem., **23**, 439–454.

Outhouse, J. and Mendel, L. B. 1933. The rate of growth. J. Exper. Zool., **64**, 257–285.

PAGE, I. H., KIRK, E., LEWIS, W. H., THOMPSON, W. R., AND VAN SLYKE, D. D. 1935a. Plasma lipids of normal men at different ages. J. Biol. Chem., **111**, 613–639.

———— 1935b. The effect of age on the plasma content of man. *Ibid.* **111**, 641–642.

PARHON, C. J. AND PARHON, M. 1923. Hypercholestérinémie de la vieillesse. C. R. Soc. Biol., **75**, (I), 231–233.

REICHARDT, E. 1870. Mitthelung von der Versuchs-Station zu Jena. Chemische Untersuchung der Knochen von Knochenbrüchigen Rindsvieh. Ann. d. Landw. Wochenbl, *X*, Jahrgang No. 40, 349–353.

REISS, E. 1909. Untersuchungen der Blutkonzentration des Säuglings. Jahrbuch. Kinderk., **70**, 311–362.

ROBERTSON, M. 1907. Metabolism and Practical Medicine. C. v. Noorden. Vol. J. Translated by I. W. Hall. W. T. Keener & Co., Chicago, Ill., 452 pp.

ROBERTSON, T. B. AND RAY, L. A. 1920. On the growth of relatively long lived compared with that of relatively short lived animals. J. Biol. Chem., **42**, 71–107.

ROFFO, A. H. 1925. Cholestérine et hemolyse. C. R. Acad., **180**, 1529–1530.

RŮŽIČKA, V. 1922. Über protoplasma-hysteresis und eine methode zur direkten Bestimmung derselben. Arch. Ges. Physiol., **194**, 135–148.

SABIN, F. R. 1928. Bone marrow. Physiol. Rev., **8**, 191–244.

SCHRODT, M. 1898. Tabulae Biological (W. Junk), Vol. III, pg. 434.

SCHWINGE, W. 1898. Untersuchungen über den Hämoglobingehalt und die Zahl der rothen und weissen Blutkörperchen in den verschiedenen menschlichen Lebensaltern unter physiologischen Bedingungen. Pflüger's Arch. f. Ges. Physiol., **73**, 299–338.

SHERMAN, H. C. AND CAMPBELL, H. L. 1924. Improvement in nutrition resulting from an increased proportion of milk in the diet. J. Biol. Chem., **60**, 5–15.

SHERMAN, H. C., CAMPBELL, H. L. AND RICE, P. B. 1937. Nutritional well-being and length of life as influenced by different enrichments of an already adequate diet. J. Nutrition, **14**, 609–620.

SHERMAN, H. C. AND MACLEOD, F. L. 1925. The Ca content of the body in relation to age, growth and food. J. Biol. Chem., **64**, 428–459.

SLONAKER, J. R. 1912. The effect of a strictly vegetable diet on the spontaneous activity and the longevity of the albino rat. Stanford Univ. Press, 26 pp.

———— 1931. The effect of different per cents of protein in the diet. Am. J. Physiol., **98**, 266–275.

SMITH, A. H. AND MOISE, T. S. 1927a. Diet and tissue growth. J. Exper. Med., **45**, 263–276.

———— 1927b. Diet and tissue growth. *Ibid.* **46**, 27–41.

SONDÉN, K. AND TIGERSTEDT, R. 1895. Die Respiration und der Gesammtstoffwechel des Menschen. Skand. Arch. Physiol., **6**, 1–224.

SSADIKOW, W. S. AND GOLOWTSCHINSKAYA, E. S. 1928. Über den Einfluss des Alters auf die Zusammensetzung der Lipoidfraktion im Tierischen Organismus. Biochem. Z., **202**, 421–438.

STEARNS, G. AND WARWEG, E. 1935. Studies of phosphorus of blood. J. Biol. Chem., **102**, 749–765.

STÖHR, R. 1932. Influence of sex and age upon the glycogen of the muscle and liver, and the alkali reserve of fasting rats. Z. f. Physiol. Chem., **212**, 121–125.

SWANSON, P. P. AND SMITH, A. H. 1932. Total nitrogen of the blood plasma of normal albino rats at different ages. J. Biol. Chem., **97**, 745–750.

THOMAS, K. 1911. (Cited by Ssadikow et al.)

TODD, J. C. AND SANFORD, A. H. 1927. Clinical Diagnosis. Philadelphia: W. B. Saunders Co., 748 pp.

TOYAMA, I. 1919. The relative abundance of serum proteins in albino rats at different ages. J. Biol. Chem., **38**, 161–166.

TRIBOT, J. 1906. Sur les chaleurs de combustion et la composition des os du squelette, en fonction de l'age chez les cobayes. C. R. **142**, 906–907.

UNDERHILL, F. P. AND PETERMAN, F. I. 1929. The relation of age to the amount of aluminum in the tissues of dogs. Am. J. Physiol., **90**, 62–71.

VANZANT, F. R., ALVEREZ, W. C., EUSTERMAN, C. B., DUNN, H. L., AND BERKSON, J. 1932. The normal range of gastric acidity from youth to old age. Arch. Int. Med., **49**, 345–359.

WATCHARN, E. 1933. The normal serum-calcium and magnesium of the rat: Their relation to sex and age. Biochem. J., **27**, 1875–1878.

WEISKE, H. 1889. Untersuchungen über Qualität und Quantität der Vogel-knochen und Federn in verschiedenen Altersstadien. Landw. Versuchsst., **36**, 81; Jahresber d. Agrikulturchem, **32**, 484–486.

WELLS, C. E. 1913. The influence of age and diet on the relative proportions of serum proteins in rabbits. J. Biol. Chem., **15**, 37–41.

WELLS, H. G. 1933. Arteriosclerosis (Editor Cowdry). New York: Mac-Millan, 617 pp.

WILDT, E. 1872. Ueber die Zusammensetzung der Knochen der Kaninchen in den verschiedenen Alterstufen. Landw. Vereuchsst., **15**, 404–454.

WILLIAMSON, C. S. AND ETS, H. N. 1926. Effect of age on the hemoglobin of the rat. Am. J. Physiol., **77**, 480–482.

WILTON, A. 1931. Die Veränderung der Bindegewebssubstanzen bei C-Hypo-vitaminose und Senilität. Acta path. et microbiol. Scandinav., **8**, 258–313.

ZONDEK, S. G. AND KARP, S. 1934. The relationship of iron with the aging of cells. Biochem. J., **28**, 587–591.

Chapter 22

AGEING OF HOMEOSTATIC MECHANISMS

WALTER B. CANNON

Boston

Homeostasis is the condition of relative constancy in the fluid matrix, i.e., the extracellular fluids in the bodies of higher animals. It is found best developed in birds and mammals. It includes steady states of temperature, glucose and calcium concentrations, acid-alkali balance, salt and water and protein content, and osmotic pressure, primarily of the blood. The general effect of these steady states is to provide the living cells of the organism with a fairly constant environment, in spite of changes in the outer world and also in spite of internal disturbances such as may be induced by muscular activity, e.g., the utilization of glucose, the evolution of heat and the production of non-volatile acid.

1. SIGNIFICANCE OF HOMEOSTASIS

Obviously, physiological mechanisms for maintaining homeostasis are not required by the developing mammal before birth. Vigorous exertion does not occur, and the immediate environment of the fetus *in utero* is kept constant by the homeostatic devices in the mother's organism. The fetus has fluid contacts which do not differ greatly from its own internal fluids. At birth, however, the infant is suddenly introduced into gaseous, cold, rough surroundings; a gasp draws into the lungs a thin, dry air and thereafter every inward breath cools by itself and by favoring evaporation, and every outward breath carries away water vapor and carbonic acid. To preserve a steady state of the fluid matrix in this strange and foreign world requires physiological operations which have not previously been exercised. Time is required to render them efficient. In the new-born, therefore, exposure to even moderate cold causes a sharp drop of body temperature. And the blood-sugar concentration of the infant oscillates from day to day and from hour to hour much more than that of the adult (Schretter and Navinney, 1930). In the course of time the homeostatic regulators, repeatedly utilized and put to test, reach a high degree of perfection.

Through childhood, youth and the early decades of adult life the capacity of the organism to meet the stresses due to external vicissitudes and internal perturbations, which might profoundly affect behavior, is remarkable. Men may ascend to heights where the oxygen tension is half that at sea level, they may expose themselves to torrid heat, they may by supreme exertion produce enough lactic acid to overwhelm quickly the buffering alkali of the blood, and yet suffer no great diminution in their ability to continue activity. Physiological adjustments occur which compensate for the low oxygen tension, protect against overheating, and burn the lactic acid to volatile carbonic acid which is readily breathed away (cf. Cannon, 1929, 1932). The admirable devices, whereby these compensatory corrective actions maintain homeostasis, will be briefly described, in order that the alterations which take place in old age may be understood. The description will be confined to the mechanisms which preserve constancy of temperature, blood sugar, and the hydrogen-ion concentration (the balance of acid and alkali). These are best known.

2. SURVEY OF SOME HOMEOSTATIC MECHANISMS

Uniformity of *body temperature* is maintained by regulation of heat production and heat loss. The continuous production of heat is dependent on the chemical processes occurring in the bodily economy— the tonic contraction of skeletal muscles, the rhythmic contractions of the heart and the diaphragm, and the functioning of glandular organs. Underlying these metabolic activities is the persistent secretion of the thyroid gland; if that fails the metabolic rate and the consequent output of heat may be reduced as much as 40 per cent.

When a normal warm-blooded animal is exposed to cold and therefore begins to lose heat, the internal temperature tends to fall. Thereupon the surface blood vessels are contracted, with the result that warm blood from the interior of the body is less exposed to cooling. Furthermore, adrenine is secreted by the adrenal medulla (Freeman, 1935), and that accelerates the burning processes in the organism (Boothby and Sandiford, 1923). And if this conservation and this extra production of heat are not sufficient to maintain a temperature homeostasis, shivering—which, like all muscular movement, liberates heat—is automatically induced. In addition to these inherent physiological adjustments there are behavioral adaptations, such as engaging in vigorous work, putting on additional covers, curling up or making contacts to reduce the bodily surface exposed to cold, or seeking a warm place. Thus, by speeding up the rate of internal combustion and reducing the outflow of heat, the fluid matrix of birds and mammals is kept relatively constant, and they are freed from the limitations imposed during the winter season on cold-blooded vertebrates, which must hibernate in sluggish inactivity.

In hot weather when the bodily temperature tends to rise the homeostatic reactions are in the opposite direction, i.e., muscular tone seems to be diminished, and certainly inactivity is the natural state; in consequence the processes of heat production are minimized. Also heat dissipation is accelerated by the outpouring of sweat which by evaporation cools the skin, and also by the dilation of superficial vessels and the attendant exposure of warm blood to the cool surface. When in a torrid, humid atmosphere the heat which is necessarily set free by functioning muscles and glands cannot be transferred to the surrounding air, homeostasis no longer prevails and the internal temperature may rise dangerously in a so-called "heat stroke."

Unlike temperature regulation, which is managed by changing the rates of continuous processes, the regulation of *blood sugar* is controlled by storage when glucose is plentifully supplied from the food, by release when there is need, and by overflow and wastage at times of excess. The greatest storage, which occurs in the liver, is dependent on proper functioning of the islet cells of the pancreas; at least, glycogen is not deposited there if those cells are absent. Normally the glycogen reserve is set free from the hepatic cells by action of the sympatho-adrenal system. Besides these factors the anterior pituitary gland and the thyroids have a regulatory influence the nature of which is not yet clear. Ordinarily the concentration of glucose in the blood is approximately 90 milligrams in 100 cc. (milligrams per cent). If the concentration becomes twice as great, glucose ordinarily begins to pass the kidney threshold and appear in the urine; if the usual concentration is much reduced a "hypoglycemic reaction" sets in, with sympatho-adrenal involvement, and the release of glucose from the hepatic glycogen reserves. This protects against a dangerously low glycemic level.

The homeostatic mechanisms for assuring a proper *acid-base balance* in the blood are called into action whenever there is a shift from the regular mildly alkaline state. Because of the continuous production of non-volatile acid in the organism the chief danger is a shift towards acidity. If the blood becomes even slightly acid, coma supervenes, and possibly death. This danger is obviated, as previously noted, by burning the non-volatile acid to volatile carbonic acid and expelling the volatile gas in the expired breath. The burning depends on an *adequate supply of oxygen* to the tissues where activity is accompanied by setting free non-volatile acid waste. A condition which puts to a test the regulatory mechanisms for maintaining the proper reaction of the blood is very vigorous muscular exertion which results in producing so much acid waste that the oxygen delivery is inadequate. In this condition the heart beats more rapidly, the blood pressure rises, the circulation rate is increased, the number of red blood corpuscles is augmented—all being changes which make the blood a more effective carrier of oxygen from lungs to active structures. Accompanying these changes is a deeper and more rapid respiration which brings a greater supply of oxygen to be taken up by the red corpuscles in the walls of the pulmonary air sacs, and which drives forth a greater amount of carbon dioxide. When in great muscular effort these mechanisms prove incapable of meeting the requirements of the organism, acid accumulates and may induce a state in which there results a lessened capacity to labor and which is commonly called "fatigue."

3. LIMITATIONS OF HOMEOSTATIC MECHANISMS

The foregoing review has illustrated the dictum that "uniformity of the internal environment is the condition for free and independent life." So long as the automatic mechanisms which preserve that uniformity are efficient, man can go about his business without much concern with the intimate circumstances which are optimum for his activity—within limits it makes little difference where he goes and what he does, those circumstances are kept fit for effective performance of bodily functions. Of course, there are limits. External temperature may be so high or so low as to overwhelm the corrective agencies of the organism, and thereby may cause death by heat-stroke or by freezing. Similarly acid may be produced in such abundance that coma results. But the rarity of these events emphasizes the extraordinary ability of the homeostatic mechanisms to maintain, inside a reasonable range, a steady state in the fluid matrix.

When the later years of life are reached evidence indicates that homeostasis is not affected to any marked degree. Body temperature is at the usual level; likewise blood-sugar concentration and the acid-base relation. What is altered is the effectiveness of the physiological factors which preserve stability. They become impaired, and consequently, although homeostasis is retained, it is retained within a narrower range. That statement will be illustrated.

4. TEMPERATURE REGULATION IN OLD AGE

That internal temperature is maintained within the usual slight variations in elderly persons has been shown by Schlesinger (1914) and confirmed by Hirsch (1926). Martsinkovski and Zhorova (1936) tested 185 individuals between 60 and 100 years of age and found no change with advancing years. The skin may feel cooler than the body temperature would lead the observer to expect, but that condition results from the poorer circulation in the skin of the aged.

Homeostasis of temperature is achieved, as already noted, by varying the rate of the continuous processes of heat production and heat loss. Fundamentally, heat production is due to the chemical changes attending the physiological processes of the organism. The common measure of these processes is the metabolic rate, determined under standard conditions of rest and absence of digestive and absorptive activity. In the later years of life the metabolic rate diminishes. The first observations by Magnus-Levy and Falk (1899) which led to that conclusion have been repeatedly confirmed by more recent, more extensive and more exact studies. The largest accumulation of pertinent data is that compiled by Boothby, Berkson and Dunn (1936) on the basis of metabolism determinations on 639 male and 828 female human subjects, selected as normal from determinations made under Boothby's direction on more than 80,000 subjects. There were fewer cases in the upper than in the lower half of the age range, which extended from 6 to 64 years among males, and from 6 to 68 years among females. The mean calories per square meter per hour at age 20 was 41.6 for men and 36.3 for women. At age 40 it had dropped to 38.3 and 35.5 respectively; and at age 60 it was down to 35.7 and 32.8—a reduction in each sex of about 9.3 per cent. Matson and Hitchcock (1934) reported that the average basal metabolic rate of 14 men with ages between 74 and 92 was 30.11, a figure not noteworthily changed by including Benedict's (1935) results from study of 5 men between ages 74 and 87. It appears that in men the fall in standard metabolism from early adulthood to late senescence might readily reach 25 per cent. Benedict's study included 36 elderly women; he found that the average metabolic rate at 66 years was 32 calories per square meter per hour—a figure close to Boothby's 32.8. At age 88 the figure in Benedict's cases was about 28—a decrease of 23 per cent in women from that at age 20. The gradual drop in basal metabolism was demonstrated also by Kisé and Ochi (1934) in an examination of 94 Japanese—44 men, 50 women—50 to 93 years old; they declare that the rate of decrease is from 3 to 5 per cent for each successive ten-year period. It is well to remember that all these figures are averages and that an old man or woman may have a metabolic rate quite close to that of middle age.

The reasons for the reduced speed of heat production in elderly persons are probably various, but pertinent among them are indications of partial involution of the thyroid gland. According to Dogliotti and Nizzi (1935) the number of follicles is reduced in the aged, and the colloid may be less and the epithelium hypertrophied in those which remain. Warren (1937), who has had large experience in examining the thyroids of people of advanced years, also has noticed clusters of very small follicles with little colloid and lined with cuboidal epithelium, but in addition clusters of colloid-distended follicles, several times the normal size, lined with flat epithelium. There is also likely to be a progressive increase of the lymphoid infiltration of the stroma of the gland together with an increase of fibrous tissue, as age advances into the seventh decade. Dogliotti and Nizzi regarded the hypertrophied follicles as a response to the low metabolism; they may be a response to the involutionary changes elsewhere in the thyroid. Obviously, on this point more information is needed.

Lessened muscular vigor is probably another reason for diminished heat output. Muscular weakness is typical of the later period of life; according to Quetelet the ability to lift has declined about 40 per cent at age 60 as compared with maximal ability between 25 and 35 (cf. Rubner, 1928). When the environment is chilly, weakness of muscles, together with habits of inaction, would render a compensatory increment of heat release in the body by physical exertion less reliable and less effective than in youth and middle age. Although all causes of reduced basal metabolism have not yet been determined, the fact that there is a lessening of the heat output reveals a limiting factor in the temperature homeostasis of the elderly person. In these circumstances, therefore, he will protect his body temperature against a fall by wearing more clothing than he used to wear, or, more characteristically than the youth, he will seek a place near a stove or open fire or other source of heat.

Besides the diminished ability to adapt themselves to cold there is not infrequently among old people a diminished ability to adapt themselves to heat. When the external temperature is high there may be real distress, much more marked in old than in younger individuals, because of difficulty of getting rid of the heat which is constantly being produced in the body. This difficulty is more marked in the *habitus corporis senilis luxus* than in the *habitus strictus* because of the layer of superficial fat under the skin in the former.

As previously noted, the process of heat loss is accelerated by sweating and by a dilation of peripheral blood vessels that allows a larger volume of blood to flow through the skin, cooled by sweating or by exposure to cool air. In old age the skin commonly undergoes a marked atrophy, attended by dryness, roughness and loss of elasticity. Also atrophy and partial disappearance of dermal capillaries have been observed (Wolbach, 1937), as concurrent degenerative changes occur in collagen and elastic tissue. "Patriarchal pallor" has been attributed to the consequent reduction of blood circulating in the surface vessels. Partial degeneration of the sweat and sebaceous glands has likewise been described (cf. Hirsch, 1926). In addition there are changes in the arteries and arterioles as age advances. Sclerosis occurs, with thickening of the intima and fibrosis of the media. Thus the size of the vascular bed, in conditions which would produce vasodilation, is reduced. All these factors, working together, interfere with a ready discharge of heat from the body. In studies on the maximal heat elimination from the hand Pickering (1936) found that under standard conditions the output in calories per minute per unit volume was about 33 per cent lower at age 70 than at age 25. Concordant with this evidence is the observation that the death rate from "heat stroke" or heat hyperpyrexia for age groups rises to a noteworthy degree after age 60 and thereafter rises sharply; in Massachusetts, between 1900 and 1930, it was about 8 per 100,000 for the age decade 70–79, about 22 for 80–90, and about 80 for 90–100. Similar results are reported for New York and Pennsylvania (Shattuck and Hilferty, 1932).

The foregoing considerations reveal gradually restricted powers of adjustment to both low and high external temperature as old age progresses. The body temperature, with moderate conditions, is maintained within its usual range of diurnal variation. But the limits of adaptation tend to become gradually narrower as one passes through the seventh decade to the later years of life.

5. REGULATION OF BLOOD SUGAR IN OLD AGE

Homeostasis of blood sugar, as already noted, is achieved by storage in times of plenty, by release in times of need and by overflow through the kidneys in times of excess. The common method of determining the efficacy of the mechanisms for storage and use of blood sugar is the "glucose tolerance" test. On an empty stomach a standard solution of glucose (100 or 50 grams, according to body size) is swallowed by the subject; at half-hour intervals thereafter the concentration of sugar in the blood is ascertained; in normal young adults the concentration follows a curve which rises sharply during the first half-hour to about 160–170 mgm. per cent, and then gradually returns to the previous level in about two hours. When the homeostatic mechanisms for glucose are defective, as in diabetes, the typical curve is altered; it rises higher than in normal individuals and persists for a much longer time.

In 1926, Porter and Langley made tests on 50 normal individuals, 10 in each decade from 30 to 80 years. They reported (1) that the basal glucose level in the blood of fasting persons tends to rise from about 80 mgm. per cent in youth to nearly 150 mgm. in the eighth decade; (2) that in the five decades represented by the subjects the maximal glycemic concentration during the test is likely to be delayed, so that it is reached at the end of an hour instead of the first half-hour after the glucose is ingested; (3) that there is an increasing delay in the return to the fasting level—it fails to return in two and a half hours; (4) that in the decade 30–40 years, the test does not result in glycosuria, i.e., overflow through the kidneys does not occur, but that in the higher decades glycosuria occurs in about 30 per cent of the tests (in the decade 60–70 years appearing in about 40 per cent); (5) that in senile cases (70–80 years old) the glycemic curve does not rise so high but is more prolonged than the curve for the cases between 60 and 70.

Observations supporting, to some degree, the foregoing results were made by Marshall (1931). In a study of 28 healthy old men the glucose tolerance test showed that 4 had quite normal glycemic curves; 20 were abnormal. Of these 20, 11 manifested a "storage deficit," i.e., a lengthening of the curve so that it did not return to the fasting level in two hours. There were 7 cases of "lag curves," with the blood sugar rising slowly but exceeding the kidney threshold, and 2 cases of "flat curves," resulting probably from slow absorption. In the group of cases 4 responded to the test with a typical diabetic curve; the maximal concentration of glucose was higher than 240 mgm. per cent and the fasting concentration was not regained in $2\frac{1}{2}$ hours. In young people, he states, this reaction to the test would justify a diagnosis of diabetes.

That the glucose tolerance test yields a higher blood sugar in elderly persons was found also by Romcke (1931). In ten cases between 61 and 70, and in cases over 70 years of age, the maximal rise was greater than in lower age groups, and in these upper age groups also appeared the most marked glycosuria. He found no noteworthy differences in the fasting blood sugar at different ages. Similar results were reported by John (1934) after 1727 tests performed on persons of different ages; the "diabetic type" of curve rose from about 10 per cent of the cases in the fourth decade to about 50 per cent in the seventh. In a study of 192 children and 1500 adults, he found that 82 per cent of the children had normal curves, as contrasted with only 62 per cent of the adults.

Nitzulescu, Ornstein and Sibi (1933), who examined 40 subjects between 50 and 85 years of age, did not find any variations of the glycemic curves corresponding to the advancement of age. With the exception of these results, the data reported indicate that there is prone to be a definite impairment of the ability of the human organism in the later years of life to use and store glucose at the rate which prevails in youth and early manhood. According to Marshall (1931), the renal threshold rises from 170–180 mgm. per cent in young adults to 200–210 mgm. per cent in the healthy aged. The overflow would therefore be less when the glycemic level rises. Even this conservative change may not be sufficient, however, to prevent a loss of sugar from the body if an amount is ingested by old people that would be quite effectively used or stored by the young.

Marshall attributed the slow descent of the curve of glycemia in the glucose tolerance tests of some aged persons to defective storage in the liver. That is an inference, however, and though it may be true, the explanation is not forthcoming. Indeed, present knowledge of the factors affecting the glycemic level is in transition, and until further progress has been made a surmise regarding the nature of the limitation of homeostatic control in the final decades would be futile. The fact of limitation appears to be well established.

6. REGULATION OF THE ACID-BASE BALANCE IN OLD AGE

The chief homeostatic mechanisms concerned in maintaining uniformity of the chemical reaction of the blood are, as already noted, the lungs, the heart and the blood vessels. Non-volatile acid, which, if allowed to accumulate, would reduce the alkaline reserve and endanger physical efficiency, is normally burned to carbonic acid and then readily eliminated. The burning process requires abundance of oxygen. The increased oxygen supply to the active tissues is dependent on an increased depth and rate of respiration and on an increased speed of the blood flow between lungs and periphery. The faster flow of blood depends, in turn, on an increased heart rate, an increased arterial pressure and dilation of vessels in active parts. An augmentation of the number of red corpuscles may also play a significant rôle. All these factors are likewise quite as important for carrying more carbonic acid from the tissues as for carrying more oxygen to them.

It has long been known that advancing age is associated with definite reduction of the respiratory functions of the lungs. In his classical studies on "vital capacity" (i.e., the measurement of the greatest amount of air which can be forced voluntarily from the lungs after the deepest intake) Hutchinson (1846) found, in 1775 healthy cases, that after the age 30–35 it gradually falls until at 60–65 it is only 80 per cent of the earlier figure. In the ninety-odd years since Hutchinson's report many investigators have confirmed his results. For the period above age 60 Levy (1933) has recently reported on examinations of 110 men 60–94 years old and on 71 women 60–92. The normal vital capacity of young adult men ranges as a rule between 3000 and 4000 cc., and of women between 2000 and 3000. The average figures, derived from a table giving the data of many tests on persons of various nationalities, were, for males 3750 cc., for females 2600 cc. (cf. Ebina, Kajiwara and Kikuchi, 1937). Levy's observations yielded the following average results:

Ages	Males	Females
60–65	2,980	1,985
71–75	2,715	1,736
81–85	2,412	1,652
86–90+	2,350	1,460

This consistent testimony of investigators in different lands and conditions has revealed that a limitation of the ability to expand and contract the thorax, and therefore a drop in the *maximal* to-and-fro movement of respired air, is a striking feature of old age, and that it is likely to be more marked the older the individual.

Associated with the limitation of vital capacity in the last decades of life is a limitation of the amount of air breathed in and out during maximal muscular work. In studies of such work, performed by men of different ages, Dill and Robinson (1938) have found that as the vital capacity is reduced in elderly men the augmented ventilation of the lungs, due to supreme exertion, is reduced correspondingly or to an even greater degree.

The lessened mobility of the thoracic wall is attributed in part to a weakening of the intercostal muscles, but especially to a stiffening of the attachments of the ribs. According to Bürger and Schlomka (1927) the water content of the costal cartilages diminishes with age, and the calcium content increases. They found that whereas the calcium of the cartilages (in mgm. per cent of dry substance) was only 125 in the second decade of life, it was 617 in the fifth, and 1399 in the seventh decade. Besides this greater rigidity of the thoracic wall there is the effect of lack of exercise and of indolent habits in the elderly which would tend to reduce the ability to engage in vigorous and ample respiratory movements lasting a considerable period.

The resting blood pressure quite commonly rises as men and women pass the age 30–40. Numerous references to observations on arterial pressure in the later years of life might be cited (see, e.g., Bowes, 1916; Richter, 1925; Sachs, 1927; Kachebries, 1933). In a statistical study of a large number of cases (about 4000) Saller (1928) found that blood-pressure measurements are more variable than other measurements because methods vary and uncontrolled disturbing conditions may influence the subjects. Nevertheless, a critical survey shows a gradual rise in average systolic pressure as years pass, with little change in diastolic pressure. His summarizing figures are as follows:

Age	Systolic-diastolic pressure	
	Men	Women
21–35	144–98	138–99
35–47	144–98	155–100
48–53	154–96	190–100
54–59	159–97	196–104
60–67	173–93	216–102
68–89	186–86	222–112

These figures are higher than those given by some other investigators (e.g., Kachebries, 1933). They are illustrative of the general testimony, however, and they indicate, furthermore, that the pressure tends to go up earlier in women than in men. The greater arterial tension may not be at all due to arteriosclerosis, though Norris and Landis (1920) express the opinion that when it rises above 160 mm. of mercury the condition is pathological, whatever the age.

Another method of learning the state of the arteries is that of determining the velocity of the pulse wave. Bramwell, Hill and McSwiney

(1923), in an examination of 74 healthy individuals with ages ranging from 5 to 84 years, found that the rate of the wave varied from 5.2 meters per second at 5 years to 8.5 at 84 years, an increase of more than 60 per cent. Using Bramwell and Hill's formula for relating the volume of the artery to the velocity of the pulse wave they estimated that the mean elasticity of the arteries expressed as 0.47 at 5 years was only 0.17 at 80. The systolic pressure rises, therefore, as the arteries become less elastic in old age; and, since the diastolic pressure does not greatly change, the pulse pressure also rises. Using a more delicate method of recording the pulse wave Hallock (1934) made observations on nearly 400 persons with ages ranging between 5 and 65 years. The figures given by him for the radial pulse, as determined in 553 records, and the figures given by Bramwell, Hill and McSwiney, from their 74 cases, show a close correspondence up to age 45. Thereafter Hallock's figures show a faster rate, indicating a greater loss of elasticity in senescence than was noted in the smaller group of subjects. If the condition of increased rigidity of the arteries in old age prevails everywhere in the body, the expansion of arterioles in active muscles, for example, would not occur in the elderly as it occurs in youths. Thus, for that reason alone, there might be a failure of muscular performance that required quick, vigorous and rapidly repeated action, such as sprinting.

It is probable that in old age the functions of the capillaries also may be impaired. In an examination of a variety of muscles Buccianti and Luria (1934) found that in old persons there is a laying down of interstitial colloid and a thickening of the sheath of elastic tissue which envelopes the individual muscle fibers. The capillaries lie in this interfibrillar region. Even if they should dilate in the usual manner when the muscle becomes active the diffusion of the respiratory gases (especially oxygen, which has a low diffusion coefficient compared with carbon dioxide) might meet obstruction because of interposed extravascular material.

In consideration of the frequency of death from "heart failure" ignorance of the ability of the heart to meet emergencies in old age is surprising. Pathologists have described both hypertrophy and atrophy of the senile heart. In Councilman's (1919) study of the hearts of 580 persons over 60 years of age, he found hypertrophy in 43 per cent. In 94 of the 580 cases the blood pressure was known; among these the average systolic level was 158 mm. of mercury in the hypertrophic cases, and only 130 mm. in the non-hypertrophic. The two conditions of high pressure and cardiac hypertrophy may be causally related (the former conditioning the latter), but that is not proved.

Few actual tests of the capacity of the old heart to adapt itself to special stress seem to have been made. Recently Dill and Robinson (1938) have subjected 91 boys and men, with ages ranging from nearly 6 to nearly 70 years, to running on a treadmill having a grade of 8.6 per cent. The speed of the mill was varied according to the ability of the individuals to run. Nearly all of them were exhausted in 3 to 5 minutes. For purposes of comparison the subjects were divided into ten groups. The mean of the maximal heart rates of a group of 9 boys having an average age of 14.2 years was 196 beats per minute; whereas in a group of 7 men with an average age of 63 the mean maximal rate was 163—a reduction of about 17 per cent. Between these two figures the records showed a continuous downward trend, i.e., a continuous failure of the heart to meet the demands of supreme exertion by as fast a beat as in youth or early adult life.

It is quite possible that even when beating at the relatively less rapid maximal rate in the late decades the heart is not working so efficiently as in the twenties and thirties. There is evidence that a vigorous heart meets an extra stress (in exercise, e.g.) by more nearly complete emptying of the ventricles with each systole rather than by great acceleration; the "hypodynamic" heart of the inactive individual, on the other hand, dilates in the same circumstances and, discharging relatively less per beat, compensates by beating rapidly (Wiggers, 1923). The slow movements of elderly people and their relative indolence as compared with the young would seem to be favorable to the development in cardiac function of that type of response to extra demand in which the burden of maintaining an increased blood flow per minute is borne by an increase in heart rate. On this point more evidence is needed. If the hypodynamic condition should be proved typical of the old, there would be a double limitation in the cardiac factor, for an inability to empty the ventricles almost completely would be added to an inability to accelerate as formerly.

A survey of the chief agencies concerned in maintaining homeostasis of the acid-base balance—lungs, blood vessels and heart—shows that as life proceeds to its later stages there is likely to be in each of these organs a narrowing of the capacity to adjust for special requirements. A routine existence within the limits of easy adaptation may continue indefinitely without revealing any weakness; but exposure to a stress which encroaches on the limits quickly discloses that they have become much restricted.

Illustrative examples will bring out the nature of the restrictions imposed by advancing years. Mori (1936) subjected men of various ages between 17 and 57 years to standard exercise for 10 minutes on a bicycle ergometer. He found that in 4 youths of the second decade there was a reduction of the alkaline reserve of the blood by about 4 volumes per cent of carbon dioxide; in 13 persons of the fifth decade the reduction was about 12 volumes per cent. Unfortunately the presence of lactic acid was not investigated. It is reasonable to assume, however, that in the circumstances the decreased alkaline reserve was due mainly to increased lactic acid. Dill and Robinson (1938), for example, have observed that when subjects of different ages are made to perform the same work (walking on a treadmill at the rate of 3.5 miles per hour, up a grade of 8.6 per cent, thus increasing basal metabolism about seven-fold), the extra amount of lactic acid demonstrable in the blood was nearly 3.5 as much at about age 60 as it was at 20. These marked changes may be interpreted as due to a larger failure in older men, compared with younger, to deliver sufficient oxygen to the active muscles to burn the non-volatile acid. Significant data bearing on this explanation have been obtained by Dill and Robinson (1938) in their study of boys and men made to perform on a treadmill the hardest work of which the subjects were capable. The ability of the respiratory and circulatory systems to supply oxygen was measured during each minute of the test. The highest figure was obtained at age 17 when the median amount of oxygen carried away from the lungs per minute by the blood was about 53 cc. per kilogram of body weight. At age 35 the figure was about 43 cc.; at 50 it was about 37; and at 63 it was down to 35 cc., a reduction of 34 per cent. This steady decline is what might be expected as the consequence of a gradual lessening of the ventilation of the lungs, a diminishing adjustment of the blood vessels, and a gradual failure of the heart to keep its rapid beat as the decades pass, though men put forth their utmost efforts.

Further evidence of the narrowing limits of adaptation of the respiratory and circulatory apparatus, when called upon in emergencies, is found in the results of competitive sports. Sprinting records are held by young men, commonly in their 'teens or early twenties; the 100-yard dash was first run in 9.4 seconds by Wykoff when he was 21. The records for distances from 1 to 5 miles are held by men whose ages range between 23 and 27 years. The 10-mile record was made by Nurmi at age 31. De Mar, who ran Marathon races many times between his twenty-second and forty-ninth year, made his best showings between 36 and 42. Thus, the figures reveal that as less speed is required, and judgment and endurance still count, the records are taken by older men. But there comes a limit. Professional base-ball players, for example, as a rule after 35 begin to "slow up," "their legs fail them,"[1] "they lose the speed they had earlier" (McGillicuddy, 1937). The same rule appears to be true for expert tennis players who, like base-ball players, have to make quick moves and sudden adjustments while in continuous action; even the most notable, who continue to be first-rate until the late thirties or early forties, usually have their peak of ability between 25 and 30. "Few have been stars in any sport after 40" (Rice, 1937). Even in the army enlistment is ordinarily limited to the years between 20 and 35; the possible heavy stresses of a campaign are not well borne by older men.

7. SUMMARY

The data presented in the foregoing pages have shown that homeostasis of the fluid matrix of the human organism is preserved in old age; no noteworthy alteration of body temperature, of the glucose content or of the hydrogen-ion concentration of the blood is manifest in senescence as compared with adolescence and middle age. There is, however, a progressive impairment of the regulatory devices which develops in most individuals as the decades pass after about the fortieth year.

The regulation of body temperature becomes more difficult in a cold environment because of a reduced metabolic rate and lessened muscular vigor, and in a hot environment because of a limited ability to dissipate heat through skin in which capillaries may be degenerated, and in which sweat glands may be deficient and arterioles contracted.

The regulation of blood sugar is impaired to a degree which may result in the glucose tolerance test yielding a high, prolonged concentration of glucose in the blood, similar to the condition in diabetes and attended by glycosuria.

The regulation of the acid-base balance, in vigorous exertion, for

[1] This expression is commonly used. Obviously running involves more than the legs. And, as shown above, the other factors which are involved in keeping the circulating blood fit for strenuous effort—the heart and lungs, especially—do not maintain in senescence the quick and effective adaptive ability manifested in youth and early manhood. For further evidence see H. C. Lehman's article, "The Most Proficient Years at Sports and Games," Reasearch Quarterly (American Association for Health and Physical Education), 1938, **9,** 3–19.

example, is affected by a reduced maximal to-and-fro movement of the air in respiration, less adaptable blood vessels, diminished ability of the heart to accelerate and probably by a "hypodynamic" state of that organ. In consequence rapidly repeated muscular efforts, involving the large muscles of the body, are not attended by so large an oxygen supply to the active muscles as is found in youth and young manhood; the alkaline reserve is reduced and the actual performance, as shown, for example, in competitive sports, which require quick responsiveness of the adjusting mechanisms of the respiratory and circulatory systems, does not match in the fourth and fifth decades that of earlier periods.

The condition of the homeostatic mechanisms in old age can be summarized in the statement that when subjected to stress they are revealed as being more and more narrowly limited in their ability to preserve uniformity of the internal environment of the living parts.

It is well to reiterate the warning that statements regarding bodily functions in old age are generalizations, based on average figures, and that many exceptions to them are found. It is well to emphasize also that more evidence is needed on numerous points considered in this chapter, before knowledge of the limitations of homeostatic mechanisms in senescence is quite satisfactory.

REFERENCES

BENEDICT, F. G. 1935. Old age and basal metabolism. New England J. Med., 212, 1111–1122.

BOOTHBY, W. M., BERKSON, J., AND DUNN, H. L. 1936. Studies of the energy metabolism of normal individuals. Am. J. Physiol., 116, 468–484.

BOOTHBY, W. M. AND SANDIFORD, I. 1923. The calorigenic action of adrenalin chloride. Ibid. 66, 93–123.

BOWES, L. M. 1916–17. Blood pressure in the aged. J. Lab. and Clin. Med., 2, 256–259.

BRAMWELL, J. C., HILL, A. V., AND McSWINEY, B. A. 1923. The velocity of the pulse wave in man in relation to age. Heart, 10, 233–255.

BUCCIANTI, L. AND LURIA, S. 1934. Trasformazioni nella struttura dei muscoli volontari dell'uomo nella senescenza. Arch. Ital. di Anat. e di Embriol., 33, 110–187.

BÜRGER, M. AND SCHLOMKA, G. 1927. Untersuchungen am menschlichen Rippenknorpel. Ztschr. f. d. ges. exper. Med. 55, 287–302.

CANNON, W. B. 1929. Organization for physiological homeostasis. Physiol. Rev., 9, 399–431.

———— 1932. The wisdom of the body. New York: W. W. Norton Company, 312 pp.

COUNCILMAN, W. T. 1919. The conditions presented in the heart and kidney of old people. Contributions to Medical and Biological Research. Dedicated to Sir William Osler. New York: P. B. Hoeber, 617 pp.

DILL, D. B. AND ROBINSON, S. 1938. (See S. Robinson, Experimental studies of physical fitness in relation to age. Arbeits physiologie, **10**, 251–323.)

DOGLIOTTI, G. C. AND NIZZI, G. 1935. The thyroid and senescence. Endocrinol., **19**, 289–292.

EBINA, T., KAJIWARA, Y., AND TIKUCHI, T. 1937. The vital capacity of the Japanese. Tohoku J. Exper. Med., **31**, 401–415.

FREEMAN, N. E. 1935. The effect of temperature on the rate of blood flow in the normal and in the sympathectomized hand. Am. J. Physiol. **113**, 384–398.

HALLOCK, P. 1934. Arterial elasticity in man in relation to age as evaluated by the pulse wave velocity method. Arch. Int. Med., **54**, 770–778.

HIRSCH, S. 1926. Das Altern der Organe in morphologischer und functioneller Hinsicht. Handbuch der normalen und pathologischen Physiologie. Berlin, J. Springer. **17**, 1204 pp. (Cf. p. 823.)

———— 1927. Beiträge zu einer allgemeinen pathologischen Physiologie des höheren Lebensalters. Ergeb. d. inn. Med., **32**, 215–266.

HUTCHINSON, J. 1846. On the capacity of the lungs and on the respiratory functions. Med.-Chir. Trans., Roy. Med. and Chir. Soc., London, **29**, 169–172.

JOHN, H. J. 1934. Glucose tolerance studies in children and adolescents. Endocrinol., **18**, 75–85.

KACHEBRIES, F. 1933. Die Norm des Blutdruckes bei Menschen im Alter von 50–70 Jahren. Ztschr. f. Kreislaufforsch, **25**, 65–74.

KISÉ, Y. AND OCHI, T. 1934. Basal metabolism of old people. J. Lab. and Clin. Med., **19**, 1073–1079.

LEVY, B. 1933. Die Vitalkapazität im höheren Lebensalter. Zentralbl. f. inn. Med., **54**, 417–420.

MAGNUS-LEVY, A. AND FALK, E. 1899. Der Lungengaswechsel des Menschen in den verschiedenen Altersstufen. Arch. f. Physiol., Suppl. Bd., 314–381.

MARSHALL, F. W. 1931. Sugar content of the blood in elderly people. Quart. J. Med., **24**, 257–284.

MARTSINKOVSKI, B. I. AND ZHOROVA, K. S. 1936. The question of distribution and regulation of heat. Acta med. Skandinav., **90**, 582–592.

MATSON, J. R. AND HITCHCOCK, F. H. 1934. Basal metabolism in old age. Am. J. Physiol. **110**, 329–341.

McGILLICUDDY, C. 1937. Better known as "Connie Mack," ex-baseball player, renowned in his later life for his wisdom and skill as a manager of baseball teams. Personal communication.

MORI, Z. 1936. Age and muscular exercise. Jap. J. of Med. Sci., Biophysics, **3**, 309–365.

NITZULESCU, J., ORNSTEIN, I. AND SIBI, M. 1933. Sur le métabolisme des sucres chez les vieillards. L'épreuve de l'hyperglycémie alimentaire. C. r. Soc. de Biol., **114**, 1136–1138.

NORRIS, G. W. AND LANDIS, H. R. M. 1920. Diseases of the chest. Philadelphia, W. B. Saunders Co. Second edition, 844 pp. (Cf. p. 164).

PICKERING, G. W. 1936. The peripheral resistance in persistent hypertension. Clin. Sci., **2**, 209–235.

PORTER, E. AND LANGLEY, G. J. 1926. Studies in blood sugar. Lancet, **2**, 947.

RICE, GRANTLAND 1937. Expert commentator on sports. Personal communication.

RICHTER, A. 1925. Über Blutdruck im höheren Lebensalter. Deutsch. Arch. f. klin. Med., **148**, 111–120.

ROMCKE, O. 1931. Der Blutzucker im älteren Alter, inbesondere bei hypertonischen Zuständen. Acta med. Skandinav., Suppl., **39**, 1–150.

RUBNER, M. 1928. Der Kampf des Menschen um das Leben. Deutsch. med. Wochenschr., **54**, 1750–1752.

SACHS, H. 1927. Der Altershochdruck und das Kreislaufsystem im Senium. Jahrsb. f. ärztl. Fortbild., **18**, 20–27.

SALLER, K. 1928. Über die Altersveränderungen des Blutdrucks. Ztschr. f. d. ges. exper. Med., **58**, 683–709.

SCHLESINGER, H. 1914. Die Krankheiten des höheren Lebensalters. Vienna and Leipzig: A. Hölder. 611 pp.

SCHRETTER, G. AND NEVINNY, H. 1930. Zur Histopathologie der Zuckerkrankheit bei Neugeborenen und Säuglingen. Arch. f. Gynäk., **143**, 465–476.

SHATTUCK, G. C. AND HILFERTY, M. M. 1932. Sunstroke and allied conditions in the United States. Am. J. Tropical Med., **12**, 223–245.

WARREN, S. 1937. Personal communication.

WIGGERS, C. J. 1923. The circulation in health and disease. Philadelphia, Lea and Febiger. 662 pp. (Cf. p. 411).

WOLBACH, S. B. 1937. Personal communication.

CHAPTER 23

AGEING OF TISSUE FLUIDS

E. V. COWDRY

St. Louis

Operation of the balancing mechanisms called homeostatic by
Cannon, provides constancy within narrow limits in the temperature
of the body, sugar content, acid-base equilibrium and other properties
of the blood. With ageing these mechanisms become more and more
restricted in their ability to maintain this essential stability. Old
men and old women adapt themselves less well to many internal and
external disturbances. In their bodies and throughout life the blood
stream is the central unifying factor. The processes of ageing can
be studied to great advantage insofar as they influence these homeostatic mechanisms.

In addition, there is some evidence that the cells outside the blood
vessels exist in tissue fluid environments which are adjusted to their
needs and are not necessarily uniform throughout the body. If this
is true the processes of ageing will manifest themselves in many different ways. It is desirable to explore the possibility in order that
the approach to the problem of ageing in this book may be from all
feasible angles. Every part of the body, all systems, all organs and
all tissues are concerned. About these no one individual is able to
speak on the basis of his own experience and research. This chapter
has been written with some hesitancy because it has little originality
since it is based almost entirely on the work of others.

The cells of our bodies have been compared with minute single-
celled creatures attached to the bed of a stream of water which itself
is likened to the blood stream. But the analogy is doubtful. Obviously, the vast majority of our bodily cells are not bathed in blood
as the single-celled organisms are in flowing water. Blood cells are
carried along in the stream, and the inner surfaces of the endothelial
cells, which line all blood vessels, are in direct contact with the blood,
but all other cells are held away from the blood stream by this vascular
endothelial barrier.

We ask ourselves what would happen if, on the contrary, all cells
were equally exposed to the circulating blood? An environment of

642

blood stabilized by the aforesaid homeostatic mechanisms would, I think, be rather uniform and very unsatisfactory. Since this condition evidently cannot be created and the results observed, all we can do is to mention certain facts which have direct bearing on the question. These may be found in the luxuriant literature on tissue culture, which is the removal of cells from the body and their growth in various fluids. Years ago Carrel and Burrows (1911) found that plasma (blood minus corpuscles) is not an optimum medium for the growth of cells planted in it. When diluted by two volumes of distilled water to three volumes of plasma, much better results were secured. It is necessary to add embryo juice and other substances to make plasma a favorable fluid environment for cells to live in. One way to obtain a pure strain of fibroblasts is to implant a tissue containing several sorts of cells and to let all except fibroblasts die off (Carrel, 1924). We are reminded by Carrel (1931) that macrophages "multiply actively in pure plasma, while fibroblasts and epithelial cells proliferate very slowly or not at all." He goes so far as to say that "The food requirements of a given cell type are as fundamental a characteristic as its morphological aspect." Few of the cells of our bodies, which have already become specialized so that they can be recognized as of different sorts, could survive if placed together in a single medium like blood plasma. Imagine the plight of nerve cells, cartilage cells, thyroid cells, ciliated cells and macrophages in this situation. A state of anarchy would ensue and some of the cells, which did live (macrophages), would act as cannibals. Frequent changing of the plasma in such cultures, so that conditions in a distant way resemble those in the circulating blood, does not make the medium a healthy one for several sorts of cells. Only a few young cells are able to realize potencies, acquired extravascularly before they were planted in plasma culture, and to differentiate to strictly limited extents. Blood cells, themselves, develop in the tissue fluid outside the sinusoidal capillaries of the bone marrow (Maximow and Bloom, 1934) and enter the blood plasma after their particular specialty has been determined. It is altogether impossible for cells, young or old, immersed in the blood stream, to provide that effective division of labor which is the mainstay of organic integration in multicellular organisms. Differential protection both chemical and mechanical from the otherwise homogenizing influence of the blood stream is essential. It is accomplished by many devices.

It is true that different species of single celled organisms (protozoa) can live for countless generations over thousands of years in a stream of water. Each breeds true to its own characteristic hereditary endowment which sometimes undergoes slow modification by sudden changes both disadvantageous and favorable known as mutations. But all the somatic cells, as distinct from the sex cells, of a multicellular organism, like man, are on a fundamentally different basis. They have the same chromosomal content and consequently the characteristic differences which they develop in a relatively very brief space of time are not due in the same way to distinctive hereditary endowments as far as nuclear material is concerned. Cytologists have often wondered, how, though this is the case, these cells differentiate, in the course of development, into so many distinct types serving different functions. They are aquatic immersed in fluid and more or less in touch with other cells which increase in number as the embryo grows. Many influences, including "organizers," operate in this complex fluid environment, which is definitely not the blood and which certainly exhibits local differences. Blood is first formed outside the embryo and only enters it later and develops within it after considerable differentiation has taken place. Actually, therefore, blood is held away from the early embryo, and, throughout life, the avascular tissues including the epidermis, the corneas, the enamel and dentin, the optic lenses and, in a large measure, cartilage, are likewise protected from direct perfusion with blood.

The endothelial surface of countless capillaries, which stand between the blood stream and the tissue fluids, is really very extensive. Landis (1934) makes use of Krogh's calculation that in humans it amounts to 6300 square meters. In other words, this thin membrane, upon which the life of each one of us depends, is equal to the surface of a plot of ground approximately 1 acre and a half in extent. Water and crystalloids are allowed to pass through the membrane freely but protein is usually held back. Return is to the blood stream and lymph. Neither the structure nor the permeability of the capillary endothelial membrane is uniform throughout its extent. The sinusoidal capillaries of the liver allow protein to enter the surrounding tissue fluid with ease. The capillaries of the intestinal mucosa take proteins, and a wide variety of other substances, not removed by the lymphatics, from the tissue fluid about them; but, perhaps, the capillaries of the limbs would do likewise if the same substances were injected subcutaneously. Almost the whole plasma of small volumes of blood is filtered into the tissue fluid of the spleen from venous sinuses (Knisely, 1936). In the bone marrow, blood cells, differentiated extravascularly, regularly enter the blood stream in large numbers through the vascular endothelial membrane. The capillary endothelia of the adrenal cortex and anterior lobe of the pituitary are distinctive and probably highly permeable. It is not unlikely that other regional differences exist. Moreover the permeability in a given area, whatever it happens to be, cannot be regarded as constant. Krogh (1929) has shown that it increases with dilatation and thinning of the wall and Hooker (1911) and Landis (1928) that it increases with lack of oxygen. Throughout life the capillary walls are subjected to a wide variety of chemical and

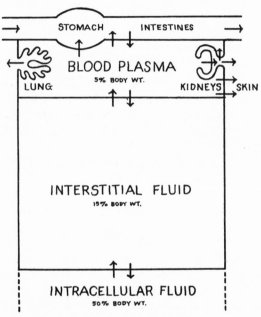

Fig. 106. Proportions of body fluids (after Gamble, 1937). The interstitial fluid includes both tissue fluid and lymph.

physical injuries, more so in some regions than in others. This likewise increases the permeability especially when the H substance of Lewis (1927), or something like it, acts. Krogh (1932) states that "The permeability of capillaries can be increased to such an extent that any colloid will pass out." Including now in our survey the vascular endothelium of other vessels, we are reminded by Cohn (Chapter 7) that the endothelial cells are largest in the veins and smallest in the arteries. Arterioles are more prone than other vessels to display intimal accumulations of hyaline material, presumably of blood protein origin

and perhaps indicative of high permeability of their endothelial walls
to protein. A gradient in permeability, which increases progressively
from arterial to venous capillary and is greatest in the venules, has been
established by Smith and Rous (1931). In view of regional differences
such as these there is ample opportunity for varied tissue fluid environments to exist outside the vascular endothelial membrane.

1. CONCEPT OF TISSUE FLUID ENVIRONMENTS

We shall proceed from large divisions of fluids to small ones, from
generalizations to specific cases and in so doing we shall try to define
our terms. Figure 106 illustrates the proportions of the three kinds
of body fluids according to Gamble (1937). The blood is above, the
interstitial fluid including lymph is between, and the intracellular
fluid is beneath. It is with the so-called interstitial fluid that we
are primarily concerned but not with all of it, for we exclude lymph.
This is one reason why the designation "interstital fluid" as commonly
employed, is not satisfactory for our purpose. It is vague and we wish
to be precise. Derived from the Latin *interstitium*, it means fluid
within "a small space, gap or hole in the substance of an organ or
tissue" (Stedman). There are many small spaces: vascular lumina,
glandular lumina, ducts and so on, which do not contain tissue fluid
as we understand it. To simply classify fluids as intracellular and
extracellular, or intercellular, is not helpful. It promotes an artificial
idea of simplicity in relationships. While the intracellular position
is definite; the extracellular and intercellular positions, from the de-
rivations of the words, can only signify locations outside of and between
cells. Fluids so located are: plasma, between blood cells; lymph,
between cells in lymphatics; secretions and excretions, between epithelial cells; and tissue fluids, between tissue cells which are extravascular and extralymphatic.

Methods devised for the investigation of the electrolyte content of
intracellular and so-called extracellular fluids give interesting results.
But analyses are often based on the assumption that chlorides do
not enter the cells depending, in part but not entirely, upon a silver
test for chlorides, which, in its application, may withdraw chlorides
from the cells. Fenn (1936) freely admits the assumption. Moreover,
the common use of dilute acids, which are applied to pieces of tissue
that are large from the point of view of histologists, introduces another
possible error. Penetration takes time, the surface is affected before
the interior and there is opportunity for the shift of electrolytes from
intracellular to extracellular positions. Unless avascular or alymphatic

tissues are used for the analysis the presence of blood or lymph will cause the results for extracellular fluids in them to depart from the real composition of true tissue fluid in proportion to the volumes of blood or lymph relative to it. No distinction is made in these analyses of the extracellular fluids between the distribution of electrolytes in the fluid ground substance and in the fibrous components of tissue fluids. We want to know about rare electrolytes, as well as the common ones, and about substances which are not to the same degree electrolytes.

The composition of tissue fluids, which can be collected in amounts permitting analysis, is naturally better known than that of those which exist in very small amounts. For the latter we have to rely on micro-chemical tests which are sometimes of questionable value and on still more dubious deductions based on information about the character and activity of the cells and the direction of fluid movements. In trying to piece together information from many sources bearing on the composition of tissue fluids we shall not arbitrarily limit ourselves to substances actually in solution in them any more than we do in con-sidering the composition of blood plasma or of secretion. The tiny droplets of fatty material (chylomicrons), which Ludlum, Taft and Nugent (1931) have investigated by physicochemical methods, occur in blood plasma, but they are not in solution. Similarly no one would think of describing the composition of milk without including fatty substances though these are not present in solution either. A person habitually selling glasses of milk, with fat content greatly reduced, might find himself in jail, since it would not be milk in the light of the law. Indeed it is common practice in the analysis of any fluid to include all substances in it. Whether they are soluble, or relatively insoluble, in solution, crystalline, or amorphous, makes no difference. Thus, in a fluid containing salts, the analysis gives the amounts and kinds of the total salts. It does not ignore those which are crystal-line and include only those in solution.

In our account of tissue fluids, we are often concerned with en-vironments which contain fibers of different sorts. These fibers are of microscopic size; some of them are much smaller in diameter than chylo-microns or fat droplets in milk. They are present in all tissue fluids which lie immediately outside of vascular endothelium. They are normally absent in blood and lymph. Histologists are not wholly agreed as to their development. They appear either in the fibroblastic (and reticular) cells of tissue fluids, or in the ground substance of the tissue fluids themselves, or in both situations. In other words, they are formed directly from tissue fluids by some process of concentration

and alignment of tissue fluid components, or by cells under the influence
of tissue fluids. The case for fibers of the collagenic variety is a little
clearer than for the rest. Wolbach (1933) believes that they are formed
from a secretion elaborated by the fibroblasts and discharged by them
into the tissue fluid in their immediate vicinity. The secretion (and
the resultant fibers) is just as truly within the tissue fluid as secreted
follicular hormone is within the follicular tissue fluid. It is safe to
conclude that, even though the origin of some fibers may be intracellular, when they become extracellular, they are all part and parcel of the
tissue fluids which contain them. Tissue fluids that possess many
elastic fibers and few collagenic ones differ from others in which the
reverse condition obtains. The difference is not simply one of the
proportions of collagen and elastin; because the fibers impede the
movement of the more fluid constituents to a greater or less degree
depending upon the closeness with which they are packed together;
and because they provide important surfaces on which adsorption
takes place. They sometimes become encrusted and impregnated with
minerals.

A fluid yields to forces which tend to change its form; a solid, by
definition, does not. This is why some people have difficulty in extending the concept of tissue fluid environments from very watery ones,
through fibrous ones, to the tissue fluid of elastic cartilage, which is
yielding, and to that of bone which is rigid. But bone is not a true
solid for its form, both external and internal, is not fixed; on the contrary, it slowly adjusts itself to deforming stresses. Moreover it is not
homogeneous. Fluids can, and do, move in and out quite freely.
The cells of bone are aquatic, like all other cells in the body, though
their tissue fluid environments are made comparatively solid by the
accumulation in them of relatively insoluble mineral crystals in an organic fibrous framework, itself, as we have said, likewise a tissue fluid
derivative. Both salts and fibers are in the fluid and are actually
parts of it. The fibers, especially the elastic ones, resist solution far
more than the dahlite crystals.

The tissue cells are also in the tissue fluid environments, but they
are not parts of it in the same sense. For hundreds of millions of
years the living substance of an unbroken line of their ancestors has
been protected by cell membranes from, and also integrated with, a
succession of tissue fluids in each and every multicellular organism.
It is a kind of partnership. Tissue cells, with the cooperation of
endothelial cells, produce tissue fluids in accordance with classical
patterns in use for ages and subject only to very gradual alteration.

The tissue fluids in turn provide environments suited to their cellular inhabitants, both as these learn their duties and discharge them. In addition the tissue fluids, by virtue of their physical and chemical properties, serve the entire body in numerous ways.

This concept of tissue fluids is in accord with the conditions that exist *in vivo* and under which the processes of ageing operate. When we separate from tissue fluid (or blood, or milk) the water and the substances in solution leaving all the rest behind we get an unnatural fluid that is not found as such in the living body. But resort must be made to experimental methods. It is done knowing that each gives us a glimpse of a part of an integrated vital whole.

2. CLASSIFICATION OF TISSUE FLUIDS

In the following very tentative topographic classification of tissue fluids we shall describe mainly histological features in mode of withdrawal or protection from the blood stream, and the outside environment, and mention chemical composition and age changes only when data are available, which, as we shall see, is frequently the case. The reader will not be able to follow us if he continues to think of tissue fluids as visible to the naked eye. It is necessary to view them at the magnification at which we ordinarily study tissue cells because their actual volume in relation to living cells is considerable.

Tissue fluids of the first order
    (separated from blood stream by vascular endothelium)
      1. Subepithelial (partly limited by epithelium)
      2. Mesenchymal
          Vascular
          Splenic
          Bone Marrow
          Bony
          Cartilaginous
          Articular
          Muscular
Tissue fluids of the second order
    (separated from blood stream by vascular endothelium, tissue fluid of
      first order and a second cellular membrane)
      1. Ectodermal (partly limited by ectoderm)
          Endolymphatic
          Cerebrospinal
          Intraocular
      2. Mesothelial (partly limited by mesothelium)
          Pericardial, pleural, peritoneal, peritesticular
          Testicular

3. TISSUE FLUIDS OF THE FIRST ORDER

1. *Subepithelial tissue fluids*

These lie between the epithelium and the vascular endothelial membrane. Three types may be recognized depending upon distance from the surface of the body: *dermal* tissue fluid which invests the body immediately beneath the epidermis; *subepithelial* tissue fluid which is under the epithelium lining the respiratory, genito-urinary and digestive tracts and their appendages which are continuous with the outside world through apertures; and *endocrine* tissue fluid in touch with epithelium, which is, however, no longer connected with the surface.

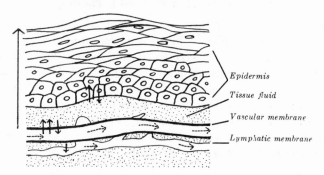

Epidermis

Tissue fluid

Vascular membrane

Lymphatic membrane

Fig. 107. Histological relations of dermal tissue fluid represented in light stipple. The broken arrows show the direction of flow of blood and lymph and the small solid arrows the movements of tissue fluid. The large solid arrow suggests the direction of a deprivation gradient in the tissue fluid.

Dermal tissue fluid can be likened to a shallow lake. Its depth appears almost negligible but in relation to cell size it is very considerable. It rests upon comparatively firm muscles, tendons and masses of subcutaneous fat. The most vitally active level is, as in a lake, near the surface immediately beneath the epidermis for it is here that the blood and lymphatic capillaries are best developed. Figure 107 is a very crude diagram in which dermal tissue fluid is represented in light stipple. It receives contributions from the blood stream (two arrows on the left) and it also gives back to the blood, but not so much, because in this situation some tissue fluid is removed by the lymphatics. Pervading the tissue fluid are connective tissue cells and fibers, the epithelial cells of cutaneous glands, occasional hair follicles and nerve endings and fibers none of which are indicated in the diagram. Some of the tissue fluid spreads between the epidermal cells, part of the way to the surface, but this likewise is not illustrated.

Whether, before entering the avascular epidermis, the tissue fluid must first pass through a basement membrane on which the epidermis lies, is uncertain. The existence of such a membrane has been both affirmed and denied. The most convincing description of a basement membrane, not beneath the epidermis but underlying the epithelial lining of the nasal passages, is given by Shambaugh (1931). He thinks, however, that it only appears after chronic irritation. The ease with which epidermis can be stripped off from the underlying corium by immersing a specimen in 0.5 per cent acetic acid for 12–24 hours suggest the existence of a thin layer of cement substance soluble in dilute acetic acid. Though I have not found (1938) distinctive changes indicative of alterations in this rather hypothetical basement membrane in the skin of a woman aged 111 years, kindly given to me by Dr. H. A. McCordock, they do occur in the testicle and it would be worthwhile to study basement membranes in all situations.

Dermal tissue fluid has been investigated by a long line of histologists so that there is considerable literature about it. The most direct observations on tissue fluid have been made by the Clarks (1933) in living rabbits. In specially constructed chambers (in which a cover glass takes the place of epidermis) inserted into the ears, they clearly demonstrated that this fluid has the consistency of a gel, in which Brownian movement of particles does not occur, and which is physically very different, both from the blood in vascular capillaries and from the lymph in lymphatic vessels. They supply significant data on alterations in the gel under the influence of transudates and exudates following injury.

By ingenious methods, Sylvia H. Bensley (1934) has studied this fluid "ground substance" in subcutaneous connective tissue of the guinea pig and in fibrosis of the pancreas after duct ligation as well as in the human uterine mucous membrane. She has investigated microscopic appearance, refractive index, consistency, extraction with NaCl and half-saturated lime water, pancreatic as well as peptic digestion, staining properties and affinity for copper salts thus providing a wealth of information. Her results confirm, with minor exceptions, the observations·made by the Clarks. They justify her conclusion that, since this gel-like, intercellular material in the tissue fluid ". . . varies with the physiological age and development of the connective tissue, it is different in different localities. Thus, in embryonic and undifferentiated tissues, such as reticular tissue, the ground substance retains its young, viscid, continuous form. In adult subcutaneous tissue it is less abundant, interrupted by tissue spaces, and chiefly encloses the connective tissue fibers."

We have strayed a little from dermal tissue fluid underlying the dermis to include tissue fluids under experimental conditions very closely approximating those normally existing *in vivo* in other localities in which the relation to connective tissue elements is comparable; because the evidence is unequivocal that the fluid differs from lymph, that it is different in different localities, varies with physiological age and mechanical injury and consequently affords diversified fluid environments for the cellular inhabitants.

Temperature of the skin at different depths and in areas of the extremities farther and farther distal (away from the heart) has been directly measured by Bazett and McGlone (1927). Interesting differences obtain. Doubtless the temperature of the dermal tissue fluid is regionally different for it must have approximately the same temperature as nearby tissue.

Particularly interesting is the fate of epidermal cells which lose touch with the tissue fluid. As those effectively nourished by it multiply, they push the more superficial cells farther away. The more these are displaced toward the surface the more they suffer from starvation and inability to evacuate waste products. They are subject to a deprivation gradient rising vertically from the capillary bed. They lose water, die and adhere very firmly together so that the outermost layers of epidermis are made up of dead cells. "While we are in life we are in death" is a true saying. We are encased in a protective armor of dead material made yielding and kept pliable by the secretions of sebaceous glands. This is partly brushed off from the surface and, at the same rate in adults, it is renewed by the moving up of generation upon generation of dying cells from within.

It is likely that rhythmic alterations occur in this dermal tissue fluid which are dependent upon changes in the activity of the cells within it and in the volume and perhaps the temperature and quality of perfusing blood. Alice Carleton (1934) has discovered that in mice there are about twice as many cell divisions in the interval between 8 p.m. and midnight as between 8 a.m. and midday. Attempts are being made to determine whether a similar 24-hour rhythm exists in human epidermis removed by circumcision.[1] If so, it would explain

[1] Cooper, Zola and Schiff, Alice, 1938. Mitotic rhythm it human epidermis. Soc. Exp. Biol. & Med. (in press).

why it is difficult to find dividing cells in tissues, in which we know that the cells are multiplying, but which, almost invariably, are collected by day. The point of practical importance is that radiosensitivity will, other things being equal, be greatest at the time of most active cell division. Activation of cholesterol by ultraviolet light to form Vitamin D in the epidermis is probably also rhythmic with alternating periods of daylight and darkness. Investigation should be made of the rhythm, if any, in the activity of cutaneous glands. In hours of activity the circulation in the dermis, and in consequence the passage of materials through the vascular endothelial membrane and their removal through it and by the lymphatics are likely to be different than in the hours of ease by night. A very leisurely pulsation on a 24-hour basis in volume and properties of this tissue fluid may take place. Rhythms are very fully discussed by Petersen (1934).

Now about the modifications in this dermal tissue fluid as old age creeps on. For one thing the circulation becomes less vigorous. Changes result in the relative amounts, and possibly also in the character, of the elastic and collagenic fibers which are immersed in the tissue fluid (see eyelids, Friedenwald, Chapter 18). Epidermal cells fail in many ways as detailed by Weidman in Chapter 12. The orderly restraint imposed upon them by a satisfactorily regulated tissue fluid wears off. This is manifested in several alterations including localized deposition of pigment and an excessive multiplication in limited areas which may be, or become, cancerous. What happens to the rhythms we do not know.

The *cornea* is a special case. The maximum effective distance of tissue fluid from the nearest vascular endothelial membrane is between 5 and 6 mm. depending on the individual. Assuming it to be 5.5 mm., or 5500 microns, it is clearly a distance to be reckoned with. It is 5500 times the distance away of a layer of tissue fluid 1 micron thick about the said membrane. Expressed differently it is equal to 657.8 red blood cells placed in line of their maximum diameters (7.6 microns). Physically the fluid is a kind of swamp in which there are many connective tissue cells and fibers. On one side (the external), it is faced by several layers of epithelial cells and the other (the internal) by Descemet's membrane and the aqueous humor. This presence of many and diverse adsorptive surfaces is important because it means that fluid passage is not as free as if it were uninfluenced physically and chemically by the cells and fibers. Probably there is a vertical gradient in composition proceeding from the vascular endothelial membrane to the most distant part in the corneal tissue fluid. The temperature of the cornea is said by Mann (1932), who quoted an earlier authority, to be 10°C lower than body temperature. This is understandable because of its avascularity and because it is always kept wet and is cooled by evaporation except when the eyelids are closed during sleep. But low temperature and avascularity do not prevent regeneration, for corneal lesions in mammals heal in the remarkably short time of 6 hours (Arey, 1936). Ageing of the cornea is discussed in detail by Friedenwald in Chapter 18.

   Teeth are partly epidermal and partly mesodermal. They supply a beautiful example of three tissue fluid environments differing among themselves yet in close apposition. The pulp, within, is highly vascularized and contains many living cells. The dentin, between, is avascular and is penetrated by the processes of cells situated in the pulp. The enamel, above, is avascular and devoid of living cells or processes. Starting with the pulp, and proceeding to the oral cavity, many interesting conditions are found some of which are indicated in figure 108.

   Noyes (1929), in commenting on the statement frequently made that the largest capillaries in the body occur in the pulp, expresses the view that "These vessels should probably not be considered as capillaries, but as veins whose walls have the structure of capillaries." This point is mentioned because the permeability of such gigantic capillaries may be different from those of the usual size and the tissue fluid about them correspondingly different. Fluid leaving such a capillary is represented by the pair of arrows near the bottom of the figure. Some fluid passes back through the vascular endothelial membrane and some enters the lymphatics. A single layer of elongated mesodermal cells (odontoblasts) is placed in the pulp next to the dentin. Their nucleated cell bodies are in the pulp and each one of them extends a long process into the dentin which may reach a distance as far as 2 mm. to the dentoenamel junction where it branches profusely. These processes are contained in dentinal tubules the nature of the walls of which is not definitely known. The tissue fluid of the pulp seeps into the dentin through the dentinal tubules along the surfaces of the processes of the odontoblasts contained within them. Particles of India ink injected into the pulp move in this direction (Fish, 1932).

   This tissue fluid, within the dentinal canals, is but a small fraction of the total tissue fluid in the dentin. Noyes (1929) has calculated that the average diameter of a dentinal tubule is 2 microns and that they

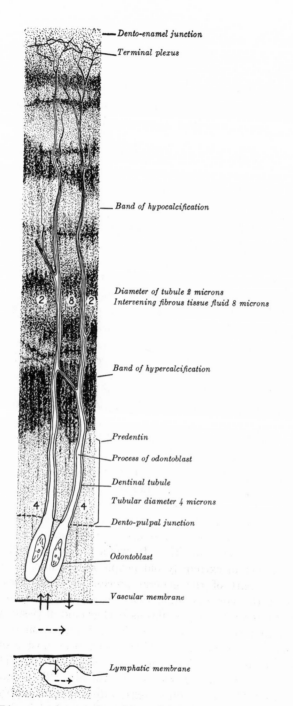

Dento-enamel junction

Terminal plexus

Band of hypocalcification

Diameter of tubule 2 microns
Intervening fibrous tissue fluid 8 microns

Band of hypercalcification

Predentin

Process of odontoblast

Dentinal tubule

Tubular diameter 4 microns

Dento-pulpal junction

Odontoblast

Vascular membrane

Lymphatic membrane

FIG. 108. Diagram of two odontoblasts in dental pulp extending processes within dentinal tubules into the dentin. Below, are portions of a giant capillary and of a lymphatic. The tissue fluid is shown in light stipple; but at levels in the dentin the stipple is denser indicative of bands of hypercalcification in the tissue fluid and not to be confused with tissue fluid of the second order for which uniformly dense stipple is used in other diagrams.

are separated by 8 microns of ground substance. This ground substance is fibrous and in it calcium salts are accumulated much as in bone. They can be withdrawn, but not with the same facility as from bony tissue fluid. They are concentrated in irregular bands of hypercalcification separated by bands of hypocalcification, but the dentin next the pulp contains less calcium than that farther removed from it and is termed predentin. Consequently there is a vertical gradient of increasing calcification in the tissue fluid passing away from the vascularized pulp. The successive bands of calcification laid down rhythmically in the rat's incisor (Schour and Steadman, 1935) are really a series of vertical gradients one on top of the other.

The shift of fluid in human dentin is not altogether through the dentinal tubules, out of them at right angles into the fluid matrix and back again; for some of it may enter the superposed enamel or the cementum, which latter limits the dentin laterally and affords attachment for fibers that hold the tooth in place. Conversely, a little fluid may move into the dentin from the enamel and rather more from the cementum. The passage of tissue fluid comparatively long distances through these myriads of extremely fine tubules possessed of living cores, in which there are currents of fluid, gives abundant opportunity for surface action and adsorption. Moreover the conditions are not altogether static; because, in addition to the vitality of the cytoplasmic processes of the odontoblasts, the dentin itself is slightly elastic since it provides an effective yielding backing for the crown of enamel. Slight alterations in the length of hundreds of thousands of dentinal tubules will cause agitation of fluid in them as well as in the tissue fluid around them.

Practically nothing is known about the ageing of dentin. New dentin, called secondary, is produced, on demand, by the odontoblasts almost throughout life. It would be worthwhile to try to discover whether in extremely old people the number of odontoblasts is reduced as part of the general process of tissue atrophy. If so the cores of the corresponding dentinal tubules will die. Also, we may expect alterations in the fibrous background of tissue fluid outside of the dentinal tubules, but there is no information on this point.

The enamel is, of all tissues of the body, the most protected from the blood stream. The dentin acts as a shield for it. This is fortunate; because, once formed it must last for life. To permit the body, in case of need, to draw upon its extraordinarily rich supply of calcium salts, in the form of dahlite crystals, would be bad business management. The incisors of rats, mice, beavers, squirrels and other rodents continue to form both dentin and enamel to compensate for wear and tear. Otherwise the owners could not survive. The tusks of the elephant are Nature's masterpieces of continuous incisor growth. The bicuspids of many carnivors act similarly.

In human enamel there is from 1 to 2 per cent of organic material which remains from parts of cells that contributed to its development. Enamel is fairly permeable to water and salts which Klein and Amberson (1929) think pass in the organic component. Many substances, especially minerals, are known to enter it, either from the oral cavity or through the dentin beneath. This permeability, according to Rosebury (1930) maintains enamel in a moist state and reduces liability to fracture. The organic material probably ages, like a colloid, and the permeability increases in advanced years (Fish). The calcium

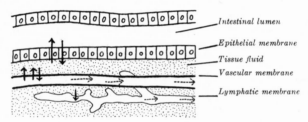

FIG. 109. Subepithelial tissue fluid. This also is one of the first order indicated in light stipple.

content of all parts of the teeth increases with ageing and the teeth become more yellow due to thickening of secondary dentin (Todd, Chapter 11).

The more deeply situated *subepithelial tissue fluids* present variations of the same problem (fig. 109). Their histological relations are highly diversified. Nothing is surely known about their microchemistry. The delicate techniques devised by Richards for the analysis of glomerular fluid should be used. The space at my disposal only allows brief reference to outstanding examples.

Consider first the fluid just within the single layer of highly permeable cells lining the *small intestine* indicated in a general way in figure 109. This is not much protected from the contents of the lumen which traverse the body but which are outside of it in a vital sense. Instead, there is an active exchange between the tissue fluid and the lumen through a delicate yet durable epithelial membrane which as far as we know does not age.   At any rate careful search should be made for age changes in it.   Accordingly this tissue fluid is less stagnant than in any others discussed thus far.   Bensley's techniques should be employed to determine whether it ever has the consistency of a gel which seems unlikely because the streams of absorption would be impeded thereby.   Here again there is a rhythm—a shorter one imposed by the absorption of products of digestion at fairly regular but unequal intervals as long as life lasts.   At times this particular tissue fluid differs from all others in chemical composition for all substances, proteins, amino-acids, carbohydrates, fats, mineral salts, vitamines and water, which are carried away in blood and lymph from the small intestine, must first pass through it.   The cells which are in and which limit small intestinal tissue fluid enjoy, therefore, a more direct supply of all materials except oxygen, internal secretions, substances released from storage and so on, which they get like the rest from the blood stream, than the cells of any other tissue fluid environment.   This holds despite the speed with which products of digestion may be removed by blood and lymph.   Some of these enter through the substance of the epithelial cells, not simply between them.

In other segments of the digestive tract, and in its glandular appendages, the epithelial cells perform different functions and the luminal contents are by no means identical.   A pleasant experiment demonstrates that alcohol passes in through the epithelial membrane of the stomach in a few seconds.   Water on the other hand is refused by this membrane but is absorbed with avidity by the epithelial linings of the gall bladder and colon in the process of concentration of their contents. The underlying tissue fluid may or may not be modified, at least for the time being, thereby.

That the epithelial linings of the respiratory tract carrying air, of the urinary tract carrying urine, and of the genital tracts transporting other materials, differ structurally and functionally cannot be denied. Whether these differences are reflected in the regional adjustments in the tissue fluid beneath, we do not know; but to discover the diversity or the similarity in the colloidal ageing of elastic fibers in these situations as well as in the walls of blood vessels and in dermal tissue fluid would be thoroughly worthwhile.   The subepithelial tissue fluid of the uterus, which is periodically reconstituted after every menstrual flow, may be different from the tissue fluid unreplaced after the menopause (see Bensley).   Many questions occur to us which have not been answered.   There is a lot said about reduction in water content with ageing. We should progress from the general to the specific, identify tissue fluid environments which suffer dehydration most and least and note the consequences in speeding up or slowing down of the ageing processes.

Endocrine tissue fluid, is also usually closely associated with epithelium, but it is ordinarily not connected with an external or internal epithelium-lined body surface. We say *usually*; because it is doubtful whether we can properly call the medullary cells of the adrenal and the follicular cells of the ovary, epithelial; while the interstitial cells of the testis are not epithelial. In any case this sort of tissue fluid does not give materials to, or receive them from, a ductlike lumen communicating with the outside. The exchange (fig. 110) is through

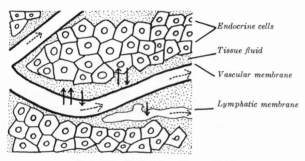

FIG. 110. Endocrine tissue fluid

the vascular endothelial membrane, in and out of endocrine cell membranes plus some absorption by the lymphatics. Hormones, produced by the cells, enter the tissue fluid, leave in the blood (or lymph) and are washed to all vascularized parts of the body. Unless they are removed from the site of origin with extraordinary speed and effectiveness, their concentration in that particular tissue fluid of origin, between secreting cells and vascular endothelium, will be greater than after dilution through admixture with blood and diffusion through other vascular endothelial membranes into a wide variety of tissue fluid environments where their stimulating or inhibiting influences are delivered. It is possible that some only become active after they are admitted to the circulation, as some enzymes do after they enter the gut. Otherwise, those hormones which act generally on cells would exercise a tremendous effect on any such cells in the endocrine tissue fluid of origin as compared with that on others in more distant regions of the body.

Examples of tissue fluids, which may safely be said to contain distinctively large concentrations of hormone, can easily be cited. Allen et al. (1930) made careful biological assays of the follicular fluid of the human ovary. They found that it contains a high concentration of the follicular hormone, theelin, second only among fluids to that of the urine of pregnant women (Doisy, 1932). Moreover this tissue fluid in the later stages of its accumulation is characteristically viscid (Robinson, 1918) so that it differs in this respect also from the general run of tissue fluids. Follicular hormone is of especial interest to us because it brings about a rapid increase in tissue fluid in female genital tissues (Allen, Chapter 14). How it does so is not clear but there appears to be a significant increase in permeability of vascular endothelium. The cells in this tissue fluid are subjected to spurts of activity.

The tissue fluid in the medulla of the adrenal gland exists in such small quantity that it is usually unnoticed, but epinephrine must pass through thin films of this fluid before it enters venous capillaries and leaves in the blood of the adrenal veins. Since its concentration in the said veins is greater than in the general circulation, or in any other tissue fluid environment, it seems to follow that the medullary tissue fluid is distinctive in its high concentration of epinephrine. Medullary tissue fluid probably differs from that in the adrenal cortex in another regard, for most of the blood which it receives must first penetrate through the cortex in delicate channels. A gradient in permeability from arterial to venous capillary and venule has been established in other situations. If there is one here also, the contribution from the blood to the cortical tissue fluid will differ from that to the medullary tissue fluid. The further we look for differences between tissue fluids in different localities the more we find. It is to be remembered that in this chapter we deal with the possibility of changes within distances measurable in microns.

An intangible, rather neglected factor in ageing may be a decrease in the tuning or responsiveness of cells to internal secretions. Hormones only act on cells tuned to react to them. The properties which determine responsiveness are beyond the scope of our present methods of examination. Epidermal cells which respond to hormone stimulation during puberty by hair formation, or during pregnancy by pigment formation, do not differ in any as yet appreciable way from similar cells in less restricted localities which do not respond. In old age the reactivity of the individual appears to decline. This is particularly true for the nervous system, though it may be due to diminution in number of cells and fibers, not to depression in responsiveness of individual ones. A feature of the ageing of homeostatic mechanisms is that the response to conditions tending to disturb equilibrium becomes less effective. Cole, Guilbert and Goss (1932) have discovered that the testicles of immature rats respond by great enlargement to the gonad stimulating hormone of mare serum while the response of the testicles of mature rats is very noticeably less. Evans and his associates (1933) observed but a feeble testicular enlargement in old rats to the gonad-stimulating hormone. Engle (Chapter 15) describes the responsiveness of the testicular interstitial cells of young rats and monkeys to the gonadotropic hormone and its decrease in older animals. Allen (Chapter 14) remarks on the well known fact "that organs which react to growth producing hormones frequently lose their reactivity. . . . It is clear that there is a decrease in the amount of ovarian hormones with age, but there may also be a loss of reactivity of the uterus." The senile ovary, after the menopause, no longer responds to anterior pituitary secretion although the gonad-stimulating-substances continue to be produced and can be found in the urine. Mammary glands cease to lactate and it would be interesting to discover whether this is due to a coincident decrease in formation of pituitary lactogenic hormone or to decrease in responsiveness.

2. Mesenchymal tissue fluid

It is hardly necessary to state that most tissue fluids are mesenchymal in the sense that they develop within the thin watery infusion or mixture of cells derived from the middle germ layer (Gr. *mesos*, middle + *enchyma*, infusion). Here we find the blood vessels, nerves and lymphatics. But some tissue fluids, which we designate, *mesenchymal*, are removed in position from all epithelial cells and in this feature differ fundamentally from those described thus far.

The first of these may be termed *vascular*, for they occur in the walls of blood vessels. They are probably far from uniform and to give even a sketchy idea of their features in a few paragraphs is difficult. We shall mention, in order, the directions of fluid movement, the structural factors involved, the known properties of the tissue fluids, how they change with ageing and emphasize their diversity, which is interesting on account of their proximity to the homeostatically regulated blood stream.

In arteries (except the pulmonary), according to Aschoff (1933), the "physiological stream of nutrition proceeds from the blood through the vessel wall toward the periphery." Arteries of a diameter greater

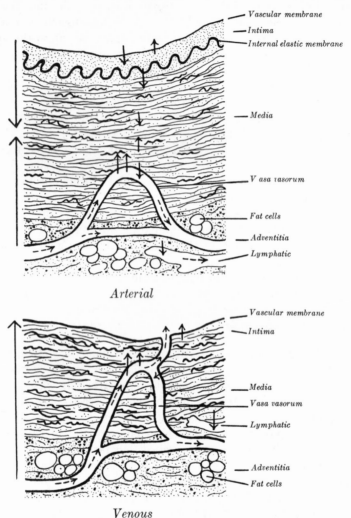

Arterial

Venous

Fig. 111. Vascular tissue fluids. In the arterial wall oxygenated tissue fluid comes both from the lumen and periphery. In the vein only from the periphery. The large arrows at the side show directions of gradients.

than 1 mm. possess, however, vessels of their own (vasa vasorum) which enter at the periphery and break up into capillaries in the outer layer (adventitia); but it is generally conceded (Maximow and Bloom, 1934) that these capillaries do not extend centrally farther than the external part of the media (fig. 111), though in special cases they may do so (Winterwitz et al. 1938). Fluid leaves by the vasa vasorum, peripheral lymphatics and probably by diffusion back into the central blood stream. In the walls of veins the directions of fluid movement are obviously different (see fig. 111). The blood in the lumen is venous (except in the pulmonary) and of little nutritive value (except in the portal). The physiological stream of nutrition enters at the periphery through the vasa vasorum, which are better developed than in the walls of arteries. It leaves by the said vasa vasorum (perhaps directly into a vein), by the peripheral lymphatics and by diffusion in a central direction into the lumen of the vein.

The structural factors involved include the vascular endothelial membranes which limit the arterial blood in the arteries, the venous blood in the veins and the blood in the vasa vasorum and capillaries, as well as the lymphatic endothelial membranes. There are no data on regional differences in permeability. The vascular endothelial cells are largest in the veins, intermediate in the capillaries and smallest in the arteries (Cohn, Chapter 7). Hydrostatic pressure is least in the veins, more in the capillaries and most in the arteries. Anitschkow (1933) thinks that the arterial vascular endothelium "is probably as permeable to the constituents of the blood as the walls of real capillaries." Innumerable barriers are presented against the freedom of movement of vascular tissue fluid. It seeps through a tissue made dense by muscle fibers, collagenic and elastic fibers, connective tissue cells and a few others. These components are arranged in layers different in size and in relative proportions of ingredients in different vessels. Very important are the elastic tissue fibers which are often merged in comparatively homogeneous sheets and bands. Thus, there are many surfaces on which adsorption takes place. In respect to composition of the tissue fluid, the vessel walls are really filters constituted partly of living and metabolically active components and partly of non-living fibers arranged in layers and the fluids passing back and forth are rhythmically shifted in arteries by contraction and dilatation of their walls.

Of the properties of the tissue fluids and of the character of the processes of ageing in veins very little is known. Both should be investigated in a contrastive way with the arteries, concerning which there is much accurate information. Schultz (1922) and Ssolowjew (1923) have shown that the homogeneous looking ground substance of arterial tissue fluid is chromotropic and stains metachromatically. We are reminded of Bensley's studies. That the fluid contains a true mucin has been abundantly demonstrated. Bjorling (1911) thinks that the particular mucin does not occur in other adult tissues but this observation awaits confirmation. The reaction of the ground substance of the tissue fluid is alkaline in young animals (Schmidtmann and Hüttich, 1928). See discussion by H. Gideon Wells (1933).

In conditions which cannot be called abnormal, several kinds of substances are found in arterial tissue fluid. Hyaline material is present in the walls of small arteries and arterioles in the spleens of 15 per cent of individuals in the first decade and of 92 per cent in the ninth decade of life (Herxheimer, 1917). It is located in the tissue fluid of the inner layer, or intima. This hyaline is of protein nature. Anitschkow (1925, 1933) believes that it passes in through the vascular endothelium from the blood stream. The fats and lipoids present in the fatty streaks of young people and adults are located both intra- and intercellularly in the intima. In the normal aorta there is a so-called "mesarterial band of calcareous impregnation" (Policard 1933). According to Policard et al. (1932) "the normal aortic intima contains much more calcium than magnesium; the normal media contains more calcium, and proportionally much more magnesium than the intima" (quoted from Wells, 1933). Data on the precise location of these minerals are lacking, though the calcium seems to be in or associated with the elastic fibers. But in medial calcification of muscular arteries, which is a statistically normal process, beginning in childhood and increasing with age, the deposition of calcium starts in the tissue fluid between the muscle fibers (Huebschmann 1906, Bell, 1933). It would appear therefore that arterial tissue fluid is invaded by blood proteins, fats, calcium and magnesium and exhibits a tendency to stratification.

Definite alterations have been reported, as resulting from ageing, in arterial tissue fluids. The mucin content increases (Wells) and there is a progressive increase in acidity (Schmidtmann and Hüttich). In various lesions, common in aged persons but occasionally encountered in adults and young people, there are increases in hyaline material particularly in the intima of small arteries and arterioles; of calcium in the media of muscular arteries; and fats, lipoids and calcium in the intima and media of elastic arteries. Exactly in what proportions the arterial tissue fluid shares in the dehydration of the body with age has not been determined. A decrease in its water content, if it occsur which is likely, would promote that decrease in flexibility and elasticity of elastic fibers which is one of the common features of ageing. These fibers, as well as the collagenic ones, are colloidal structures bathed in tissue fluid and influenced both by it and by mechanical forces of stress and strain. Bell (1933) says: "In the case of the elastic arteries, it is commonly assumed that degeneration of the elastic tissue is the primary change, and that the new formation of collagenous tissue is a compensatory process to maintain the strength of the vessel wall. Similarly, in the muscular arteries, we may assume a primary degeneration of muscle, and a secondary formation of collagenous tissue."

But the problem is far from simple. Indeed the processes of ageing of arteries will only be understood if, with Kast (1933) we appreciate that the tissue fluids in their walls "develop different properties in different situations." This view is entirely reasonable. Cohn, in chapter 7, emphasizes the lack of uniformity "not only in arteries of different sizes but also in arteries of the same size"; between those which serve as reservoirs (elastic) and as passages (muscular); and between others depending on their position in the body and unknown factors. Uniformity of their tissue fluids is not to be expected in the face of this diversity and in view of the local structural factors listed in a previous paragraph.

Differences in vascular tissue fluid environments both actual and potential may in some measure condition the vulnerability, or the reverse, of certain vessels to ageing. A vast amount of evidence, presented in a cooperative volume on Arteriosclerosis which I edited, shows unmistakably that the burden of years is not evenly felt by blood vessels of all sorts. In addition to such local differences in *susceptibility* remarkable differences in *speed* of operation of the ageing processes are noted. To cite only a few instances, the umbilical artery lasts but a short time, the ductus arteriosus becomes senile a few months after birth and the uterine arteries are rejuvenated with each pregnancy. That a man is as old as his arteries is part of the story and the tissue fluid environment in his vessels, part of "—the milieu interieur of Claude Bernard—seems worthy of intensive investigation" (Kast).

Of all the tissue fluids in our bodies that of the *spleen* is perhaps the most interesting in the light of recent investigations by Knisely (1936). He has managed to observe directly in the spleens of living animals contributions being made to the splenic tissue fluid by the venous sinuses. The spleen is divisable into thousands of lobules and the

structural relations at the side of one nodule are illustrated diagrammatically in figure 112 with many details omitted. The white pulp is on
the left. It is separated by a broken line from the red pulp on the right.
The course of the blood stream is indicated by arrows. The venous
sinuses are sausage-shaped bodies in the red pulp. Stages in their
cyclic activity are represented from above downward.

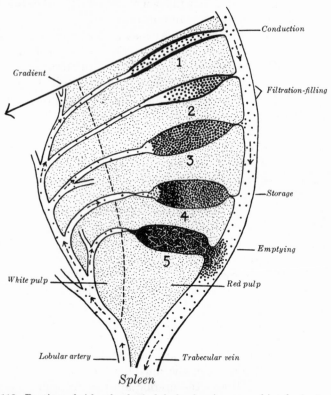

Spleen

FIG. 112. Portion of side of splenic lobule showing some histological relations
of mesenchymal splenic tissue fluid of the first order. The blood cells are here
represented as tiny spherules in the blood stream. They become closely packed
together in the venous sinuses as plasma is filtered off.

In the *first* (1), called conduction, blood flows through quickly and
the wall is thick and consequently not very permeable. In the *second*
(2, 3), known as filtration-filling, the efferent sphincter, which guards
the opening into the trabecular vein, closes. The sinus gradually fills,
the wall thins, plasma filters into the surrounding tissue fluid and the
cells become more closely packed together. In the *third* (4), the

afferent sphincter closes, prevents more blood from entering and the stage is termed storage. After an interval the *fourth* phase of emptying begins by opening of the efferent sphincter. The cheezy mass of blood cells breaks up, the afferent sphincter opens and the contents are flushed into the trabecular vein. Then the cycle begins again with free conduction of blood through the sinus.

This is a situation in which almost all of the plasma filters into the tissue fluid, but it is possible that some substances remain adsorbed on the surfaces of the blood cells. Since the filtration is mainly in the red pulp, and the capillaries in the white pulp, show no signs of being as permeable as the venous sinuses, it follows that a gradient in composition of the tissue fluid is probably established. This extends from the region where the plasma contribution is largest to where it is least as suggested by the large solid arrow at the top of the figure. Another factor, likely to produce such a gradient, is the difference, both qualitative and quantitative, in the cell content of red and white pulp and the resultant differences in metabolic requirement. The tissue fluid is shifted by passive and rhythmic contractions of the whole spleen.

It cannot therefore be doubted that the cells of the spleen enjoy a tissue fluid environment all their own in which it is to be observed that there are no epithelial elements. The presence of so much plasma protein, which diffuses into the white pulp in the direction of the gradient, may contribute to the hyaline infiltration of the arterioles in the white pulp, which is a conspicuous feature of ageing of the spleen. It is however not the sole cause, for similar infiltration occurs in a less marked degree in other organs.

The spleen is not essential to life. The first English translation of Pliny contains the following passage. "This member hath a proprietie by itselfe sometimes, to hinder a man's running: whereupon professed runners in the race that bee troubled with the splene, have a devise to burne and wast it with an hot yron. And no marveile: for why? They say that the splene can be taken out of the bodie by incision and yet the creature live neverthelesse" (McNee, 1930-31).

The tissue fluids of *bone marrow* afford an instructive contrast to the vascular and splenic ones. They are within rigid walls and are not shifted rhythmically back and forth over similarly adsorptive fibrous filters; neither are they in a soft organ the volume of which changes in the manner related. Alterations in volume take place gradually by operation of factors reviewed by Drinker and associates (1922). Like all tissue fluids they are based on the blood stream. Their separation from the blood stream is peculiar. In these localities blood flows through what Maximow and Bloom (1934) call venous sinusoids which are limited, they say, not by endothelium but by "littoral cells of the macrophage system" through which pass out from the tissue fluid into the blood stream not only granular leucocytes but also non-motile red blood cells by a mechanism "probably regulated by changes in the permeability of the walls of the vessels and in the surface energy." The possibility is therefore created of a difference between these bone marrow tissue fluids and other tissue fluids limited by the usual endothelial membrane.

Bone marrow itself is not of uniform properties. There exist two main kinds, red and yellow. The red variety is a blood cell producer and the yellow is loaded with swollen fat cells. It can be safely assumed that the metabolic rate is higher in richly cellular red than in yellow marrow. Huggins, Blocksom and Noonan (1936) have discovered that in mammals there is a temperature gradient extending from centrally placed marrow to distal marrow, near the ends of the extremities, where it is 4 to 8°C. lower. Huggins and Blocksom (1936) observed that the red marrow decreases in amount and the yellow increases in passing from deep to peripheral tissues. They performed numerous experiments such as bending rats' tails and inserting them into abdominal cavities, thus increasing the temperature, and found that red marrow was increased in amount by elevation of temperature. Evidently the tissue fluid environment of developing blood cells must be maintained at a high temperature just as that of the testicle, which we shall describe later, must be held at a low temperature in order to produce sperms.

Because of these differences in cell and fat contents, in rate of metabolism and in temperature we would not look for uniformity in hydrogen ion concentration and in composition of tissue fluids of red and yellow marrow. More data are needed. A definite age change, is replacement of red by yellow marrow. Sometimes the latter assumes a gelatinous consistency as a result of wasting diseases—a phenomenon which should be sought in very old people.

Bone is abundantly supplied with blood vessels. To illustrate this fact a blood vessel and a lymphatic are depicted passing between two rows of spider-like bone cells (fig. 113). The space containing them is known as an Haversian canal. Materials leave as usual through the vascular endothelial membrane and enter the tissue fluid occupying the lumen of the canal. This is limited on the sides by a layer of cells (not shown) backed by bony matrix made rigid by the accumulation of mineral salts mostly of calcium, phosphorus and magnesium. It is reinforced by fibrous components. From the mesenchymatous tissue fluid in this matrix, materials are picked up by the processes of the cells and into it waste is discharged.

To arrive at tentative conclusions as to composition of bony tissue fluid is difficult because most analyses relate to the bone as a whole consisting of cells, plus tissue fluid. Valuable data, however, are given in Chapter 11 by Todd and by Huggins (1937). The latter believes that "Many if not all substances present in the body fluids and difficultly soluble in a faintly alkaline aqueous medium are deposited in new bone." The composition of bone of different ages will be to some extent different depending upon the availability of substances in the circulation at the time that it is formed. Without specifying the age, but presumably for both old and young bone of adults, Maximow and Bloom (1934) say that the interstitial substance (our tissue fluid), which includes everything but cells, contains 30–40 per cent of organic material (chiefly collagen, called ossein, plus small amounts of osseo-mucoid and osseo-albuminoid) and 60 to 70 per cent of inorganic material of which the calcium exits in the form of dahlite. The question for us is where, in a histological sense do the depositions occur? This, in order of decreasing likelihood, seems to be in ground substance of the tissue fluid, within the fibers in it, and within the bone cells. About all we can say is that calcium salts and other minerals, though of limited solubility are deposited in bony tissue fluid, perhaps free or adsorbed on the surfaces of the fibers or in their substance at a concentration higher than in most tissue fluids with the exception of enamel and the possible exception areas of calcification (not ossification) in cartilaginous and other tissues.

Bony tissue fluid is certainly a reservoir of calcium and other minerals of great importance to the organism. Throughout life calcium may be withdrawn on demand. There are indications that the amount of calcium in the bones of old people is somewhat reduced. The bones appear to become more brittle. Fracture of the hip is a calamity suffered chiefly by persons of advanced years whose coordination is not very good and who fall very hard. Significant results might be obtained by an investigation of the ageing of the organic components of bone which are as a rule forgotten though there is a decrease in collagen. They consist of the cells and fibers in the tissue fluid.

The topographic relations of the several membranes serving *cartilage*

are represented in figure 113. The blood stream is held away from the
cells for cartilage is practically avascular, though some so-called vascular canals do appear about the 3rd fetal month and attain a maximum
development at 30 years of age (Todd in Chapter 11). The tissue
fluid immediately outside the vascular endothelial membrane is small
in volume and of thin consistency. The amount is exaggerated in the
diagram and the perichondrium is indicated only by a single row of

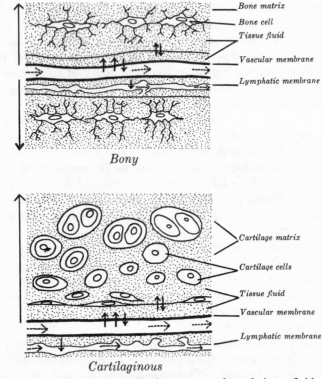

Bony

Cartilaginous

FIG. 113. Bony and cartilaginous mesenchymal tissue fluids

flattened cells. Diffusion inward is to some extent retarded by a firm
matrix of variable physical properties depending upon the number and
character of the contained fibers which are not shown in this diagram or
in any of the others. Still the cells, enclosed singly or in pairs in little compartments in the matrix, are surrounded by mesenchymatous
tissue fluid (with its fibers) from which they take up nutriment and
into which they discharge waste. Too close association with the

homeostatically regulated blood might indeed be inconsistent with the development and maintenance of cartilage as a useful component of the body. When blood vessels do penetrate into the substance of young cartilage, as in endochondral ossification, the cartilaginous matrix is absorbed and the cells degenerate. It is probable that a gradient exists in the properties of the tissue fluid as one passes deeply into cartilage in a direction vertical to the blood vessels which are some distance away. Bürger and Schlomka (1927) found that in ageing costal cartilages water decreases and calcium increases. This leads to loss of elasticity and in some cases to actual calcification. A different age modification in costal cartilages exposed to forces of twisting and shearing is, Aschoff (1933) states, " . . . an actual splitting and loosening; the cementing matrix disappears, and the fibers which had been concealed in it become again visible. This is called fibrous degeneration of the intercellular substance." He writes, further, "It will have to be conceded . . . that in some parts of the body the intercellular substance becomes so important for the function of the organ concerned that the processes of ageing seem to take place principally or exclusively in it while the cells are affected only secondarily." His intercellular substance is our tissue fluid.

The *joint fluids* are called synovial because they have the consistency of slippery white of egg. They contain mucin. The word is derived from the Greek, *syn*, together and the Latin, *ovum*, an egg. They are formed by fluid which enters the joints through synovial membranes which stretch on the sides between the opposed bones (see fig. 114). These membranes are, in the view of the best authorities, simply concentrations of mesenchymatous cells and fibers. They are not built of orderly arranged epithelial cells. Fluid seeps in through them and back again into the more watery tissue fluid next to the vascular endothelial membrane. The articulating surfaces are faced by special articular cartilage. Old people are less agile than young ones. They often complain of an increasing stiffness of the joints. How much this is occasioned by ageing of nerve and muscle on the one hand and by failure in lubrication on the other should be discovered though it will be a difficult task. Apparently there are no data available on age changes in the composition of the joint fluids or in the total and differential counts of the cells in them, but alterations have been frequently reported in the articular cartilages.

A universal manifestation of ageing is decrease in height. Extremely tall people in the prime of life notice that when they rise in the morning they are taller than when they go to bed at night. That we, on the average, become about 30 mm. shorter by day and regain our length by night is well-known to physiologists. The critical discussion by Martin (1928) is recommended. It would be interesting to ascertain what happens in extremely old people and the relation to senile alterations in the water content of the intervertebral discs (Todd, Chapter 11).

Intramuscular tissue fluid, between muscle fibers, also requires consideration for the sake of the completeness of our survey. It is

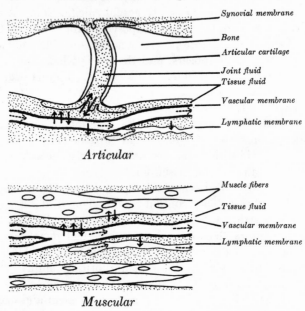

Articular

Muscular

Fig. 114. Articular and muscular mesenchymal tissue fluids

mesenchymal insofar that it contains the connective tissues derived from mesenchyme that accompany the blood vessels which supply the muscle fibers. But it is far distant from epithelium. Fluid enters through vascular endothelium, bathes muscle fibers and a few connective tissue cells and fibers and leaves by passing back into the blood vessels or lymphatics (see lowest diagram in figure 114). In skeletal muscle there are few if any lymphatics. This intramuscular tissue fluid is more subject to mechanical pressure with muscular contraction than any other but it obviously does not circulate in the way that blood does. The balance of forces concerned in maintaining its stability are shown diagrammatically by Adolph (1933). If it were present in any considerable amount it might interfere with the efficiency of muscle.

When microscopic preparations are made of muscle from a recently killed animal we find spaces between the muscle fibers which are only partly occupied by connective tissue cells, fibers, nerves and blood vessels. These apparently vacant areas are occupied by tissue fluid. They are never large, yet when added together they comprise a fraction of the total volume of muscle which gives food for thought. The fraction seems to be larger in cardiac than in a skeletal muscle. Wearn (1928) estimated that the capillary bed per sq. mm. of ventricular wall is about twice that calculated by Krogh for skeletal muscle. Perhaps the vascularity and the amount of tissue fluid are here related though there are instances where this does not obtain. More tissue fluid may occur in muscle than histological preparations indicate, because the shrinkage of the muscle, occasioned by the technique, includes dehydration and is more likely to decrease the size of the spaces than to increase it.

The bearing of all this on the problem of the ageing of muscle remains, like so much in this chapter, purely a matter of speculation until well controlled experiments are performed. As muscles age they decrease a little in size and become quite flabby. Smooth muscles do not age as skeletal ones do. In the latter Bucciante and Luria (1934) observed an increase in size of muscular fibers correlated probably with a decrease in number since the size of the muscles does not increase. Between the muscle fibers they found an increase in connective tissue elements particularly elastic fibers. Close examination of their figures appears to reveal an increase in the areas occupied by tissue fluid. But we ordinarily expect dehydration in advanced age. Todd suggests in Chapter 11 a decrease in intracellular fluid, containing potassium and protein, and an increase in intercellular fluid, containing sodium and chloride with ageing. See new techniques for quantitative measurements suggested by Baker, 1938.

4. TISSUE FLUIDS OF THE SECOND ORDER

These are anatomically farther removed from the homeostatically regulated blood stream by the interposition of special cellular membranes. Though the distances may be small, the degree of separation is not the same for all members of the order. In all the diagrams of figures 115–117, tissue fluids of the second order are indicated in dense stipple. Here also the diagrams are not drawn to scale but are intended to illustrate the microscopic features of the structural environments. Unlike the tissue fluids of the first order, they do not contain connective tissue cells and fibers so that they lack important factors in creating diversity of tissue fluid environments. Membranes intervene between them and the tissue fluids of the first order. The latter are represented in the usual light stipple. For convenience we divide this second order into two classes depending upon whether the membrane is ectodermal or mesothelial.

1. *Ectodermal tissue fluids*

The endolymph of the internal ear is typical (fig. 115). It is shown in the uppermost diagram and is separated from the perilymph, next the vascular endothelial membrane, by a membrane of ectodermal origin. Fluid enters and leaves through the ectodermal membrane but the principal exit, according to Guild (1927), is by way of the endolymphatic duct and sac. Investigations on alterations in the composition and circulation of endolymph in aged persons are much needed.

The ventricular *cerebrospinal fluid* belongs in the second order because it, likewise, is set apart from tissue fluid of the first order by the choroid plexus membrane constituted of ectodermal cells. The principal avenue of drainage is through the roof of the fourth ventricle into the subarachnoid space. The fluid in this space can be listed as belonging to the first order for the reason that it comes partly from the perineuronal spaces existing between the nerve cells and the vascular endothelial membrane. This contingent is represented by the arrow entering from the left side. Fluid returns to the venous stream mainly *via* the arachnoidal villi which project into the lumina of large venous sinuses. The concentrations of diffusible organic solutes are regularly less than in blood serum (Peters, 1935). A search for data on ageing of the mechanisms involved in stabilization of the cerebrospinal fluid is disappointing. The last word on this important tissue fluid is contained in a book by Merritt and Fremont-Smith (1937). There are almost no changes in the cerebrospinal fluid associated with senescence. The volume of the fluid is smallest in infancy and increases as one grows from adulthood into old age. This parallels the shrinkage in the volume of the brain. Whether there is a steady increase in fluid volume during adult life, or whether there is a flat plateau during this stage, there are no data. Excepting in the cadaver, measurements of volume are quite rough. The cerebrospinal fluid pressure increases from a range of 15 to 80 mm. of water in the new-born to a range of 70 to 180 in adult life. Adult pressure seems to have been reached, however, at six to eight years of age, and we have no evidence of increase thereafter. The vast majority of normal pressures lie between 100 and 160 mm. with the mean in the neighborhood of 140 to 150. It is extremely difficult to get

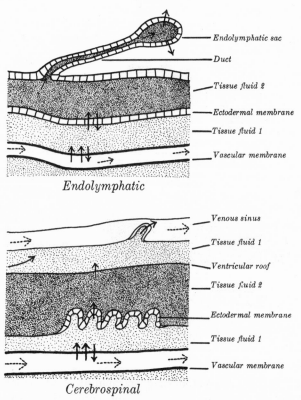

Endolymphatic sac
Duct
Tissue fluid 2
Ectodermal membrane
Tissue fluid 1
Vascular membrane

Endolymphatic

Venous sinus
Tissue fluid 1
Ventricular roof
Tissue fluid 2
Ectodermal membrane
Tissue fluid 1
Vascular membrane

Cerebrospinal

FIG. 115. Endolymphatic and cerebrospinal tissue fluids of the second order. Tissue fluid of the first order (light stipple) always intervenes between them and the vascular endothelial membrane.

data in aged individuals who are known to be normal. However the findings of Merritt and Fremont-Smith in 277 cases of cerebral arteriosclerosis are of interest since this group includes a large number of old people. The cells were normal in 85 per cent, the pressure normal in 81 per cent, the protein normal in 75 per cent and the colloidal gold reaction normal in 80 per cent. Normal values for sugar and chloride were also obtained in relatively few cases.   Apparently there is no progressive change in these constituents with age.   Fremont-Smith went over the records of the Massachusetts General Hospital with special reference to the protein content of the fluid with regard to age, and found that the majority of fluids in patients of 70 years of age and over had entirely normal protein values as compared with young adults (personal communication).

Intraocular tissue fluid (aqueous humor) is on a slightly different anatomical basis (fig. 116).   Interposed between it and tissue fluid

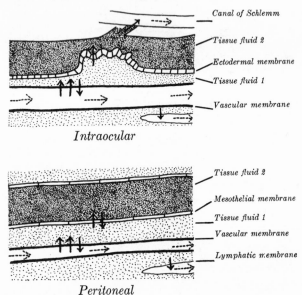

FIG. 116.   Intraocular and peritoneal tissue fluids of the second order (dense stipple).

of the first order is the ectodermal epithelium of the ciliary process. The fluid passing through this membrane enters the posterior chamber and flows between the iris and the lens into the anterior chamber. From the sulcus circularis it leaves by the endothelium lined spaces of Fontana and in some way discharges by the Canals of Schlemm into the venous blood stream.   Glucose, urea and other diffusible organic solutes are regularly present in concentrations less than in blood serum (Peters, 1935).   But the concentration of lactic acid is greater than in blood serum (Wittgenstein and Gadertz, 1926; Fischer, 1934).   Duke-Elder's (1934) carefully prepared account contains no reference to ageing of this fluid; but alterations probably occur in advanced years and may perhaps be correlated with modifications in the lens described by Friedenwald in Chapter 18. The vitreous body deserves more study.

The central parts of the *optic lenses* are perhaps of all tissues in the body the most protected from the homeostatically regulated blood stream. They are suspended in aqueous humor. According to Friedenwald (1930) the permeability of the lens capsule exceeds that of the capillaries. In cows a significant decrease in permeability occurs with ageing. The vitamin C content is interesting (Fischer, 1934). The metabolism of the lens is considerable. Critical discussion by Bourne (1937) on this point is recommended. Cataract formation is not uncommon in the aged. See Chapter 18 by Friedenwald.

2. *Mesothelial tissue fluids*

In the same way the peritoneal, pericardial, pleural and peritesticular tissue fluid are not in direct contact with vascular and lymphatic endothelia. Between them are small amounts of tissue fluid of the first order and a delicate layer of mesothelial cells which forms a distinct membrane. Entering fluids must pass through vascular endothelium, tissue fluid of the first order and a mesothelial membrane; while those leaving must traverse a mesothelial membrane, tissue fluid of the first order and vascular endothelium or lymphatic endothelium before they can be drained off (fig. 116). These fluids obviously play a different rôle in bodily integration. They provide lubrication by which yielding surfaces can move on each other. In contrast to those just mentioned they contain the same concentrations of glucose, urea etc. as blood serum (Peters, 1935).

The layer of mesothelium limiting the peritoneal cavity is carried down into the scrotum when the testicles descend. In this situation it forms two separate, lubricated, mesothelium lined cavities in which the testicles have slight freedom of movement. Tissue fluid environments are thus provided for the testicles in which the temperature is from 1.5 to 3°C less than in the peritoneal cavity. These are the extremes within which the temperature in the scrotum is regulated. To cool the testicles the muscles in the wall of the scrotum relax, so that a larger surface is exposed to the air and heat may be lost by radiation. To warm them the muscles contract, the surface is reduced and the heat derived from the blood stream is conserved.

When the testicles in the scrotum are kept for a sufficient length of time at the temperature to which they would have been subjected

had they remained in the abdominal cavity, they cease to manufacture sperms. Conversely, when abdominally retained testicles,
which do not form sperms, are dragged down into the scrotum they may
acquire the ability to produce sperms. All this is well presented by
Moore (1939). In other words, a temperature lower than that of the
peritoneal cavity is essential to manufacture sperms. It is a good
example of protection against uniformity of temperature which necessitates shifting of the particular organs almost outside of the body.

So much for the difference in temperature in the scrotal and peritoneal cavities. That within the substance of the testicle, where the
sperms are formed, is probably a little higher than in the scrotum but
nevertheless lower than in the peritoneal cavity. The ageing of the
testicle has been discussed by Engle in Chapter 15. It is probably
linked with alterations in tissue fluid as all vital activities are, but,
again, we need more information and to distinguish between cause and
effect is very difficult. Sperms often continue to be formed in advanced old age. Possibly a decrease in tissue fluid of the first order
immediately surrounding the seminiferous tubules—a part perhaps
of the progressive dehydration of the body—may constitute a factor in
preventing the sperms from getting out. The line of argument would
be as follows. The sperms, when shed into the lumina of the tubules,
must find themselves in a watery medium. If this were present in
insufficient amount, or if it were too viscous in consistency, the passage
of the sperms through tubes of many sorts into the vas deferens might
be impeded. We know very little about the production of this fluid
medium. There is no reason to believe that it is a secretion by either
the Sertoli or sperm forming cells, but we cannot definitely exclude
secretion. An internal secretion of the tubular epithelium may pass
out into the tissue fluid. Probably it accumulates simply by passage
of the surrounding tissue fluid into the lumina of the tubules impeded
more or less by the basement membrane which ages as is well described
by Engle in Chapter 15. It is quite possible, therefore, that reduction
in formation and transfer of this tissue fluid in very old men may
lead to a condition in which, though potentially active sperms develop,
they die without ever being included in an ejaculate of semen.

5. DIVERSITY OF TISSUE FLUID ENVIRONMENTS

Before listing their properties as compared with those of the blood
it is necessary to recall that the range in normal temperature of the

blood, that is to say its degree of stability in this regard, is not uniform throughout the body but different in different localities. The same holds for acid-base equilibrium and for composition. Obviously the arterial blood, first offered in the capillaries in different regions, is fairly uniform in these respects. But the nutritive arterial blood in the second set of renal capillaries, after it has passed through the glomerular capillaries, is probably different from what it was to start with. When capillaries are stretched out in one main direction, as from the cortex to the medulla of the adrenal, the contained blood will be modified in consequence of a gradient in permeability and a difference in environment. That the venous blood differs in certain localities is to be expected and has been repeatedly observed. This may be a matter of consequence for tissue fluids in the walls of vessels that carry venous blood and in organs which possess venous portal veins—the liver, the anterior lobe of the pituitary (Wislocki, 1937) and perhaps for others. Until we know the range in properties in the main parts of the circulation, and the tissue fluids are systematically investigated, it will be difficult to be sure how far the tissue fluids differ from the neighboring blood stream although the differences among themselves may be definite.

It is safe to say that *temperature* of the tissue fluid in the cornea is lower than that of the nearest blood to it and that, by its avascularity, it is protected from regulation by some of the homeostatic mechanisms controlling temperature.

By vital staining with phthalein indicators Rous (1925) and Drury and Rous (1926) have discovered marked lack of uniformity in *acid base equilibrium* of the tissues which they divide into two groups. In the most cellular ones there is a relative and probably an absolute acidity while in the others, composed mostly of tissue fluid with its fibers and a few cells, the reaction is less acid or faintly alkaline. Thus the ground substance of the tissue fluid of connective tissue is of all the most alkaline. The reaction is conditioned by the character of the tissue in any given area. Consequently the acid base equilibrium is likely to be different from that of the nearest flowing and therefore constantly changing blood.

The *composition* of certain tissue fluids is individualistic and exhibits a range in properties far exceeding that of the blood as a whole. Space only permits review of outstanding examples described in the foregoing pages.

1. The cerebrospinal fluid and the aqueous humor of the eye, which are tissue fluids of the second order, contain regularly less diffusible organic solutes than blood serum. This, Peters attributes to the distinctive features of the living membranes of the choroid plexus and ciliary body.

2. Subepithelial tissue of the small intestine receives all absorbed substances from the lumen and as a result differs somewhat periodically from other tissue fluids which do not receive them.

3. Tissue fluids separated from the blood stream by highly permeable endothelium resemble blood plasma more closely than do the others. During the cyclic filtration by venous sinuses of the spleen, the splenic tissue fluid receives most of the contained blood plasma leaving only a mass of closely packed cells behind (Knisely). Here again there is a rhythm.

4. "Loose, fine-meshed connective tissue" provides storage by inundation for water, salts and sugar (Cannon, 1932). When passing into this tissue their concentrations will be greater in the blood and when leaving less in the blood than in the tissue fluid. Unless the other kinds of connective tissue act in the same way, this particular sort of tissue fluid differs from that in the others.

5. The distinctive gel-like consistency of connective tissue fluid in some localities has been demonstrated by the Clarks and by Bensley.

6. The concentration of lactic acid in aqueous humor is greater than in blood serum.

7. Since epinephrine in the adrenal vein is more concentrated than in the general circulation it follows that its concentration in the adrenal medullary tissue fluid is also greater.

8. The follicular hormone, theelin, exists in a particularly high concentration in follicular tissue fluid, which is also, before ovulation, characteristically viscid.

9. The tissue fluids of bone and dentin are resevoirs for crystalline mineral salts particularly calcium. They can be removed easiest from bone.[2]

10. The vascular tissue fluids of veins and arteries differ in numerous

---

[2] Meyer, Smyth and Dawson (Science, 1938, **88**, 129) have recently discovered in bovine synovial tissue fluid ". . . a sulfur- and phosphorus-free polysaccharide acid of high molecular weight, containing per equivalent weight one equivalent each of nitrogen, hexosamine, acetyl and hexuronic acid." It is not bound to protein but occurs as a salt.

respects. Arterial tissue fluid regularly contains a mucin which is said to differ from all other mucins in the body; in the aorta it normally shows calcium and magnesium, and, in limited areas, an intimal fatty deposit. Protein hyaline material appears in the intimal tissue fluid of arterioles. The amount of hyaline, and the number of vessels exhibiting it, increases with age.

In many situations, especially subepithelial, the tissue fluid is present in such small amounts that analyses cannot be made. To increase its volume by causing injury leading to edema and to analyse the edema fluid is not satisfactory. Moreover the analyses made thus far of almost all available tissue fluids are limited in scope and cannot be said to cover the range of possible contents. They should include all substance entering or leaving the cells as well as others which may conceivably exist in the tissue fluid without action on the cells or adsorbed on their surfaces or on fibers. Histospectrographic analyses by the method of Scott (1937) might prove useful for both common and more rare minerals. When the electron microscope (McMillen and Scott, 1937) is further improved it should be used. Vitamine, enzyme, immune body, hormone and trephone analyses of the smaller tissue fluids have not been made. The difficulty of heterotransplantability of tissue cells from one organism to another, as contrasted with the ease of homiotransplantability, depends upon the fact that they find themselves in a tissue fluid environment which is different from that to which they are accustomed and they proceed to modify the environment in ways which are not acceptable to their hosts who treat them as foreign invaders, but how they do so is beyond our ken. The chemist as yet sees no difference in the tissue fluid environment of the invaders and of the invaded.

The matter simmers down, in some localities, to individual opinion as to probabilities based on very little evidence. To assert that all minute tissue fluids are really the same, except perhaps for changes in the amounts of protein in different regions, is in my opinion more arbitrary than to hold that at least a few of them are probably different. The composition of the blood stream, on the other side of the endothelial membrane, is far from uniform in different regions. Neither is the permeability of the limiting vascular endothelium uniform. This view of the probability of local differences is shared by many cytologists. Carrel (1931) writes: "Each tissue or organ certainly manufactures in some measure its own medium which, in turn, acts on the cells. It is only through the analysis of the physicochemical and chemical conditions of the local medium that the state of the tissue *in vivo* can be completely understood." His "local medium" is our tissue fluid.

6. DIVISIONS OF THE MILIEU INTERNE

We have classified tissue fluids on the basis of the structural features of the environments in which they occur. We have indicated the special properties which some exhibit, and have noted what little is known of the modifications that occur in advancing years. But the tissue fluids are only part of the *milieu interne* of Claude Bernard and it seems proper before concluding this chapter to turn to it as a whole. It is "the totality of circulating fluids of the organism," includes all fluid that is not intracellular and is divisible into lots possessed of distinctive properties. Yet, according to him, "It is the fixity of the *milieu interieur* which is the condition of free and independent life"

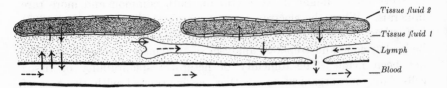

FIG. 117. Horizontal divisions of the *milieu interne*

(quoted from Cannon 1932). *Fixity* seems to be too strong a term. It is incompatible with that variation within physiological limits, which occurs in all living things. It would be better to say "constancy within certain limits of different fluid environments within higher organisms is the condition of free and independent life."

Any description of the position of the divisions of the *milieu interieur* in space is bound to be inadequate. It will be agreed however that the blood stream, which circulates yet moves in all directions with respect to the force of gravity, provides a good base line or plane which we may consider as physiologically (not geophysically) horizontal with reference to the cells and fluids, often in layers, which border it. The blood stream is limited everywhere by endothelium and it is our first and basic horizontal division of the *milieu interne* (fig. 117). It is paralleled by tissue fluids which constitute the second major horizontal division. A third horizontal division, the lymph, makes its appearance with the evolution of the vertebrates. It is insinuated into the tissue fluids and is surrounded by them though limited, like the blood, by an endothelial membrane in the lymphatic capillaries and vessels and by littoral cells in the lymph nodes. The lymph provides drainage of tissue fluid supplementary to that afforded by the blood. It parallels the blood, but its horizontal extent is definitely less than that of the blood, for there are many parts of the body, particularly most of the nervous system, where there are no lymphatics.

Vertical divisions exit to a minor degree in the blood and lymph, because these are not uniform either in their chemical or physical properties throughout their extent, but show regional differences. It is in the tissue fluids that the vertical divisions are most pronounced topographically. The movement of fluids in those of the first order is directly from and into the blood stream and into the lymph (where that is present) and therefore in a sense vertical in respect to both, and not so much lateral as in the horizontal divisions of blood and lymph. These vertical divisions of the tissue fluids merge with each other laterally. Their limits are usually not clearly defined except in encapsulated organs.

Tissue fluids of the second order have different structural environments. They are separated from those of the first order by delicate ectodermal or mesothelial membranes. The fluids pass directly, we say vertically, by the shortest route, from the blood through the vascular endothelial membrane, across thin films of tissue fluid of the first order, and enter through these special membranes. There is more lateral, or horizontal, movement than in those of the first order, indeed reference is frequently made to a sluggish circulation in a definite direction or directions of the ocular, endolymphatic and cerebrospinal fluids. But the spread of all fluids of the second order is sharply defined by the particular membranes which surround them.

Briefly stated the main factors that determine the properties of vertical divisions of tissue fluid of both orders include differences both quantitative and qualitative: (1) in association with the horizontal division of the blood stream; (2) in association with the external environment both surface and penetrating into the body; and (3) in their cellular and fibrous contents.

Gradients in composition are created as one passes from the vascular endothelial membrane up into the several tissue fluid environments. Some of them are suggested by the large arrows in figures 107, 111–113. These depend upon the effectiveness of factors modifying the tissue fluid in a given distance. Thus, in the tissue fluid beneath and within the epidermis, the hold of the blood stream becomes less and less as one approaches the surface of the skin. Similarly, in the dentin of teeth there is a somewhat irregular gradient of increase in mineral, matter based upon the vascularized pulp and moving vertically through the avascular predentin and dentin. In the walls of arteries, receiving fluids from the blood stream within and from the vasa vasorum without, levels in composition or gradients are established, witness the intimal hyaline and the mesarterial band of calcarcous deposit. In avascular tissues, like cartilage, the optic lens and perhaps in the cornea, others are formed passing away from the blood stream. Probably also there is a gradient in the splenic lobules, for the permeability of the peripherally placed venous sinuses, in the red pulp, is much greater than of the centrally placed capillaries, in the white pulp.

It is difficult to conceive of any tissue fluid environment in which a gradient of some sort vertical to the vascular endothelial membrane, or general plane occupied by the nearest capillaries, sinusoids, or venous sinuses, will not be set up. Equal distribution of substances in such an environment could only be achieved if it were homogeneous, in the sense that it were wholly fluid and contained no metabolically active cells, or dead cells, or fibers, or other structures, on which adsorption could take place; and if the passage in and out of water, salts etc. through the vascular endothelial membrane were constant. There is no tissue fluid environment of this sort anywhere in the body. That in dental enamel comes nearest to it in that it is metabolically inactive; but the entry of fluid from the oral cavity and from the dentin is not constant and the mineral components are not uniformly distributed.

The homeostatic regulation of tissue fluids is little understood. Though some tissue fluids have been known and studied for a long time, there are few data on the extent of normal disturbances of balance in them. This may be due to constancy of the fluids or to failure to look for alterations by adequate methods. Because the particular properties of the cerebrospinal fluid are remarkably constant, it does not mean that others are equally constant. For example the tissue fluid in the female genital system decreases in amount in the absence of follicular hormone; but, when this is supplied, it increases to a very striking degree (Allen, Chapter 14). It is possible that the change is qualitative as well as quantitative. Perhaps the greatest swing in properties of tissue fluid takes place in the uterine mucosa during the menstrual cycle. Are, we may ask, the distinctive special temperatures, acid base equilibria and other features regulated by the same mechanisms which Cannon has so well described in homeostasis of the blood? Yes, to a large extent, but not entirely. It would be unwise to ignore local factors, for, as we have said, the amplitude of range of property difference is often greater in the tissue fluid environments, taken as a whole, than in the blood stream itself. Thus the temperature of the cornea is much lower, the concentrations of epinephrine and of follicular hormone are higher, the viscosity of synovial fluid and of some subcutaneous connective tissue fluids is greater and the range of hydrogen concentration of various tissue fluids is wider than in the blood.

The tissue fluids intervene between the tissue cells and the homeostatically regulated blood stream from which they are separated by the vascular endothelial membrane. Obviously there are two main influences to be balanced: the closeness of the secondariness of the tissue fluids to the blood and the closeness of their dependence on the tissue cells and fibers in and about them. When the influence of the blood is very direct the tendency will be for them to share the homeostasis of the blood. When, on the contrary, the blood is held at a distance, in ways which we have specified, the influence of the tissue components will be increased and the homeostasis of the blood will be less potent. In the equilibrium of fluid exchange between blood plasma and tissue fluid four main factors are concerned. Hydrostatic pressure of the blood and effective osmotic pressure of the plasma on one side, and deformation tension, or tissue resistance, and effective tissue fluid osmotic pressure on the other. But the system is not so simple. The tissue fluid in turn is in more or less equilibrium with the intracellular fluid. There is, as Adolph (1933) states, the cellular membrane to consider as well as the vascular endothelial one. And the cells are of many kinds in different functional states. Well known local rhythms of different sorts are manifest in most physiological activities. The chances are that these will affect local, cell-rich tissue fluid environments more directly than the blood stream which is constantly moving and of much larger volume.

If vascular intermittency turns out to be a phenomenon manifested in several regions of the body, we may expect other rhythms in minute areas of particular tissue fluids immediately adjacent to capillaries. Richards (1935), believes that the blood flow through the capillary tufts (glomeruli) of the kidney is intermittent. He suggests that after closure of the afferent arteriole an asphyxial change occurs in it which causes the muscle to become relaxed and to be for a time "refractory to the continuing constrictor stimulus." In other words there is an intermittent, local oxygen-lack in the tissue fluid about the muscle cells. Confirmation is needed. Wearn et al. (1934) have observed intermittency in flow of blood in arterioles and capillaries about the air sacs of the lungs where they think it unlikely that lack of oxygen is a factor. There is strong evidence that in resting muscle as many as 90 per cent of the capillaries are closed (Krogh, 1932). But we do not know whether in muscular activity the previously closed ones are more likely to open than the previously open ones to remain open—whether there is intermittency or rhythm. Doan (1922) has reported collapsed blood capillaries in bone marrow. If they open and close, it is a case of intermittency; if they remain closed, and the open capillaries in the immediate vicinity of the closed ones do not compensenate for the lack of blood flow, the local tissue fluid environments outside of the closed capillaries will differ from those outside of open ones.

Finally it is evident that to visualize these horizontal and vertical divisions of the *milieu interne* is extraordinarily difficult. Some are visible to the naked eye but many are not. Histologists are prone to think of cells, fluids and contained fibers as they are seen at a magnification of several hundred diameters, while biochemists and physiologists are not so reliant upon a microscope, yet take into careful consideration important structural components which are much smaller, such as monomolecular layers. Any description is bound to be of limited scope and is likely to be one-sided. To speak of their uniformity, or fixity, or even of their constancy, without qualification is unwise. They are the changing fluid environments in which the processes of ageing become manifest. There is movement everywhere and there are numerous rhythms of different lengths. To ascertain the extent of normal changes in each and every one of them from birth through senility to death is a task which will require the best efforts of generations of investigators.

7. SUMMARY

The problem of ageing is one of great complexity. The living human body is a wonderful creation of which the central integrating mechanism is the homeostatically regulated blood stream. Most of the vital units, or cells, perform their duties outside the blood vessels in the tissue fluids all which are not of uniform temperature, acid-base equilibrium, composition or fiber content throughout the body. It is already evident that some of these tissue fluid environments are fairly characteristic and exhibit special properties. Space does not permit review of each but taken as a whole the following deviations from blood serum are found in particular tissue fluid environments: (1) less diffusible organic solutes; (2) presence of mucin and hyaline material; (3) higher concentration of hormones; (4) more lactic acid, mineral salts, etc; (5) greater range in fluidity and hydrogen-ion concentration; (6) variable amounts of water, salt and glucose depending upon storage and release from storage; and (7) occurrence in different proportions, depending on their nature, of non-vital, but surface active, colloidal fibrous components.

These and other differences in local tissue fluid environments are partly occasioned by regional inequality in the operation of some factors which can be identified and probably by many unknown ones. Among the former, differences, both quantitative and qualitative may be mentioned: (1) in association with the blood stream; (2) in association with the external environment, both surface and penetrating into the body; (3) in the cells and fibers, either in them or about their margins.

As investigation proceeds it may be discovered that the properties of other tissue fluids are adjusted to special needs, or those about which little is known at present may be found to constitute a group in which a fair degree of uniformity prevails.

With progressive impairment of the regulatory devices of homeostasis of the blood, as old age creeps on, it is logical to suppose that decrease in metabolic rate, decrease in ability to use and store glucose, reduction in alkali reserve of the blood, increased blood pressure, ageing of colloids, progressive dehydration and other changes discussed in this book, will be felt differently in the different tissue fluid environments. Some may prove more susceptible than others to the same change and the speed and kind of reaction may also differ.

There are some progressive alterations in the properties of the blood in advancing years, which are therefore not held relatively uniform during this time by homeostatic mechanisms. McCay in Chapter 21 refers to *decrease* in specific gravity and serum calcium and to *increase* in refractive index, total nitrogen, lactic acid, indoxyl and urea. Obviously these alterations in old age, as well as changes in amounts of growth inhibiting and growth promoting factors studied by Carrel and his associates, will not be without influence on the tissue fluid environments outside the vascular endothelial membrane.

On the very important question of alterations in permeability of capillary endothelium with age, there is a good deal of speculation but a dearth of facts. Drinker and Field (1931) write: "Is it not possible that an old man owes his loss in weight, and dried up appearance, to a progressive decrease in the permeability of his blood capillaries, which is only partially compensated by an increase in capillary blood pressure? Such an individual is perhaps unable to hold water in his tissue spaces because the permeability of his capillaries for protein has in large degree been lost, and he has nothing extravascular to retain water when his capillary blood pressure falls in even slight degree. One may look to some condition such as maintenance of the volume of extravascular water for an explanation of the normal increase of blood pressure in old age, and indeed hypertension in general, and it does not seem extravagant to suggest that decreased capillary permeability, with a consequent lowered supply of extravascular protein, is at the root of the problem." Landis (1934) in discussing the manner in which protein leaks through the capillary wall says: "Protein might pass in very low concentration through the entire endothelial surface or unmodified plasma might leak through a few capillaries which are abnormally permeable owing to trauma, or to a natural process of ageing." In the first quotation a decreased capillary permeability is hypothecated as an ageing process and in the second an increased permeability.

Cohn in Chapter 7 notes that capillary permeability "is said" to decrease with age but adds that "there is no literature as yet on this point." He suggests that the capillaries may share in the loss of elasticity with age that occurs in the aorta even without loss in distinctive staining reaction of the elastic fibers. If dilatation becomes less effective, that increase in permeability, which accompanies increase in spread and decrease in thickness of the wall, will also be less effective. On the same basis, where there is endothelial proliferation and thickening as sometimes happens in vessels usually of larger girth than capillaries, permeability would be decreased. On the other hand, if there is an appreciable oxygen lack, or accumulation of H substances, we would look for increase in permeability in areas where these alterations occur. It is possible, of course, that capillary endothelium retains its youthfulness in extreme old age for new capillaries can develop normally and tumors become vascularized. The partial disappearance of dermal capillaries (Cannon, Chapter 21) and the progressive decrease in the number of renal glomeruli (Moore, 1931) may not be primary senile changes but an expression of decrease in functional demand for them with general tissue atrophy often expressed by loss of weight in the aged which is probably not altogether due to dehydration.

With the wasting, or partial involution, of lymphoid tissue (see Chapter 8 by Krumbhaar), there may be an alteration in the lymphatic capillaries. Should Pullinger and Florey's (1935) conception of the mechanism of dilatation prove correct then the ageing of collagenic fibers will be a factor. If the lymphatic capillaries fail, the drainage of tissue fluid will be modified differently in different regions owing to diversity in distribution of lymphatics and in the character of lymph they carry. But it does not necessarily follow that the character of the tissue fluids will be altered.

Muscular tissue fluid, containing sodium and chloride, increases with ageing while intracellular fluid of muscle containing protein and potassium decreases (Todd, Chapter 11). The sodium of the blood does not change (McCay, Chapter 21). The connective tissue fluid varies with physiological age (Bensley). In the embryonic and undifferentiated tissues, which have been investigated, it is young viscid and continuous. In adults, it is less abundant and interrupted by spaces presumably containing more fluid material; observations on the aged are needed. In the arterial tissue fluids there are increases in acidity and mucin content with age, the amounts of hyaline material, lipoids and calcium salts tend to increase, and the colloidal elastic fibers age with gradual depression of electric charges on their particles so that dispersion is decreased, condensation increased and chemical reactivity decreased. These age changes are prone to occur in definite, often quite restricted, local tissue fluid environments.

In the outlying tissue fluids, which are present in avascular areas, the action of the processes of ageing is clearly manifest. The mesenchymal tissue fluids of cartilage may remain about the same, increase in firmness by calcification, or become looser by removal of minerals again depending upon local conditions mechanical and otherwise. In the optic lenses cataracts often form in aged persons. In the epidermis, regulation appears to become less effective. Though there may be a slight general atrophy, local foci of cellular proliferation are commonly met with which may turn out to be malignant.

The study of rhythms in the epidermis has only been commenced. Cohn (Chapter 7) reports that in ageing of the heart "as time progresses there is a marked tendency for abnormalities of rhythm to multiply." The suppression of the menstrual rhythm is an early age change. There are numerous other rhythms, some of which we have mentioned, with which the processes of ageing may interfere for the rhythms are conditioned by many factors. Indeed, when more information becomes available, this may prove to be one of the main features of ageing. Another is decrease in responsiveness of cells to stimuli (or to inhibitions). All we have at present is evidence of decrease in reactivity to certain hormones.

We may hope to find clues as to the nature of the processes of ageing by balancing local alterations in cells and fibers against changes in fluid environment. If similar cells or fibers age in the same way in different tissue fluid environments, that would be significant. For example, elastic fibers in the dermis, and in walls of the bladder, respiratory passages, arteries and veins, are subjected to different physical strains. It would also be interesting if different cells or different fibers age differently in the same fluid environment. The systematic microscopic investigation of the processes of ageing has barely been commenced. Many techniques are available, yet have not been applied. Cooperation between cytologists and biochemists is essential.

REFERENCES

ADOLPH, E. F. 1933. The metabolism and distribution of water in body and tissues. Physiol. Rev., 13, 336-370.

ALLEN, E., PRATT, J. P., NEWELL, Q. U., AND BLAND, L. J. 1930. Hormone content of human ovarian tissues. Am. J. Physiol., 92, 127-143.

ANITSCHKOW, W. 1925. Zur Histophysiologie der Arterienwand. Klin. Wchschr., 4, 2233-2235.

———— 1933. Experimental Arteriosclerosis in Animals in Cowdry's Arteriosclerosis. New York: The Macmillan Co., 617 pp.

AREY, L. B. 1936. Wound healing. Physiol. Rev., 16, 327-406.

ASCHOFF, LUDWIG 1933. Introduction to Cowdry's Arteriosclerosis. New York: The Macmillan Co., 617 pp.

BAZETT, H. C. AND McGLONE, B. 1927. Temperature gradients in the tissues of man. Am. J. Physiol., 82, 415-450.

BELL, E. T. 1933. Arteriosclerosis of the Abdominal Viscera and Extremities in Cowdry's Arteriosclerosis. New York: The Macmillan Co., 617 pp.

BENSLEY, SYLVIA H. 1934. On the presence, properties and distribution of the intercellular ground substance of loose connective tissue. Anat. Rec., 60, 93-110.

BJORLING, E. 1911. Ueber mukoides Bindegewebe. Virchow's Arch., 205, 71-100.

BOURNE, M. C. 1937. Metabolic factors in cataract production. Physiol. Rev., 17, 1-27.

BUCCIANTE, L. AND LURIA, S. 1934. Transformazioni nella struttura dei muscoli volontari del—l'uomo nella senescenza. Arch. Ital. Anat. e. Embriol., 33, 110-187.

BAKER, H. 1938. Estimation of fiber, fat cells and connective tissue in muscle. Science, **87**, 555–556.

BÜRGER, M. AND SCHLOMKA, G. 1927. Untersuchungen am menschlichen Rippenknorpel. Ztsch. f. d. ges. exper. Med., **55**, 287–302.

CANNON, W. B. 1932. The Wisdom of the Body. New York: W. W. Norton Company, 312 pp.

CARLETON, A. 1934. A rhythmical periodicity in the mitotic division of animal cells. J. Anat., **68**, 251–263.

CARREL, ALEXIS 1924. Tissue culture and cell physiology. Physiol. Rev., **4**, 1–20.

———— 1931. The New Cytology. Science, **73**, 297–303.

CARREL, ALEXIS AND BURROWS, M. T. 1911. On the physiochemical regulation of the growth of tissues. J. Exper. Med., **13**, 562–570.

CLARK, E. R. AND CLARK, E. L. 1933. Further observations on living lymphatic vessels in the transparent chamber in the rabbit's ear—their relation to the tissue spaces. Am. J. Anat., **52**, 273–305.

COLE, H. H., GUILBERT, H. R. AND GOSS, H. 1932. Further considerations of the properties of the gonad-stimulating principle of mare serum. Am. J. Physiol., **102**, 227–240.

COWDRY, E. V. 1938. Textbook of Histology, Philadelphia: Lea & Febiger, 600 pp.

DOAN, C. A. 1922. The circulation of the bone-marrow. Contrib. to Embryol. (Carnegie Inst. Wash.) **14**, 27–46.

DOISEY, E. A. 1932. Biochemistry of the Follicular Hormone, Theelin, in Allen's Sex and Internal Secretions, Baltimore: Williams & Wilkins, 481–498.

DRINKER, C. K., DRINKER, K. R. AND LUND, C. C. 1922. The circulation of the mammalian bone-marrow. Am. J. Physiol., **62**, 1–91.

DRINKER, C. K. AND FIELD, M. E. 1931. The protein content of mammalian lymph and the relation of lymph to tissue fluid. Am. J. Physiol., **97**, 32–39.

DRURY, D. R. AND ROUS, PEYTON 1926. The relative reaction of living mammalian tissues. J. Exp. Med., **43**, 669–701.

DUKE-ELDER, W. S. 1934. Physico-chemical factors affecting intraocular pressure. Physiol. Rev., **14**, 483–605.

EVANS, H. M., MEYER, K., SIMPSON, M. E. 1933. Biology of gonad-stimulating hormone in males. Memoirs Univ. California, **2**, 207–228.

FENN, W. O. 1936. Electrolytes in muscle. Symposia on Quantitative Biology, **4**, 252–259.

FISCHER, F. P. 1934. Über das C-Vitamin der Linse. Klin. Wchnschr., **13**, 596–597.

FISH, E. W. 1932. An experimental investigation of enamel, dentine and the dental pulp. London: John Bale, Sons and Danielsson, 48 pp.

FRIEDENWALD, J. S. 1930. The permeability of the lens capsule to water dextrose and other sugars. Arch. Opth., **4**, 350–360.

GAMBLE, J. L. 1937. Extracellular fluid. Bull. Johns Hopkins Hosp., **51**, 151–173.

GUILD, S. R. 1927. The circulation of the endolymph. Am. J. Anat., **39**, 57–81.

HERXHEIMER, G. 1917. Ueber das Verhalten der Kleinen Gefässe der Milz. Berl. Klin. Wchnschr., **54**, 82–84.

HOOKER, D. R. 1911. Effect of exercise upon the venous blood pressure. Am. J. Physiol. **28**, 235–248.

HUEBSCHMANN, P. 1906. Beitrag zur pathologischen Anatomie der Arterien-verkalkung. Beitr. z. path. Anat. u. z. allg. Path., **39**, 119–130.

HUGGINS, C. 1937. The composition of bone and the function of the bone cell. Physiol. Rev., **17**, 119–143.

HUGGINS, C. AND BLOCKSOM, B. H., JR. 1936. Changes in outlying bone marrow accompanying a local increase of temperature within physiological limits. J. Exper. Med., **64**, 253–274.

HUGGINS, C., BLOCKSOM, B. H., JR. AND NOONAN, W. J. 1936. Temperature conditions in the bone marrow of rabbit, pigeon and albino rat. Am. J. Physiol., **115**, 395–401.

KAST, LUDWIG 1933. Foreword in Cowdry's Arteriosclerosis, New York: The Macmillan Co., 617 pp.

KLEIN, H. AND AMBERSON, W. R. 1929. A physico-chemical study of the structure of dental enamel. J. Dental Res., **9**, 667–688.

KNISELY, M. H. 1936. Spleen studies. Anat. Rec., **65**, 23.

KROGH, A. 1929. Anatomie und Physiologie der Capillaren. Berlin: Julius Springer.

——— 1932. The Capillaries in Cowdry's Special Cytology, New York: Paul B. Hoeber, Inc., **1**, 477–503.

LANDIS, E. M. 1928. The effects of lack of oxygen on the permeability of the capillary walls to fluid and to plasma proteins. Am. J. Physiol., **83**, 528–542.

——— 1934. Capillary pressure and capillary permeability. Physiol. Rev., **14**, 404–481.

LEWIS, T. 1927. The blood vessels of the human skin and their responses. London: Shaw, 322 pp.

LUDLUM, S. D., TAFT, A. E. AND NUGENT, R. L. 1931. The chylomicron emulsion. J. Physical. Chem., **35** (1), 269–288.

MANN, IDA 1932. Cowdry's Special Cytology, New York: Paul B. Hoeber, Inc., **3**, 1305–1331.

MARTIN, R. 1928. Lehrbuch der Anthropologie. Jena: Gustav Fischer, **1**, 578 pp.

MAXIMOW, A. A. AND BLOOM, W. 1934. Textbook of Histology, Philadelphia: W. B. Saunders Co., 662 pp.

McMILLEN, J. H. AND SCOTT, GORDON H. 1937. A magnetic electron microscope of simple design. Rev. Sci. Instruments, **8**, 288–290.

McNEE, J. W. 1930–31. The Lettsomian lectures on the spleen: its structure, functions and diseases. Trans. Med. Soc. London, **54**, 185–236.

MERRITT, H. H. AND FREMONT-SMITH, F. 1937. Cerebrospinal fluid, Philadelphia: W. B. Saunders Co., 333 pp.

MOORE, CARL 1939. Allen's Internal Secretions in Relation to Sex, Baltimore: Williams & Wilkins Co. (in press).

MOORE, R. A. 1931. The total number of glomeruli in the normal human kidney. Anat. Rec., **48**, 153–168.

NOYES, F. B. 1929. Dental histology and embryology. Philadelphia: Lea and Febiger, 527 pp.

PETERS, J. P. 1935. Body water. The exchange of fluids in man, Springfield: Charles C. Thomas, 405 pp.

PETERSEN, W. F. 1934. The Patient and the Weather, Ann Arbor: Edwards Bros. Inc., **2**, 530 pp.

POLICARD, A. 1933. Mineral constituent of blood vessels as determined by the technique of microincineration. (Chapter in) Cowdry's Arteriosclerosis, New York: Macmillan, 617 pp.

POLICARD, A., MOREL, A. AND RAVAULT, P. P. 1932. Étude histospectrographique de la localisation du calcium et du magnesium dans l'aorte humaine et de leur variations au cours de l'athérome. C. Rend. Acad. d. Sc., **194**, 201–203.

PULLINGER, B. D. AND FLOREY, H. W. 1935. Some observations on the structure and functions of lymphatics: Their behavior in local oedema. Brit. J. Exper. Path., **16**, 49–61.

RICHARDS, A. N. 1935. Berglund and Medes' The Kidney in Health and Disease, Philadelphia: Lea & Febiger, 754 pp.

RIDDLE, OSCAR 1935. Contemplating the hormones. Endocrinology, **19**, 1–13.

ROBINSON, A. 1918. The formation, rupture, and closure of ovarian follicles in ferrets and ferret-polecat hybrids and some associated phenomena. Trans. Roy. Soc., Edinburg, **52**, 85.

ROSEBURY, T. 1930. A biochemical study of the protein in dental enamel. J. Dental Res., **10**, 187–213.

ROUS, PEYTON 1925. The relative reaction of living mammalian tissues. J. Exper. Med., **41**, 739–759.

SCHMIDTMANN, M. AND HÜTTICH, M. 1928. Die Bedeutung der Gefässwandreaktion für die Arteriosklerose. Virchow's Arch., **267**, 601–624.

SCHOUR, I. AND STEADMAN, S. R. 1935. The growth pattern and daily rhythm of the incisor of the rat. Anat. Rec., **63**, 325–333.

SCHULTZ, A. 1922. Ueber die Chromotropie des Gefässbindegewebes in ihrer physiologischen und pathologischen Bedeutung, insbesondere inhre Beziehungen zur Arteriosklerose. Virchow's Arch., **239**, 415–450.

SCOTT, GORDON H. 1937. The distribution of inorganic salts in adult and embryonic cells and tissues. Occasional Pub. Am. Assoc. Adv. Sci., **4**, 173–180.

SHAMBAUGH, G. E. 1931. The basement membrane of the mucosa of the upper respiratory passages. Arch. Otolaryngol., **13**, 556–569.

SMITH, F. AND ROUS, P. 1931. The gradient of vascular permeability. J. Exper. Med., **54**, 499–514.

SSOLOWJEW, A. 1923. Über die Zwischensubstanz der Blutgefässwand. Virchow's Arch., **241**, 1–15.

WEARN, J. T. 1928. The extent of the capillary bed of the heart. J. Exper. Med., **47**, 273–316.

WEARN, J. T., ERNSTENL, A. C., BROMER, A. W., BARR, J. S., GERMAN, W. J. AND ZSCHIESCHE, L. J. 1934. The normal behavior of the pulmonary blood vessels with observations on the intermittance of the flow of blood in the arterioles and capillaries. Am. J. Physiol., **109**, 236–256.

WELLS, H. GIDEON 1933. The Chemistry of Arteriosclerosis in Cowdry's Arteriosclerosis, New York: The Macmillan Co., 617 pp.

WINTERNITZ, M. C., THOMAS, R. M., AND LeCOMPTE, P. M. 1938. The Biology of Arteriosclerosis. Springfield: Charles C. Thomas, 142 pp.

WISLOCKI, G. B. 1937. The vascular supply of the hypophysis cerebri of the cat. Anat. Rec., **69**, 361–387.

WITTGENSTEIN, A. AND GAEDERTZ, A. 1929. Über den Milchsäuregehalt des Kammerwassers. Biochem. Ztschr., **176**, 1–16.

WOLBACH, S. B. 1933. Controlled formation of collagen and reticulum. A study of the source of intercellular substance in recovery from experimental scorbutus. Am. J. Path., **9** (suppl.), 689–699.

CHAPTER 24

AGEING PROCESSES CONSIDERED IN RELATION TO TISSUE
SUSCEPTIBILITY AND RESISTANCE

WM. DEB. MACNIDER

Chapel Hill

Considerations of senescence and the ageing process have been of
interest and speculation in a philosophical sense for an indefinite period
which at least antedates the classical discussion by Cicero. Such
processes were in a measure transferred for thoughtful analysis to the
domain of science by August Weismann in his essay on longevity
which appeared in 1882. Prior to this time, individuals eminent in
physiology and pathology had arrived at certain very general conclusions concerning the basic causes involved in the development of
senescence. Both Johannes Muller (1844) and Cohnheim (1882) came
to the conclusion that conditions which determine senescence, the time
of the appearance of such changes, and the rapidity with which they
developed, culminating in such general alterations in an organism
and such organ defects in function that physiological or senile death
was the result, were to be found in the physiological constitution of
the individual. Any interest in the ageing process, whether it be
solely one of cytomorphosis or of such cell changes considered in the
capacity of their functional effectiveness, resistance, or susceptibility to injury, has to concern itself with an attempt to understand,
not only what this "physiological constitution" is, but how it operates
in a given species of animal or in family groups or in organ systems
to bring about at various age spans certain rather characteristic modifications in such large or small aggregates of organisms as to be designated ageing or senescence.

In 1889 certainly a definite step forward was made by Richard
Hertwig (1903) in his cytological studies of depressed function and
physiological degeneration of cells, cell states which he supposed closely
resembled the development of senescence and death. He was observant
of nuclear changes and alterations in cell cytoplasm which at least
localized his conception to an intracellular maladjustment which expressed modified function. Commencing with a publication in 1909
in connection with cytological studies at first concerned with surgical

shock, Dolley (1909, 1910, 1911) both continued and amplified the work of Hertwig, emphasizing the significance of changes in the nucleus-plasma relationship of cells, not only in various states of exalted and depressed function, but also of this fundamental intracellular structural relationship as it occurred in youth and in senility. A cytological change correlated with function, as expressed at the extremes of the age span of an organism, at least opened the cell for future study. About the same time of Dolley's publication, there appeared certain investigations of Minot (1908, 1913) in which he, with great wisdom and breadth of understanding, as was his custom, emphasized the early date at which ageing commenced, the association of this state with cell differentiation, and its constant association with morphological cell changes designated by him as a process of cytomorphosis. Change, specialization, movement, took their place with groups of cells as a part of the ageing process. Even though Minot's conceptions were far from explaining what senescence is, they brought into this domain of understanding two fundamental factors which have to be considered in this process, time and change—change not as an intracellular adjustment but as shifts in cellular morphology, organ structure, and the generalized changes in an organism as a whole as transitions are made as a result of the time factor which perhaps we should best consider as tissue adaptations at different periods of the life span. Such changes should not be looked upon as morphological shifts steadily progressing to a terminal end reaction but as changes which tend for a period of hours, days, or years, depending upon the species of animal, to effect an adaptation and stabilization of the organism at certain periods in the age span as youth, maturity, and senescence. In considering ageing as a product of the life span, both susceptibility and resistance enter into this process of transitory adaptation to the factor of time expressing itself in the reaction of tissues to it.

Any preamble to a consideration of the ageing process would be far from complete without reference to two monographs: the first by Morgan (1901) with his understanding of repair and regeneration as cells and organs pass through one period of life to another and withstand, with normal or modified function, injury; the second a volume by Child (1915) in which both senescence and rejuvenescence are approached in a masterful fashion as they occur in low, multicellular forms of life, and in which he points out differences which occur in metabolic gradients, dependent upon the age of the organism which influence both the rapidity and perfection to which the senescent state may develop, and furthermore, how these differences influence in senescence the process of rejuvenescence. Such metabolic shifts in cells as they live in highly specialized organs may be factors of a chemical nature responsible for cell stabilization and for the functional effectiveness of the cells at different age periods. Behind changes in cellular morphology which may represent periods of susceptibility or resistance there must be chemical modifications in cell life responsible for these states. More recent than these contributions is the monograph by Pearl (1922) which takes into its consideration as a part of its scope the allimportant genetic factor in ageing, as well as other factors of a biological order which constitute "The Biology of Death."

In the foregoing introduction brief mention has been made to certain contributions to the subject of ageing in order, through the diversity of their nature, to indicate that any consideration of this process, even in one organ or system or organs, in terms of tissue resistance and susceptibility has, if possible, to be seen not in a state of isolation but as a local expression of biological phenomena which also influence the organism as a whole. Cellular changes dependent upon time as a determining factor as they occur in very low forms of life may very likely be found, as modified expressions of the process, to occur in the life span of the higher organisms. Such basic studies as those of Loeb (1906), Jennings (1912), and Woodruff (1908) give students of ageing and senescence fundamental conceptions of such processes. Finally, the processes of ageing which connote both functional and structural change on the part of an organism have, if possible, to be furthermore seen not only in an ontogenetic sense but, in states of advanced senescence as such or associated with disease, in a phylogenetic sense in which certain organ changes and cell metaplasias may represent a reversion to a type of cell or structure normal for an ancestral type of animal. Such changes, though not specifically designated as such, have been observed in investigations by Grafflin (1933), MacNider (1933), and Oliver (1935).

Two questions arise when ageing is considered in the higher animals which are difficult if not impossible to answer and which force a student of the subject away from the accuracy which he desires to accept in its place an age lattitude, in which he may work, represented by animals which fall in certain age groups. Even such a grouping must be of an elastic nature. The questions referred to are first, the age of a cell or groups of cells in an organ under investigation and second, as to whether or not cell changes observed in organs during the process of ageing are due to this factor expressing itself either locally or diffusely as such, or whether such changes must be considered as primary expressions of disease or as disease secondary to other structures in a given organ. Is there such a state as expressed by changes in the structure of cells which may be considered a normal physiological retrogression?

Concerning the first question, it is impossible in the multicellular organisms of any extensive organ differentiation to say that a given group of cells has had a definite life span. Such cells as they advance in age, on the basis of Dolley's work, effect nuclear readjustments which lead to recuperation and a continuation of normal function. Furthermore, if we are permitted to see the ageing process as one common to all forms of animal life, the possibility at least offers itself that as cells age they may at a certain point in the process undergo a nuclear change akin to endomixis in certain unicellular forms which results in a reconstitution and rearrangement of their chromatic material and with this, cellular rejuvenation. In the higher forms of animal life accurate information can not be obtained as to the age of a group of cells related in similar function unless it be for certain ganglion cells, cells of the central nervous system and blood cells.

The second question which has been raised concerning cell changes as an animal ages is even more difficult to answer, for it has to be considered in a relative sense. Are such changes as they occur with ageing normal, physiological retrogressions, or should such changes be classed as essentially degenerative changes, processes of disease ever tending without halt to such modification in organ resistance and function as to lead to organ death? To admit that all such changes fall in the category of disease is a way to obtain a ready answer to a difficult question. When, however, one observes such changes in an organ of a senescent animal associated with modified function and likely with an acquired resistance which both stabilizes for a period at this level and maintains the life of the animal, the question becomes more difficult to answer. From one point of view an adaptation in structure has developed from some cause associated with the ageing process which enables the life of an organ to continue to operate for a period in a state of acquired protection. Such changes in an organ location may enable an animal to age and function effectively for its senile needs as it ages. The foregoing discussion has been indulged in for the purpose of pointing out at least two of the major difficulties which one encounters when an attempt is made to investigate the ageing process either as a whole or as a localized organ expression in the higher animals.

During the past thirty years a large number of animals (dogs) have been used in this laboratory for purposes of investigation. Fortunately, in one of the early series of experiments (MacNider, 1913) the factor of the age of the animal appeared to exert a definite influence on the type of reaction manifested by the members of the group. Since this time a record has been kept of the age of all animals used for experimental purposes. In some instances such a record is of doubtful accuracy and has been so interpreted. However, a continuous record is available of at least one factor, that of age, which may exert an influence over a variety of reactions occurring in such animals whether these be expressed locally in an organ, indicating cytological susceptibility or resistance, or whether the reactions may be of a more generalized order as shown by disturbances in the stabilization of the acid-base equilibrium of the blood. The present study is based on an analysis of the factor of age as expressed by dogs reacting to a variety of experimental procedures. The animals under review were either bred in the laboratory kennels, in which case the age record is accurate, or were obtained from other reliable sources, in which case the record is relatively accurate with an assured discrepancy of only a few months. These dogs may be divided into three groups: an immature or young group, varying in age from puppies of six weeks old to animals of one year of age; the adult group, dogs between two years and seven years of age; and a senescent group of animals varying in age from seven years to fourteen years and four months. Such a grouping is sufficiently elastic to permit the factor of age to express itself as a part of the response of such animals to various injurious agents which damage may or may not be followed by such cell changes as to develop a resistance on the part of such tissues to subsequent injury. There is, however, a variable which should be stated. The animals under consideration were of different breeds and mixed breeds. Such factors may influence the rate with which the ageing process develops.

1. SUSCEPTIBILITY OF KIDNEY OF AGEING ANIMALS TO URANIUM NITRATE, ETHER AND CHLOROFORM

The susceptibility of the kidney to the action of uranium as influenced by the age of the animal is beset by the difficulty that as the animal ages certain changes may take place in the vascular tissue which, whether they be regarded up to a certain stage as an ageing process or as disease, influence by modifying the circulation through the kidney the specific epithelial response to this poison. On the other hand, the fact that the salts of uranium have a selective affinity for the cells in the proximal convoluted segment of the tubule enables one to observe the type and extent of the injury which such a substance may effect as animals age and the influence of age as expressed by the severity of the injury on the type of epithelial repair process which develops both in terms of cell morphology and resistance. It would be fortunate in considering the relative toxicity of uranium nitrate in the animals of the three age groups if definite cytological differences could be determined to exist in such cells which were dependent upon the age of the animals. Except for certain animals in the senescent group of dogs such differences though suggestive are probably too ill-defined to be of any determining significance. In the senescent animals referred to, a very definite cytological change develops in the epithelium of this segment of the tubule which imparts to it resistance against an amount of uranium which is cytotoxic for normal cells found in this segment of the tubule in adult animals. Such kidneys would appear to fall in that group of renal modifications definitely associated with senescence which have been discussed by Kaufman (1911). In so far as differences in the cytological structure of the epithelium in the proximal convoluted tubules is concerned in the young or immature and adult group of animals, it becomes difficult to make any accurate statement. This in turn affords an opportunity for research. From a histological study of a very large number of kidneys in such groups of animals my impression is that in the immature group the epithelium in the convoluted segment is more flattened and shows less differentiation than in the adult group. In the younger animals the brush border of these cells is imperfectly developed and they fail to show stainable lipoid material in the cytoplasm. In the adult group, cell differentiation is usually clean cut, the cells are higher, even columnar in configuration, and the brush border is well defined. Lipoid material as dust-like particles or small droplets can usually be demonstrated in the cell cytoplasm.

When animals in these respective age groups are intoxicated by uranium nitrate (MacNider, 1914, 1917) in the amount of two to four mgs. per kilogram the factor of the age of the animal is shown as a local reaction in the kidney, and as a more generalized reaction. The convoluted tubule injury in the young and immature animals is slight when compared with the changes observed in the adult animals and in a certain number of the senescent group. The changes in the younger group consist of cloudy swelling of the epithelium, the appearance of stainable lipoid material, a moderate grade of edema, faulty staining of the nuclei, and rarely any extensive necrosis. The repair process which develops in these young animals results in the formation of a normal type of epithelial cell which fails to have any acquired resistance

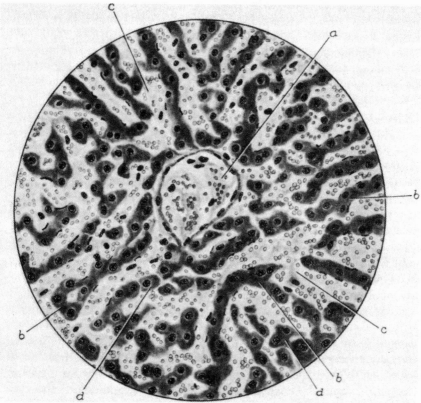

FIG. 118. Camera lucida drawing from the liver of a dog, age eleven years. The liver lobules have an atypical epithelial structure consisting mainly of such tissue in syncytial formation showing in areas imperfect cell differentiation. The syncytia appear as flattened cords which show branching and budding. This type of naturally acquired metaplastic epithelium has only been observed in senile animals. The liver of this animal was subjected to the action of chloroform for one hour and forty-five minutes. Such atypical epithelium is resistant to chloroform which is certainly hepatoxic to normal hepatic epithelium. At a, is shown a large central vein. At b, are shown syncytial cords of atypical liver epithelium with intensely staining nuclei, while at d, is shown an area with partial cell differentiation. The large hepatic sinusoids appear at c.

to secondary intoxications by uranium (MacNider, 1929a). The relatively resistant epithelium of the younger animals appears to be insufficiently injured by the poison to develop in the repair process a cell of such an altered order both morphologically and chemically as to acquire resistance. When adult animals, and a certain number of the senescent group which show a greater degree of specialization in cell structure are intoxicated by the same amount of uranium per kilogram, the same general type of epithelial injury develops but it is of a severer order. Their cells become vacuolated and necrotic, the nuclei are fragmented or appear as shadows, and stainable lipoid material as as droplets or fused masses makes its appearance in the cytoplasm of the cells which are sufficiently preserved. The repair process which develops in such animals is characterized by the formation of a flattened, atypical type of cell or by the formation of definite syncytial structures. This type of repair process in the older animals which have participated in a severer type of epithelial injury has a marked degree of resistance to an increased amount of uranium. Apparently the age of the animal not only expresses itself in the degree of epithelial injury but also in the type of repair process which is instituted by the animal. If this repair process is effected by an order of cell which shows poor cell differentiation, syncytial formation, or epithelium of an embryonic type, such tissue acquires a resistance to subsequent injury.

In the senescent group of animals two types of epithelial reaction develop from the use of uranium. The usual response is characterized by such extensive necrosis and sloughing of the epithelium in the tubules that the institution of any form of repair process becomes impossible. Animals thus affected fail to survive. In another group of such animals there has occurred, as a result of the ageing process or definitely attributable to glomerular disease, the formation of the same atypical type of cell which has been described as the usual process of repair for the adult group of animals. When this type of cell predominates in the convoluted segment of the tubule they have been shown to be resistant to secondary intoxications by uranium. This type of cell or syncytial structure when produced as a reaction of repair from uranium has been furthermore shown to be resistant to bichloride of mercury (MacNider, 1937a).

The foregoing observations would indicate that there exists a resistance to uranium on the part of the epithelium in the proximal convoluted segment of the nephron in puppies and young animals, and furthermore, that an injury of the order of severity which is induced in such animals by this substance is followed by a process of repair in which cells normal for this segment are formed and which fail to have any acquired resistance to this poison in excess of their natural resistance. In contrast to this type of response the epithelium in the same location of the tubule in older animals shows the ageing process of the animal by an increased susceptibility to the toxic action of this poison which is followed usually by an atypical type of epithelial

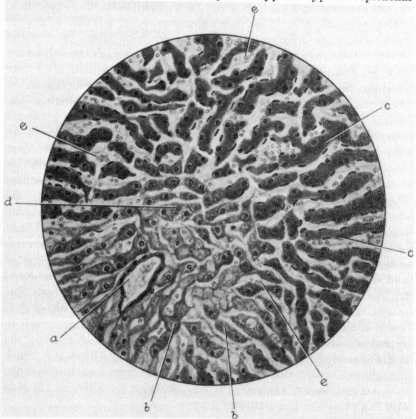

Fig. 119. Camera lucida drawing from the liver of the same animal two weeks later, at which time the animal was anesthetized with chloroform for a longer period of three hours and forty-five minutes. The atypical epithelium shows evidence of a commencing injury in a narrow, central zone of the lobule. Cell resistance is a relative and not absolute value. At *a*, is shown the central vein. At *b*, and *d*, the area of incomplete injury to the epithelium. At *c*, are shown the well-preserved syncytial cords of hepatic epithelium. Cell differentiation is very imperfect. At *e*, liver sinusoids of reduced diameter.

repair, resembling in certain particulars epithelium of an embryonic nature, which is resistant to uranium. In a final group of senescent animals the epithelium shows such a susceptibility to this substance that a repair process of any kind fails to develop. However, falling in this group of senescent animals there are instances of resistance on the part of the epithelium to uranium in which the cells in the convoluted segment have either changed their morphology as a result of ageing to the atypical type of cell or the change has been induced as a result of disease manifesting itself as a major tissue reaction in the glomeruli.

Reference has been made to a difference in the general reaction of these animals of different age groups to an intoxication by uranium nitrate, a reference which on the basis of its type might be considered of a metabolic nature. The animals as a whole, regardless of the age grouping, become polyuric, there is a loss in weight, a reduction in the reserve alkali of the blood and the urine contains both albumin and glucose. In addition to these changes, the older members of the younger group of dogs, the adult and senile groups exhibit ketone bodies in the urine. The percentage concentration of these bodies in the urine increases with the age of the animal as does the degree of the disturbance in the acid-base equilibrium of the blood. The composite effect resembles the reaction which may be obtained in animals from the use of a cyanide, the action of which is to inhibit intracellular oxidations. Arguing from these observations with no ascertained facts for the basis of the argument, one might infer that youthful tissue has a greater oxidizing capacity than senescent tissue and that the same degree of inhibition of tissue oxidations in youthful animals by uranium would find less expression in terms of the hyperglycemia, ketone body formation, and in the reduction of the reserve alkali of the blood than would be the case in the adult and senescent group of animals. Such an hypothesis may apply to processes of intracellular oxidations in the epithelium of the proximal segment of the convoluted tubules. Such thoughts are rather closely connected with the differences in metabolic rate in youth and senility as have been observed by Aub and Du Bois (1917) and by Du Bois (1916).

The significance of the ageing process in animals intoxicated by uranium nitrate is also seen when an attempt is made to protect animals of different ages against the toxic action of this poison by giving intravenously a solution of sodium carbonate (MacNider, 1916). When such solutions are employed, the degree of protection which the animals develop both as a local reaction in the kidney and as shown by the general reaction on the part of the animal depends very definitely on the age factor. As the animals advance in years the degree of protection lessens so that in the majority of the senescent animals such solutions are entirely ineffective. The degree to which protection can be influenced is associated very definitely with the ability of such a solution to stabilize and maintain a normal acid-base equilibrium of the blood. This becomes more difficult as the animals advance in years. The

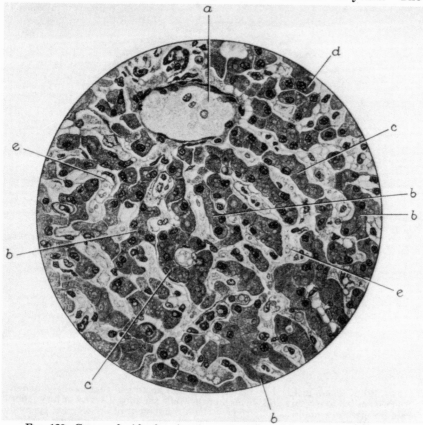

FIG. 120. Camera lucida drawing from the liver of an animal that has been been under observation for two years and four months since the initial severe injury from uranium nitrate which was followed by the development in the liver of an atypical type of epithelial cell, or epithelial syncytial formations, which were resistant to chloroform. The animal was anesthetized with chloroform for one and one-half hours without developing evidence of the typical hepatic injury. The atypical epithelial structure has maintained its resistance to this agent. At a, is shown the central vein of a liver lobule. At b, is shown the narrow, syncytial epithelial structures which at c, show a beginning cell differentiation. At d, is shown a group of hepatic cells of normal polygonal configuration.

animals of the various age groups as normal animals are able to stabilize and maintain this fundamental equilibrium, but when it becomes subjected to the strain of an intoxicant such as uranium the factor of age shows itself by the older animals giving evidence of a more ready disturbance in the balance and a greater degree of reduction in the

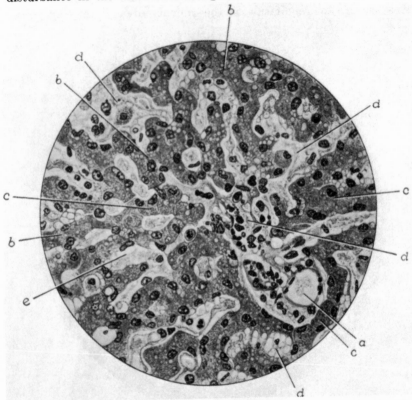

FIG. 121. Camera lucida drawing of the liver of an animal that has been under observation for four years and seven months since the initial severe injury from uranium nitrate which was followed by the development of an atypical type of epithelium or syncytia which were resistant to chloroform. The liver of this animal shows a definite reversion to a normal type of epithelial cell. When the animal was given chloroform by inhalation for one and one-half hours, areas of necrosis of epithelium appeared in certain areas in which such a change in epithelial type has occurred to that of a normal order of cell. At a, is shown the central vein of a liver lobule. At b, is shown liver epithelium in syncytial formation, while at c, the epithelium shows definite cell differentiation of a normal order. At d, are shown foci of partial and complete necrosis. The changes in epithelial type illustrate the loss of resistance which occurs when the undifferentiated or imperfectly differentiated tissue reverts to a type of epithelial cell normal for the liver.

equilibrium than is the case with the younger animals. As definitely as is the influence of the ageing process on both the readiness and extent to which the acid-base equilibrium of the blood may be interfered with by the use of uranium nitrate, it must be recalled that the injury to both the liver and the kidney in such animals by uranium may in part explain the susceptibility of this balance to such an interference. It would therefore strengthen the conclusion that the acid-base equilibrium of the blood is stabilized with more difficulty in an aged animal than it is in a youthful animal if such an observation could be made in normal animals at different age periods under the influence of some physiological process in which neither the liver nor the kidney participate in an injury.

Extending over a period of ten years, seventy-three pregnant dogs of different age periods and at different stages of the gestation period have been studied in this laboratory (MacNider, 1926a, 1928). These animals have varied in age from eleven months to ten years and four months and the duration of gestation of from three to ten weeks. The average length of gestation in the dog is nine weeks. Studies of these pregnant animals have been controlled by observations on a group of animals of the same relative age which were not pregnant. In both groups studies of the urine and the use of renal functional tests gave no evidence of renal injury. A study of the normal animals from periods of youth into senescence has shown that these animals are able to maintain a normal acid-base balance of the blood. This does not mean that the balance is perfectly stabilized for in two of the older animals in which there was no evidence of renal disease there occurred such variations in the reserve alkali of the blood as to indicate very clearly a lack of stability in this equilibrium.

Studies of the stability of this equilibrium as influenced by the ageing process and the duration of the gestation period demonstrate that the young animals tend to maintain a normal acid-base equilibrium of the blood during and to the termination of the gestation period. As the animals in this state advance in years there is a progressive tendency for a larger number to show an instability of the equilibrium, and furthermore, a reduction in the reserve alkali of the blood occurs earlier in the gestation period in the older than it does in the younger animals. These observations on the influence of the ageing process would appear to be of definite importance for they show how such a fundamental equilibrium is not only influenced by ageing but also the effect of a physiological state, gestation, when it is permitted to exercise its influence as the animal ages. Such observations are furthermore strengthened when the influence of a uranium intoxication is studied in such animals of various ages during the gestation period (MacNiher et al., 1927). The toxicity of uranium as expressed by its ability to reduce the reserve alkali of the blood and lead to the development of an acid intoxication shows a rather definite parallel with the age of the respective animals and the duration of the period of gestation. As the animals increase in age and as the duration of the gestation period progresses, the ability of uranium to reduce the reserve alkali becomes intensified.

The ageing process, certainly as it expresses itself in advanced senility, has been looked upon as a type of physiological anesthesia becoming a completed process in death. Processes of oxidation, the completeness with which such reactions are accomplished, the degree to which organs and organ systems function show a retardation in the senescent state which may be compared to the influence of such substances as the general anesthetics on tissues in general, as well as to the localization of their influence in various organs. When the general anesthetics, ether or chloroform, are employed in pregnant animals of different age periods it has been found that the older animals are more susceptible to the action of such anesthetic bodies as is shown by a reduction in the reserve alkali of the blood, and that the duration of the gestation period increases this suceptibility. Furthermore, the use of such substances in pregnant animals is more apt to induce, as a local expression of tissue damage, a renal injury as the animal advances in years. Finally, when an attempt is made to protect such animals against either the localized or general toxic expression of these bodies by the use of a solution of glucose, the degree of protection diminishes as the age of the animal advances (MacNider, 1926b). In those animals in which chloroform was employed as an anesthetic agent, virtually no evidence of protection was obtained in animals of any age period (MacNider, 1929b). Many years ago it was demonstrated that associated with the ageing process there occurred an increase both in the amount and distribution of stainable lipoid material in renal epithelium (MacNider, 1921). The increase of this material with its appearance in the cells of the proximal segment of the convoluted tubule was associated with the ageing process and in turn influenced the susceptibility of this epithelium to the toxic action of both ether and chloroform. Whether or not such a change in the lipoid content of the epithelium takes place during gestation in an exaggerated form which in turn determines the susceptibility of the epithelium to the general anesthetics and the degree to which such animals can be protected by the use of a solution of glucose is entirely unknown.

2. SUSCEPTIBILITY OF LIVER OF AGEING ANIMALS TO URANIUM NITRATE AND CHLOROFORM

In discussing the ageing process as shown by various changes in the kidney and the influence which such states might have in determining susceptibility or resistance, reference was made to the fact that on account of the specialization in the vascular tissue of the kidney and the susceptibility of this tissue to injury that these states might by reflecting their influence on the epithelial tissue interfere with the proper interpretation of the epithelial changes. A difficulty of this sort is not encountered when the liver is studied in an attempt to investigate the ageing process and states of susceptibility or resistance which may appear at such periods or be induced by experimental procedure.

In the liver there is no specialization in structure of the vascular tissue which sets aside a tissue to show evidence of injury, as is the case with the kidney. The liver receiving its blood supply from both the hepatic artery and portal vein, which supplies are united at some point in the liver, afford this organ blood which comes in intimate contact with its epithelial tissue without the intervention of any specialized structure which may influence its distribution operating in a physiological manner or under the influence of pathological changes. For these reasons the liver is a more appropriate organ in which to study the ageing process of its epithelial tissue, the susceptibility of this tissue to injury as influenced by the age of the animal, and the development of epithelial changes which may impart resistance to such tissue.

The observations which have been made on the liver have extended over a period of fourteen years, thus enabling such studies to be made on a large number of animals at ages varying from six months to over fifteen years. In these studies the same latitude has been taken in the age grouping as was employed for the dogs in which the ageing process was observed as a localized reaction occurring in the kidney. The animals now under consideration may be divided into an immature or youthful group with ages varying from six months to between one and two years, an adult group of from two to eight years old, and a senescent group from eight years to a few months over fifteen years in age. Histological studies of the livers of animals in the respective age groups made by obtaining biopsy material, except for certain of the senescent animals which will be referred to later, have shown even less evidence of cytological changes dependent upon age than have similar studies which were carried out in connection with the kidney. In the very young animals one gains the impression that cell differentiation in the epithelial cords is less perfect than in the adult animals and certain of the senescent animals. In the young animals stainable lipoid material is difficult to demonstrate. It is present as small or coalesced droplets in the adult animals and especially in those senile animals in which a complete change in the type of epithelium has not occurred. The intoxication by uranium is expressed by a more diffuse and a severer degree of epithelial injury in the adult animals and in senescent animals with a normal type of cell than it is by the epithelium of young animals. Following such degrees of injury there develops a difference in the type of repair process. The adult animals with the severer order of epithelial injury institute a process of repair by the formation of an atypical, flattened type of cell or by cell structures which are definitely syncytial and which are of functional value in that they can remove phenol-tetrachlorphthalein from the plasma and have acquired a definite resistance to uranium. The very young animals which have shown resistance to uranium repair the epithelial injury by the formation of a normal type of cell which has no resistance to secondary intoxications by the poison (MacNider, 1936a). If those animals of the adult and senescent groups which have effected an epithelial repair by the formation of an atypical type of epithelium be subjected to a period of starvation for twenty-four hours and then be given chloroform by inhalation for a period of one and one-half hours, there fails to occur a necrosis of the epithelium around the central veins of the lobules. When animals with a normal type of epithelial repair process in the liver or adult and senescent animals which have not been subjected to injury and which have an epithelium of the usual order are starved for twenty-four hours and anesthetized with chloroform for one and one-half hours, there develops the usual necrosis of the epithelium which involves the inner one-half to two-thirds of the liver lobules (MacNider, 1936b). The ageing process reflects itself in the liver by an increase in its susceptibility to the toxic action of uranium and by a modification in the type of epithelial repair process which in turn determines whether or not the livers of such animals have acquired a resistance not only to uranium but also to chloroform.

Reference has been made to a group of senescent animals that have shown, as a naturally acquired process not dependent upon experimental injury followed by repair, a change in the type of epithelial structure in the liver. Twenty-four senescent animals have been studied in which from some unknown cause but always associated with advanced senescence the type of epithelial structure of the liver has undergone a diffuse change in cell type. Such epithelium occurs as flattened, syncytial cords with rarely cell differentiation. The cytoplasm of such structures stains evenly and intensely. The nuclei are large in proportion to the surrounding cell cytoplasm and often appear hyperchromatic. Mitotic figures have not been observed. Between such syncytial cords are large venous sinusoids. This type of epithelium resembles that which develops in an adult animal following a severe injury from uranium except that its syncytial nature is more marked and there is more evidence of syncytial branching and budding. The naturally acquired, atypical epithelium which has only been observed in senescent animals shows an even greater degree of resistance to chloroform than the atypical cells and syncytia which have developed as a repair process secondary to a severe injury from uranium (MacNider, 1936c). The atypical epithelium occurring in the senescent animals is of definite functional value.

A final group of animals should be discussed not on the basis of the age of the animals but for the purpose of illustrating how changes in cell types in the liver of the same animal may be associated with states of resistance or susceptibility at different periods of observation. The livers of such adult animals were severely injured by uranium nitrate. The repair process, as was shown by a study of biopsy material, was effected by the formation of the atypical type of epithelial structure which has been described. At this period of observation the liver was resistant to chloroform when given by inhalation for one and one-half hours. It failed to induce a central necrosis of the lobules. Two years later than this a study of biopsy material from the liver showed in areas a reversion of the flattened, atypical type of cell to a normal cell of polyhedral contour. At such a period of cell type change, the inhalation of chloroform for one and one-half hours induced a partial necrosis in those areas composed of cells of a normal order. The atypical cells remained resistant.

These experiments not only serve to emphasize variations in susceptibility and resistance associated with different cell types and an assumed difference in chemical constitution but also the significance of the time factor in such cellular transitions (MacNider, 1937b).

3. SUMMARY

In the preceding analysis of a rather wide variety of experiments in which the age factor has been taken into consideration, an attempt with a fair degree of accuracy has been made to ascertain how the process of ageing expresses itself in terms of susceptibility to injury on the part of organs and certain specialized cells in them, the influence of the same factor as expressed by an organ in acquiring a fixed cell tissue resistance, and, finally, certain more generalized reactions on the part of the organism as a whole which are modified by the ageing process. In summarizing the results, the following conclusions would appear to be warranted, ever remembering that the age groupings of the animals were of an elastic order and that the breed of the animals, if pure, as well as the mixed breed status of other animals, might influence not only the rapidity but the extent to which the ageing process develops.

1. Young animals, in which epithelial differentiation may be imperfect and in which epithelial specializations in structure have failed to appear in a state of perfect development, appear to be more resistant to injurious agencies than those possessing a type of epithelium which is perfected in its differentiation and specialization of structure, as represented by an adult group of animals. The occurrence of stainable lipoid material in such cells influences in a favorable manner their susceptibility to injury.

2. When epithelial tissue in young animals in certain organ locations participates in a process of repair, the type of cell formed is predominantly of a normal order for such locations and has no acquired resistance to injury. When a similar type of injury is produced in the more susceptible epithelium of an adult animal and in senescent animals that retain a normal type of epithelial structure, there is shown by such animals either an inability to participate in any type of repair process or the process is effected by an atypical type of cell resembling in certain respects, especially in its lack of differentiation, embryonic epithelium which, though of functional value, has acquired a resistance to injury. It would appear that in adult and certain senescent animals the power of instituting a normal type of repair for epithelium in certain locations has been modified or lost, and that the difference in the readiness with which repair is effected and the type of cell employed in the process is associated with the age of the animal more than it is with the severity of the injury in the animals of the different age groups. As an animal advances in its life span, the cytology of the repair process becomes modified and associated with such changes there may develop an acquired resistance for certain chemical substances. This is especially true both for the kidney and the liver in animals in advanced senility in which a type of abnormal epithelium

may appear either as a result of the ageing process or may be produced as a reaction of repair in the senile state which is resistant to injury and, though of less functional value, tends for a period to stabilize the animal as a senescent animal and protect these organs against an extension of injury. The experiments would indicate the significance of time expressed as ageing in not only influencing cell susceptibility but also the ability of certain tissues to so modify their process of cell repair as to acquire resistance. Such a resistance acquired as a result of ageing or as a result of artificial injury followed by repair is of changing order. Resistant cells may so change their morphology and likely at the same time so modify their chemical structure that susceptibility to injury again develops. These observations emphasize the changing, shifting character of even fixed cells. They have been of a very gross order. Changes of a finer nature, impossible or difficult at present to detect, when accompanied by chemical modifications may explain in part not only the ageing process but also the susceptibility and resistance of fixed cells at various age periods to the effect of outside agencies and to chemical bodies produced in cells as products of the life process.

3. An observation of significance in connection with the ageing process and which does not confine itself to one organ or group of organs is the effect of age on the stability of a fundamental equilibrium in the organism, the acid-base equilibrium of the blood and tissue juices. As normal animals advance in age this equilibrium becomes of an unstable order and in advanced senility the organism may be unable to maintain it within the range of normal variations. Such an instability may be demonstrated when animals of different ages participate in the physiological process of gestation and when they react to various intoxications. Furthermore, it becomes increasingly difficult as the age of the animal advances to restore to the normal as well as to stabilize this fundamental equilibrium. A tendency to, or the actual development of, a reduction in the reserve alkali of the blood as the animal ages appears to be a definite characteristic of the ageing process which, in turn, by influencing chemical reactions of an intracellular nature during life, may in part determine the rate with which the ageing process develops.

The ageing process as shown by various studies which have been reviewed is not one which proceeds from a certain peak of perfection in an uninterrupted downward course to its termination. The process is characterized as it progresses by variations in cell susceptibility and by the development of transitory states of cell resistance which give to the downward progress of the curve, representing ageing, an irregular course; points of depression, indicating periods of susceptibility, and points of elevation in the curve, variable in their duration at which resistance is acquired. As ageing progresses such transitory states of cell adaptation to it become less and less effective, finally manifesting their inability in terms of such depressed function or lack of function on the part of an organ or organ system that the life of the organism as a whole comes to an end.

REFERENCES

Aub, Joseph C. and Du Bois, Eugene F. 1917. The basal metabolism of old men. Arch. Int. Med., **19**, 823–831.

Child, C. M. 1915. Senescence and rejuvenescence. Chicago: Univ. Press, 000 pp.

Cohnheim, J. 1882. Vorlesungen über Allgemeine Pathologie, II. Auflage, Band II, Berlin: A. Hirschwald.

Dolley, David H. 1909. Alterations occurring in the Purkingje cells of the dog's cerebellum. J. Med. Res., **20**, 275–295.

———— 1910. The numerical statement of the upset of the nucleus-plasma relation in the Purkinje cells. *Ibid*, **22**, 331–337.

———— 1911. Studies on the recuperation of nerve cells after functional activity from youth to senility. *Ibid*, **24**, 309–343.

Du Bois, Eugene F. 1916. The metabolism of boys 12 and 13 years old compared with the metabolism at other ages. Arch. Int. Med., **17**, 887–901.

Grafflin, A. L. 1933. Glomerular degeneration in the kidney of the Daddy Sculpin (Myoxocephalus Scorpius). Anat. Rec., **57**, 59–79.

Hertwig, Richard 1903. Über Korrelation von Zell- und Kerngrösse und ihre Bedentung für die geschlechtliche Differenzierung und die Teilung der Zelle. Biol. Centralbl., **23**, 49–62, 108–119.

Jennings, H. S. 1912. Age, death and conjugation in the light of work on lower organisms. Pop. Sci. Monthly, **80**, 563–577.

Kaufman, E. 1911. Lehrbuch der speziellen Pathologischen Anatomie fur Studierende und Arzte. Berlin, 6 Aufl., **11**, 815–818.

Loeb, Jacques 1906. The dynamics of living matter, New York: Macmillan, 233 pp. Columbia University Press.

MacNider, Wm. deB. 1913. On the difference in the effect of Gréhant's anesthetic and of morphine-ether on the total output of urine and composition of the urine in normal dogs. Proc. Soc. Exp. Biol. and Med., **10**, 95–96.

———— 1914. On the difference in the response of animals of different ages to a constant quantity of uranium nitrate. *Ibid*, **11**, 159–162.

———— 1916. The inhibition of the toxicity of uranium nitrate by sodium carbonate, and the protection of the kidney acutely nephrophatic from uranium from the toxic action of an anesthetic by sodium carbonate. J. Exp. Med., **23**, 171–187.

MacNider, Wm. deB. 1917. A consideration of the relative toxicity of uranium nitrate for animals of different ages. *Ibid*, **26**, 1–17.

———— 1921. A preliminary paper on the relation between the amount of stainable lipoid material in the renal epithelium and the susceptibility of the kidney to the toxic effect of the general anesthetics. J. Pharm. and Exp. Therap., **17**, 289–323.

———— 1926a. The factor of age in the chemical stability of the blood during gestation. Science, **66**, 479–480.

———— 1926b. Studies concerning the value of a solution of glucose in maintaining the acid-base equilibrium of the blood in pregnant animals. I. The effect of a period of ether anesthesia in pregnant animals. The protection conferred by a solution of glucose. J. Pharm. and Exp. Therap., **29**, 381–396.

———— 1928. Concerning the stability of the acid-base equilibrium of the blood in pregnant animals. J. Exp. Med., **43**, 53–59.

———— 1929a. The functional and pathological response of the kidney in dogs to a second subcutaneous injection of uranium nitrate. *Ibid*, **49**, 411–433.

———— 1929b. II. The effect of a period of chloroform anesthesia in pregnant animals. The lack of protection conferred by a solution of glucose. J. Pharm. and Exp. Therap., **35**, 31–48.

———— 1933. Pathological changes in the dog kidney resembling the normal histological structure in the aglomerular fish kidney, Opsanus Tau. Proc. Soc. Exp. Biol. and Med., **31**, 293–295.

———— 1936a. A study of the acquired resistance of fixed tissue cells morphologically altered through processes of repair. I. The liver injury induced by uranium nitrate. A consideration of the type of epithelial repair which imparts to the liver resistance against subsequent uranium intoxications. J. Pharm. and Exp. Therap., **56**, 359–372.

———— 1936b. II. The resistance of liver epithelium altered morphologically as the result of an injury from uranium, followed by repair to the hepatoxic action of chloroform. *Ibid*, **56**, 373–381.

———— 1936c. III. The resistance to chloroform of a naturally acquired atypical type of liver epithelium occurring in senile animals. *Ibid*, 383–387.

———— 1937a. Development of an acquired resistance to bichloride of mercury by renal epithelium in proximal convoluted tubule. Proc. Soc. Exp. Biol. and Med., **37**, 90–91.

———— 1937b. IV. Concerning the persistence of an acquired type of atypical liver cell with observations on the resistance of such cells to the toxic action of chloroform. J. Pharm. and Exp. Therap., **59**, 393–400.

MacNider, Wm. deB., Helms, Samuel T., and Helms, Selina C. 1927. The course of uranium nitrate intoxications in pregnant dogs. Bull. Johns Hopkins Hosp., **40**, 145–159.

Minot, C. S. 1908. The problem of age, growth and death. New York: p. 280.

———— 1913. Moderne Probleme der Biologie. Jena: p. 111.

Morgan, T. H. 1901. Regeneration, New York: 1901.

MULLER, JOHANNES 1844. Handbuch der Physiologie des Menchen, IV. Auflage, Band II, Coblenz.

OLIVER, JEAN AND LUEY, ANN SEWARD 1935. Plastic studies in abnormal renal architecture. III. The aglomerular nephrons of terminal hemorrhagic Brights Disease. Archiv. Path., **19**, 1–23.

PEARL, RAYMOND 1922. The biology of death. Philadelphia: J. B. Lippincott Co., 275 pp.

WEISMANN, AUGUST 1882. Über die Dauer des Lebens. Jena:

WOODRUFF, L. L. 1908. The life cycle of paramecium when subjected to a varied environment. Am. Naturalist, **42**, 520–526.

Chapter 25

AGEING FROM THE POINT OF VIEW OF THE CLINICIAN

LEWELLYS F. BARKER

Baltimore

In his premedical and medical training, the prospective clinician studies physics, chemistry, biology, human anatomy and histology, embryology, physiology, pharmacology and pathology and, later, is instructed in the symptomatology, diagnosis and treatment of the diseases to which human beings are subject. During this training, he must perforce become familiar with the form and functions of the human body in health and in disease from the time of fertilization of the ovum onward through the periods of growth, maturity, senescence, and old age.

In his everyday work, the clinician, and especially the general practitioner of medicine, sees patients at all stages of life (infancy, childhood, adolescence, adulthood, and old age). His intimate personal relations with these patients make it possible for him to acquire a better knowledge of their bodies and a truer insight into their minds than is practicable for the majority of non-medical observers.

The conscientious clinician makes it a point, too, to secure autopsies upon as many as possible of those of his patients that die and careful macroscopic and microscopic examinations of the organs and tissues of persons dying at different ages afford a knowledge of the gross anatomy and finer histology of the body in disease and also reveal the more characteristic changes that the human body undergoes in successive periods of life.

Though the clinical and pathological studies are individualized, the physician can, after long experience, form a general and composite picture of the *average* conditions that exist in human beings at different ages of life and thus arrive at fairly valid conclusions regarding the processes that are characterisic of ageing.

1. PHYSIOLOGICAL (OR NATURAL) AND PATHOLOGICAL (OR ABNORMAL) AGEING

Though it has been maintained that some (not all) unicellular organisms are "potentially immortal" in favorable environments, all are agreed that individual human beings (like all other multicellular organisms) are limited as to length of life, no matter how good the heredity nor how favorable the environment may be.

Man is, by Nature, predestined after growth and development to decline and finally to die. His structure and functions are more complex than those of any other living creature. The intricacies of his make-up and the specialization of the component cells of the body have made possible extraordinary capacities for adjustment to environment. Thanks especially to the evolution of his brain, functions of intellect, emotion and will have emerged in unprecedented measure and have made possible writing, printing and reading, and a truly marvelous individual and social life. What can be more astounding to the thoughtful person than the recognition of what man is and whence he has been evolved? When we contrast the narrow limitations of lower forms of life with the widely extended activities of thought, feeling, and action of human beings, we cannot but be amazed that such a development ever became possible. That our modern civilization (with its physical and material comforts, its intellectual and emotional interests, its opportunities for personal freedom, its economic organization, its social institutions, its expansion of human knowledge and human power, its political relationships—local, national and international—its achievements in the realms of art, literature and science and its creation of ethical values) presents one of the greatest enigmas of the universe as known to us, all will agree. But the greater richness of life enjoyed by the many-celled animals, and especially by man, must be paid for; and the price exacted for the reciprocal interdependence of the cells, tissues and organs of the body includes (1) an inevitable decline in function after a certain age has been reached and (2) ultimately, the death of the organism.

In "physiological" or "natural" old age, there is a gradual involution of the body as a whole; the body-cells slowly atrophy and in the organs there is relative increase of the interstitial tissues with corresponding decrease of the parenchymatous elements. This "major involution" that occurs in later life after the fundamental biological functions have been fulfilled, is for the whole organism comparable to the "minor involutions" that occur in single parts of the organism at certain stages of life when parts are no longer of use (e.g., branchial clefts; ovaries); it must, I believe, be considered to be as physiological as is growth at earlier periods, the tendencies both to growth and to ageing processes being inherent in the qualities of the germ-plasm inherited.

In "pathological" or abnormal old age, there is premature breakdown of one or more of the organs or organ-systems owing to disease or to trauma.

The "human life span" has been fully dealt with by Louis I. Dublin in Chapter 6. I shall therefore merely summarize the main points concerning it in as far as they are of interest to the clinician.

During the past one hundred and fifty years, the *average duration of human life* has undergone great increase. Thus at the end of the eighteenth century the average expectation of life at birth seems to have been about thirty years. Between 1800 and 1850 this was increased by eight or nine years, and between 1850 and 1900 by about as many more years, so that at the beginning of the present century a male new-born babe had at birth an average life expectancy of some forty-five years, a female babe of some forty-seven years. By 1910 the average expectation of life for males had increased to 49.33 years, for females to 53.06 years; by 1920, for white males to 54.07 and for white females to 56.56; by 1930, for males to 59.48 and for females to 62.74 years. Thus, between 1900 and 1930 the average life expectancy was increased by about $13\frac{1}{2}$ years for each of the two sexes— a rapidity of advance never before witnessed.

The *maximal span of human life* is met with only among those who go on to a "physiological" old age, though it is true that many who become subjects of a "pathological" ageing process may outlive "average expectancy." Centenarians and nonagenarians are not numerous. A quarter of all those who are born die before they are 50, a half before they are 65, three-quarters before they are 78, and the majority of the remainder before they are 90.

It would seem to be quite possible (with further advances in the application of knowledge of curative and preventive medicine) that the average expectancy of human life at birth may ultimately be extended to the age of seventy. That the maximal span of life will be increased much beyond 100 years would seem to be doubtful even though some investigators in Moscow who are conducting experiments with the prolongation of life in view are said to entertain the ideal of 180 years duration for the normal span of human life! The extremely long lives of certain individuals reported by ancient authors are, of course, now regarded as mythical.

Unless intellectual and moral decay can be prevented, as well as the tedious diseases of old age, great longevity might be a calamity rather than a blessing. It is probably better for the race that human individuals should not live too long, for, as Goethe said, "Death is Nature's device for securing abundant life." Exemption from death, unless it could be associated with permanent health and vigor, would not be desirable for man. I cannot help but recall the ancient legend according to which the goddess Aurora becoming enamored of a mortal, Tithonus, begged Zeus to make him immortal. Her prayer was granted but Aurora forgot to ask for continuance of his youth as well as for his immortality. He finally grew so old and decrepit that she had to confine him to his chamber. His feeble voice was, however, incessantly heard, so that, ultimately, out of compassion for him she changed him into an insect—a cicada! A good story—even if it isn't true! Those who know the writings of Jonathan Swift will remember his description of the "Struldbruggs" who though immortal soon grew to be melancholy, were faced with the dreadful prospects of never dying, and discovered that death was less an evil than undue prolongation of life.

2. CAUSES OF DEATH AMONG THE OLD

In about half of our older people, *diseases of the circulatory system* are responsible for death. Circulatory insufficiency due to disease of the heart muscle and arteriosclerosis, with or without high blood pressure, are common causes of death among the old. Cerebral apoplexy and cerebral thrombosis are frequent fatal complications of arteriosclerotic disease. Coronary thrombosis may be the cause of sudden death soon after middle life (see Chapter 7).

About one-eighth of the deaths among older people are due to diseases of the *respiratory system*. Of these, acute lobar pneumonia and acute or subacute bronchopneumonia are by far the most common, for these maladies are far more often fatal in older people than in younger people. Pulmonary tuberculosis, the cause of many deaths in earlier life, is only occasionally responsible for death among the old. Pulmonary emphysema may lead in later life to overburdening of the right side of the heart and to death from circulatory insufficiency.

Another eighth of the deaths among the old are due to *cancer* in one or another part of the body (stomach, rectum, prostate, lung, breast, uterus, etc.).

About 8.5 per cent of the deaths among the old are due to *diseases of the kidneys* (especially "chronic Bright's disease"), about 6.5 per cent to *diseases of the digestive system other than cancer* (see Chapter 9), and the remaining 10 per cent to *diseases of other organ systems* or to *traumata.* In obscure cases of death among the old, some physicians report "deaths from senility"; this is ill-advised and it is better to report such deaths as due to "unknown cause." *Suicide* occasionally occurs among the old but it is far less common among the aged than among adolescents; the majority of the old desire to live on—indeed in many the wish for the continuance of life seems to increase with age.

In the winter more old people die than during the summer. During the latter half of the night more old people die than during the day and the first half of the night.

Luckily, only rarely, do either young people or old people, when on their death-beds, know that they are about to die. I have seen many people die and in relatively few instances has the patient been aware of the close proximitity of the Great Silencer. This observation is in accord with the experience of my predecessor at the Johns Hopkins Hospital, the late Sir William Osler, who, in his "Science and Immortality" published in 1904, mentions his findings with reference to the modes of death and the sensations of the dying in his careful records of some 500 deathbeds. He stated that about 90 of the 500 suffered bodily pain or distress, 11 showed mental apprehension, 2 were positively terrified, 1 expressed spiritual exaltation, and 1 suffered from bitter remorse. But, he continued: "the great majority gave no sign one way or the other; like their birth, their death was a sleep and a forgetting. The Preacher was right; in this matter man hath no preeminence over the beast—'as the one dieth, so dieth the other'."

3. CHANGES THAT ACCOMPANY PHYSIOLOGICAL AGEING IN LATER LIFE

Theoretically, the processes of ageing begin with the fertilization of the ovum and continue until the death of the organism. As C. S. Minot emphasized, even during the development of the body to its maximal structure and function, "minor involutional processes" are continually going on; after the highest physical and mental powers have been reached, the "major involution of the organism as a whole" gradually sets in, leading ultimately to a cessation of those powers. Minot's studies of animals convinced him that the best method of measuring vitality is the rate of growth, which steadily diminishes throughout life and finally ceases. He said that "life is growth, the retardation of growth is old age, and its cessation is death." Perhaps he was somewhat too dogmatic in his statements for, though growth is one measure of vitality, function must be regarded as another.

Clinicians are prone to think of the latter half of life as the "period of ageing"; they think of "senescence" as the climacteric period (beginning in the early forties or even earlier in women), and of "senectitude" as a post-climacteric period or old age proper. Ordinarily, the doctor does not really think of "old age" until after the patient's 65th or 70th year has been passed. It is interesting that in human beings the vascular system and the nervous system are as a rule the parts of the body most frequently affected and the earliest to suffer from the ageing process. Thus it is now well-known that even in normal persons there is atrophy and gradual decrease of the weight of the brain from mid-life onward though these changes progress more rapidly after the age of 70.

The general physical and psychical changes common in later life were long ago described by intelligent laymen; in the Bible, in the literature of the Greeks and Romans, in the writings of Shakespeare and of other wise authors before and after him, these changes did not escape notice but were often vividly pictured and with considerable accuracy. In the 90th Psalm, we are told that "the days of our years are threescore years and ten; and if by reason of strength they be fourscore years, yet is their strength labour and sorrow; for it is soon cut off and we fly away." One writer on old age has said that no passage in all the literature of the world has had such influence as this; it is pathetic, he said, to see how incessantly it is quoted and "how bibliolatry has made it accepted almost as a decree of fate." Almost as influential has been the view of old age as pictured in Ecclesiastes where one is exhorted to remember his creator in the days of his youth "while the evil days come not, nor the years draw nigh, when thou shalt say, I have no pleasure in them; while the sun, or the light, or the moon, or the stars be not darkened, nor the clouds return after the rain; in the day when the keepers of the house shall tremble, and the strong men shall bow themselves, and the grinders cease because they are few, and those that look out of the windows be darkened, and the doors shall be shut in the streets, when the sound of the grinding is low, and he shall rise up at the voice of the bird, and all the daughters of music shall be brought low; also when they shall be afraid of that which is high, and fears shall be in the way, and the almond tree shall flourish, and the grasshopper shall be a burden, and desire shall fail; because man goeth to his long home and the mourners go about the streets." The best-trained clinician might well envy this Preacher in Ecclesiastes for his ability so wonderfully and figuratively to characterize some of the outstanding features of old age—

the tremor of the hands, the tendency to stoop, the loss of teeth, the inclination to early rising, the failing eyesight, the developing deafness, the growing apprehensiveness regarding environmental dangers, the graying of the hair, the increasingly felt burden of slight irritations and inconveniences, and the waning of sexual desire and potency, as man approaches his long home (the grave). The bodily machine is breaking down; the dust is to return to the earth as it was, and the spirit unto God who gave it. All seems to be merely transitory to the Preacher who exclaimed: "Vanity of vanities; all is vanity."

In Ancient Greece, old people, except perhaps for Homer's Nestor, and for the "gerousia" or council of 28 old men (all over 60), were in general looked upon as useless and even harmful to those who were younger. Old men were hated by boys, despised among women, and dishonored by nearly all. Hesiod said: "Work for youth; counsel for maturity; prayers for old age." One pleasing aspect of life in Greece, however, was the frequent establishment of close friendly relationships between older men and youths (e.g., Socrates and Char-mides), whereby youths could profit by the experiences of their elders and youth and age could inspire one another with courage. But, unfortunately, these relationships had their dangers, for homosexual activities sometimes developed when the elders had not, like Socrates, entirely sublimated eroticism into the passion for truth. The sombre view of old age among the ancient Greeks is well illustrated also by the gloomy accounts given of it by Aristotle. He said that the old through experience were forced to be doubtful and suspicious; they were never positive about anything, tended to be uncharitable and selfish, to be cowardly and alarmistic, and to live in memory rather than by hope. Their self-control was due to the abatement of desires and because self-interest was their leading passion. No wonder that suicides were not uncommon in Ancient Greece; even Socrates drank hemlock at the age of 70, though Plato lived to be 80.

Among the Romans, the views of later life were less pessimistic than those that prevailed in Greece. The Roman Senate (as its name suggests) was composed of a group of old men. As a schoolboy in Canada, I had to read Cicero's *De Senectute* in which old Cato in a long monologue refers to many important things that had been ac-complished by old men. Cato, himself, began to study Greek when he was already an old man of 80 years. The loss of business ability, the infirmity of the body, the curtailment of the enjoyments of earlier life and the approach of death complained of by many old persons were all discussed by Cato, who urged that everyone should prepare himself for old age and learn how to mitigate its natural infirmities. Many old persons still perform tasks that are useful to society. Though certain pleasures are no longer available to the old, there are, Cato continued, still many that can be enjoyed, especially the charms of country life, companionship with persons of different ages and the reading of good books.

In re-reading Shakespeare least summer, I was struck with the numerous and remarkable descriptions of both normal and pathological old age (the period of "the lean and slippered pantaloon") in the several plays. Especially intriguing was the account of Adam in *As You Like It* who attained to a physiological old age; he looked old but was still strong and lusty because in youth he had lived hygienically, never wooing "the means of weakness and debility"; hence his age was "as a lusty winter, frosty but kindly." On the other hand, in *King Lear* there are masterful descriptions of pathological old age (senile dementia). Lear knew that he had become a "foolish, fond old man, fourscore and upward," feared that he was not in his perfect mind, was ignorant of where he was, did not know where he had lodged the night before, nor whence the very garments that he wore had come from; the old fool had become a babe again!

There is a vast literature upon old age and the changes that accompany it, derived partly from lay, partly from medical writers. Though I have no intention of reviewing that literature here, I do desire to point out that, in it, there are very many records of persons who have reached advanced years and yet have been normal enough to do important work in the later part of life. The pessimism expressed in Anthony Trollope's novel *The Fixed Period* (in which a community is described in which euthanasic death was compulsory in the latter part of the 6th decade of life), as well as that in Dr. William Osler's (partly jocular) remarks in his Farewell Address on the "relative uselessness of persons over 60," is by no means justified. Normal old age is desirable, not only for the individual, but also for the race. It should not be forgotten that Sophocles wrote his *Oedipus* at 90; Pope Leo XIII inaugurated most of his enlightened policy after he was 70 and lived to be 94; L. Cornaro published books and essays until he was 95; Titian who lived to be over 99 had painted his masterpiece, the bronze doors of the sacristy at St. Mark's, at the age of 85. In England, many examples of normal old age could be cited, including Newton who lived to be 85. And in our own country the distinguished

American diplomat, statesman and scientist, Benjamin Franklin, was born in 1706 and lived to be 84 years old. By the time he was 70 he was "one of the most talked about men in the world" besides being most highly esteemed and beloved. At the age of 72 he was appointed sole plenipotentiary to the French court and at the age of 75 was appointed a member of a commission to make peace with Great Britain. After his return to America at the age of 79 he became the chief executive officer of the State of Pennsylvania, serving in that capacity until he was 82 years old. His "last days were marked by a fine serenity and calm." Heredity doubtless played an important part in his health and longevity (his father had lived to be 89 and his mother to be 85, neither of them having had any sickness but that of which they died). W. D. Howells who believed the golden age to be between the fiftieth and sixtieth years of life exhibited a normal old age; he wrote a paper for Harper's in 1919 entitled *Eighty Years and After*. Oliver Wendell Holmes lived to be 85, and six years before his death began the series of papers that he happily designated *Over the Tea Cups* and concerning which the Encyclopoedia Britannica has said "as a *tour de force* on the part of a man of nearly fourscore years, they are very remarkable." One of the most distinguished scholars America ever produced was the late Paul Shorey, Professor of Greek at the University of Chicago. He was a great admirer of Plato and especially of Plato's masterpiece, the *Republic*. Shorey's last major work, *What Plato Said*, was published in 1933, when he was 75 years of age. In a recent article one of his admirers and a former student of his at Bryn Mawr, Mrs. Emily James Putnam, has authoritatively said of this work: "It is not an old man's book. The immense learning drawn upon is as readily available as if it had been acquired the week before, and he is ready to fight the old battles at the drop of the hat." Every clinician must be deeply impressed with this evidence of the mental health and vigour of Paul Shorey in his seventies. Elihu Root died in 1937 at over 98 years of age; he was one of the greatest statesmen America ever produced, and continued his activities and interests until well over 90 years of age. Our distinguished pathologist at the Johns Hopkins Hospital, the late Dr. William Henry Welch, lived in good health until over 80 and up to the end of his life continued to give wise counsel to great foundations. Thomas A. Edison, the great American inventor, born in 1847, lived to be nearly ninety years of age; he greatly enriched the life of the world by devising methods of quadruplex and sextuplex telegraphic transmission, the microphone, the phonograph, the incandescent lamp, and motion pictures, and he did excellent work even between his 70th and 80th year. Florence Nightingale, the nursing heroine of the Crimean War and the subject of Longfellow's beautiful poem, *Santa Filomena*, lived to be 90 and until late in life was active in health crusades. Cardinal Gibbons, who was well known in Baltimore as one of the greater representatives of Catholicism, worked steadily throughout life, avoided worry, exercised regularly, was moderate in the use of food and drink and in 1919 published an article entitled, *Why I Am Well at Eighty.* Robert S. Brookings, born in 1850, lived to be 82 years old; after a successful career as merchant and manufacturer he became noted as a philanthropist, placed Washington University of St. Louis and its medical school in the front rank among institutions of its kind, and in still later life founded the Brookings Institution for Economic Research in Washington, D. C., and married happily at the age of 77. President G. Stanley Hall, after retiring from University work (his resignation from the presidency led to press notices that sounded to him like obituaries), wrote, as a septuagenarian, one of the best treatises on old age ever produced, his *Senescence: The Last Half of Life*, published when he was 74. Though the journalist "Dorothy Dix" (Mrs. Gilmer) was born in 1870 her syndicated newspaper column still brings wise counsel to hundreds of thousands who read it daily; one hopes that it may be conitnued for still many years to come. These few examples (and hundreds more could be cited) will suffice to show the advantages of long life both for individuals and for society when later life is not too abnormal.

Women recognize the approach of senescence much earlier, as a rule, than do men. The first wrinkles in front of the ears, the appearance of the first gray hairs, the fading of the complexion and the change of bodily figure are noticed with poignant apprehension; the occurrence of the menopause is often felt by women to be a real tragedy. Some women will do all they can to try to deceive themselves and others regarding their increasing age; this fact accounts for much of the money spent on dress, jewels, care of the hair and other means of compensating for declining charms of the body itself. Indeed, women continue to be interested in dress as long as they live. Dale Carnegie has said that his grandmother who died at 98 was shown, shortly before her death, a photograph of herself that had been taken a third of a century earlier; though her eyes had failed so that she could not see the picture very well, she at once asked "What dress did I have on?" The clinical symptoms of ageing of the female reproductive system and the underlying endocrine mechanisms are fully described in Chapter 14 of this volume, and the changes in the male reproductive system are epitomized in Chapter 15. The so-called "male climacteric" is of far longer duration than the menopause of women. Sexual desire and sexual potency in men wane far more slowly than in women, though after the age of fifty the decline in both inclination to and power of sexual activity is usually progressive, notwithstanding the fact that octogenarian and even nonagenarian paternity may, in a few instances, still be possible. The changes in personality and especially in psychosexual phenomena in later life are thoroughly dealt with in Chapter 16. The psychoanalysts, as Hamilton points out, are of the opinion that if the sex urge persist into later life, and especially if it be frustrated, there is a tendency to fall back upon the major erotic satisfactions· of infancy but in inverse order of development—masturbation, urethral, anal and oral. Clinicians are well aware that masturbation frequently occurs among sexagenarians. In my clinical experience it is much more common in late life among men, however, than among women. The increased frequency of urination in older men I have always attributed to beginning prostatic disturbance rather than to frustration of heteroerotic desires. Moreover, the development of over-anxiety concerning bowel movements and the over-indulgence in food and increased pre-occupation with eating exhibited by many persons past middle life, as well as the garrulity of old age, are not looked upon by most internists as manifestations of regressive anal and oral eroticism.

Clinicians attribute what we call "normal" old age largely to good fortune in both heredity and environment. If a person comes from long-lived parents, and has not suffered too severely from infections, intoxications or traumata especially in early life, he has a very good chance of living long and of enjoying a relatively healthy old age.

The histological changes that accompany the ageing process in the various bodily systems have been discussed in preceding chapters. Alterations in the finer structure of the nervous system and sense organs, in the endocrine glands, and in the musculature seem to be, in the main, responsible for the symptoms that clinicians observe in "normal" old people (Chapters 13 and 17). In how far these changes are dependent upon normal and unavoidable involutional processes and in how far they are due to preceding infections, intoxications, and the general "wear and tear of life" are subjects that have been much discussed; to me, as a clinician, it seems probable that involutional processes are inherent in the organism itself, that they represent, as

Warthin thought, inherited qualities of the germ-plasm. Even the chemical changes that accompany ageing (Chapter 21) would also seem to be constitutionally determined.

Undoubtedly a career of activity, rather than a life of idleness, predisposes to length of life, and no definite chronological age can be safely predicted as the time for retirement or for sudden and marked reduction of activities. Each person should carry on full activities as long as he can do so without over-fatigue or other injury to his constitution. The matter is individual and personal; no hard and fast rule can or should be laid down. At the same time, the active man must know when in the latter part of life to begin "to take in sail" and how to delegate progressively more of his duties and responsibilities to others if he wishes to prolong his life into a healthy and useful old age. Self-control, poise, and calmness of mind are also very conducive to length of life. Any tendency to narrow the horizon of interest to the immediate environment should be combated as age advances.

The psychology of normal old age is probably never very well understood except by those who, remaining healthy, live to be old themselves. In normal old age, though the emotional experiences are less vivid than in earlier life and though the egoistic interests have become less urgent than they were, the intellectual pleasures continue and may increase, even despite beginning impairment of memory for names and for recent events. In healthy old age, the interest in current events may still be keen, and judgment as to their significance may be sounder than ever before; an increasing altruistic trend may come with advancing years and the present and future welfare of others may receive ever greater consideration. There are, too, certain joys of meditation and of contemplation that are greater than those experienced in youth and in middle age. Reconciliation to the idea that death may not be many years away (rather than fear of death or avoidance of the thought of it) is characteristic of the more philosophic among the old, for, as Hall emphasized, facing the Great Enemy squarely is far better than cowardice or self-deception and "to have once deliberately oriented ourselves to death before our powers fail gives us a new poise, whatever attitude toward it such contemplation leads us to."

4. PATHOLOGICAL OLD AGE AND THE MORE SERIOUS DISEASES OF LATER LIFE

Space will permit of only a brief mention of senile dementia and of other serious pathological conditions among the old. Great age in itself does not necessarily entail the development of a senile dementia, as was shown by a person at least 109 years old (perhaps 118) who exhibited no signs of dementia during life and whose brain, later carefully studied by Kucynski, showed no more atrophy of brain cells than did brains of persons dying at a much earlier age and there were very few arteriosclerotic changes and almost no deposits of cholesterin or lime.

Senile dementia and other senile psychoses. I have already referred to King Lear as depicted by Shakespeare as a pathetic example of senile dementia. Clinicians (see E. A. Strecker) have described several forms of mental deterioration occurring in the aged, especially among those from 65 to 75 years old; in all of them there are defects of memory and of orientation, often a marked change of temperament with increasing irritability, obstinacy, and distortion of the personality that may lead to troublesome behavior. Arrangements for permanent care in a psychiatric hospital frequently become necessary. Early recognition and the timely institution of proper custodial and palliative care are most important, for otherwise such patients may easily become the victims of designing persons, may waste their resources, or may exhibit behavior that brings disgrace to their families. Special forms of senile psychoses include (1) the so-called "Alzheimer disease" (see descriptions by Barrett and others in this country) and (2) the so-called Pick's disease (circumscribed senile brain atrophy). The several forms of senile and presenile psychoses are described by W. Runge in Bumke's *Handbuch*.

Recurrences of psychoneurotic states and of affective disorders (exaltations and depressions) to which patients were subject in earlier life are not infrequently met with between the ages of 60 and 80.

The clinician must be on the look-out for the development of the so-called "involutional psychoses" during and after the climacteric period.

Arteriosclerotic disease. So-called "essential arterial hypertension" without definite clinical signs of arteriosclerosis is quite common after the 60th year. Thickening of the arteries, with or without the development of increased blood pressure, is very common among the aged and may result in serious impairment of the functions of the heart, of the kidneys or of the nervous system. Cerebral hemorrhage (apoplexy) and cerebral thrombosis are most often the results of arteriosclerosis and are responsible for many of the paralyses, aphasias, and agnosias of later life. Any one of several varieties of arteriosclerotic psychoses may be met with in old age (cf. F. Stern).

Diseases of the coronary arteries. Attacks of *angina pectoris* are usually associated with arteriosclerosis of the coronary arteries and of the aorta. Sudden death from the formation of a clot in one of the coronary arteries (*coronary thrombosis*) is not uncommon after middle life. Many of the cardiac irregularities and myocardial insufficiencies of later life are secondary to coronary disease.

Cancer. This form of malignant tumor rarely develops before middle life but is very common afterward. Early recognition and prompt surgical removal of the tumor and of the regional lymph glands are most important if life is to be saved or prolonged.

Benign prostatic hypertrophy. Enlargement of the prostate gland is common among men over 60 years of age. It is prone to lead sooner or later to obstruction of the urethra and difficulty in urination. Formerly many old men were forced to carry catheters about with them to be passed into the bladder in order to draw off the urine. Fortunately, in recent years operations have been devised for the safe removal of the prostate (or of parts of it), thus relieving many elderly males of a most troublesome malady.

Parkinson's disease (paralysis agitans). This form of "shaking palsy" is a disease of later life characterized by marked tremor, rigidity of the muscles, slowing of movements, a characteristic body-attitude ("Parkinsonian stoop"), a tendency on walking to go suddenly forward ("propulsion") or suddenly backward ("retropulsion"), and loss of the associated movements of swinging of the arms on walking. Though the disease is slowly progressive, life may not be shortened. The malady is incurable but considerable relief can be obtained by the cautious administration of scopolamin hydrobromide. In early life, lethargic encephalitis may be followed by a similar clinical picture ("post-encephalitic Parkinsonism").

Joint diseases of later life. In addition to the various types of inflammation of the joints (*arthritis*) that may occur at any age, there is a form of disease of the bones and joints that is relatively common in later life, namely *hypertrophic osteoarthropathy.* It is not an inflammatory disorder, but is due to degeneration of joint cartilages and to new bone formation at the edge of the cartilage. Pains in the affected joints with some restriction of movements are common symptoms. Hips, knees, shoulders, or the joints of the spine may become involved. The small bony enlargements so often seen in older people at the bases of the terminal phalanges and known to medical men as "Heberden's nodes" seem to be a part of this hypertrophic osteoarthropathy. True *gouty arthritis*, not uncommon among older people ("high livers"), is an entirely different process and is due to a disturbance of uric acid metabolism. An acute attack of gout often first attacks the joint of one great toe (severe pain, sudden swelling, dusky-red color). The presence of "tophi" in the ears and an excess of uric acid in the blood are confirmatory of the diagnosis of gouty arthritis. Preparations of colchicum may promptly ameliorate the symptoms. The cautious use of cincophen (or of neocincophen) may be advantageous, but the physician must take great care to avoid the occurrence of cincophen poisoning. Between attacks the diet should be largely purin-free and alcohol should be avoided.

The pneumonias. Acute lobar pneumonia or acute broncho-pneumonia may occur at any time of life. In old age, it is often a terminal event—one reason why the late Sir William Osler sometimes spoke of pneumonia as "the old man's friend."

Recurrent Bronchitis. Many older persons have prolonged attacks of bronchitis during the colder half of the year. "Catarrhal vaccine" given at the end of the summer may prevent the attacks. Some patients, however, are forced to spend the autumn and winter in warm climates.

5. WHY ELDERLY PERSONS NEED TO CONSULT PHYSICIANS AND THE RESULTS OF THOROUGH GENERAL DIAGNOSTIC STUDY

In the Group Clinic in which I work we have records of complete group studies of more than 16,000 patients. With the help of one of my associates, Dr. J. H. Trescher, and of our secretarial staff, we have studied the histories of some 300 new patients over 60 years of age applying to us for group diagnosis and treatment during the past seven years in order to ascertain (1) the commoner symptoms of which these elderly persons complained and (2) the more outspoken abnormal findings in them as determined by physical examination, X-rays and laboratory tests. It must be remembered that the clientele does not perhaps represent a cross-section of the more aged population since we are presumably consulted as general internists (and neurologists) rather than as surgeons or as practitioners in more specialized domains. Moreover, the majority of the patients come from the relatively well-to-do classes.

The results of the analyses of the findings yielded some surprises. In the first place it was rather astonishing to find that approximately one-tenth of the new patients who now apply for group studies have reached the age of 60 or older; one wonders whether our clinic is coming to be known as having an especial interest in geriatrics! Of the 300 patients mentioned 240 were between 60 and 70 years of age, 57 were between 70 and 80, and 3 were over 80.

In the *age group 60–70*, the chief symptoms complained of by the 240 patients at the beginning of the diagnostic study suggested, in by far the majority of cases, disturbances in (1) the nervous system, (2) the digestive system, (3) the circulatory system, or (4) the locomotor apparatus; in relatively few instances did the chief complaint suggest disturbance of the respiratory system, the haemopoietic system, the urogenital system or the endocrine apparatus.

Thus, in this age group (60 to 70) the commoner complaints suggesting disturbance of the *nervous system* were (1) depression, in 29 instances (2) nervousness in 26, (3) fatiguability in 23, (4) insomnia in 20, (5) acroparaesthesias in 11, (6) headaches and "odd feelings in the head" in 10, (7) dizziness in 9, (8) visual disturbances in 9, (9) tremor in eight, (10) worrying tendency in 7, (11) failing memory in 5, (12) "fainting spells" in 5, (13) deafness in 5, (14) disturbance of speech in 3, (15) fears in 3, (16) "anxiety" in 3, (17) tinnitus in 3, (18) difficulty in walking in 2, and "sciatica" in 2.

In the same age group, the commoner complaints suggesting disturbances of the *digestive system* were (1) abdominal pain in 22, (2) "poor digestion" in 16, (3) constipation in 16, (4) "gas" in 15, (5) nausea (and sometimes vomiting) in 12, (6) loss of appetite in 7, (7) diarrhoea in 5, and (8) difficulty in swallowing in 1.

The commoner complaints suggestive of disturbances of the *circulatory system* in the same age group (60–70) were (1) precordial pain or oppression in 21, (2) shortness of breath in 20, (3) palpitation in 9, (4) rapid pulse in 2, and (5) disturbed blood supply to the lower extremities in 1.

The commoner complaints suggestive of disturbances of the *locomotor system* between 60 and 70 were (1) "joint trouble" in 30, (2) disturbances of locomotion in 13, and (3) "backache" in 13.

Outside of the four systems mentioned the patients registered very few other symptoms as their main complaint, though underweight, overweight, recent unexplained loss of weight, pruritus and urticaria should be mentioned as occasional initial complaints.

In the 60 patients over 70 years of age, the relative incidence of the initial complaints was very similar to that of the larger group between the ages of 60 and 70, though the following deviations were noticeable: (1) a relatively smaller number of patients whose first main complaint pointed to the circulatory apparatus and (2) a relative increase in the number whose initial complaint was difficulty in swallowing (4 of the 60 patients).

The members of our diagnostic group, while paying due attention to the main complaint made at the beginning of the study, are careful not to allow themselves to be over-influenced by it, realizing that it is only after a general diagnostic survey has been made and the results of it analyzed that the true relative importance of the patients' main complaint can be properly evaluated. In every case, therefore, after registration of the main complaint and of a full anamnesis, a thorough general physical examination is made, certain routine laboratory tests and indicated X-ray tests are ordered, and when deemed necessary reports from practitioners in certain special domains are arranged for. After collection of all the data, the positive and negative findings are arranged under the several bodily systems upon a special summary sheet. The diagnostician can then very rapidly make a brief multi-dimensional diagnosis, placing the several items in the order of their relative importance.

We turn next to a *summary of the more important diagnostic features* that emerged after the completion of the studies in the 300 patients mentioned.

In the age group 60–70, the most numerous maladies discovered were in the domain of the *circulatory apparatus*. They included 42 cases of "cardio-vascular-renal disease" as well as 27 cases of so-called "essential hypertension," 8 cases of angina pectoris, 2 cases of coronary thrombosis and 2 cases of Raynaud's disease. Under these diseases of the circulatory apparatus were included general arteriosclerosis (with or without hypertension), myocardiopathies, and the various arrhythmias revealed on electrocardiographic examination.

Next in order of frequency were the maladies in the domain of the *nervous system*. They included 43 cases of functional emotional and nervous disturbances (affective disorders; psychoneuroses), 7 cases of Parkinson's disease (paralysis agitans), 4 cases of senile psychosis (3 of senile dementia and 1 of paranoid type), 3 cases of paralysis secondary to organic brain disease, and 3 cases of organic encephalopathy of doubtful nature. Many of the patients were found to have refraction errors that needed better correction; only one patient had definite cataract.

Diseases of the *locomotor system* came next in order of frequency and importance. In the 60–70 group, 40 suffered from joint lesions (nearly all of them hypertrophic osteoarthropathy rather than any actual inflammation of the joints) and there were two cases of Paget's disease of the bones.

Despite the large incidence of initial symptoms suggestive of disturbances of the *digestive system* (see above) we found only 3 cases of gall-bladder disease, 2 cases of ulcer of the pylorus, and 2 cases of duodenal ulcer. Achylia gastrica and gastric hyperacidity, spastic colon, inguinal hernia and relatively severe hemorrhoids were occasionally encountered. Oral sepsis (abscessed teeth and pyorrhoea alveolaris) were relatively common findings.

Of other maladies found in this age group (60–70), I may mention (1) 11 cases of tumor, chiefly cancer (colon, liver, esophagus, pylorus, prostate, breast), (2) 5 cases of diabetes mellitus, (3) 5 cases of lues and (4) several cases of severe obesity as well as of marked undernutrition. Aside from the above, thyroid disturbances, dermatopathies, chronic bronchitis, and asthma were occasionally encountered. In not a few, faulty hygiene was discovered (inappropriate diet; overwork; excessive tabagism; potatorium; drug habits).

In the group of patients over 70, relatively fewer severe disorders were found than in the age-group 60–70; cardiovascular renal disease predominated, though essential hypertension and angina pectoris were relatively less frequent; the incidence of cancer however increased (6 of the 60 patients manifesting it); organic diseases of the digestive tract were relatively decreased (none of the 60 having gall bladder disease nor ulcer of the pylorus or duodenum); benign prostatic hypertrophy showed no change in relative incidence; organic osteopathies (Paget's disease, etc.) were somewhat more frequent relatively, though the relative incidence of hypertrophic osteoarthropathy was practically unchanged. It was rather surprising to find no senile psychoses in the 60 patients over 70, though in the 60–70 age-group 4 of 240 patients manifested them.

6. PLEA FOR GREATER INTEREST AMONG CLINICIANS

Following upon the great advances that have recently been made in the prevention and treatment of diseases of childhood and of early life, the relative number of older people has been rapidly increasing and doubtless will continue to increase during the decades ahead of us. Unfortunately people over 60 have not received from clinicians the attention that they merit. This has been partly due to the idea that most if not all of the infirmities of old age are inevitable and irremediable and that "Nature must take her course." This idea has been prevalent among the old themselves and has had its corresponding psychological malevolent effect upon many of them; too often it has been harbored also by some of the physicians under whose care such older people would naturally fall. Moreover old people are prone to lose faith in doctors, most of whom are younger than they are and often incapable of understanding fully their mental reactions to the environment; such older people except for traumata and for serious acute illnesses are prone to "doctor themselves."

Luckily, during recent years, as knowledge of the importance of preventive medicine has spread, more and more young and middle aged people have been trained to report to their physicians (as well as to their dentists) at least once or twice a year for a so-called "health check-up." The advantages of such periodic health examinations have been so conclusively proven that it seems likely that the practice will be carried over into the later years of life. In my own clinical work we have had an ever increasing number of persons over 60 who return regularly once or twice a year for a 'health examination,' whether they are bothered by any symptoms at the time or not. The cultivation of this procedure makes it possible for the clinician timely to modify the activities and habits of his patients to their great advantage as their years increase. The duration and intensity of the daily work may be gradually lessened, the diet can be adjusted carefully to the nutritional needs, and the optimal amount of diversion, recreation and social participation can be duly estimated. When the time for retirement comes, the physician can often be very helpful to the patient in making necessary readjustments. Sudden cessation of all activities and the assumption of a life of "innocuous desuetude" is not only disheartening but is often disastrous and undoubtedly shortens many lives. The wise clinician will study the interests and capacities that still exist and will help to plan the life after retirement in the best way possible. Many elderly people turn to various altruistic, social or literary interests as surrogates for earlier business or professional activities. Some may be encouraged to write (or to dictate) their autobiographies, even if they are not to be published. Some will do well, as did the late John D. Rockefeller, Sr., to spend their winters in the south and their summers in the north. Those who have not travelled widely during early or middle life may enjoy "seeing the world" during the sunset of their lives. I have known many elderly men and women who have with enjoyment undertaken extensive voyages, even trips around the world, after the age of 70. Travelling is now made so easy, especially by sea, that long voyages may safely be made by fairly healthy aged persons without danger of the necessity of over-exertion.

The treatment of diseases occurring in the old often has to be somewhat different from the treatment of the same maladies in younger persons. Fortunately, certain diseases (notably the acute exanthemata) to which the young are subject occur only rarely among old people. Moreover, many disorders of earlier life often terminate either in cure or in death before old age is reached (e.g., tuberculosis, sarcomata, dementia paralytica, pernicious anaemia, and leukaemia).

Cardio-vascular renal disease, so common in the later decades of life, must be even more cautiously treated in the old than in the young; the amount of rest enjoined should be relatively greater, the dangers of physical and mental over-exertion of any kind should be more strongly emphasized, and the dietetic and hygienic regimes should be more rigid and more closely supervised. No matter how carefully elderly patients with cardiovascular renal disease are cared for, a large proportion of them will in time succumb to myocardial insufficiency, coronary thrombosis, cerebral apoplexy, or uraemia.

The *diseases of the joints* that occur in later life are for the most part, as we have seen, of the type of hypertrophic osteoarthropathy. Much can be done to ameliorate the condition by treatment at suitable spas or in the physical therapy division of modern hospitals and pain can be lessened by the continued use of small doses of sodium iodide or when more severe by the administration of acetosalicylic acid.

The *diseases of the digestive apparatus* occurring in old people require essentially the same treatment as in young people, though naturally one would hesitate to subject septuagenarians or octogenarians to intraabdominal surgery unless the pathological conditions are such as seriously to threaten the lives of the patients and even then the choice between surgical intervention and non-interference may often be such as to warrant the physician in leaving the decision to the patient.

Among the *diseases of the nervous system* that occur among the old, the general principles of treatment are about the same as for similar diseases in younger persons. Thus, among the psychoses, elations and depressions may be merely repetitions of similar states in earlier life, and according to their severity may be treated either inside or outside psychiatric institutions. Paranoid states and senile dementia should have permanent institutional care. In the treatment of psychoneurotic states it may not be wise to make use of the complete rest and the isolation that are often so helpful to psychoneurotics in early and middle life, though some increase of rest and partial isolation may be safely enjoined. After paying due attention to any physical abnormalities found to be associated with the psychoneurotic state and after relieving insomnia and undue restlessness by suitable drugs (bromides, phenobarbital, nembutal), much can be done by simple psychotherapeutic conversations with the patient. The physician should listen carefully to the complaints and especially to the worries that are reported as well as to the causes to which the patient ascribes them, even if considerable time is necessary to tell the whole story, for it does the patient a vast deal of good to "unburden his soul" to someone in whom he has confidence. Old people are often more reluctant than younger persons to make such full confessions, but if they can be induced to do so, much will be gained and the physician can then re-assure and encourage. Any attempt at deeper psycho-analytic procedures in the treatment of psychoneuroses among the old is to be deprecated; Freud, himself, long ago said that they were worthless. The general practitioner of sympathy, tact and good common sense, if he be acquainted with psychoneurotic manifestations can do all that is necessary. He should it is true have sufficient prestige to make elderly persons willing to follow his counsel.

Women of psychoneurotic trend may easily be upset in later life through the folly of selfish and wayward husbands. One such woman at one time complained to me that her husband (older than she) had so gotten on her nerves that she couldn't sleep and that she felt forced to talk the matter out with me as her physician and to get my advice. She was of the retiring, over-conscientious type, her husband was of the egoistic "hail fellow-well met" type who at periods showed signs of somewhat pathological elation. She had inherited a moderate fortune and had made provision for her children, had paid the family expenses, and had given her husband a liberal allowance. Both husband and wife had reached the age when sexual desire and potency naturally wane and when sex interests are best "sublimated" by both marital partners. Unfortunately, after a prostate operation, the elderly husband had had a sudden flare-up of sex-interest and had sought the companionship of various gay young women and frequented parties that were rather "lively." To make matters worse, he made many unwise expenditures and had the bills paid out of funds that were provided for the maintenance of the family and for the care of his wife's property. And though he was generally cheerful and good natured, he was capable of being disagreeable if any adverse comment upon his conduct or expenditures was made. The wife resented all this and moreover was rather fearful that this abnormal behavior might become matter of gossip that would be hurtful to family pride. The question was put up to me as to what she should do. Had I not been personally fairly well acquainted with the situation, I might have been inclined to advise her to consult a good lawyer, to place her affairs at once in the hands of a reliable trust company, and to have a psychiatrist consult with her family physician as to the best treatment of her husband's condition. But I was of the opinion that less drastic measures might suffice. So I told her that I thought that she had been worrying too much about the situation, that the mere talking it out fully with me would prove to a great relief to her, and that, temporarily, she might be helped in sleeping by taking a $1\frac{1}{2}$ grain tablet of phenobarbital at bed time and if awake an hour later a $1\frac{1}{2}$ grain capsule of nembutal. I advised her to be "hard boiled" about expenditures, to have vouchers kept and to have a good accountant give her a monthly audit. Otherwise, I advised her to ignore her husband's conduct, to let him be as "frisky" as he wanted to be (time would soon "cure" him), and to trust to her grown up sons and daughters to keep an eye on the general situation and upon the protection of the family reputation. Only in case these measures were not successful need the more drastic plan be put into operation.

A psychasthenic trend persists in some persons until late in life. The management of the fears, the indecision and the obsessions of the psychasthenic is the same at all periods of life though the management may be more difficult in the elderly than in the young since the psychasthenic has practically to be given "orders" by his physician what to do and the old are less apt than the young to receive such orders graciously. In this connection I may be permitted to recall an instance in my own practice in which a strange psychasthenic "quirk" was overcome to the patient's advantage late in his life. On a Friday in June, 1927, a wealthy man (of international eminence as a business man, economist, philanthropist and educator) who lived in a neighboring city asked if he could have a private professional interview with me with regard to a personal matter that concerned him deeply. I arranged for him to lunch with me in a small room at the club where he told me his story. Born in 1850, he had had a happy and a very successful career except that he had not been able to marry the woman that he loved. She was 22 years younger than he and when she was 27 years of age he had asked her to marry him and she had accepted as she loved him devotedly. Because he was so many years her senior and had dandled her as a little girl upon his knee, he felt compunctions about marrying her and felt that he must break the engagement. On two occasions later, he renewed the invitation to marriage, was accepted, but broke off the engagements quickly because of some psychic obstacle. Though able to engage decisively in large financial matters, he seemed unable to meet the particular new situation of getting married. Their warm friendship continued. When near this woman he showed such devotion that she thought that since he could not bring himself to the point of marrying her it would be less embarrassing for her to live in Europe, so as to see him only occasionally when she revisited America. Though the patient had had a serious heart attack in 1926 he felt better again and he told me that he had come to the conclusion that he must marry the woman of his choice in the hope of having at least a few years of relatively good health and loving companionship. After hearing his story I told him that before giving my consent from the medical side I must first have an interview with the lady concerned and this was arranged for two days later (on Sunday), when he brought her to my house and I had a long frank talk with her alone. The whole matter was thoroughly ventilated and I learned that she had continued to love this man for over 25 years and was perfectly willing to marry him, though she felt sure from previous experience that he could not possibly bring himself to the point of marriage. She said that since his interview with me two days earlier he had spent two sleepless nights and that she was convinced that the same peculiar psychic condition that had prevented his marriage on three earlier occasions was again developing in him! I told her of the heart attack he had had and of the possibilities of serious illness during the few years he might have ahead of him and asked her if visualizing all the circumstances she would still be willing to marry him if I could arrange for it. She said that she would, especially because of his present feeling of urgent need for her companionship and aid; she felt sure, however, that neither I nor anybody else could really get him to marry. I then saw the two of them together and asked him if he still felt as he did two days earlier. He replied that he did but that the only objection to the marriage was his fear that he might become a burden upon, and be harmful to, the woman he loved. Excusing myself from them for a few moments I found out by telephone how to get a marriage license on Sunday,

got the consent of the Rev. Dr. Kinsolving "to marry two people who
were at the time in my office and who should by all means be married
at once" and then called a taxi. I asked them to go into town with me.
The patient immediately asked, "What does this mean?" I told him
that I was taking them into the city to be married. He immediately
protested, said it was impossible, and that he must have a certain
time to prepare. My reply was that he had had some 27 years to
prepare and hadn't yet got ready; this time, I had made the preparations
and I was going to see to it that they were married that afternoon.
We secured the license, Dr. Kinsolving married them, and his daughter
and I witnessed the marriage! The patient lived until mid November,
1932, dying at the age of 82. It is interesting that the symptoms of
disease of his heart passed off after his marriage in a remarkable way.
He and his wife had 5½ years of happiness and increasing contentment
that they would have missed entirely if that psychasthenic "quirk"
of the man had not been handled clinically in the right way. I was
much gratified when his wife wrote me on the second anniversary of
their marriage: "I wonder if any two human beings have ever owed
another as much as we owe you."

7. SUMMARY

In his introduction to this volume, a great American philosopher,
Professor John Dewey, has discussed briefly but in a most admirable
way the biological bases of the ageing process on the one hand and the
educational and social aspects of that process on the other. His
introduction should be carefully read by every practicing physician.
That he is right in attributing the contemporary status of the old
partly to inescapable biological processes and partly to modifiable
social and cultural processes every discerning clinical worker will agree.
He admits, however, that, as yet, no one knows just how important
relatively these contrasting processes are. He seems rather to lean
to the view of a marked preponderance of the social and cultural
factors; clinicians, as a result of their experience, while granting the
real need of a change in educational, social, and political patterns,
will be inclined I believe to attribute rather more of the present unsatisfactory conditions prevalent among the aged to determining
biological factors than does perhaps Professor Dewey. In any case,
both sets of factors are of great importance and the problems that now
confront human society in connection with old age are unprecedented since it is estimated that by 1980 the number of persons over
65 years of age will be more than double that of today. These problems

should be attacked in a scientific way in order that true causes may be determined and that rational measures (preventive and mitigative) may be devised and instituted. The present volume illustrates an excellent start in the right direction. But as knowledge of the ageing process develops further, we shall need ever greater coöperation not only among physicists, chemists, biologists, psychologists and medical men but also among educators, sociologists, and politicians who can modify social and cultural patterns to meet the newly-discovered needs.

In medicine, we shall require an increasing number of men (so-called "gerontologists") who will specialize in geriatrics but their number need not be nearly so large as those who specialize in pediatrics. But every student in the medical schools should attend at least a short course in geriatrics and in this he should be taught to train his patients of middle age to prepare themselves for later life so that in old age they can be contentedly occupied themselves and, as far as possible, also continue to be socially useful. He should be told to point out to them the growing tendency of elderly people to live apart from their children, either in homes of their own or in homes for the aged, and that people of middle age should therefore make timely provision for their later lives by the establishment of trust funds or by the purchase of annuities. The old age security laws are unlikely soon to make adequate provision for the majority of elderly people, though they may be expected to mitigate the hardships now suffered by the aged poor. Each physician should, from the time of his graduation onward, keep in mind the nature of the problems that are associated with old age, and should do everything in his power to aid in their solution from the biological as well as from the social-cultural side.

During the past few decades there has been an enormous improvement in child care, especially in the placing of orphans through the activities of the Child Welfare League of America. I would suggest that it might be very helpful to form an American League for the Promotion of the Health and Welfare of Elderly People as a national organization with local branches in the different states. If such a league could be organized one might expect to see most valuable results for the older section of our population within a very short time.

REFERENCES

BARKER, L. F. 1933. The senile patient. Ann. Int. Med., **6**, 11125–1135.
BARKER, L. F. AND SPRUNT, T. P. 1925. The degenerative diseases; their causes and prevention. New York: Harper & Co., 254 pp.

BARRETT, A. M. 1913. A case of Alzheimer disease with unusual neurological distrubances. J. Nerve. & Ment. Dis., **40**, 361.

HALL, G. STANLEY 1922. Senescence: the last half of life. New York: D. Appleton & Co., 518 pp.

KUCYNSKI 1925. Von den körperlichen Veränderungen beim höchsten Alter. Krankheitsforschung, **1**, 85 (cited by W. Runge).

NASCHER, I. L. 1916. Geriatrics. Philadelphia: Blakiston 2 ed.

PICK, A. 1908. Die umschriebene senile Hirnatrophie als Gegenstand klinischer und anatomischer Forschung. Arb. a. d. deutsch.-psychiat. Univ. Klin. in Prag. Berl., **20–29**.

PUTNAM, EMILY JAMES 1938. Paul Shorey. Atlantic Monthly, **161**, 795–804.

ROLLESTON, H. 1922. Some medical aspects of old age. New York: Macmillan, 205 pp.

INDEX

AGING AND OLD AGE

An Arno Press Collection

(Armstrong, John). **The Art of Preserving Health.** 1744

Canstatt, Carl. **Die Krankheiten des Hoheren Alters Und Ihre Heilung.** 1839

Carlisle, Anthony. **An Essay on the Disorders of Old Age, and on the Means for Prolonging Human Life.** 1818

Cavan, Ruth Shonle, et al. **Personal Adjustment in Old Age.** 1949

Charcot, J(ean) M(artin). **Clinical Lectures on Senile and Chronic Diseases.** 1881

Cheyne, George. **An Essay of Health and Long Life.** 1724

Child, Charles. **Sensecence and Rejuvenescence.** 1915

Cicero, M(arcus) T(ullius). **Cato Major.** 1744

(Cohausen, Johann Heinrich). **Hermippus Redivivus.** 1771

Cornaro, Luigi. **The Art of Living Long.** 1917

Cowdry, E. V., ed. **Problems of Ageing.** 1939

Cumming, Elaine and William E. Henry. **Growing Old.** 1961

Day, George E. **A Practical Treatise on the Domestic Management and Most Important Diseases of Advanced Life.** 1849

Department for the Aging, City of New York. **Older Women in the City.** 1979

Floyer, John. **Medicina Gerocomica.** 1724

Gruman, Gerald J., ed. **The "Fixed Period" Controversy.** 1979

Gruman, Gerald J., ed. **Roots of Modern Gerontology and Geriatrics.** 1979

(Hufeland, Christoph Wilhelm). **Art of Prolonging Life.** 1854

Jameson, Thomas. **Essays on the Changes of the Human Body at Its Different Ages.** 1811

Kirk, Hyland Clare. **When Age Grows Young.** 1888

Kleemeier, Robert W., ed. **Aging and Leisure.** 1961

Lessius, Leonard and Lewis Cornaro. **A Treatise of Health and Long Life With the Future Means of Attaining It.** 1743

MacKenzie, James. **The History of Health, and the Art of Preserving It.** 1760

Martin, Lillien J(ane) and Clare de Gruchy. **Sweeping the Cobwebs.** 1933

Minot, Charles S. **The Problem of Age, Growth, and Death.** 1908

Nascher, I(gnatz) L(eo). **Geriatrics.** 1914

Pearl, Raymond and Ruth DeWitt Pearl. **The Ancestry of the Long-Lived.** 1934

Ramon y Cajal, S(antiago). **El Mundo Visto a Los Ochenta Anos.** 1934

de Ropp, Robert S. **Man Against Aging.** 1960

Stieglitz, Edward J. **The Second Forty Years.** 1946

Sweetser, William. **Human Life.** 1867

Thoms, William J. **Human Longevity.** 1873

Tibbitts, Clark, ed. **Living Through the Older Years.** 1949

Tolstoy, Leo. **Last Diaries.** 1960

Vercors (pseud. Jean Bruller). **The Insurgents.** 1956

Warthin, Aldred Scott. **Old Age.** 1929